26.50

A COMPANION TO DENTAL STUDIES
Volume 1 Book 2

# Editorial Board

*A.G. Alexander*   MDS FDSRCS
Dean of Dental Studies and Professor of Conservative Dentistry, University College Dental School, London

*W.G. Armstrong*   MSc MSc PhD
Professor of Biochemistry in Relation to Dentistry, Royal Dental Hospital of London School of Dental Surgery, London

*R. Duckworth*   MD BDS FDSRCS FRCPath
Professor of Oral Medicine, The London Hospital Medical College Dental School, London

*R. Haskell*   MRCP FDSRCS
Consultant Dental Surgeon, Guy's Hospital, London

*R.B. Johns*   PhD LDSRCS
Professor of Restorative Dentistry, University of Sheffield

*J.W. Osborn*   PhD BDS FDSRCS
Professor of Oral Biology, The University of Alberta, Canada

*A.H.R. Rowe*   MDS FDSRCS
Professor of Conservative Dentistry, Guy's Hospital Dental School, London

*J.H. Sowray*   LCRP MRCS FDSRCS
Professor of Oral Surgery, King's College Hospital Medical School, London

*R.L. Speirs*   BSc PhD
Professor of Physiology in Relation to Dentistry, The London Hospital Medical College, London.

A COMPANION TO DENTAL STUDIES
Editors in Chief / A.H.R. Rowe & R.B. Johns
Volume 1 Book 2

# Dental Anatomy and Embryology

Edited by
J. W. OSBORN

Blackwell Scientific Publications
OXFORD LONDON EDINBURGH
BOSTON MELBOURNE

© 1981 by
Blackwell Scientific Publications
Editorial offices:
Osney Mead, Oxford OX2 0EL
8 John Street, London WC1N 2ES
23 Ainslie Place, Edinburgh EH3 6AJ
Three Cambridge Center, Suite 208
  Cambridge, Massachusetts 02142,
  USA
667 Lytton Avenue, Palo Alto
  California 94301, USA
107 Barry Street, Carlton
  Victoria 3053, Australia

All rights reserved. No part of this
publication may be reproduced, stored
in a retrieval system, or transmitted,
in any form or by any means,
electronic, mechanical, photocopying,
recording or otherwise
without the prior permission of
the copyright owner

First published 1981
Reprinted 1988

Set by Santype International Ltd
Salisbury, Wiltshire
Printed and bound in Great Britain
by Billing and Sons Ltd, Worcester

DISTRIBUTORS

USA
Year Book Medical Publishers
200 North LaSalle Street,
Chicago, Illinois 60601

Canada
The C.V. Mosby Company
5240 Finch Avenue East
Scarborough, Ontario

Australia
Blackwell Scientific Publications
(Australia) Pty Ltd
107 Barry Street, Carlton
Victoria 3053

British Library
Cataloguing in Publication Data

A Companion to dental studies.
  Vol.1
  Book 2: Dental anatomy and embryology
  1. Dentistry
  I. Rowe, A.H.R. II. Johns, R.B.
  III. Osborn, J.W.
  617.6     RK51

ISBN 0−632−00799−0

# Contents

Contributors to Volume 1 Book 2, viii
Contents of *A Companion to Dental Studies*, x
Foreword, xii
Preface, xiii

### 1  Embryology and Development   1
Introduction/*J.W. Osborn*
Early embryology/*J. Joseph*
Embryology of different systems and organs/*J. Joseph*
The branchial (pharyngeal) arches/*J. Joseph*
Craniofacial development/*P. Sullivan & A.G.S. Lumsden*

### 2  Genetics   47
Genes, chromosomes and genetic variation/*J.A. Sofaer*
Genotype and phenotype/*J.A. Sofaer*
Patterns of inheritance/*J.A. Sofaer*
Quantitative and population genetics/*J.A. Sofaer*

### 3  Growth and Ageing   62
Introduction/*C.L.B. Lavelle*
Skull and jaws/*J.W. Osborn*
Ageing/*A.E.W. Miles*

### 4  Evolution and Adaptation of the Vertebrate Mouth   88
Agnatha: jawless fishes/*A.G.S. Lumsden*
Placodermi: early jawed fishes/*A.G.S. Lumsden*
Chondrichthyes/*A.G.S. Lumsden*
Osteichthyes/*A.G.S. Lumsden*
Amphibians; reptiles; birds/*A.G.S. Lumsden*
Synapsid reptiles/*A.G.S. Lumsden*

### 5  Tooth Morphology   118
Tooth morphology/*B.K.B. Berkovitz & B. Moxham*
Racial differences of tooth morphology/*J.A. Sofaer*

| 6 | Dental Tissues | 155 |

**Evolution:** comparative development of dental tissues/*P. Shellis*
Comparative histology of dental tissues./*P. Shellis*
**Human tissues:** dentine/*P. Shellis*
Enamel/*J.W. Osborn*
Pulp/*A.F. Hayward*
Sensory mechanisms of dentine and pulp/*B. Matthews*
Cement/*S.J. Jones*
Biochemistry of the dental tissues/*W.G. Armstrong & R.L. Speirs*

| 7 | Tooth Support | 210 |

Types of tooth support and their properties/*P. Shellis*
Formation of attachement tissues/*P. Shellis*
Adaptive radiation of tooth supporting structures/*P. Shellis*
Alveolar bone/*J.W. Osborn*
Periodontal ligament/*B.K.B. Berkovitz*
Gingiva/*G.C. Cowley*
Innervation, blood supply and lymphatics/*B.K.B. Berkovitz & B. Moxham*

| 8 | Development of Dentition | 246 |

Early stages of tooth development/*B.K.B. Berkovitz & B. Moxham*
Developmental controls/*J.W. Osborn*
Dentine and pulp formation/*B.K.B. Berkovitz & P. Shellis*
Enamel development/*J.W. Osborn*
Cuticles/*J.W. Osborn*
Development of the peridontium/*B.K.B. Berkovitz*
Cement/*S.J. Jones*
Developmental abnormalities/*F. Ingram*

| 9 | Development and Maintenance of Occlusion | 299 |

Evolution/*J.W. Osborn*
Occlusion/*J.R. Mills*
Tooth eruption/*B.K.B. Berkovitz*
Establishment of dentition/*D.C. Picton*

| 10 | Dentition in Function | 329 |

Functions of teeth/*P. Butler*
Chewing; evolution of mammalian molars/*P. Butler*
Developments from the tribosphenic pattern/*P. Butler*
Jaw muscles/*P. Butler*
Jaw joints/*P. Butler*
Functional aspect of development/*P. Butler*
Ageing/*J.W. Osborn*

| | | |
|---|---|---|
| 11 | Evolution of Man | 357 |

    The primates/*K.M. Hiiemae*
    The hominids/*K.M. Hiiemae*
    Modern man/*C.L.B. Lavelle*

| | | |
|---|---|---|
| 12 | Comparative anatomy of dentition | 399 |

    **The dentition of mammals:** the orders of placental mammals/*A.G.S. Lumsden*
    The order primates/*K.M. Hiiemae*
    The dentition of laboratory rodents and lagomorphs/*P. Shellis & B.K.B. Berkovitz*

Index, 440

# Contributors to Volume 1 Book 2

*W.G. Armstrong* MSc MSc PhD
Professor of Biochemistry in Relation to Dentistry, Department of Biochemistry, Royal Dental Hospital of London School of Dental Surgery, Cranmer Terrace, London SW17 0RE.

*B.K.B. Berkovitz* MSc PhD LDSRCS
Senior Lecturer, Department of Anatomy (Oral Biology), Bristol University Medical School, Bristol BS8 1TD

*P.M. Butler* BSc MA PhD
Honorary Research Fellow, Department of Zoology, Royal Holloway College, 'Alderhurst', Bakeham Lane, Englefield Green, Surrey TW20 9TY.

*G.C. Cowley* BDS DDS
Professor of Periodontology and Community Dentistry, University of Dundee Dental School and Hospital, Park Place, Dundee DD1 4HR.

*A.F. Hayward* BSc MB BS PhD
Reader and Head of Department, Department of Anatomy, Royal Dental Hospital of London School of Dental Surgery (Royal Dental School), Cranmer Terrace, London SW17 0RE.

*K.M. Hiiemae* BSc BDS PhD
Professor and Head of Department of Oral Anatomy, College of Dentistry, and Professor of Anatomy, School of Basic Medical Sciences, University of Illinois at the Medical Center, 801 South Paulina Street, PO Box 6998, Chicago, Illinois 60680, USA.

*F.L. Ingram* DMRD LDSRCS MRCS LRCP
'Little Wildwood', 44 Heathfield Way, Barham, Canterbury CT4 6QF.

*S.J. Jones* PhD LDSRCS
Senior Lecturer, Department of Anatomy and Embryology, University College London, Gower Street, London WC1E 6BT.

*J. Joseph* MD DSc FRCOG
Professor and Head of Department of Anatomy, Guy's Hospital Medical School, St Thomas' Street, London SE1 9RT.

## Contributors to Volume 1 Book 2

*C.L.B. Lavelle*   MDS DSc FRCD
Professor and Head of Oral Biology, The University of Manitoba, 780 Bannatyne Avenue, Winnipeg, Canada R3E 0W3.

*A.G.S. Lumsden*   MA PhD
Unit of Anatomy in Relation to Dentistry, Department of Anatomy, Guy's Hospital Medical School, St Thomas' Street, London SE1 9RT.

*B. Matthews*   BDS PhD
Professor of Physiology, Bristol University Medical School, Bristol BS8 1TD.

*J.R.E. Mills*   DDS MSc FDSRCS DOrth
Professor of Orthodontics, Institute of Dental Surgery, Eastman Dental Hospital, Gray's Inn Road, London WC1X 8LD.

*A.E.W. Miles*   DSc LRCP MCRS FDSRCS
Emeritus Professor of Oral Pathology, The London Hospital Medical College Dental School, and Honorary Curator of the Odontological Collection, Royal College of Surgeons of England, 1 Cleaver Square, London SE11 4DW.

*B.J. Moxham*   BSc BDS PhD
Lecturer, Department of Anatomy (Oral Biology), Bristol University Medical School, Bristol BS8 1TD.

*J.W. Osborn*   PhD BDS FDSRCS
Professor and Chairman of the Department of Oral Biology, Faculty of Dentistry, The University of Alberta, Edmonton, Canada T6G 2N8.

*D.C.A. Picton*   JP BSc PhD FDSRCS
Professor of Experimental and Preventitive Dentistry, University College Dental School, Mortimer Market, London WC1E 6JD.

*R.P. Shellis*   BSc MSc PhD
MRC Dental Unit, Dental School, Lower Maudlin Street, Bristol BS1 2LY.

*J.A. Sofaer*   BDS PhD
Senior Lecturer, Departments of Oral Medicine and Oral Pathology, and Human Genetics, Department of Oral Medicine and Oral Pathology, Old Surgeon's Hall, High School Yards, Edinburgh EH1 1NR.

*R.L. Speirs*   BSc PhD
Professor of Physiology in Relation to Dentistry, The London Hospital Medical College, Turner Street, London E1 2AD.

*P. Sullivan*   PhD FDSRCS DOrth
Reader in Orthodontics, Department of Child Dental Health, The London Hospital Medical College Dental School, Turner Street, London E1 2AD.

# A Companion to Dental Studies

## Volume 1 Book 1  Anatomy, Biochemistry and Physiology

1. Biological Variation and its Measurement
2. The Basis of Scientific Investigation
3. The Biopolymers
4. The Cell and its Metabolism
5. Nerves
6. Muscles
7. Supporting Tissues
8. Lining Tissues
9. Secreting Tissues
10. Locomotor System
11. Respiratory Passages
12. Upper Alimentary Tract
13. The Remainder of the Alimentary Tract
14. Liver
15. The Cardiovascular System
16. Urinary and Genital System
17. The Endocrine System
18. Nutrition
19. Nervous System
20. Vision and Hearing

Appendix. The Fundamentals of Physics and Chemistry in Biochemistry

## Volume 2  Clinical Methods, Medicine, Pathology and Pharmacology

1. General Introduction
2. Pharmacology and Therapeutics
3. General Pathology
4. Hereditary and Congenital Abnormalities
5. Inflammation and Inflammatory Disease
6. Physical and Chemical Injury
7. Neoplasms
8. Organ System
9. General

# Volume 3     Clinical Dentistry

1. Disorders of the Masticatory Apparatus
2. The Masticatory System
3. Tooth Abnormalities
4. Injuries
5. Dental Plaque
6. Dental Caries
7. The Pulp
8. Diseases of the Supporting Structures
9. Psychology in Dental Practice
10. The Dental Surgery—Equipment—Operating Positions
11. Meeting the Demand for Dental Care
12. Primary Assessment and Stabilization
13. Local Analgesia
14. General Anaesthesia and Sedation
15. Choice of Anaesthetic Method
16. Periodontal Diagnosis and Treatment
17. Restorations of Teeth
18. Treatment Following Damage to Dental Pulps in the Permanent Dentition
19. Paedodontics
20. Replacement of Missing Teeth
21. Bridges
22. Partial Dentures
23. Immediate Replacement and Complete Dentures
24. Implants
25. Orthodontics
26. Oral Surgery
27. Management of Cleft Lip and Palate
28. Management of the Special Patient
29. Community Health
30. Dental Materials Science

# Foreword

*A Companion to Dental Studies* has been written to provide both the undergraduate and the recent graduate with a comprehensive and integrated text of dentistry. We hope that the series will provide the background for an appreciation of the scientific foundation of dentistry, as well as the techniques and philosophies necessary for its practice.

The Companion will be published in three volumes and integrated in a manner which it is hoped will give balance to the increasing complexity of the undergraduate dental course. The Editors and authors are all experienced teachers and well qualified to understand the needs of the students and can help them explore the plethora of information now available.

While there are many excellent texts on the different elements of the dental course, these have inevitably led to much duplication of subject matter. Furthermore, it is difficult for the student to assess the relative importance of each discipline, each teacher tending to feel that his particular subject is at the heart of dentistry. The Companion seeks to avoid unnecessary repetition and yet to provide the reader with an opportunity to appreciate the many facets within the subject and their relevant importance and perspective.

The authors and contributors have shown the utmost forebearance in having their texts modified and revised in order to conform to the overall style and limitations that a project of this complexity requires. The Editors, however, take responsibility for any errors or imbalance which have persisted into the final text.

At the end of each chapter there is a short reading list which is to be regarded as a stimulus to further study of a particular subject.

There have been important changes in nomenclature in some fields, such as anatomy, and the modern terminology has been adopted throughout. SI units have been used, except in a few instances, for example for blood pressure where the old unit still appears to be appropriate.

The idea that a sister publication to the successful *Companion to Medical Studies* should be written was that of Per Saugman, and he should be given full credit for this inspiration.

The Editors-in-Chief wish to acknowledge the invaluable support of the publishers, particularly Miss Helen Varley, who has been responsible for the sub-editing, under the guidance of Mr Peter Saugman. The artists have diligently drawn and redrawn many of the illustrations and Mr Frank Wallis has been responsible for preparing the indices.

Finally we wish to express our appreciation to the many secretaries who have been responsible for producing innumerable drafts of the texts.

*A.H.R. Rowe* *July* 1981
*R.B. Johns*

# Preface

The majority of what is known about the structure and physiology of teeth is included in courses given to dental students, but some contain little reference to comparative anatomy apart from evidence derived from experimental studies of laboratory animals. This is a pity because the true significance of any design, including that of the human dentition and jaws, can only be understood in any depth by comparing it with other designs, and different designs abound in the dentitions of other animals. With this in mind we have liberally sprinkled the text with comparative anatomy and include an appendix which describes in outline the dentitions of most mammals, and more detailed descriptions of those of primates and laboratory rodents. The result is that this book probably contains enough information on dental anatomy and physiology for students of zoology and anthropology as well as the students of dentistry to whom it is primarily directed. A study of human dentition, about which far more is known than any other dentition, should benefit the former two groups of students.

It has been convenient to add chapters on embryology, genetics, and ageing. The embryology of the face and jaws fits well with their evolution; genetics with human dental variation, general ageing with ageing of the dentition.

The decision was made to depend largely on line drawings because, in our view, more can be learned by a student from a diagram which selects key points, rather than a photomicrograph which inevitably includes confusing distractions. Few planes of section are ever as perfect as those constructed in diagrams.

Finally, we hope that where the reader finds within the text a new idea or point that is particularly well explained, he will make the effort to credit the contributor of the relevant section. We would like to thank several contributors for generously permitting us to make alterations which led to some uniformity of style and hope that we have not thereby muddied the excellence of their contributions.

*J.W. Osborn* *July* 1981

# CHAPTER 1

# Embryology and Development

Most of the text presented here describes the facts of normal development. However, these facts are introduced by an elementary survey of some interpretations which have been suggested by experimental embryology.

## DNA

The discovery of the DNA double helix is now a familiar story. However, molecular details apart, the double helix has a relationship to embryology which can be likened to that between the neurone and behaviour. All behaviour ultimately depends on the discharge of neurons; a knowledge of the structure of a neuron gives as much information about locomotor behaviour as the present knowledge of DNA tells us about the development of an embryo.

Observations of cell structure and behaviour are the 'meaning' of DNA. But our ignorance of the method by which this 'meaning' is represented in the enigmatic polymers of DNA makes inadequate any but the most elementary analysis of embryogenesis in terms of DNA. To state that the shape of a cell, its products or its movement are genetically controlled by DNA merely informs us that it is not entirely controlled by the environment.

## Cell differentiation

### THE PROBLEM

The adult human body contains about $10^{14}$ cells. Because all these cells have been derived from a single fertilized ovum it can be calculated that each cell in the adult is the descendant of about 45 cell generations (remembering that this is only an average figure).

A simplified lineage for some human cells is shown in Fig. 1.1 (the numbers of cells recorded are estimates which are only intended to give an idea of the magnitudes involved). The successive cell divisions within each lineage create increasingly more specialized (differentiated) cells, terminating in fully differentiated cells. When a cell has reached any of the stages shown in Fig. 1.1, it cannot normally regress to an earlier stage but either remains at its present stage or advances to the next. The final stage is the fully differentiated cell. For example, basal cells in adult skin can divide to generate prickle cells; there is some evidence from rabbits that they may be able to generate new hair rudiments leading to new hair follicles and possibly sweat glands. Therefore they are not fully differentiated. In contrast, the glandular cell in a sweat gland can probably do nothing other than maintain the synthesis and secretion of sweat; it is a fully differentiated cell. These two examples indicate a very common finding in embryology and development: if a cell is able to divide it is usually capable of further differentiation whereas a cell which cannot divide is usually incapable of further differentiation.

### DIFFERENTIATION

The astonishing similarity between all members of a species indicate that there exist stringent developmental controls over the myriads of cell divisions which eventually generate an adult. Even so, during the most complex period of development, the period in which an embryo develops all the miniature organs of the fetus that will later grow into the adult, there appears to be no central control (hormones may be involved at later stages). However, if an aggregate of what appear to be identical cell types is isolated in tissue culture, it is usually incapable of any further specialization: either the cells stay at the stage of development reached prior to their isolation or they degenerate. If these isolated cells are now cultured along with those of a different germ layer it is often found that they proceed to a further stage of differentiation. These results indicate that adjacent tissue layers interact during development to progress to further stages of differentiation. The controls cannot be centralized: they must be localized at the cellular level because

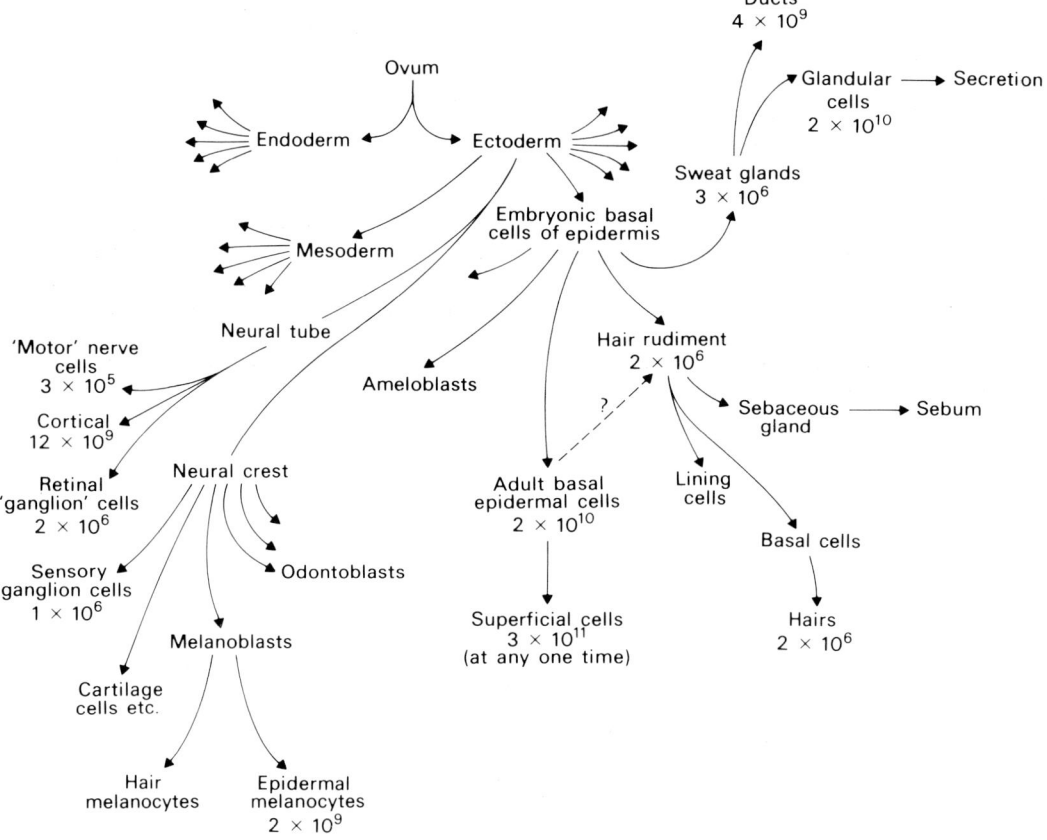

**Fig. 1.1.** A simplified lineage for some human cells.

differentiation takes place in the culture medium. It is concluded that differentiation proceeds by a (predetermined) sequence of reciprocating interactions between different tissue layers.

INDUCTION

A cell at a particular stage of differentiation may have several alternatives for further differentiation. For example (Fig. 1.1), at the gastrula stage, the ectodermal cells foster lineages which, amongst others, may become neural tube, neural crest or basal cells of the embryonic epidermis. At a later stage in development, these basal cells foster lineages which may become sweat glands, hair rudiments or ameloblasts or remain as basal cells. In each example, the alternative followed by the descendant cells is probably dictated by the subjacent tissue layer. Thus, at a particular stage of development, neural crest cells from the mandibular process of a newt embryo can be transferred to a site beneath the epidermis of the abdomen: in this position they are able to induce the overlying basal cells to differentiate into ameloblasts. The process is known as induction. In all the above examples, whether it is the effect of the chordamesoderm (presumptive notochord) inducing the formation of neural tube, mesoderm inducing sweat glands or hair rudiments and so on, it is not known how the inducing cell manages to initiate changes in the differentiating cell.

In different circumstances the cell which differentiates appears to have its fate already determined. For example, if cells from the endodermal outgrowth which will later produce the pancreas are cultured with mesenchyme from a rudiment of a salivary gland, the endodermal cells differentiate into cells producing pancreatic amylase. In this interaction, presumptive pancreatic epithelium is non-specifically induced by salivary mesenchyme; whereas the differentiation of embryonic epithelium from the oral mucosa into salivary acini in response to salivary mesenchyme is specifically induced.

We can visualize that each path along which a cell may differentiate is closed by a locked gate. Different cells progress along different paths blocked sometimes by only one gate and sometimes by a choice of several gates. A successful induction is a key which unlocks a gate. Obviously, if there is only one gate then the next stage of differentiation is already determined, any successful induction can only unlock the one gate. Such an induction is non-specific—it does not specify a gate. However, where there is a choice of several gates the stimulus specifies which gate: this is a specific induction. Some locks can only be opened by a single key. Other, less complicated, locks can be opened by several different keys.

COMPETENCE

If mandibular neural crest cells transplanted beneath abdominal epidermis induce the epidermis to differentiate into ameloblasts, it is said that the abdominal epidermis is competent to react to the inducing stimulus. During embryogenesis the competence of each particular cell aggregate to react to different inducing stimuli rises and later falls. If the cell aggregate is not induced during the period of its competence, it has 'missed the boat'. For example, human adult oral epithelium is no longer competent to react to induction by mandibular neural crest cells and develop new teeth.

MECHANISMS

It would be satisfying if it could be demonstrated that an inducing cell secretes a substance which causes a competent cell to differentiate. This requires; (a) a stimulus to cause the inducing cell to manufacture and secrete the substance, (b) the absorption by the competent cell of this substance and (c) the reaction by the competent cell to the substance. In such research, attempts are made to purify the active ingredient from either the inducing cell or the extracellular substance. The purified substance is tested by challenging competent cells and observing whether they differentiate. Either RNA or protein, for example, secreted by an inducing cell, may be absorbed by a competent cell and induce its differentiation-specific induction. Alternatively, a circulating protein such as a hormone may cause a change in the plasma membrane of the competent cell, which releases internally a substance causing its own differentiation. This is a non-specific induction, provided only one such substance is available for release, since any stimulus causing the release induces the same differentiation.

**Morphogenesis**

From the influence of nuclear DNA at the molecular level, to differentiation at the cellular level, we pass to the development of shape. A heart consisting of randomly arranged muscle, endothelium, valves and pericardium would be useless. Obviously the cell types must differentiate but so also must they be arranged into the functionally appropriate shape. The development of shape, whether of a gastrula or an organ such as a limb, is known as morphogenesis.

During embryogenesis cells differentiate, move and divide to develop different growing shapes. Although differentiation can be understood as the result of an interaction between two different cell types it is necessary to visualize a more widespread coordination between many different types of cell in order to understand how a limb bud can generate an arm. But even in this example, coordination is largely independent of the rest of the body. For example, if a leg bud from a chick is transplanted to the wing region it continues to grow into a leg; it also develops into a recognisable leg if it is grown *in vitro*. A limb bud is self-regulating.

It is clear that different parts of a limb bud must grow at different rates in order to change from a flattened bud into an arm and hand. This is referred to as differential growth. The elementary and predictable observation of differential growth sometimes appears to be thought of as an explanation for the development of shape. All too often a term coined to describe an observation eventually comes to be considered by some as an explanation.

Very little is known about the control of morphogenesis (development of shape). However, studies of isolated cell aggregates in tissue culture have revealed several mechanisms by which their behaviour might be regulated in developing systems.

CELL RECOGNITION

In order to react in a way which permits a continuation of normal development it is clear that cells must recognize their immediate environment. For example, if during normal development apparently identical osteoblasts on one side of a bone are laying down tissue at twice the rate of those on another side it can be assumed that the cells are responding, or have responded, to differences in their environment. In different circumstances cells may 'recognize' changes in their extracellular environment or they may 'recognize' and react to adjacent plasma membranes.

The above 'short range' recognition, which is very localized, can now be extended to chain reactions passing through large aggregates of cells. For example, in an elegant series of experiments, it has been shown that a layer of cells can be in electrical continuity, a change in potential of one cell leading to a simultaneous 'awareness' of this change by all the other cells. This might be thought of as 'medium range' recognition.

A circulating hormone causing a non-specific induction (see 'Mechanisms') is an example of 'long-range' recognition.

## CONTACT INHIBITION

It is possible to remove a piece of tissue surgically and, by immersing it in trypsin or a chelating agent, to separate all the cells. Subsequently a particular cell type can be isolated from the aggregate and cultured *in vitro*. The cells grow and divide on the culture plate and may move around. It is observed that those cells which are normally separated from each other *in vivo*, such as fibroblasts and mesenchyme cells, move about until they contact another cell, then they stop moving and later move in a different direction. This phenomenon is known as contact inhibition of movement. Presumably, the change in direction of cell movement is a response to the activation of receptors in their plasma membranes.

In contrast, cells which pile up on each other, such as the cells in a stratified squamous epithelium, do not 'contact inhibit' each other's movement *in vitro*.

## CELL ADHESION

Instead of separating when cultured, many cells adhere to each other. In general, it is found that like cells adhere together more strongly than unlike cells. This property leads to an interesting phenomenon when two different types of cell are mixed together. For example, if liver and kidney cells are mixed in culture, they move around until like meets like and after some time it is found that they have re-arranged themselves into histologically organised fragments.

It is interesting that cells in a carcinoma (cancer) are not strongly adhesive. They readily break away from the primary tumour and get passed via lymphatics to new regions where they may initiate a secondary tumour.

## CONTACT GUIDANCE

In tissue culture it has been observed that fibroblasts move along grooves or along lines of stress introduced in the substrate. Although the evidence is not conclusive, it seems probable that one tissue layer may often provide a surface which guides the movement of cells in an adjacent tissue layer. Once again the plasma membranes of the relevant cells can be thought of as containing some form of receptor which enables them to be guided in a particular direction. A possible example of contact guidance is the growth of the enamel organ around the dental papilla (Fig. 8.6). The cervical loop of the enamel organ does not grow out into the surrounding mesoderm: throughout the 6 or so years taken for a human permanent tooth to develop, the cervical loop continues to grow over the surface of the dental papilla.

## CHEMOTAXIS

It is possible that motile cells, particularly those in very early embryos, may be guided to or from a region by attraction or repulsion in response to chemical substances.

## MOVEMENT FOLLOWING CELL DIVISION

Continued, unrestrained and random cell divisions would produce a growing ball of cells whose surface approximated that of a sphere. If the cell aggregate is growing between two other layers of tissue, it becomes a sheet of cells whose growing margin migrates between the restraining layers.

## CELL DEATH

In some situations the final shape only appears after certain cells have died. For example, in a particular developmental anomaly the fingers and thumb of the hand are not separated but are connected together by 'webs', as in the webbed feet of ducks. This seems to be due to the tissues between the digits failing to die. In several other situations, particularly in the survival of only one of two embryonic bilateral structures, planned cell death seems to be important.

## GENERAL

All the above mechanisms have been proposed in order to account for observations of the behaviour of cells *in vitro*. It is not known which, if any, are important for normal development. However, following any description of cell movement, or changes in shape or growth of an embryo, it is often worth considering whether it is possible that one or other of the above mechanisms is responsible. For example, it is known that during development cells of the neural crest migrate into the mandibular process. There are several ways in which this movement could be guided. First, it is possible that chemotaxis is involved, either repulsion away from the neural tube or attraction into the mandibular process. Second, the neural crest cells proliferate between the neural tube and the ectoderm. These restraining layers could mechanically channel the growing margin of the neural crest aggregate ventrally into the gill arches. Third, it may be that contact guidance is involved, either the surface ectoderm or the mesoderm of the mandibular process being the source of 'information'.

## Embryogenesis

It must be remembered that only in a restricted sense does nuclear DNA control the activity of a cell. Certainly, an enucleated cell rapidly dies; from which it can be concluded that nuclear DNA is essential for the life of the cell; however, a plasma membrane is equally essential. The activity of a cell must be closely related to those segments of nuclear DNA which are being transcribed. But the cytoplasm of a cell plays a vital role in controlling which segments are being transcribed. And, by processes such as diffusion, the contents of the cytoplasm are partly controlled by the environment. It must always be remembered that DNA is only information.

During embryogenesis we can observe tissues moving, splitting, changing shape, reacting, depositing matrix, swelling, folding, and so on, in the countless different ways which finally generate a full complement of correctly arranged and shaped tissues and organs. Each step is explicable in terms of the chemistry and physics of single cells but the complexity of the whole is formidable. All activity must rely on reciprocating interactions and biological clocks.

## EARLY EMBRYOLOGY

### Germ cells

It is thought that the primitive germ cells are distinguished from the other cells of the developing embryo at a very early stage of development and can be recognized in the human embryo at about 4 weeks. These germ cells, larger than the other cells, develop in the endoderm near the yolk sac (Fig. 1.10) at the caudal end of the embryo but subsequently are found on the posterior wall of the upper part of the abdominal cavity (the mesonephric ridge). As is the case with other tissues and organs, so-called migration is due largely to differential growth, although amoeboid movement of cells cannot be excluded. A recognizable gonad appears at about the 5th week due to a thickening in one area of the surface cells. Whether the gonad becomes an ovary or a testis is determined genetically.

THE OVUM

There are several million ovarian germ cells in the fetus at about 20 weeks. This number is considerably reduced before birth and up to the age of puberty, so that there are, at maturity, about 400 000 germ cells left in each ovary, of these only about 400 are required during the fertile period of the average woman. Germ cells are called oogonia in the developing gonad. When the oogonia multiply they are called primary oocytes, which are found in the ovary.

A general description of the changes which occur before ovulation is given in Book 1. These involve the formation of an ovarian follicle (Fig. 1.2). At ovulation the ovum is released and enters the uterine tube. Before fertilization takes place the ovum undergoes maturation, which includes an increase in size and a reduction in the normal number of chromosomes (diploid number) to half

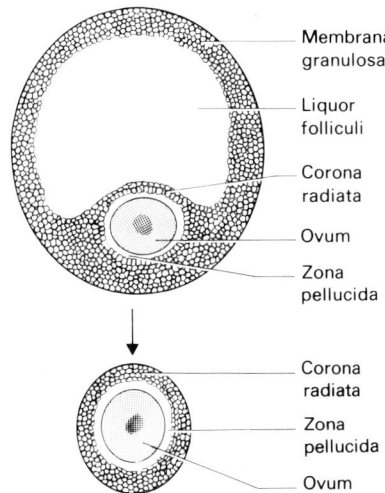

Fig. 1.2. Ovarian follicle (above) and primary oocyte (below).

(haploid number). The reduction in the number of chromosomes is called meiosis and occurs when a primary oocyte divides and forms a secondary oocyte. Initially (Fig. 1.4a) the primary oocyte contains the usual 23 pairs of homologous chromosomes. At the onset of meiosis each chromosome is duplicated, so each then consists of two chromatids (Fig. 1.4b). Homologous chromosomes come together (Fig. 1.4c) and material is exchanged between homologous chromatids, never between sister chromatids. One homologous chromosome from a pair passes to each daughter cell (Fig. 1.4d). The daughter cells therefore contain half the usual number of chromosomes (a reduction in the number of chromosomes) but each cell contains the same volume of DNA as the original cell (cf. Figs. 1.4a and d). One of these two cells enlarges and is the secondary oocyte; the other degenerates and is the first polar body (Fig. 1.3). Occasionally there is an

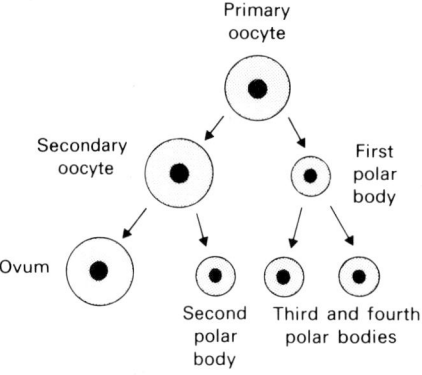

**Fig. 1.3.** Formation of ovum and polar bodies.

unequal division of the chromosomes at this stage of development which results in genetic abnormalities. During the formation of the ovarian follicle the primary oocyte increases in size, from about 30 to 130 $\mu$m. It also becomes surrounded by a clear area called the zona pellucida which separates the oocyte from the layers of cells which form the follicle. A cavity appears in the layers of follicular cells and is filled with fluid (Fig. 1.2). The oocyte is now surrounded by the zona pellucida and a covering of cells which is attached at one place to the wall of the follicle. When ovulation takes place the primary oocyte has already undergone its meiotic division and the first polar body lies within the zona pellucida which is surrounded by cells called the corona radiata (Fig. 1.2).

The final stage of maturation of the secondary oocyte begins before, but is completed after, fertilization. It is called the second meiotic division (Fig. 1.4d and e) in which the number of chromosomes remains the same but the quantity of chromosome material is halved. As in the first meiotic division, two unequal sized cells are formed; the larger is called the ovum and the smaller, the second polar body. The first polar body may divide equally so that three polar bodies

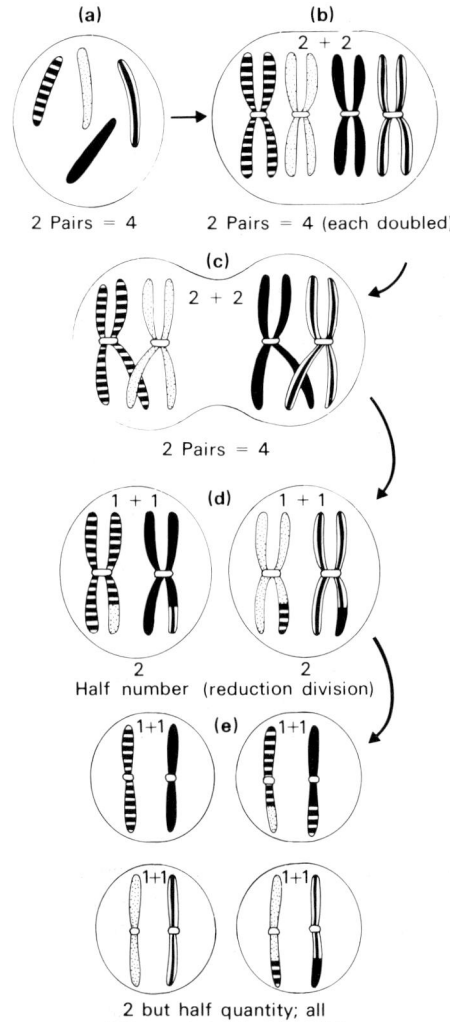

**Fig. 1.4.** First and second meiotic divisions of oocyte. (a) Four chromosomes. (b) Two pairs of chromosomes, each of which has doubled in quantity. (c) Interchange of chromosome material between individual chromosomes of a pair. (d) First meiotic division reducing number of chromosomes in each cell to two. (e) Second meiotic division in which each daughter cell has two chromosomes but each chromosome has half the quantity of genetic material; because of this and the interchange in (c), each cell is different from but related to (a).

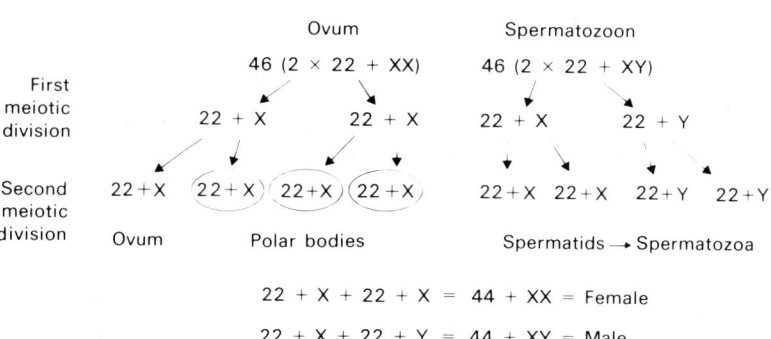

Fig. 1.5. Diagram to illustrate the reduction in the number of chromosomes and the determination of genetic sex.

are formed (Fig. 1.3) within the zona pellucida: all degenerate.

Maturation of the oocyte thus involves a reduction in the number of chromosomes and the storage of nutritive material (yolk) required for the early stages of development following fertilization. One of the 23 pairs is the sex pair of chromosomes, designated as XX in the female and XY in the male. A mature human ovum always contains 22 + X chromosomes. During the first meiotic division, as well as their number halving, genetic material is exchanged between the chromosomes as is shown in Fig. 1.4c. This explains why brothers and sisters are often alike and resemble their parents. Each child has some genetic material which is the same as that of the other, but due to the transference before the first meiotic division and the reduction in the amount of chromosome material, the genetic endowment of individual brothers and sisters is different.

SPERMATOZOA

Although maturation of the spermatozoa from the germ cells (spermatogonia) involves a number of changes similar to those seen in the maturation of the oogonia, the end result is strikingly different. Mature spermatozoa are motile, numerous, elongated (50 $\mu$m), narrow (4 $\mu$m) structures as compared with mature ova. There are approximately 100 million spermatozoa per cm$^3$ of seminal fluid and about 3 cm$^3$ of seminal fluid in an ejaculation.

In the course of the changes which occur during spermatogenesis the spermatogonia multiply by frequent mitotic division. Some of the cells undergo nuclear changes and form primary spermatocytes. These divide and form secondary spermatocytes which divide and form spermatids. Thus, the first meiotic division halves the number of chromosomes (Figs. 1.4b and c) and the second reduces the quantity of chromosome material (Figs. 1.4d and e). Human primary spermatocytes contain 46 chromosomes (2 × 22 + XY). The first meiotic division results in cells with 22 + X or 22 + Y chromosomes. If a spermatozoon with 22 + X chromosomes fertilizes the ovum, a cell containing 2 × 22 + XX results. This is a genetic female (Fig. 1.5). Fertilization by a 22 + Y spermatozoon results in a genetic male (2 × 22 + XY chromosomes).

Spermatids undergo a series of changes which result in the formation of spermatozoa. The nucleus, forming the head of the spermatozoa (Fig. 1.6), is covered by the acrosomal cap and the centriole lies behind the nucleus. Behind the centriole is a cylindrical part about 7 $\mu$m long and 1 $\mu$m in diameter which contains a large number of mitochondria. The rest of the spermatozoa consists of the tail, by means of which motility is achieved.

The secretions of the epididymis, seminal vesicle and prostate have a marked effect on increasing spermatozoa motility. Passage through the tubular structures of the male sex organs is due to ciliary activity and muscular contraction rather than movements of the tails of the spermatozoa.

**Fertilization**

This is the process whereby the male and female sex cells fuse and consequently make possible the development of a new individual. Unless fertilization occurs the ovum does not complete its second meiotic division and dies. An ovum is fertilizable for only 24 hours after ovulation. Spermatozoa are capable of fertilization for about 3 days after entry into the female genital tract, although they may remain motile for as long as 21 days.

The ovum is usually fertilized at the lateral end

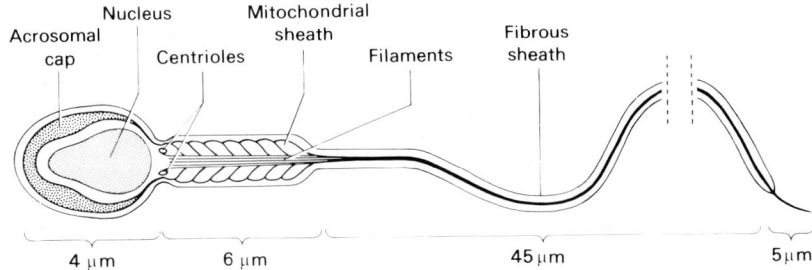

**Fig. 1.6.** Diagram of a spermatozoon.

of the uterine tube. This requires the spermatozoa to move from the upper end of the vagina or lower part of the cervical canal to the lateral end of the tube (Fig. 1.7). It is believed that this passage is assisted by contractions of the uterus and tube.

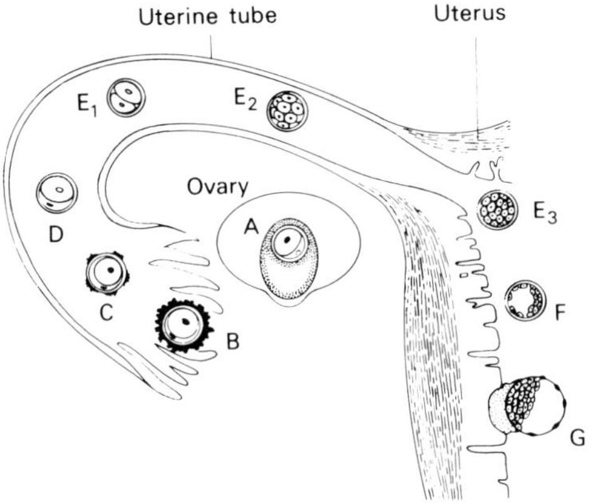

**Fig. 1.7.** Diagram to illustrate ovulation, fertilization and implantation: (A) Ovarian follicle; (B) ovulation; (C) ovum in uterine tube; (D) fertilization; $E_1$, $E_2$, $E_3$, dividing fertilized ovum becoming a morula; (F) blastocyst; (G) embedding into wall of uterus.

When spermatozoa reach the ovum only one penetrates its cell membrane although several may pass through the corona radiata and even the zona pellucida. There appears to be a species-specific reaction which allows this penetration to take place. Enzymes in the acrosomal cap of spermatozoa are responsible for the breakdown of the cell membrane, allowing entry into the cytoplasm of the ovum. Changes immediately occur in the ovum preventing the entry of further spermatozoa. The head and adjacent part containing the centriole separate from the rest of the spermatozoon and enter the ovum. The head becomes the male pronucleus. The ovum with its female pronucleus now contains the diploid number of chromosomes. Two centrioles, probably derived from that of the spermatozoon, appear and the zygote undergoes mitotic division. The next phase in the development of the embryo is called cleavage or segmentation.

### Cleavage, formation of the blastocyst and implantation

The first division of the zygote into two equal sized cells smaller than the ovum, the blastomeres, takes place within 24 to 36 hours. The blastomeres divide and form 4, 8, 16 and 32 cells, all of which are smaller than their predecessors and are contained within the zona pellucida (Fig. 1.8). The term morula is used to describe an embryo consisting of more than four cells but with no

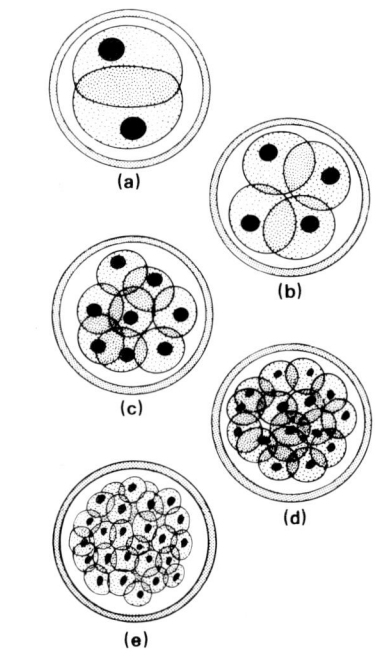

**Fig. 1.8.** (a–e) Formation of morula of 32 cells.

cavity in its centre. As the blastomeres increase in number the morula moves towards the cavity of the uterus which it is believed to reach about 72 hours after fertilization.

Shortly before the zona pellucida disappears fluid accumulates in the centre of the morula and a blastocyst is formed. In one region of the wall of the blastocyst there is a thickening of cells. This thickening projects into the cavity of the blastocyst and forms the inner cell mass from which the embryo and part of its membranes will develop (Fig. 1.10a). The cells forming the rest of the wall of the blastocyst form the trophoblast.

About 5 or 6 days after fertilization the trophoblast, which has spread over the outer surface of the inner cell mass, becomes attached to the lining of the uterus, usually its posterior wall, and destroys the uterine tissue. The blastocyst thus penetrates the uterine wall and comes to lie in the thickened, vascular mucosa. The lining of the uterus is called the decidua and normally the blastocyst does not penetrate the wall beyond the decidua basalis, the decidua adjacent to the uterine muscle (Fig. 1.9).

While the blastocyst is implanting, the trophoblast cells form syncytial masses (syncytiotrophoblast). Subsequently the inner part of the trophoblast develops as a cellular layer (cytotrophoblast). The syncytiotrophoblast breaks down the endometrium so that spaces are formed which receive maternal blood from the eroded uterine veins. The trophoblast can now be referred to as the chorion.

The inner cell mass by the 12th day consists of a layer of columnar cells, the embryonic ectoderm adjacent to the cytotrophoblast and a layer of cubical cells, the embryonic endoderm adjacent to the cavity of the blastocyst. Between the 12th and 20th day the inner cell mass forms two cavities and is joined to the wall of the blastocyst by a mass of cells, called the connecting stalk (Fig. 1.10). The cavity related to the ectoderm is called the amniotic cavity and its walls, other than the ectoderm, the amnion. The cavity related to the endoderm is called the secondary yolk sac. (The primary yolk sac is the name given to the cavity surrounded by the cytotrophoblast, which is lined by a layer of flattened cells continuous with the endoderm and called the primary mesoderm.)

While the amniotic and yolk sacs are being formed, the trophoblast develops extensions into the blood spaces in the endometrium of the uterus. These processes are called villi and consist of syncytiotrophoblast lined by cytotrophoblast. The primary villi branch and form secondary and tertiary villi which acquire a core of mesoderm

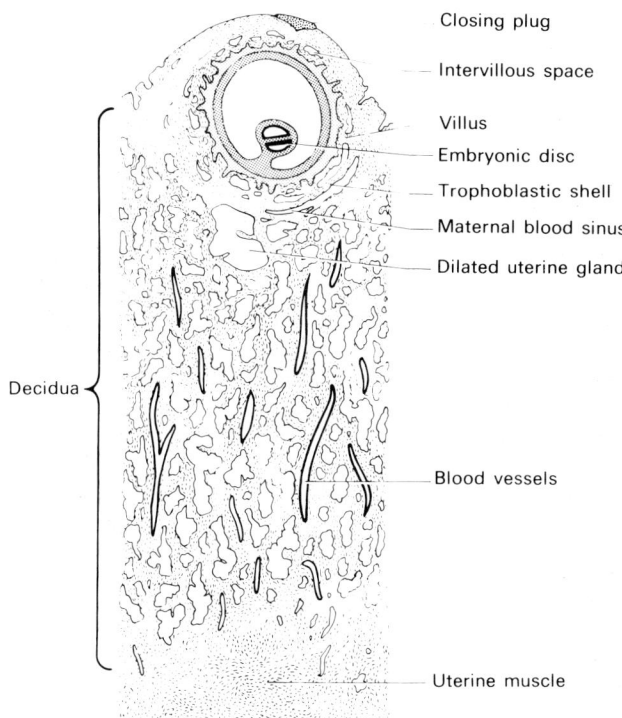

**Fig. 1.9.** Embedding of ovum.

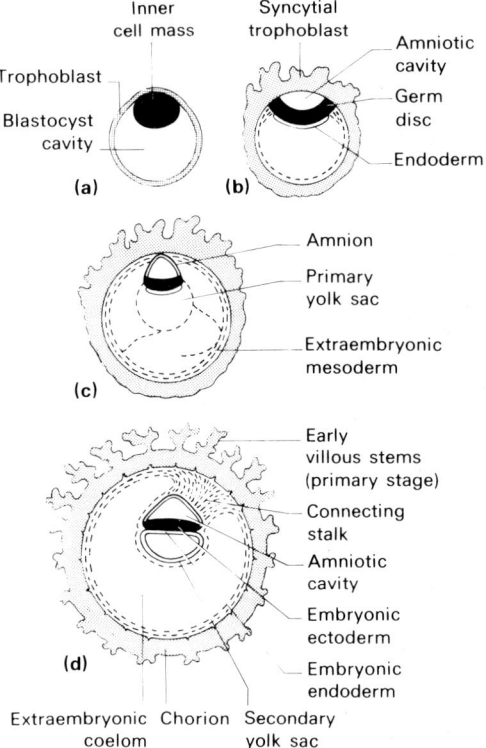

**Fig. 1.10.** Development of embryo. (a) Blastocyst in section, (b) formation of germ disc and amniotic cavity, (c) formation of primary yolk sac and mesoderm, (d) formation of secondary yolk sac, embryonic plate and chorion.

derived from the wall of the primary yolk sac. Blood vessels develop in this mesoderm. The villi which develop from the surface next to the connecting stalk are larger than those over the rest of the surface of the blastocyst and ultimately form the placenta. The villi over the rest of the surface disappear by the 3rd month (Figs. 1.11 and 1.12).

The trophoblast is able to penetrate almost any tissue with which it comes in contact. If for some reason the developing embryo is delayed in its passage along the uterine tube and trophoblast develops in its surface the embryo will embed in the wall of the tube. This is called an ectopic or tubal pregnancy. After about 6 weeks the tube ruptures with serious abdominal haemorrhage. Sometimes the developing embryo is extruded from the lateral opening into the abdominal cavity and the embryo may implant there and even go on to term (40 weeks). If diagnosed, a live fetus may be obtained by abdominal operation. Usually however the pregnancy is thought to be intra-uterine and after a false labour, the fetus dies.

## Placenta

At term the fully developed placenta is round and flat, about 15–20 cm in diameter and 3 cm thick in its middle. It weighs about 0.5 kg and has a fetal surface which is smooth and shiny due to the covering amnion. The umbilical cord is usually attached to the middle of this surface. The umbilical vessels can be seen branching and passing peripherally from this attachment. The maternal surface is rough and divided into a number of round lobes or cotyledons (about 20) of varying size. The umbilical cord at term is about 50 cm long and 2 cm in diameter. It is covered by amnion and contains a viscid, mucoid connective tissue called Wharton's jelly in which the tortuous umbilical vein and arteries run. The remains of the yolk sac, vitello–intestinal duct and vitelline vessels as well as the allantois are also found in the umbilical cord near its fetal end.

The placenta is the means by which substances pass from the mother to the fetus and vice versa. The fetal blood is always separated from the maternal blood by the tissues forming the villi. During the second half of pregnancy, although there is an increase in the diameter of the placenta, there is no increase in thickness. This is due to a cessation of growth in depth of the villi. There is a thinning of the tissues separating the fetal from the maternal blood, especially the cytotrophoblast and the connective tissue. In this way the nutrition of the fetus can be maintained because the passage of substances is facilitated.

Gases such as carbon dioxide and oxygen, water and salts can pass through the placenta by simple diffusion. Large molecules such as those of proteins and lipids are transferred by pinocytosis. The trophoblast also manufactures hormones such as oestrogens, progestogens, lactogens and chorionic gonadotrophins.

Many drugs pass readily from the mother to the fetus and some of these may be harmful. Organisms and viruses from the mother are also able to infect the fetus. The effects which drugs and viruses may produce on the embryo or fetus are related to the stage of development it has reached. Thalidomide and the German measles virus will produce developmental abnormalities during the first 8–10 weeks of pregnancy. The Rhesus factor is considered in Book 1.

After the birth of the baby, the placenta and membranes (the chorion and the amnion) are separated from the wall of the uterus and expelled by its contractions. The placenta separates in the plane of the blood spaces in the uterine wall and bleeding from the uterus is prevented by a marked

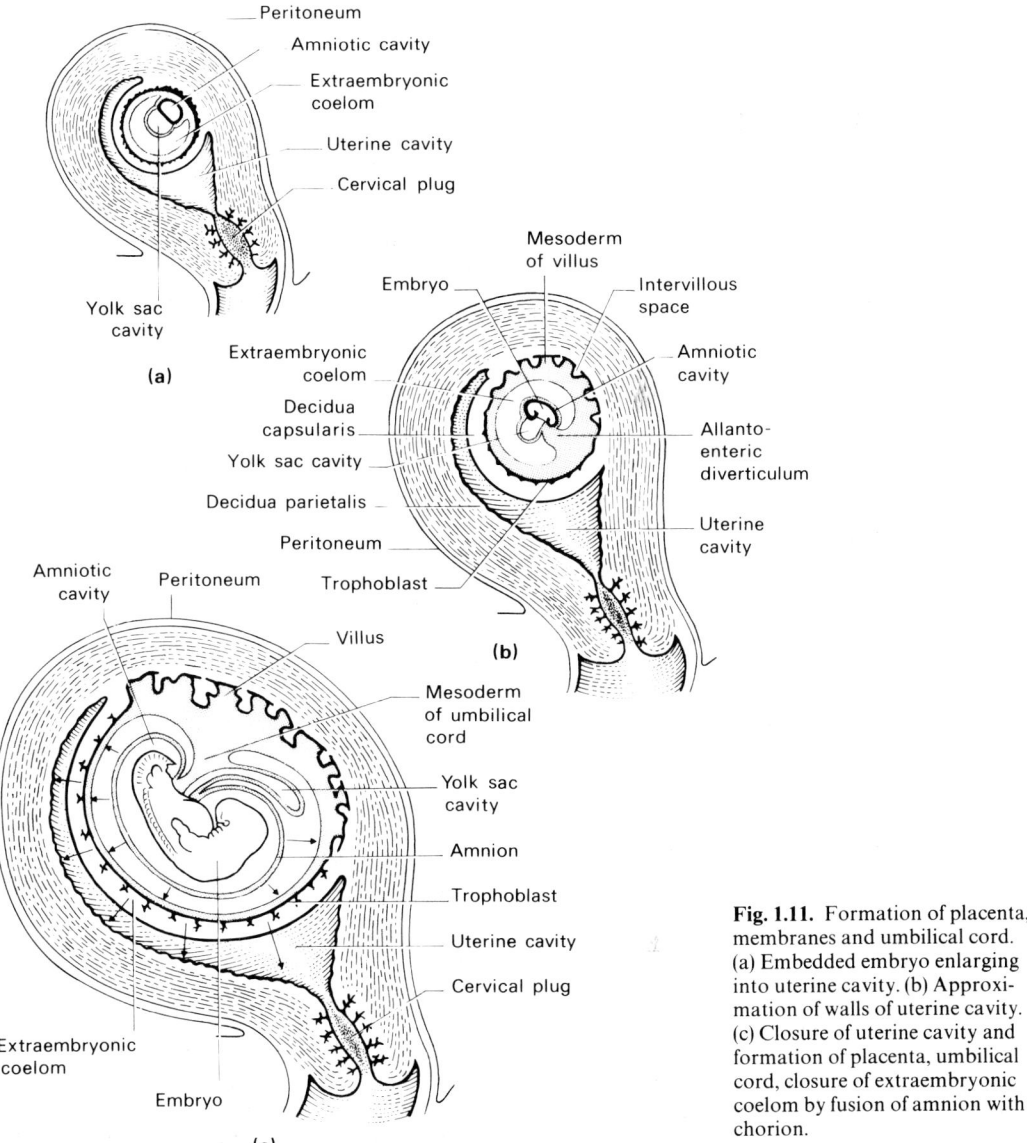

**Fig. 1.11.** Formation of placenta, membranes and umbilical cord. (a) Embedded embryo enlarging into uterine cavity. (b) Approximation of walls of uterine cavity. (c) Closure of uterine cavity and formation of placenta, umbilical cord, closure of extraembryonic coelom by fusion of amnion with chorion.

contraction of the uterine muscle. Unfortunately, the contraction of the uterus may be intermittent and careful supervision is required for several hours after delivery in order to prevent post-partum haemorrhage.

**Early development of the embryo**

Up to this point the word embryo has been used to describe the whole of the structure which has developed from the fertilized ovum, the term from now on will be used to describe the bilaminar structure consisting of ectoderm and endoderm. At about 14 days this structure is roughly circular. The ectoderm consists of about three layers of columnar cells and the endoderm consists of only one layer of cuboidal cells. Mesodermal cells cover the amnion and yolk sac. There is no mesoderm between the ectoderm and endoderm. The connecting stalk is related to what will be the caudal end of the embryo. A thickening of the endoderm at the opposite end of the embryo forming the prechordal plate, indicates the cephalic end of the embryo. As it elongates and becomes pear-shaped, with the wide part at the cephalic end, a midline linear thickening of ectoderm in the

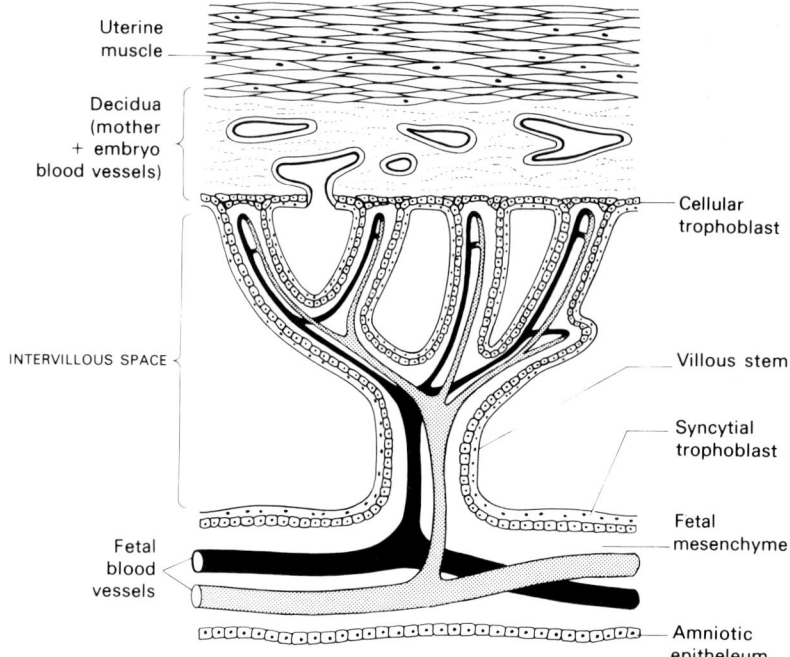

**Fig. 1.12.** Structure of placenta.

caudal part of the embryo is seen. This is called the primitive streak and its cephalic (anterior) end the primitive knot (Fig. 1.13a, d).

INTRAEMBRYONIC MESODERM

From the primitive streak, cells stream laterally, backwards and forwards between the ectoderm and endoderm: these cells become the intraembryonic mesoderm and thus a trilaminar embryo is formed (Fig. 1.13a, d). In the midline however the primitive knot extends forwards as a rod-like process of cells (the head process) between the ectoderm and endoderm and reaches the prechordal plate: it does not extend into it. The area of the prechordal plate where there is no mesoderm forms the buccopharyngeal membrane (Fig. 1.13b). There is a similar area in the midline at the caudal end of the embryo, the cloacal membrane, which consists of only ectoderm and endoderm (Fig. 1.13e). The head process, after a series of changes, becomes the notochord, the primitive vertebral column (Fig. 1.13a, c, f).

The intraembryonic mesoderm spreads laterally and fuses with the extraembryonic mesoderm. It also passes forwards on either side of the head process (the notochord) and the prechordal plate, and then medially from both sides in front of the plate where the mesoderm fuses. In this mesoderm the heart will develop and its most anterior (cephalic) part will form the septum transversum (Fig. 1.13f). In a similar manner the mesoderm passes on either side of the cloacal membrane and fuses in the midline behind it at the caudal end of the embryo.

NEURAL TUBE

While the above events are taking place the ectoderm in front of the primitive streak and overlying the notochord thickens and forms the neural plate (Figs. 1.13c and 1.14). The edges of the neural plate become raised and form the neural folds. These are more prominent at the anterior end of the plate and indicate the enlargement which will form the brain. Even at this early stage (2nd–3rd week) this enlargement shows two constrictions which indicate the future fore-, mid- and hindbrains. Eventually the neural folds fuse and the neural tube is formed (Fig. 1.14).

SOMITES

The mesoderm during the 4th week becomes thickened at the side of the notochord and forms the paraxial mesoderm (Fig. 1.14b). Lateral to the thickening is the intermediate mesoderm and more lateral still is the lateral mesoderm which is

# Embryology and Development

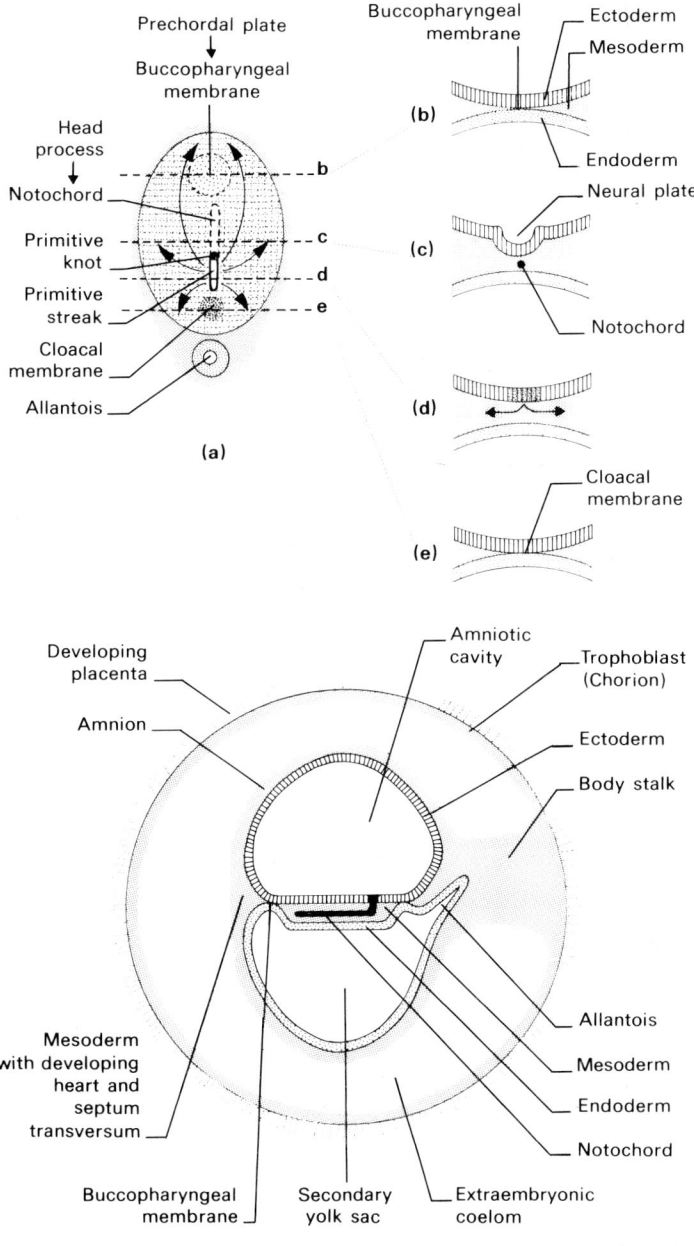

Fig. 1.13. (a) Surface view of embryonic plate (arrows indicate growth of mesoderm). (b) Section of (a) at b–b to show buccopharyngeal membrane, (c) section of (a) at c–c to show notochord and neural plate, (d) section of (a) at d–d to show origin of mesoderm from primitive streak (ectoderm), (e) section of (a) at e–e to show cloacal membrane, (f) sagittal section of embryo.

continuous with the extraembryonic mesoderm. The paraxial mesoderm becomes divided by transverse grooves so that a series of blocks of mesoderm is formed. This begins at the level of the hindbrain and extends backwards until about 45 blocks or somites are formed (Fig. 1.15). The number of somites present is used to describe the stage of development of an embryo (6 somite, 10 somite, 20 somite etc.) (Fig. 1.15). The mesoderm of the somites differentiates into a ventromedial part (the sclerotome) from which develops the vertebral column and a dorsilateral part (the dermomyotome) from which develop most of the skeletal muscle (myotome) and the dermis (dermatome) of the skin. Since the spinal cord is segmented in a similar manner, the innervation of

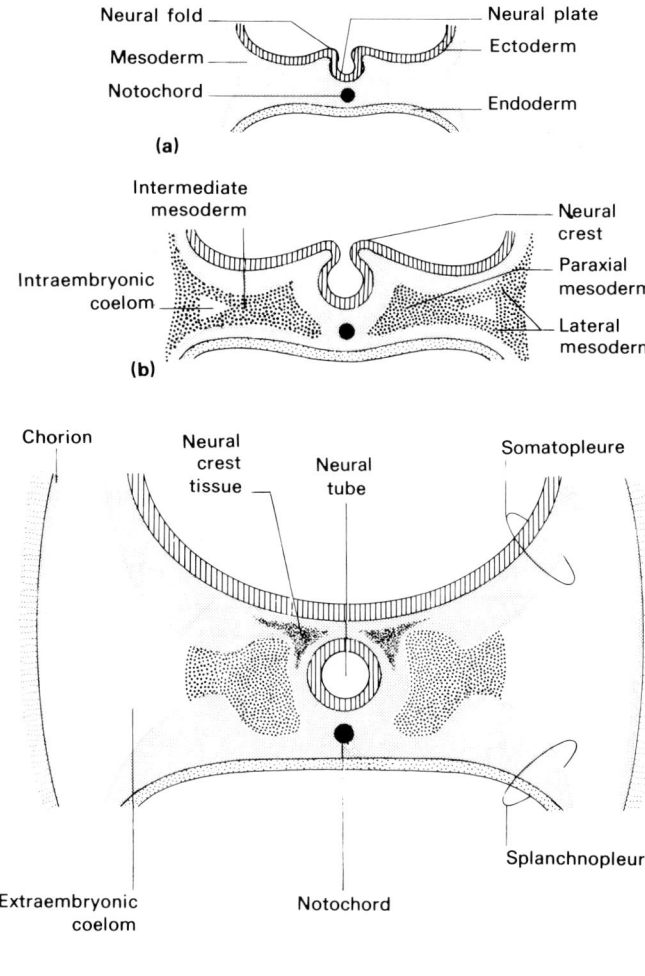

Fig. 1.14. Formation of neural tube and differentiation of the mesoderm. (a) Transverse section through middle of notochord; (b) similar section at later stage to show formation of neural tube; (c) similar section at later date showing the neural tube, the position of the neural crest tissue and the formation of the somatopleure and splanchnopleure. The intraembryonic coelom is continuous with the extraembryonic coelom.

the individual muscles and areas of the skin will correspond with the myotomes and dermatomes from which they are derived. (The muscles of the tongue are derived from the occipital myotomes and are therefore supplied by the motor nerve of the corresponding segments of the neural tube, namely the hypoglossal nerve.)

COELOM AND ITS WALLS

Most of the urogenital system develops in the intermediate mesoderm. The lateral mesoderm is divided into two layers due to the coalescence of a number of clefts in the mesoderm. The cavity thus formed becomes continuous with a cavity which develops in the cardiogenic mesoderm, anterior to the buccopharyngeal membrane. This results in the formation of an inverted U-shaped cavity which is called the intraembryonic coelom (Fig. 1.14b). From this the pericardial, pleural and peritoneal cavities develop. The mesoderm at the lateral edges of the lateral mesoderm breaks down so that the intraembryonic coelom becomes continuous with the extraembryonic coelom, the cavity surrounding the yolk sac and amniotic cavity and contained within the chorion. The lateral mesoderm and ectoderm are together called the somatopleure and the lateral mesoderm and endoderm are called the splanchnopleure (Fig. 1.14c). The somatopleure forms, together with dermatomes, the skin and subcutaneous tissues of the body wall. The splanchnopleure forms the walls of the heart and the alimentary tract.

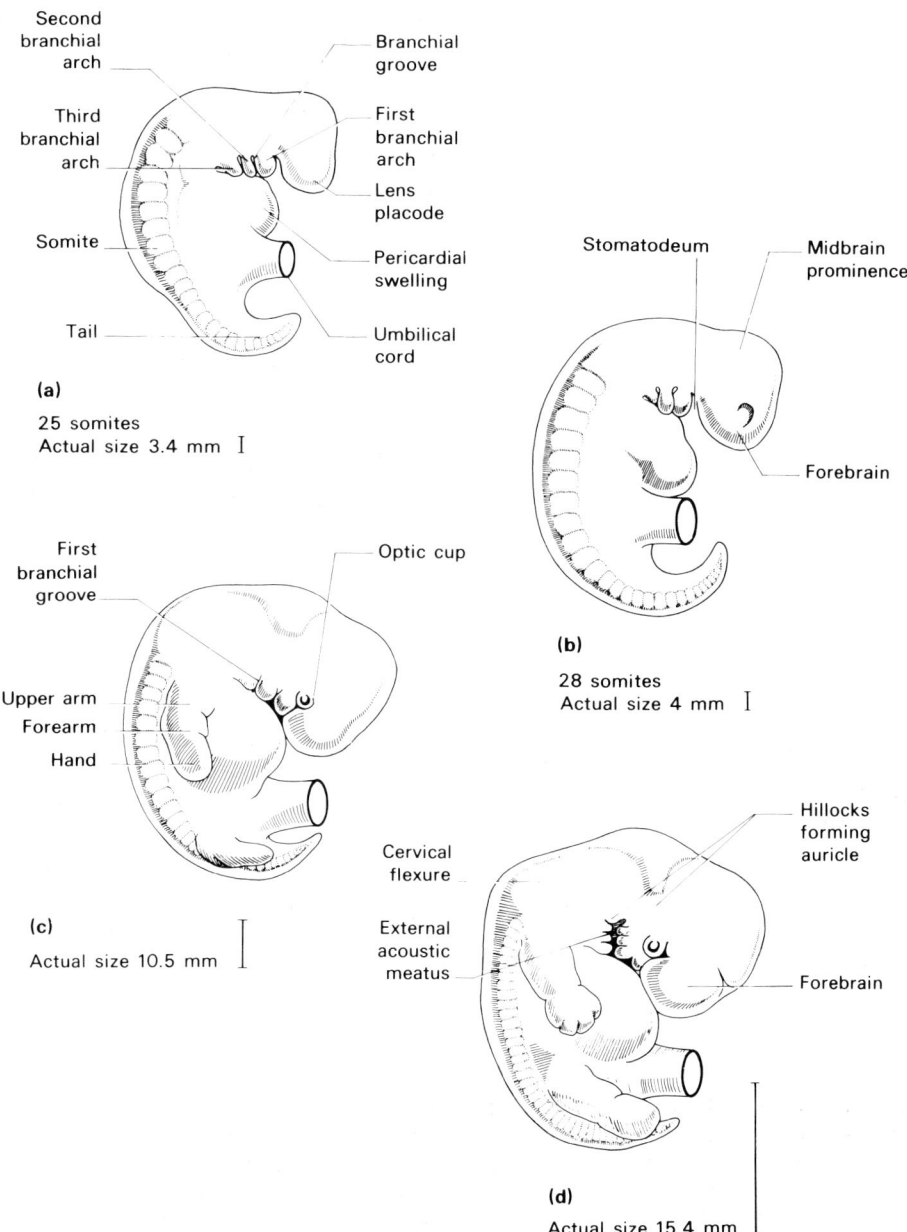

**Fig. 1.15.** External appearance of embryo at (a) 28 days; (b) 30 days; (c) 37 days and (d) 40 days.

EMBRYONIC FOLDS

During the 4th week, the embryo begins to change its shape as the inner parts are growing more rapidly than the peripheral (Fig. 1.16). The head fold is largely due to the expansion of the forebrain and results in the cranial end of the embryo being formed mostly by the forebrain. The bucco-pharyngeal membrane, pericardium and septum transversum come to lie on the ventral surface of the embryo. The membrane lies in a depression called the stomatodeum (primitive mouth). The tail fold brings the body stalk and cloacal membrane ventrally. The lateral folds, together with the head and tail fold, result in part of the yolk sac being enclosed in the embryo. This forms the enteron or gut which communicates with the yolk sac through a channel called the vitello–intestinal

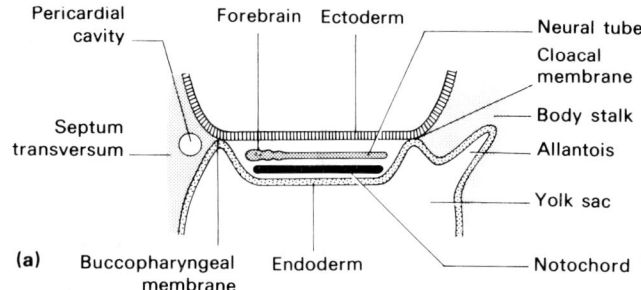

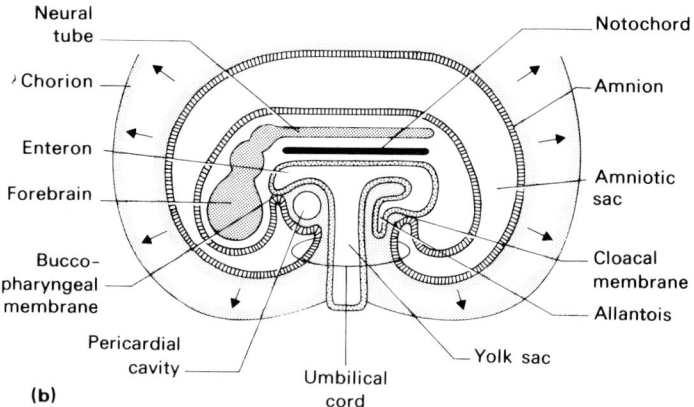

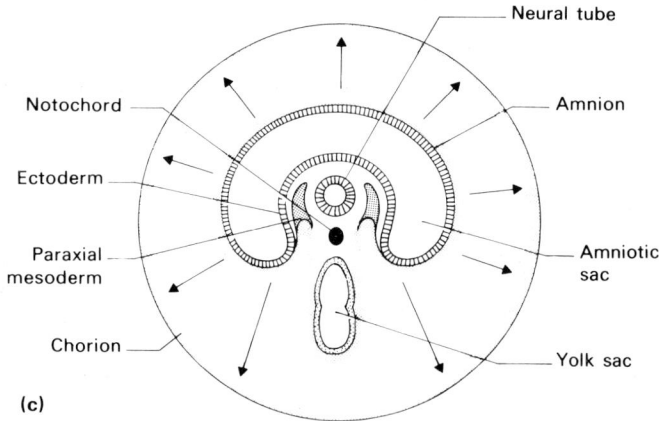

**Fig. 1.16.** Diagram to illustrate the head, tail and lateral folds of the embryo. (a) Sagittal section through embryo before folds. (b) Sagittal section after head and tail folds (note the new position of the septum transversum, pericardial cavity and forebrain bulge, and the formation of the enteron from the yolk sac). (c) Transverse section during the formation of the lateral folds.

duct. Before the tail fold develops a diverticulum from the yolk sac, the allantois, passes into the body stalk. With the development of the tail fold the allantois comes to lie anterior to the cloacal membrane and communicates with the cloacal part of the hindgut.

FORMATION OF AMNIOTIC CAVITY

One of the consequences of the folding of the embryo is the formation of the umbilical cord which now replaces the body stalk, the connection between the embryo and the developing placenta (Fig. 1.16). The wall of the amniotic sac expands (Fig. 1.16) at the same time and lines the chorion and placenta. The amnion continues over the umbilical cord and is continuous with the ectodermal covering of the body wall at the umbilicus. The amnion and chorion constitute the membranes. The amniotic cavity contains the amniotic fluid (liquor amnii) which consists largely of water (98%) (urea and organic salts are also present).

# Embryology and Development

## DERIVATIVES OF THE THREE GERM LAYERS (TABLE 1.1)

**Table 1.1.** Structures which develop from the three basic layers of the trilaminar embryo.

*Ectoderm*
1   The epidermis and its derivatives—the sweat glands, hairs, sebaceous glands and nails.
2   Nervous tissue, including the neural crest (see below), the neurohypophysis (the posterior lobe of the hypophysis cerebri) and the neuroepithelium of the special sense organs.
3   The epithelium of the roof of the mouth, cheeks, gingivae, nasal cavity and paranasal sinuses; the enamel; the epithelium and secretory cells of the salivary glands.
4   The epithelium lining the terminal part of the anal canal and urethra.
5   The epithelium of the conjunctiva and cornea; the epithelium and secretory cells of the lacrimal gland; the lens; the smooth muscle of the iris.
6   The adenohypophysis (anterior lobe of the hypophysis cerebri).

*Endoderm*
1   The epithelial lining of the alimentary tract except for that of its beginning and end as indicated in the ectoderm derivatives (3) and (4).
2   The epithelial secretory cells of all ducts and glands derived from the epithelium of the alimentary tract, including the liver and pancreas but excluding the salivary glands.
3   The epithelium of the auditory (Eustachian) tube, middle ear, thyroid and parathyroid glands and thymus.
4   The epithelium of the whole of the respiratory system.
5   The epithelium of urinary bladder and most of the urethra, and the secretory epithelium of the prostate.

*Mesoderm*
1   Connective tissues including cartilage and bone apart from those derived from the neural crest.
2   All skeletal and smooth muscle except that of the iris.
3   The heart and all blood and lymphatic vessels including their lining and blood cells.
4   The urogenital system except the endoderm derivative (5).
5   The serous membranes (pleura, pericardium and peritoneum).
6   The cortex of the suprarenal gland.

## EARLY BLOOD VESSELS

About the 15th day blood tissue begins to develop in the mesoderm of the yolk sac, chorion and connecting stalk and vessels develop in the chorion and embryo. In the latter, two longitudinal channels, the dorsal aortae, develop dorsilaterally. At the same time the heart tube develops ventral to the pericardium. As the head fold develops, the surfaces of the heart tube are reversed and the ventral surface becomes dorsal (Fig. 1.16). Thus the heart tube is dorsal to the pericardium. At the same time the dorsal aortae curve ventrally round the most cephalic part of the enteron and enter the tubular heart. The caudal ends of the dorsal aortae extend into the body stalk and become continuous with the umbilical arteries which have developed there. Before the folds are formed the right and left umbilical veins develop in the somatopleure near the edge of the embryo, run towards the heart tube and enter its caudal end. The umbilical veins pass through the connecting stalk and connect with the vessels of the chorion. The right umbilical vein disappears about the 8th week of pregnancy.

## NEURAL CREST

When the neural tube is formed (Fig. 1.14) many of the (ectodermal) cells at the neural crest migrate into the mesoderm (Fig. 1.14c). Some of these cells give rise to:
1   The ganglia and associated fibres of the cranial and spinal nerves.
2   Sympathetic ganglia.
3   The adrenal medulla.
4   The melanocytes of the pigmentary system.

Other cells differentiate along pathways typical of mesodermal cells and give rise to:
1   The branchial arch cartilages.
2   The tooth tissues apart from enamel.
3   Satellite (Schwann) cells.
4   The meninges.

## FROM 27 DAYS TO 8 WEEKS

Near the end of the 4th week when the embryo is about 27 days old and about 4 mm long, the head, tail and lateral folds have been completed, the neural groove is closed, the heart is represented by a simple tube, and the beginning of the development of a considerable number of structures can be seen. After 4 weeks it is necessary to follow the development of individual parts, organs and systems but it is important to appreciate that this development of the different parts is taking place at the same time. By the end of the 8th week, the embryo is recognizably human and thereafter the term fetus is used. After the 3rd month most of the changes are in size (and proportion) although individual organs may not be fully developed.

## AGE AND CR MEASUREMENTS

The following are some embryonic and fetal lengths at various times during pregnancy. These are usually measured from the top of the head to the buttock (crown–rump length = CR) (Fig. 1.15). At 21 days the embryo is about 2 mm long, at 28 days about 3.5 mm, at 35 days about 8 mm, and at 42 days about 14 mm. During the 7th and 8th weeks, that is at the end of 2 lunar months, the length increases to about 30 mm and the weight to 3 g. During the fetal period from the 8th to the 40th week the length increases to 50 cm and the weight to 3000 g. (Pregnancies in terms of time are best measured in weeks because of the confusion between calendar and lunar months.)

## EMBRYOLOGY OF DIFFERENT SYSTEMS AND ORGANS

### Cardiovascular system

#### THE HEART

As has already been pointed out, the earliest indication of the developing heart is the appearance of blood tissue in the mesoderm of the region between the pericardium and endoderm anterior to the prechordal plate (Fig. 1.16a, b, c). The blood tissue develops into two tubes which fuse to form a tubular heart during the formation of the head fold. The dorsal aortae curve ventrally on either side of the gut and enter the cranial end of the heart tube. The heart tube becomes divided by two deepening grooves into the bulbus cordis, ventricle and atrium (Fig. 1.17a). The atrium receives on each side an umbilical vein and a vitelline vein (from the yolk sac) by means of a common trunk, the sinus venosus which therefore has a right and left horn. All these changes take place during the 3rd week.

In the 4th week the heart grows more rapidly than the surrounding tissue and forms a U loop so that the bulbus cordis comes to lie to the right and the ventricle to the left (Fig. 1.17b). By the end of the 4th week the truncus arteriosus appears due to the lengthening of the connection between the dorsal aortae and the bulbus cordis. The arteries of the developing arches pass from the dorsal aortae round the sides of the gut to the truncus arteriosus.

Behind the developing heart (Fig. 1.17b) the right sinus venosus enlarges and carries into the atrium the blood from the umbilical and vitelline veins (later joined to become the termination of the inferior vena cava), and both the common cardinal veins (the right forms the superior vena cava). The left horn of the sinus venosus persists as the coronary sinus.

The sinus venosus opens into the atrium which

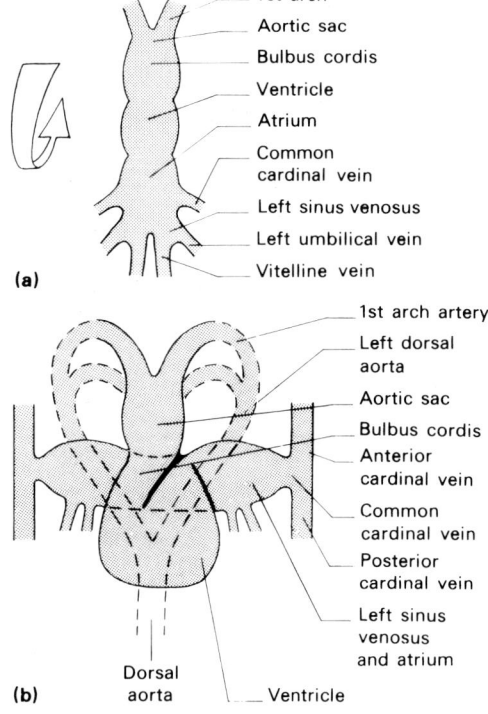

**Fig. 1.17.** (a) The subdivision of the tubular heart; (b) the change in position of the subdivisions of the heart, and the development of the right and left sinus venosus and artery of the first arch.

in turn opens into the ventricle via the atrioventricular canal. Swellings on the ventral and dorsal walls of the canal enlarge and fuse with each other so that these develop right and left atrioventricular openings (Fig. 1.18a). The free communication between the right and left halves of the atrium is reduced by the growth of a septum between the dorsal and ventral walls of the atrium, the septum primum (Fig. 1.18a). This septum remains patent so that the blood can pass from the right to the left part of the atrium. The opening is called the foramen ovale. There also develops a septum secundum to the right of the septum primum. The septum secundum remains patent so that blood can pass from right to left through the foramen ovale (Fig. 1.18d). The arrangement of the two septa allows the septum primum to act as a flap valve when the pressure in the left atrium is equal to or greater than that in the right atrium. Since in the fetus the right atrial pressure is greater than the left the blood is able to pass through the foramen ovale until after birth when the pressure in the left atrium rises and closes the foramen. The fused septa become the interatrial septum. The septum

# Embryology and Development

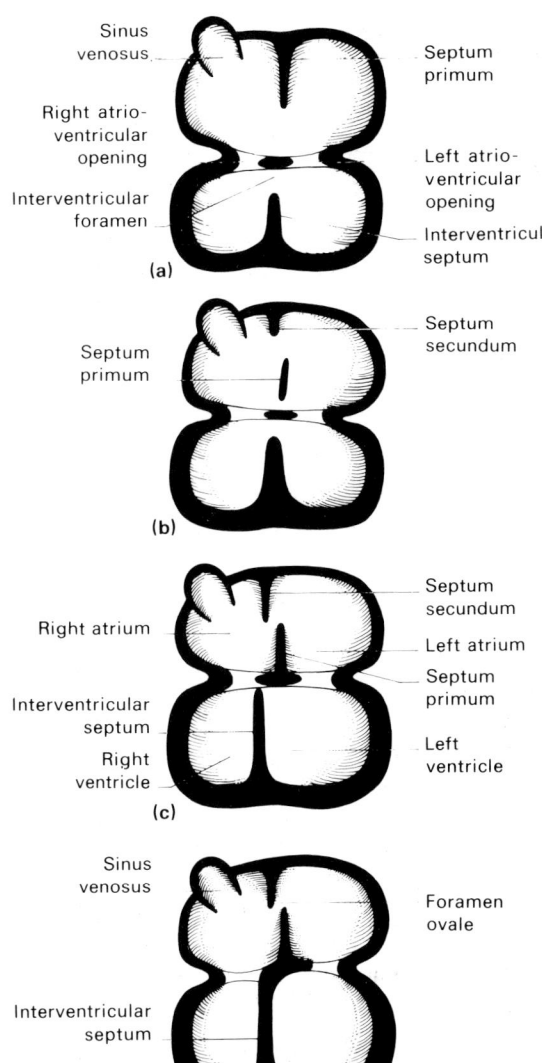

**Fig. 1.18.** The development of the four chambers of the heart. (a) The formation of the interatrial septum from the septum primum and the development of the interventricular septum. (b) The septum secundum and the septum primum. (c) and (d) The formation of the foramen ovale in the interatrial septum.

primum fuses with swellings in the atrioventricular canal so that the right atrium opens into the right part of the ventricle and *vice versa*.

The ventricle becomes divided into right and left parts by the growth of a septum which fuses with the swellings in the atrioventricular canal (Fig. 1.17). While this septum is developing the bulbus cordis, and aortic sac are being divided into two channels by a spiral septum with the result that the ascending aorta and pulmonary trunk are developed (Fig. 1.19).

All the above developments are usually completed by the end of the 8th week.

Left and right pulmonary veins, each formed by the union of two veins, join to become the common pulmonary vein which opens into the back of the left atrium. The left atrium enlarges by incorporating first the common pulmonary vein and then the left and right pulmonary veins with the result that four veins open into it.

CONGENITAL ABNORMALITIES OF THE HEART

It is now possible to understand some of the common congenital abnormalities of the heart associated with a high mortality in infancy.

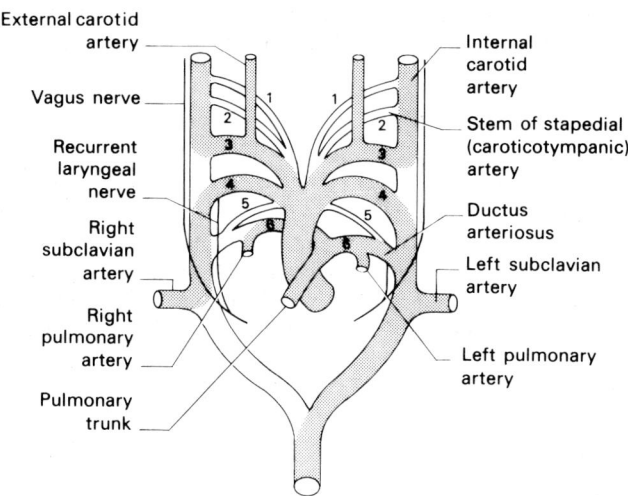

**Fig. 1.19.** The fate of the branchial arch arteries (non-shaded vessels disappear). The relation of the recurrent laryngeal nerve to the subclavian artery on the right and its relation to the ductus arteriosus and aorta on the left is shown.

Fallot's tetralogy, as the name implies, has four features: (a) an interventricular septal defect in the part near the atrioventricular opening; (b) an aortic orifice which lies over the interventricular septum; (c) pulmonary stenosis (narrowing); (d) hypertrophy of the right ventricle. Interatrial septal defects are due to faulty closure of the foramen ovale. Minor communications between the right and left atria are of little significance. Large ones result in one type of blue baby, due to shunting of the deoxygenated blood from the right to the left side of the heart. The truncus arteriosus may not divide correctly into the pulmonary trunk and aorta so that the aorta comes from the right ventricle and the pulmonary trunk from the left ventricle. In dextrocardia the apex of the heart points to the right and all the large vessels and aortic arch present a mirror-image as compared with the normal.

### THE AORTA

The large blood vessels develop as definitive channels in a capillary network which appears in the mesoderm. This network is connected to the aortae and large veins so that eventually the large arteries and veins are seen as branches of the aorta or tributaries of the venae cavae. The two ventral aortae arise from the truncus arteriosus and at a very early stage they fuse and form the aortic sac. As the branchial arches appear each develops an artery passing from the aortic sac into the dorsal aorta (Fig. 1.19). There are six arches and therefore six arch arteries but as the more caudal arches develop the cranial arches disappear.

### THE BRANCHIAL ARCH ARTERIES

Each of the six branchial arches contains an equivalent artery. The fate of each artery is represented in Fig. 1.19. The first, second (except for a small part which becomes the stapedial artery) and fifth arteries, together with the part of the dorsal aorta between the third and fourth arteries, disappear. The third, together with part of the dorsal aorta, becomes the internal carotid artery. An extension from the third artery becomes the external carotid artery. The fourth, on the right side becomes the subclavian artery, and on the left side becomes part of the arch of the aorta. By the time the sixth artery appears the spiral septum has already divided the pulmonary trunk from the aorta; the sixth artery joins the pulmonary trunk. On each side a branch of the sixth artery passes to the lung and forms the pulmonary artery. On the right side the dorsal part of the sixth artery disappears: on the left side the connection between the pulmonary artery and the aorta remains as the ductus arteriosus. This acts as a shunt for some of the blood from the heart to the aorta so that the blood does not pass through the lungs. There are therefore two pathways for bypassing the lungs: one from the right to the left atrium through the foramen ovale; and the other from the left pulmonary artery to the aorta through the ductus arteriosus.

The rest of the two dorsal aortae fuse to form a single descending aorta at about the 4th week.

REMAINING ARTERIES

The dorsal aortae give off transverse segmental branches to the rest of the body. These branches anastomose longitudinally. The vertebral and internal thoracic arteries, for example, are persistent anastomoses following the degeneration of the segmental arteries. The abdominal arteries develop from three sets of segmental branches of the dorsal aorta: ventral to the gut, lateral to the urogenital system and somatic to the body wall.

VEINS

Venous development has to be considered in relation to both the vitelline and umbilical veins, which convey nutrition to the embryo, and to the veins of the rest of the body. The sinus venosus receives the left and right umbilical veins and the left and right vitelline veins; the latter have several cross anastomoses (Fig. 1.20a). The right umbilical vein disappears. The developing liver surrounds the remaining three veins with the result that their blood passes through the liver sinusoids (Fig. 1.20b) before entering the developing heart. A new and large channel, the ductus venosus, bypasses the liver sinusoids and carries blood directly from the placenta to the heart. The right vitelline vein and its dorsal anastomosis with the left vitelline vein (Fig. 1.20a and b) become the portal vein which is formed by the union of the superior mesenteric and splenic veins (Fig. 1.20c).

The common cardinal vein, formed by the union of the precardinal and postcardinal veins joins the sinus venosus (Fig. 1.21a). With the preferential growth of the right sinus venosus, blood from the left precardinal vein enters an anastomotic channel, the left branchiocephalic vein, and joins the right precardinal vein (Fig. 1.21b). In this way blood from both left and right sides of the head, neck and upper limbs drains into the superior vena cava, which is on the right side.

Blood in the postcardinal veins is transferred from the common cardinal veins mainly to the longitudinal subcardinal veins (Fig. 1.21a) which establish communication with the developing inferior vena cava. Only a few remnants of the postcardinal veins remain, in particular the termination of the azygos vein which opens into the superior vena cava (Fig. 1.21b). The azygos and hemi-azygos veins develop from longitudinal anastomoses between transversely running segmental branches of the postcardinal veins.

FETAL CIRCULATION

The fetal circulation is established by the end of the 12th week. Blood leaves the placenta by the left umbilical vein which passes to the umbilicus in the umbilical cord. It enters the fetus and runs via the ductus venosus into the inferior vena cava (see Figs. 1.20c, 1.22). From here, blood enters the right atrium and most of it passes through the foramen ovale into the left atrium (Fig. 1.22) on to the left ventricle and then into the aorta. Most of this blood goes to the heart, head, neck and upper limbs via aortic branches and returns in the superior vena cava to the right atrium. This blood passes into the right ventricle and then into the pulmonary trunk. From there the blood passes via the ductus arteriosus into the aorta beyond the origin of its large branches. The blood then passes in the aorta to the common iliac and internal iliac arteries. The internal iliac arteries continue into the umbilical arteries which pass to the umbilicus and thence to the placenta. A small quantity of blood passes into the lower limbs via the external iliac arteries.

Some blood does pass through the non-functioning organs, especially the liver (Fig. 1.20c). It also appears that although blood enters the right atrium via both the superior and inferior venae cavae, the two streams of blood remain separate. The blood going to the heart, head, neck and upper limbs has more oxygen and nutrients than that going to the rest of the body.

At birth, with the onset of respiration, more blood passes through the lungs and therefore more blood returns to the left atrium through the pulmonary veins. The pressure in the left atrium rises. In addition the pressure in the right atrium falls due to occlusion of the umbilical vein. With the equalization of pressure in the two atria, the septum primum and septum secundum are forced together and blood no longer passes through the foramen ovale from right to left. The ductus arteriosus, which contains in its wall a considerable amount of smooth muscle, closes due to contraction. It is finally sealed by proliferation of its lining endothelium and forms a fibrous cord, the ligamentum arteriosum. The umbilical vessels and the ductus venosus also close and become fibrous cords.

**The alimentary tract and respiratory passages, including diaphragm**

It is convenient to consider these together since the respiratory passages develop from the gut. It will be recalled that with the folding of the embryo,

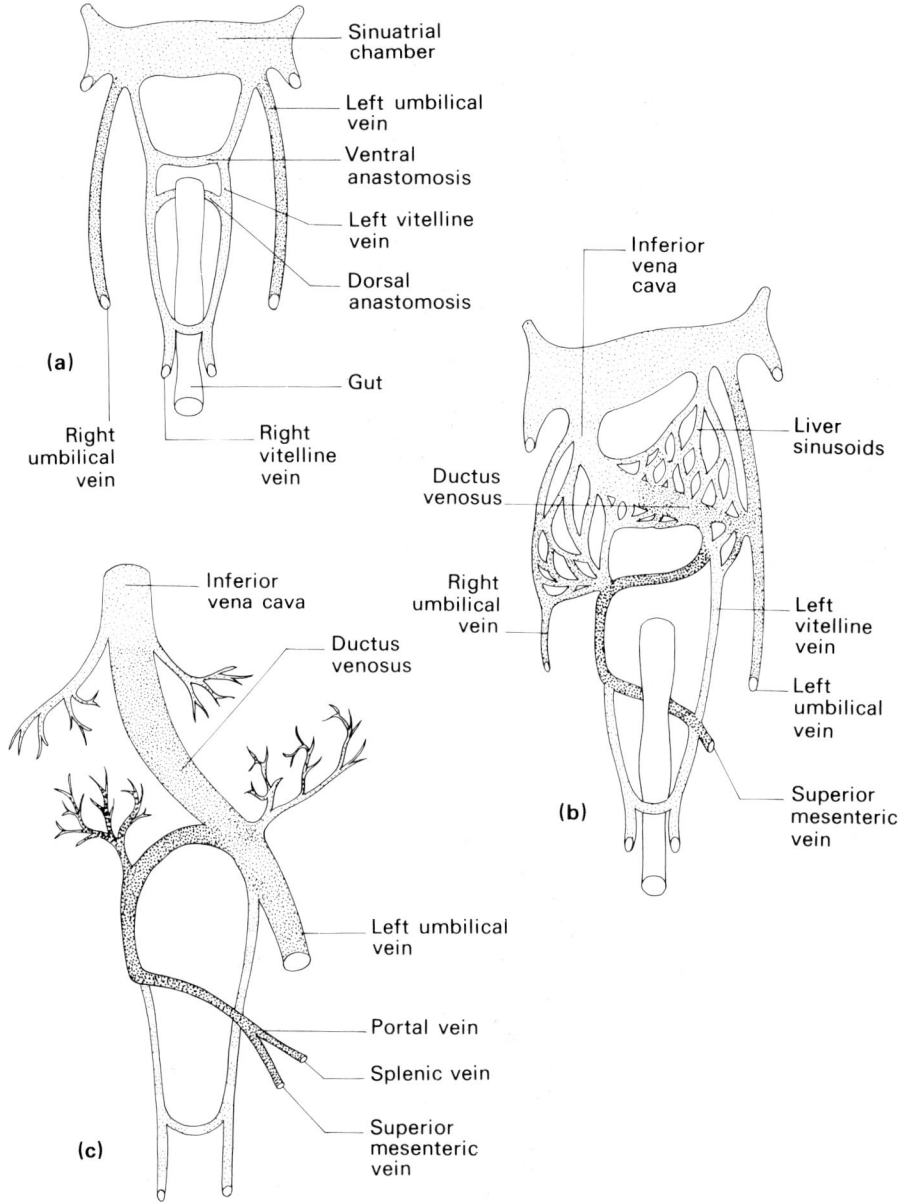

**Fig. 1.20.** (a) Early arrangement of the vitelline and umbilical veins, (b) development of the ductus venosus and portal vein, (c) final arrangement in the fetus of the vitelline and umbilical veins.

part of the yolk sac was enclosed within the embryo and for a time remained in communication with the rest of the yolk sac through the vitello–intestinal duct (Fig. 1.16). The yolk sac within the embryo can now be called the enteron or gut, comprising the foregut, the midgut and the hindgut. These are more precisely defined later on.

It will also be recalled that in two places the endoderm of the yolk sac was attached to the ectoderm without any mesoderm intervening. The cranial area is called the buccopharyngeal membrane and the caudal, the cloacal membrane. The buccopharyngeal membrane, after the formation of the head fold, lies in a recess called the

# Embryology and Development

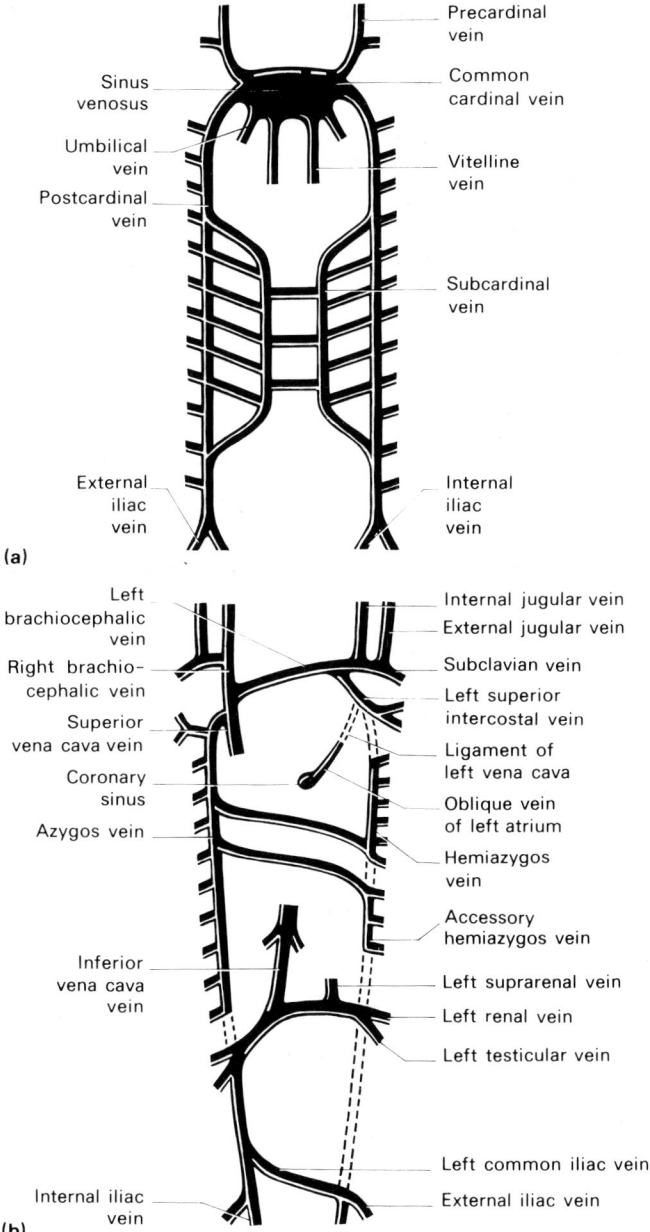

**Fig. 1.21.** (a) Early arrangement of main veins of the body; (b) final arrangement of these veins.

stomatodeum. At this stage the bulge of the forebrain is cranial to the stomatodeum and the pericardial bulge is caudal. There is no neck or face and their development is described elsewhere. The branchial arches (often called pharyngeal) develop round the cranial end of the foregut (the mouth and pharynx). Caudal to this region the foregut elongates and forms the oesophagus.

Distal to the septum transversum the foregut dilates and forms the stomach which at first is in the midline with right and left surfaces. The stomach, due to differential growth, is displaced to the left. The midgut elongates rapidly and for a time (from the end of the 5th to the end of the 12th week) it is extruded into the proximal part of the umbilical cord because of lack of space in the abdominal cavity, due to the enlargement of the liver and mesonephros (fetal umbilical hernia)

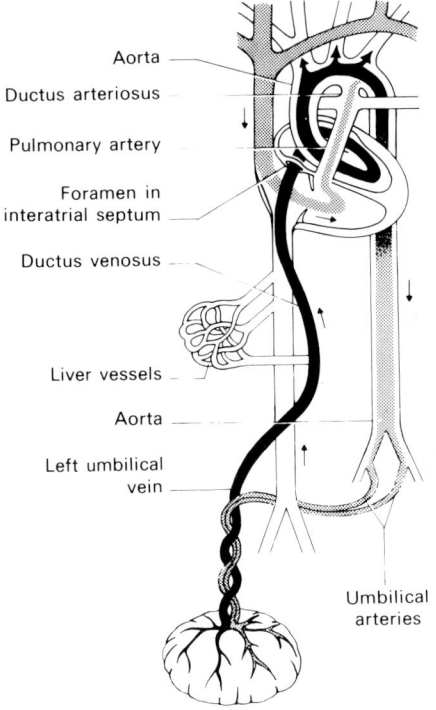

**Fig. 1.22.** The fetal circulation.

The liver develops in the 4th week as a diverticulum of endoderm from the foregut. The liver cells become surrounded by blood-filled sinusoids derived from the mesoderm of the septum transversum (see Fig. 1.20). The fetal liver is proportionately larger and occupies a much bigger volume of the abdominal cavity than in the adult. It is haemopoietic.

The cystic duct and the gall bladder develop from an outgrowth of the original liver diverticulum which canalizes and becomes the bile duct.

The pancreas develops in two parts in the 4th week; one is a diverticulum from the dorsal wall of the duodenum, the other is a diverticulum from the bile duct. The two parts gradually grow and fuse together.

The spleen develops on the dorsal wall of the coelom at the level of the stomach. It is not connected with the endoderm of the gut wall.

The respiratory passages distal to the pharynx develop from the ventral wall of the pharynx. At about the 4th week the laryngotracheal groove appears and forms a tube which passes caudally, ventral to the pharynx (Fig. 1.24). The tube of endoderm grows into the pleural part of the coelomic cavity and is covered by splanchnopleure (visceral mesoderm). The epithelium of the respiratory passages is thus endodermal in origin and the rest of the tissues (visceral pleura, blood vessels, cartilage, etc.) is mesodermal. Early on the tube which is ventral to the pharynx divides into two lung buds from which the lungs develop (Fig. 1.24c). The right lung bud divides into three and the left into two, so that the three lobes of the right lung and two of the left are indicated as early as the 5th week and the lungs extend into the pleural part of the coelom. The lobar lung buds keep dividing and by the 25th week the air sacs are formed. The alveoli are formed during the last 12 weeks.

The diaphragm develops from the septum transversum: the intraembryonic coelom (p. 12) passes dorsal to the septum. This part of the coelom is the communication between the cranial part which develops into the pleural cavity and the caudal part which becomes the peritoneal cavity. This communication is called the pleuroperitoneal canal. The two cavities become completely separated by the growth of the edges of the canal towards the septum transversum. That part of the septum transversum above the developing liver forms the ventral and middle parts of the diaphragm and the tissue which closes the pleuroperitoneal canals forms the dorsal part. A peripheral contribution to the diaphragm is also made from the chest wall of the embryo.

(Fig. 1.23). At first the loop has an upper exiting limb and a lower entering limb. The loop rotates counterclockwise so that the upper limb passes to the right and the lower to the left. In the 6th week a protrusion of the loop from the lower limb appears and develops into the caecum and vermiform appendix, thus differentiating the small from the large intestine (Fig. 1.23b). The original proximal limb of the loop elongates and forms the small intestine. In the 12th week the gut returns to the abdominal cavity. As it does so it continues to rotate in a counterclockwise direction so that what was the lower loop crosses over the upper loop at the part which becomes the duodenum (Fig. 1.23c). This explains why the transverse colon crosses the duodenum and the superior mesenteric vessels are anterior to it.

The caudal end of the hindgut is called the cloaca and is separated from the surface of the embryo by the cloacal membrane. The cloaca becomes divided into dorsal and ventral parts by the growth of a mesodermal septum. The dorsal part remains continuous with the hindgut and becomes the rectum. The ventral part, known as the urogenital sinus, develops into the bladder and part of the urethra. Later the rectal part of the cloacal membrane breaks down.

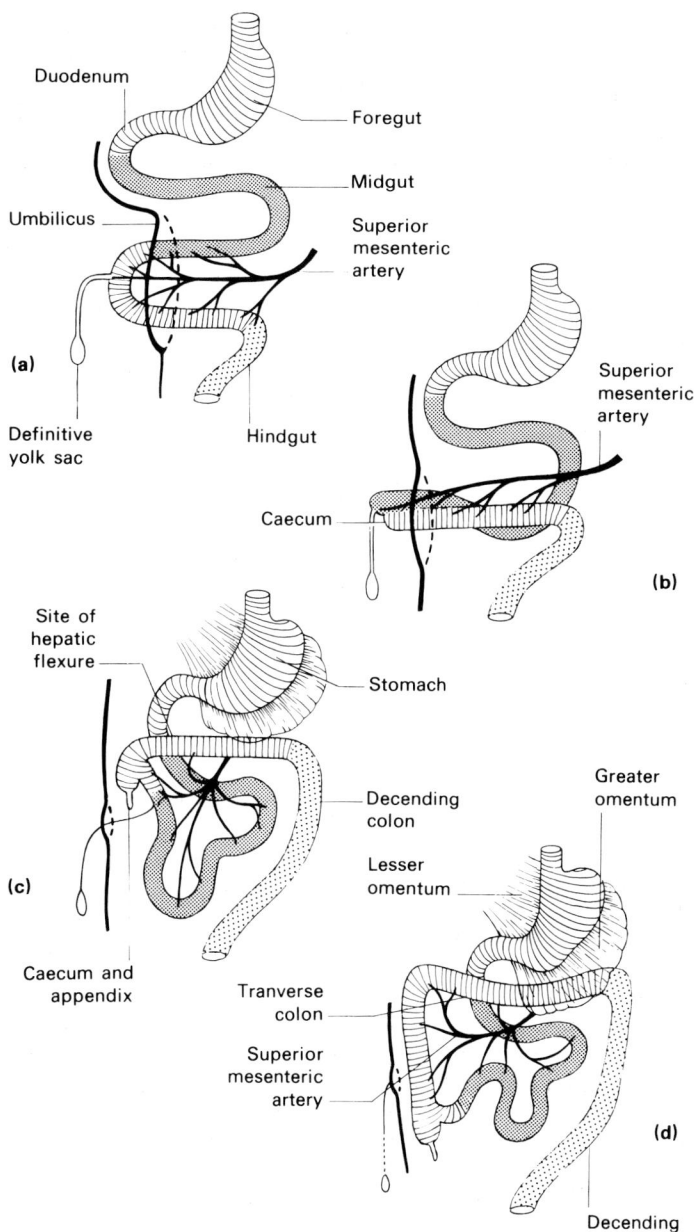

Fig. 1.23. The development of the gut. (a) The formation of the U-shaped temporary umbilical hernia, (b) the counterclockwise rotation of the gut so that the upper limb of the 'U' moves to the right, (c) the continuing rotation of the gut and reduction of the hernia, (d) the final position of the gut in which the lower limb of the loop has crossed the upper limb.

## Urogenital organs

The intermediate mesoderm (p. 12) grows and differentiates to produce the reproductive and urinary organs.

### GENITAL SYSTEM

A region on the medial side of the lumbar part of the intermediate cell mass rapidly proliferates and becomes separated from the remainder. It differentiates into the ovary of the female, and the seminiferous tubules and rete testis of the male.

Throughout its length, the lateral part of the intermediate cell mass differentiates into a repetitive sequence of horizontal tubules from which developed the kidney of ancestral vertebrates. These connect with a longitudinally running duct, the mesonephric duct, which opens into the urogenital sinus, the ventral part of the cloaca.

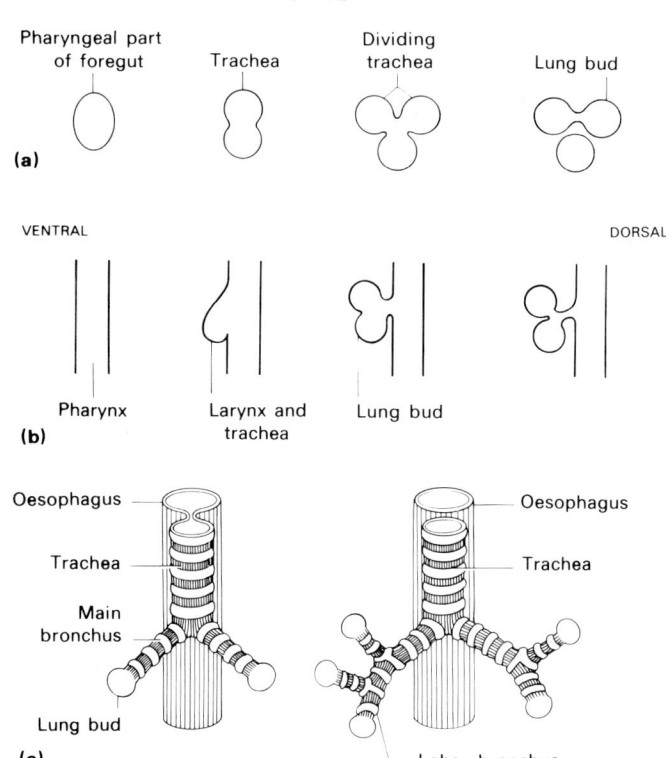

Fig. 1.24. Development of the trachea and lungs. (a) Cross-sectional view, (b) sagittal section view, (c) as seen from the ventral surface.

Only in the male do these structures persist and differentiate: the caudal (mesonephric) horizontal tubules become the epididymis and the duct becomes the ductus deferens, seminal vesicle and ejaculatory duct. In the female all the tubules normally degenerate. In both the male and female embryo the paramesonephric (Mullerian) duct develops within a column of cells which grows on the lateral part of the mesonephric ridge from the wall of the coelomic cavity. In the female this duct develops into the uterine tubes, uterus and part of the vagina. The peritoneal cavity is continuous with the lumen of the tube. In the male most of it degenerates.

KIDNEY

The kidney develops from the ureteric bud which is an outgrowth from the caudal end of the mesonephric duct. The bud comes in contact with mesoderm which is called the metanephrogenic cap, which forms the nephrons and the glomeruli. The ureteric bud forms the collecting tubules, collecting ducts and ureter.

## THE BRANCHIAL (PHARYNGEAL) ARCHES (Figs 1.15, 1.16, 1.25)

The ventral aspect of the cranial end of the embryo shows the depression forming the stomatodeum with the bulge of the forebrain above and the cardiac projection below. Neither the face nor neck is present. The foregut extends cranially to the buccopharyngeal membrane which separates it from the stomatodeum. The membrane consists of only ectoderm and endoderm but around the periphery of the membrane there is also a layer of mesoderm. The anterior end of the foregut can be called the pharynx. During the 4th week the mesoderm forms a series of rod-like thickenings which extend ventrally from the lateral side of the pharynx. These thickenings are called the branchial or pharyngeal arches (Fig. 1.25). Between the thickenings there is no mesoderm, so that the arches are limited by grooves. The external grooves are called clefts and the internal ones are called pouches.

The mesoderm of each arch gives rise to a skeletal element, muscles and an artery (Fig.

# Embryology and Development

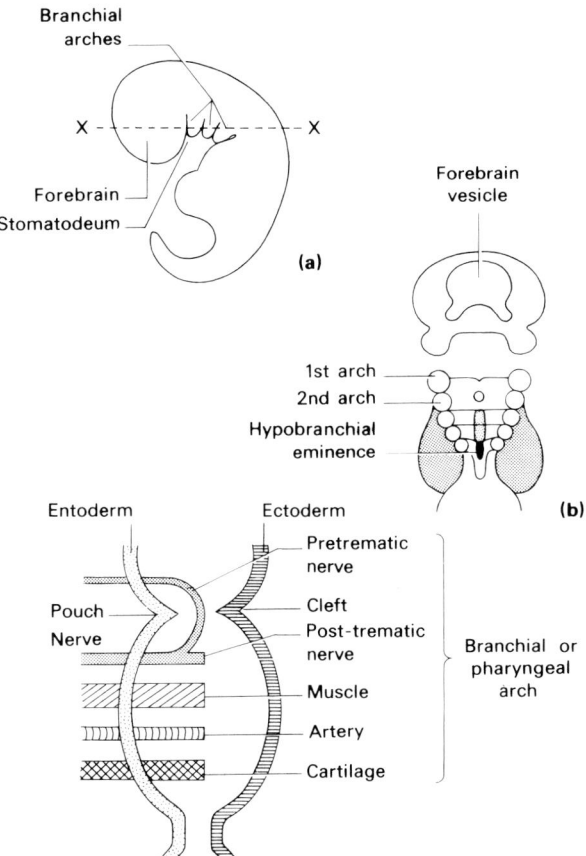

**Fig. 1.25.** (a) External form of a 20-day embryo, (b) section of (a) along X–X (the ventral part of the branchial arches are seen from behind, (c) diagram of structures which develop in an arch.

1.25c). It is also supplied by a nerve which innervates the muscles and the surface epithelium derived from the arch. If the muscles migrate away from their arch they take their nerve supply with them. In man the most anterior arch is called the first, or mandibular arch and the second the hyoid. These are much more prominent than the remaining arches, especially the fifth and sixth.

## Face and nasal cavities

The development of the face is related to that of the branchial arches. The buccopharyngeal membrane breaks down at a very early stage (at the end of the 4th week) so that the pharynx communicates with the exterior. At about the same time the mandibular process on each side, formed by a thickening of the mesoderm of the first arch, grows ventrally round the side of the pharynx (Fig. 1.26). The two processes meet in the midline, caudal to the stomatodeum. During the 4th week the mesoderm in the midline, in front of the bulge of the forebrain, thickens and forms the frontonasal process. In the 5th week the ectoderm on each side ventrolateral to this process thickens and forms the olfactory placode (Fig. 1.26b). The edges of the placode become elevated and form the lateral and medial nasal processes and the depressed area between the processes is called the olfactory pit. The medial nasal process is less prominent but extends more caudally than the lateral.

At the same time as the olfactory pits develop, a thickening of mesoderm grows from the cranial side of the dorsal part of the mandibular process. This is called the maxillary process (Fig. 1.26b). This grows ventrally above the stomatodeum and fuses with the lateral nasal process. The maxillary process continues to extend medially between the ectoderm and endoderm, and fuses with the medial nasal process. There is a difference of opinion as to whether the maxillary process continues to grow towards the midline and bury the lower part of the frontonasal process (Fig. 1.26c, d, e): if it does, the central part of the upper

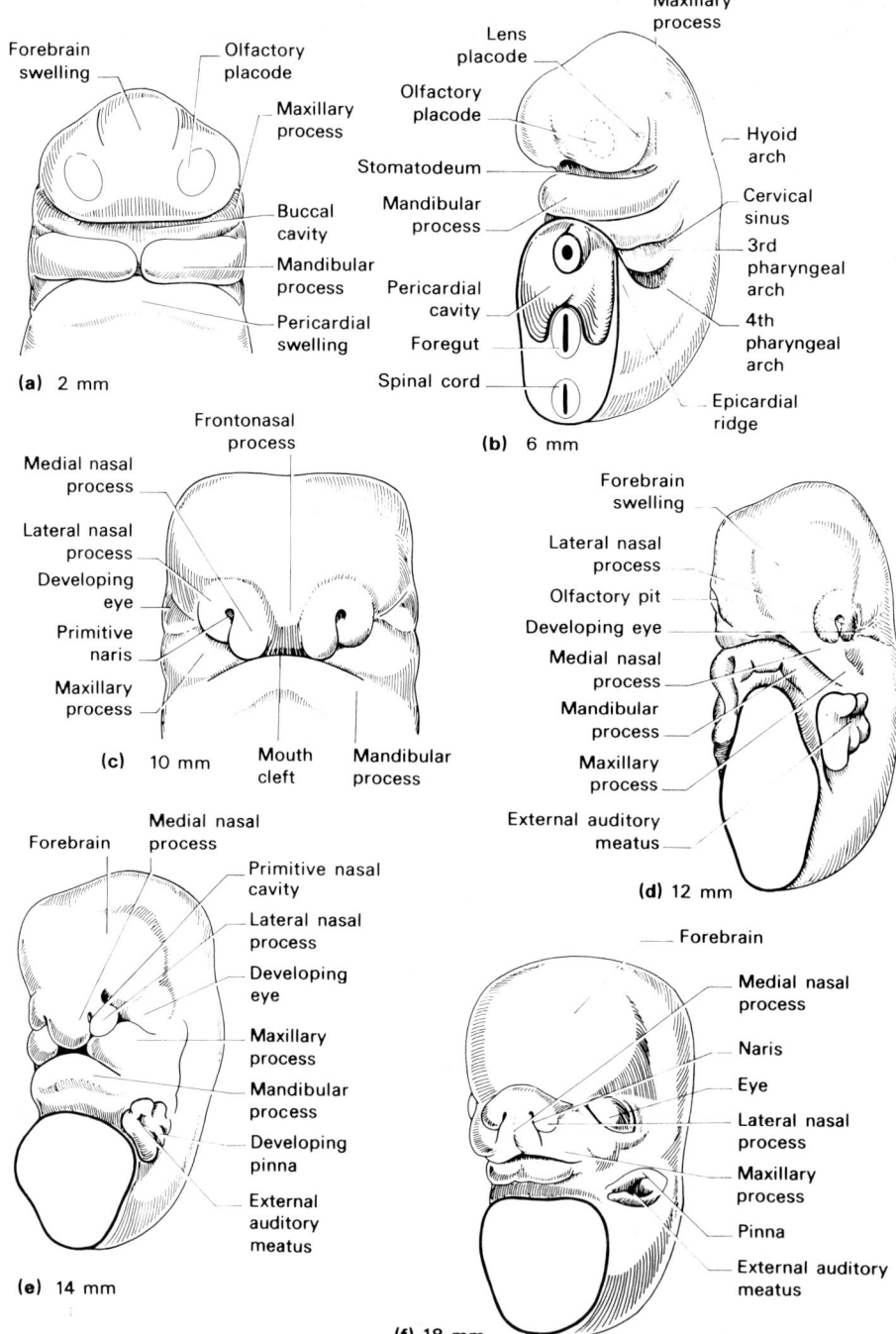

**Fig. 1.26.** Development of the face.

lip would be derived from the maxillary process and not from the frontonasal process. The term premaxilla can be used to describe the mesoderm of the frontonasal process in the midline above the stomatodeum. This mesoderm may be derived from a medial extension of the mesoderm of the medial nasal process. At about 25 days the developing eye can be seen on the side of the forebrain bulge cranial to the maxillary process (Fig. 1.26). As the face develops due to the changes described the eye moves towards the front of the face. The ventral, later medial, angle of the eye lies above a thickening of ectoderm between the maxillary process and the lateral nasal process. This thickening sinks below the surface and lies in the line of the nasolacrimal duct. The solid rod of ectoderm becomes canalized and communicates above with the medial angle of the eye and below with the lateral wall of the nasal cavity. It forms the nasolacrimal duct (Fig. 1.29).

By the fusion of the maxillary process with the medial nasal process the lower boundary of the external nasal aperture (the naris) is formed. The continued growth of the mesoderm round this opening deepens the olfactory pit which can now be called the primitive nasal cavity (Fig. 1.26e). The deepest part of the ectodermal lining thins and breaks down, so that the nasal cavity communicates with the oral cavity. At this stage there is no roof to the mouth. However, a palate is defined as

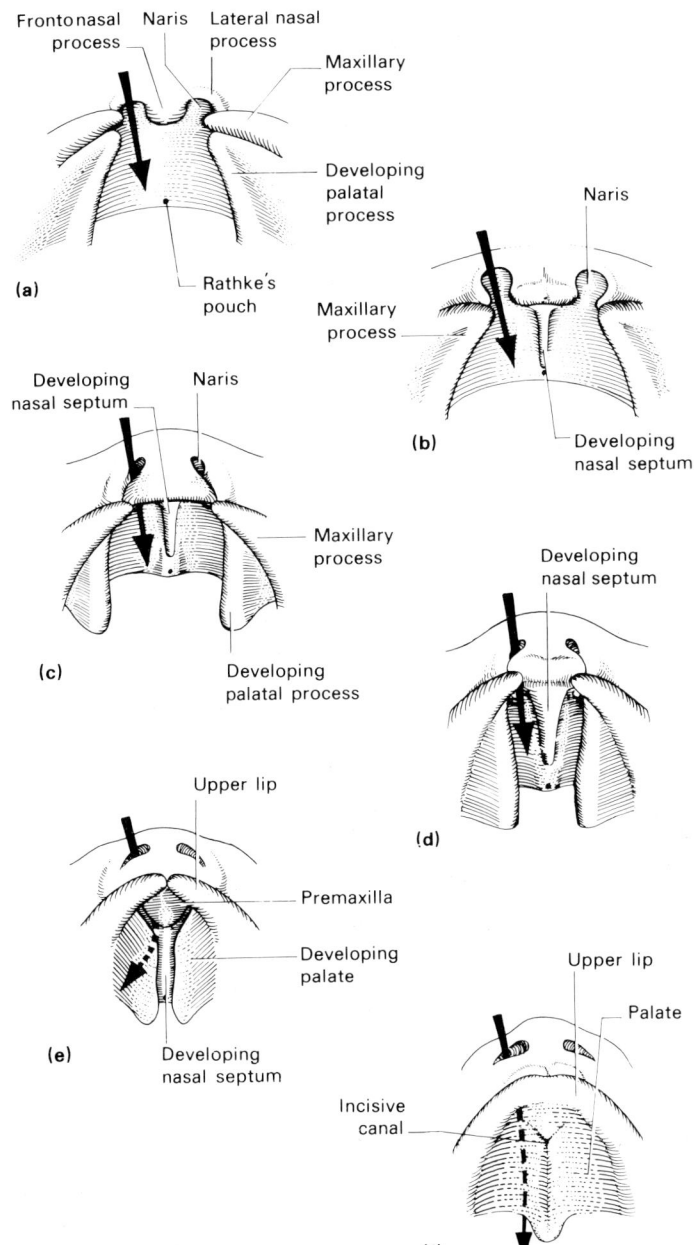

**Fig. 1.27.** Development of the palate and nasal septum viewed from below (the arrow passes through one naris and into that part of the buccal cavity) which becomes the nasal cavity.

horizontal tissue between the oral and nasal cavities, therefore the deeper part of the premaxilla can be described as the primary (primitive) palate (Fig. 1.27). Similarly if the nasal septum is defined as the tissue between the two halves of the cavity then the tissue in the midline between the two deepening olfactory pits is the primary (primitive) nasal septum. Mesoderm, which has infiltrated between the developing brain and the endoderm lining the roof of the pharynx, grows into the buccal cavity to produce a posterior extension of the primary nasal septum (Fig. 1.27b, c, d and Fig. 1.28) which now becomes the definitive nasal septum.

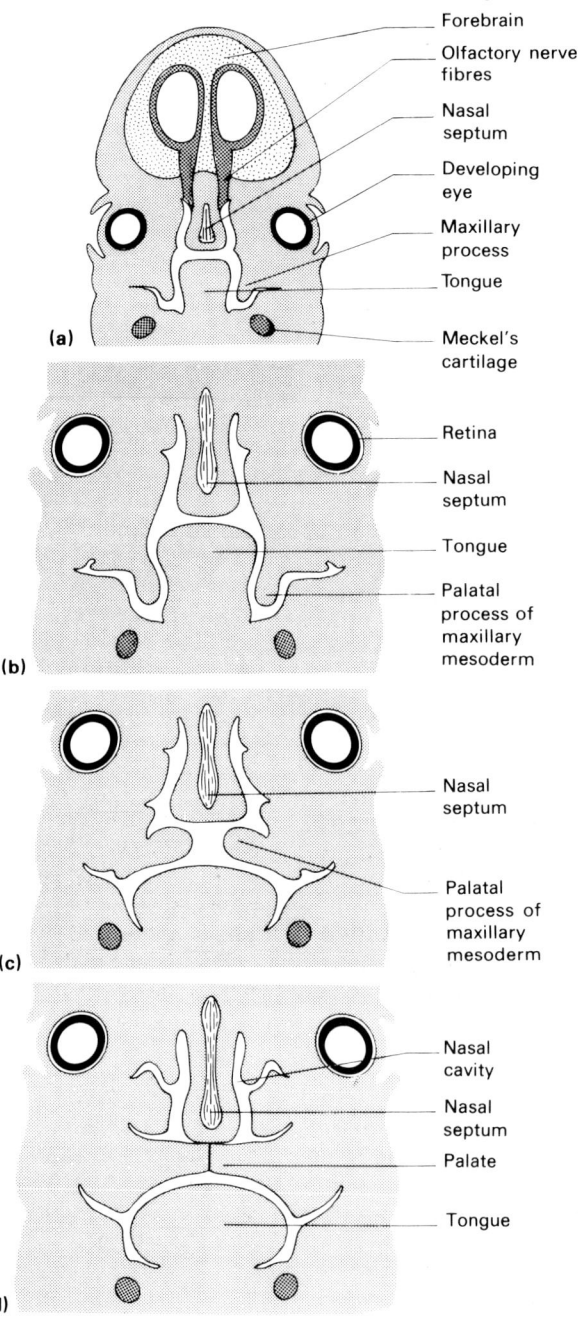

**Fig. 1.28.** Development of the palate and nasal septum (coronal sections through the buccal cavity).

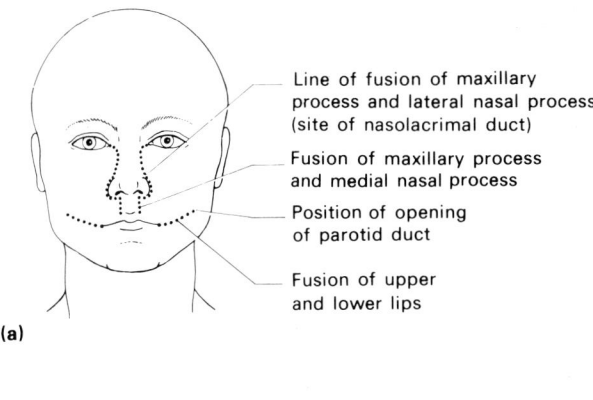

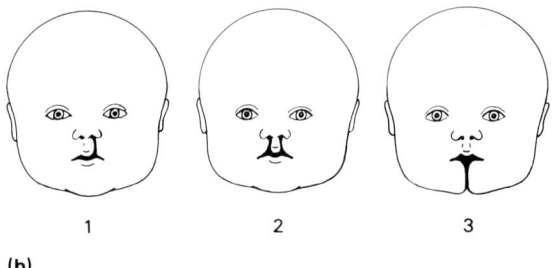

**Fig. 1.29.** (a) Lines of fusion on the face. (b) Some congenital abnormalities of the face: 1, unilateral cleft lip; 2, bilateral cleft lip; 3, median cleft of lower lip and jaw.

Between 35 and 40 days the palatal processes grow out horizontally towards the midline from the maxillary processes. The developing tongue projects upwards from the floor of the mouth and reaches the primitive palate (Fig. 1.28a, b). With the ventral growth of the mandibular region the tongue descends and the palatal processes, which at first lie at the sides of the tongue, now rise and meet in the midline where they fuse, from before backwards, with each other and the inferior free edge of the nasal septum (Fig. 1.28b, c, d). The nasal cavities are now separated from the oral cavity.

If the maxillary process fails to fuse with the medial nasal process (or premaxillary region) a cleft lip results (Fig. 1.29). A unilateral or bilateral cleft lip may or may not be associated with a cleft palate (p. 58). Cleft palates vary in degree. The smallest cleft is limited to the uvula or the uvula and the soft palate. The most marked is a failure of fusion of the two palatal processes with each other and with the septum. Sometimes one palatal process fuses with the septum so that a unilateral cleft palate is seen. When there is a complete cleft palate with a bilateral cleft lip, it is almost impossible for the baby to suck and food is frequently regurgitated through the nose. An immediate bilateral temporary closure of the cleft lip is carried out to allow sucking and a definitive repair of both the lip and palate postponed until the child is about 18 months old, that is before talking begins.

**Mouth and tongue**

The oral (buccal) cavity is thus formed partly from the ectoderm of the stomatodeum (Fig. 1.25a) and partly from the endoderm of the pharynx. The inner surface of the gingivae can be regarded as the dividing line between the ectoderm and endoderm (Fig. 1.31b). The opening into the oral cavity becomes bounded by the fused maxillary processes above and fused mandibular processes below. (The middle part of the upper boundary may be derived from the premaxilla.) The lips and cheek become separated from the gingivae by a growth of ectoderm (the vestibular lamina) which subsequently breaks down and forms the labiogingival sulcus (Figs. 1.31 and 8.11).

The ventral part of the floor of the pharynx is formed by the fused ventral ends of the first, second and third branchial arches, which are covered by endoderm (Fig. 1.30a). The anterior part of the tongue develops as a thickening of the first (mandibular) arch from a median and two lateral tongue buds (The median was called the tuberculum impar) which fuse. Behind the median tongue bud, the second, third and fourth arches

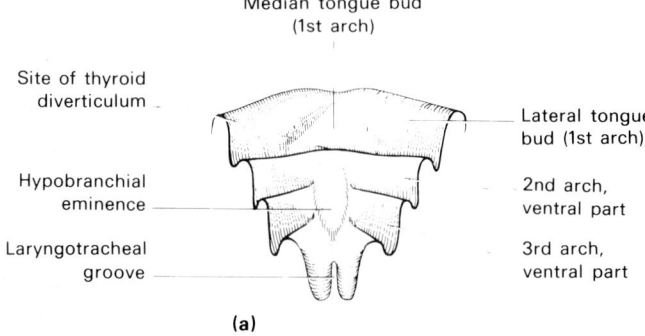

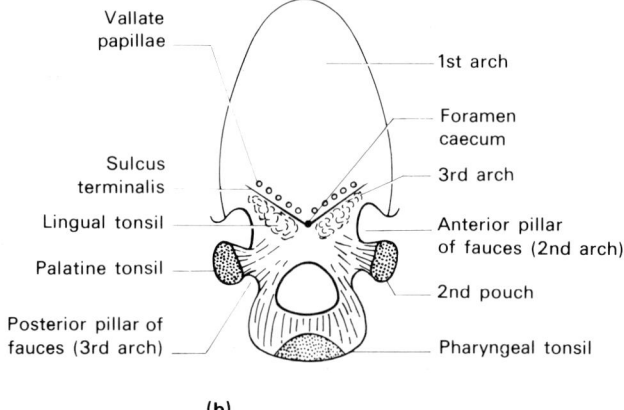

**Fig. 1.30.** (a) Ventral ends of the branchial arches seen from behind (i.e. the developing floor of the mouth). (b) The tongue and posterior part of the buccal cavity seen from behind and above.

thicken and form a projection called the hypobranchial eminence (Fig. 1.30a). Its caudal part is separated off by a groove and forms the epiglottis: cranially it grows towards the anterior part of the tongue. While this is taking place the endoderm of the third arch overgrows that of the second which is excluded from the tongue. The line where the posterior part of the tongue meets the anterior part is indicated by the V-shaped sulcus terminalis (Fig. 1.30b). The apex of the sulcus is marked by a depression from which the thyroglossal duct develops. After the disappearance of the duct the depression is called the foramen caecum. The tongue is separated from the floor of the mouth by a downgrowth of ectoderm between it and the developing gingiva (Fig. 1.31). The ectoderm subsequently degenerates with the formation of the linguogingival sulcus.

The mesoderm of the tongue is invaded by the muscle fibres of the occipital myotomes which grow ventrally round the side of the pharynx. They take their nerve supply with them, the hypoglossal nerve. The mucous membrane of the anterior part of the tongue is supplied by the nerve of the first arch, the mandibular nerve. It is also supplied by the pretrematic branch of the nerve of the second arch (Fig. 4.4), the facial nerve through one of its branches, the chorda tympani. The mucous membrane of the posterior part of the tongue is supplied by the nerve of the third arch, the glossopharyngeal nerve. It is more difficult to explain the glossopharyngeal innervation of the vallate papillae which are on that part of the tongue in front of the sulcus terminalis. This may be due to a ventral migration of that particular part of the mucous membrane.

### Salivary and thyroid glands and hypophysis cerebri

The parotid gland is the first of the salivary glands to develop (at about the end of the 4th week). It first appears as a solid cord of ectodermal cells burrowing into the mesoderm of the cheek from the angle of the mouth, between the mandibular and maxillary processes. The tip of the cord grows

# Embryology and Development

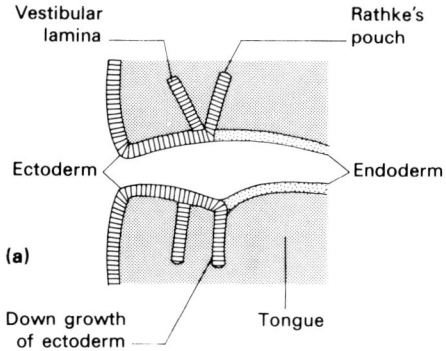

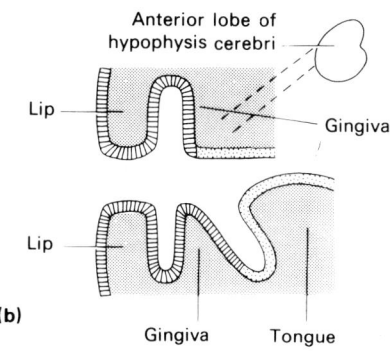

**Fig. 1.31.** (a) Sagittal section through the buccal cavity before the separation of the lips, gingivae and tongue. (b) The separation of the lips, gingivae and tongue.

hollow tube, the thyroglossal duct, which grows in a caudal direction ventral to the second and third arch mesoderm (Fig. 1.32). The duct divides and forms cellular plates from which the isthmus and lobes of the thyroid gland develop. The thyroglossal duct disappears. Its origin is marked by the foramen caecum of the tongue (Fig. 1.30b). Part of the duct may remain anywhere along the line of its growth and form aberrant thyroid tissue or a midline cyst. A cyst of this type remains attached to the tongue by a cord of fibrous tissue and moves upwards on protrusion of the tongue.

The anterior lobe of the hypophysis cerebri develops from the roof of the stomatodeum just ventral to the buccopharyngeal membrane (Fig. 1.31). It begins as a recess (pouch of Rathke) which deepens and reaches the floor of the forebrain. The diverticulum is closed off by mesodermal growth leaving a hollow clump of cells at the base of the brain. These cells proliferate and form the anterior lobe. A small cavity, the remains of the diverticulum, persists within the anterior lobe and separates the major part of the lobe from a smaller posterior intermediate lobe. The posterior lobe of the hypophysis cerebri (the neurohypophysis) develops as a hollow diverticulum from the floor of the forebrain, that is, it develops from neuroectoderm. The diverticulum meets the anterior lobe which extends dorsally on both sides of the posterior lobe. The stalk of the diverticulum becomes solid by cell growth into its lumen and

backwards towards the ear region where it repeatedly branches to form a tree-like system. The cords canalize and salivary acini develop at the ends of the twigs in response to induction from the adjacent mesoderm. The maxillary and mandibular processes unite medially from the site at which the gland originated with the result that the parotid duct opens well behind the definitive corner of the mouth. The extent to which these processes fuse determines the transverse dimension of the mouth. Conditions of macrostoma (abnormally large mouth) and microstoma (abnormally small mouth) are recognized (Fig. 1.27a).

The submandibular gland develops during the 5th week from the linguogingival sulcus as an epithelial cord. Its subsequent development is similar to that of the parotid gland.

The sublingual gland develops somewhat later as a number of epithelial cords from the linguogingival sulcus. Many of these connect with what subsequently becomes the submandibular duct.

The thyroid gland is first seen in the 3rd week as a thickening of endoderm caudal to the median tongue bud (Fig. 1.30a). The thickening becomes a

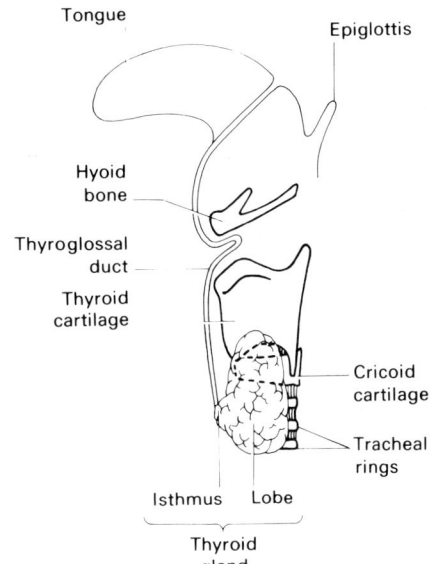

**Fig. 1.32.** Diagram to show the development of the thyroid gland.

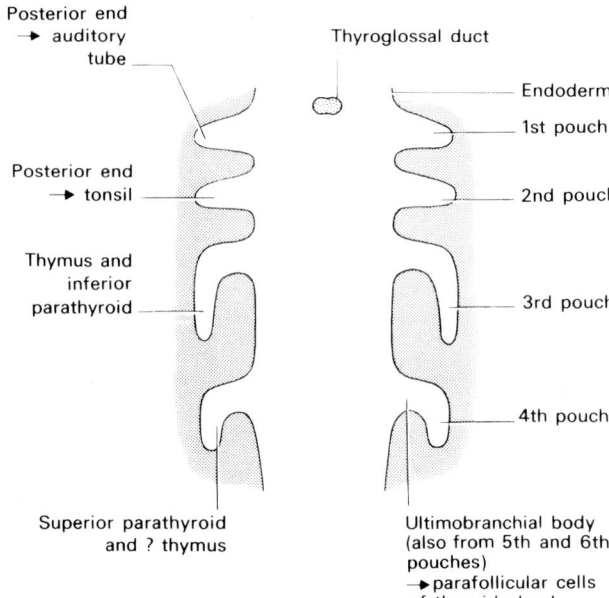

**Fig. 1.33.** The derivatives of the pharyngeal (branchial) pouches.

forms the infundibulum (stalk) of the hypophysis cerebri. The cells of the anterior lobe grow along the infundibulum towards the floor of the third ventricle where they form the tuber cinereum.

**Pouch (endodermal) derivatives** (Fig. 1.33)

It will be recalled that a branchial (pharyngeal) pouch is the depression between two branchial arches where the endoderm and ectoderm meet without any intervening mesoderm. The posterior end of the first pouch deepens and forms the tubotympanic recess from which the auditory tube, middle ear, mastoid antrum and some of the mastoid air cells develop. The posterior end of the second pouch may contribute to the tubotympanic recess. The palatine tonsil develops in relation to the second pharyngeal pouch. It begins as solid downgrowths of endodermal cells. These downgrowths become hollowed out and form the crypts of the tonsil. Accumulation of lymphocytes round the crypts form the tonsillar lymphoid follicles. The intratonsillar cleft in the upper part of the tonsil may be a persistent part of the second pharyngeal pouch.

The thymus develops in the 6th week from the endoderm of the ventral parts of the third pouch. It develops as a diverticulum on each side which grows caudally in the mesoderm. The diverticula become solid by multiplication of the cells. Ventral to the aortic sac the two cords of cells meet. The connection with the third pouch is lost. There may be a contribution to the thymus from the ventral ends of the fourth pouch. The endodermal part of the thymus is invaded by vascular tissue including lymphoid stem cells from the bone marrow. The endodermal derivatives form the cells of the concentric (Hassall's) corpuscles and the reticulum and the lymphocytes form the greater bulk of the thymus. The thymus is relatively large at birth.

The superior parathyroid glands develop from the fourth pouch. As they develop they become attached to the thyroid gland and retain this relationship. The inferior parathyroid glands develop from the third pouch. They are attached to the developing thymus gland and therefore pass caudally, with the thymus, before becoming attached to the thyroid gland caudal to the superior parathyroid glands.

The ultimobranchial body is the name given to a diverticulum from the fourth pouch which may or may not develop in the human embryo. The endodermal cells which form this body become associated on each side with the developing lobes of the thyroid gland and the superior parathyroid glands. These cells form the parafollicular cells of the thyroid gland and produce calcitonin.

**Cleft (ectodermal) derivatives**

The dorsal part of the first pharyngeal cleft deepens and forms the external auditory (acoustic) meatus and the outer epithelium of the tympanic membrane (Fig. 1.26). It may be added that projections due to proliferation of the underlying mesoderm at the dorsal ends of the first and second branchial arches contribute to the formation of the auricle. The ventral part of the first branchial cleft is obliterated.

At the end of the 5th week the cervical sinus is seen behind the hyoid (second) arch. This is a depression bounded above by the hyoid arch, below by the epicardial ridge (Fig. 1.26b) and dorsally by developing muscle partly derived from ventral extensions of the occipital myotomes and partly from developing muscle *in situ*. The epicardial ridge has this name because it separates the cervical sinus from the pericardium. The ridge can be followed cranially towards the first arch. It is thought that the occipital myotomes grow along this ridge to the mesoderm of the mandibular arch and form the muscle of the tongue. The hypoglossal nerve accompanies the muscle. This explains why this nerve is superficial to both the internal and external carotid arteries. By caudal growth of the hyoid arch over the sinus the rest of the arches are excluded from forming any part of the outer surface of the neck.

In the neck, sinuses (epithelial tracts communicating at one end with an epithelial surface but ending blindly at the other) and fistulae (epithelial tracts communicating at both ends with an epithelial surface) may occur as a result of the persistence of parts of branchial clefts and pouches. For example, the cervical sinus may remain with an opening on to the surface of the neck. If the sinus is closed but its ectodermal wall remains, a cyst may develop. If the ectoderm of a cleft and the endoderm of the corresponding pouch break down a fistula may form.

**Mesodermal derivatives** (Table 1.2)

# CRANIOFACIAL DEVELOPMENT

The human skull develops from several elements whose phylogeny is reviewed in Chapter 4. The separate identity of many of these elements has been lost during evolution, either by fusion with other components, or by total disappearance.

The progression from early mammal to *Homo sapiens* is marked by a large increase in brain size. This increase is associated not only with increase in the size of the bony vault of the skull, but also with its relocation within the skull structure. Whereas in more primitive mammals the brain capsule lies at the back of the skull, in man it occupies a most prominent position. In association with this change the skull components concerned with prehension and mastication, which were found in front of the brain capsule, have become repositioned underneath the forebrain.

Before considering the contribution made by different components of the skull to its overall development, the mechanisms of bone formation should be appreciated.

## Mechanisms of bone formation

ENDOCHONDRAL BONES (primary cartilage)

At the time of merging of the facial processes the head consists of soft tissue layers of ectodermal, mesodermal and endodermal origin. The mesodermal layers contain undifferentiated mesenchyme cells which give rise to the primordial framework of the skull consisting of primary cartilage and fibrous tissue sheets. The primary cartilage framework is presaged by a condensation of mesenchyme cells in which chondroblasts differentiate. The matrix of hyaline cartilage secreted by these cells is the primary cartilaginous skeleton which, by endochondral ossification (Book 1), contributes to part of the bone structure of the skull.

The cartilage precursor for each long bone of the appendicular skeleton differentiates into a miniature model of the eventual adult bone. The model increases in length by interstitial growth of the cartilage in the epiphyseal region (note that the replacement of cartilage by bone does not lengthen the model) and increase in width by the surface deposition of bone. During growth the bone is remodelled to become a recognisable enlarged version of the original cartilage model.

The evolutionary history of the skull is complex and most of its primary cartilage structures fuse together and are modified by development in such a way that the adult bones are not large scale reproductions of the original cartilage models. In certain areas the first formed or primary cartilage is not fully replaced by bone until well after birth. The remaining cartilage acts as a growth centre which increases the size of the bone. An example of such an area is found between the sphenoid and occipital bones at the spheno-occipital synchondrosis which has an important part to play in the later growth of the base of the skull.

DERMAL BONES

Bone formation may take place without an intervening cartilage stage, in this case by differentiation of the mesenchyme cells directly into osteoblasts which lay down mineralized bone

**Table 1.2.** The derivatives of the cartilages, muscles, nerves and arteries of the branchial (pharyngeal) arches.

| Branchial arch | Skeleton | Muscles | Nerve | Artery |
|---|---|---|---|---|
| 1 (mandibular) | Quadrate cartilage —incus Meckel's cartilage —malleus Anterior ligament of malleus, sphenomandibular ligament, central core of body of mandible | Muscles of mastication (temporalis, masseter, medial and lateral pterygoids) Mylohyoid and anterior belly of digastric Tensor veli palatini and tensor tympani | Mandibular division of trigeminal nerve (post-trematic) Chorda tympani branch of facial nerve (pretrematic) | Disappears |
| 2 (hyoid) | Stapes, styloid process, stylohyoid ligament, lesser cornu and upper part of body of hyoid bone | Facial (including buccinator, extrinsic and intrinsic auricular muscles, occipito-frontalis and platysma) Posterior belly of digastric and stylohyoid Stapedius | VII Facial (post-trematic) | Disappears |
| 3 | Greater cornu and lower part of body of hyoid bone | Stylopharyngeus Probably part of upper pharyngeal muscles | IX Glossopharyngeal (post-trematic) | Common and internal carotid |
| 4, (5) and 6 | Laryngeal cartilages | Pharyngeal, laryngeal and palatal muscles (except tensor veli palatini) | Superior laryngeal and pharyngeal branches of vagus (cranial accessory) | 4 Right—subclavian Left—arch of aorta 6 Right—pulmonary artery Left—pulmonary artery and ductus arteriosus |

tissue (Book 1). Bones formed in this way (intra-membranous ossification) are called dermal or membrane bones and they play an important role in growth of the skull particularly in the formation of those bones found in the skull vault such as the frontal and parietal bones as well as the upper and lower jaw.

SECONDARY CARTILAGE

In some cases areas of cartilage develop in association with dermal bones. These cartilages do not develop from, or have any connection with, the primary cartilage of the first-formed skull framework and are termed secondary cartilages. They are associated with growth, a particularly important example being the secondary cartilage of the mandibular condyle which may persist until the beginning of the third decade.

## Development of the bones of the skull

ORIGIN OF THE BONES (Fig. 1.34)

The terms given to the various parts of the skull differ depending on whether they are being described by palaeontologists and comparative anatomists, (who each seek to understand the relationship between the bones of animals as diverse as bony fish and porpoises), or by primatologists and orthodontists (who confine their studies to a single order of mammals). For the latter workers that part of the skull surrounding the brain is the cranium and the remainder is the face (Fig. 1.35). The cranial vault (calvaria) covers the brain and the cranial base is the floor. Comparative anatomists are more concerned with the homologies between the different bones of all vertebrates and designate the parts of the skull according to their development and evolution (Fig. 1.34). During evolution some bones have moved from the facial region to the cranium (e.g. the malleus) while others have moved from the cranium to the face (e.g. the nasal bones). The neurocranium consists of those bones and cartilages which originally evolved to support and cover the brain and special sense organs. The viscerocranium consists of the anterior branchial arch cartilages and those bones which originally evolved to surround them. Ancestrally, both the neuro- and viscerocranium were cartilage and are together known as the chondrocranium. It can be seen from Fig. 1.34 that all that remains of the cartilaginous viscerocranium is incorporated in the cranial base of mammals. During evolution many dermal bones have been added to both the neurocranium and the viscerocranium (Fig. 1.34).

It is now convenient to consider the development of the skull under three headings; the cranial base, cranial vault and face.

CRANIAL BASE

The first sign of an organized framework supporting the brain is seen at about the 2nd month of fetal life when the cartilaginous skeleton is differentiated. Centres of chondrification develop in the mesenchyme capsule associated with the cranial extremity of the notochord (Fig. 1.36). Lateral to the notochord are the parachordal cartilages and the cartilages formed from the occipital somites; anterior are the polar cartilages and alisphenoids (roots of the greater wing of the sphenoid) which come from the viscerocranium (arch 1), and further anteriorly is the trabecula (arch 0; Fig. 4.6) also from the viscerocranium. These centres enlarge and eventually coalesce to form a cartilage platform supporting the developing brain. Around the platform are added cartilages associated with the three paired sense organs; the nasal capsule, orbital plate (orbitosphenoid = lesser wing of the sphenoid: Fig. 1.37) and otic capsule (Fig. 1.38).

The cartilages grow and encircle the nerves and vessels passing to and from the brain (Fig. 1.36). While the cartilage mass is growing its older parts are replaced by bone so that at birth only the region separating the occipital and sphenoid bones (the important spheno–occipital synchondrosis) and part of the nasal septum remain as cartilage. Further growth of the cranial base is permitted by the development of sutures between the bones which have developed from the cartilage (mesethmoid, sphenoid, temporal and occipital) and between the four parts of the occipital bone which contribute to the cranial base; the basiocciput from the parachordal cartilage, and the two exoccipitals and the lower squamous part of the occipital (supraoccipital) developed from the occipital somites. The supraoccipital is equivalent to the neural arch of a vertebra surrounding the spinal cord (Fig. 1.37).

CRANIAL VAULT

In addition to bone formation at the skull base ossification takes place in the layer of connective tissue surrounding the vault of the brain. This becomes organized into two layers. From the inner layer are derived the pia mater and the arachnoid mater. The outer layer itself differentiates into two layers which comprise the dura mater and an outer fibrous capsule in which the calvarial bones develop.

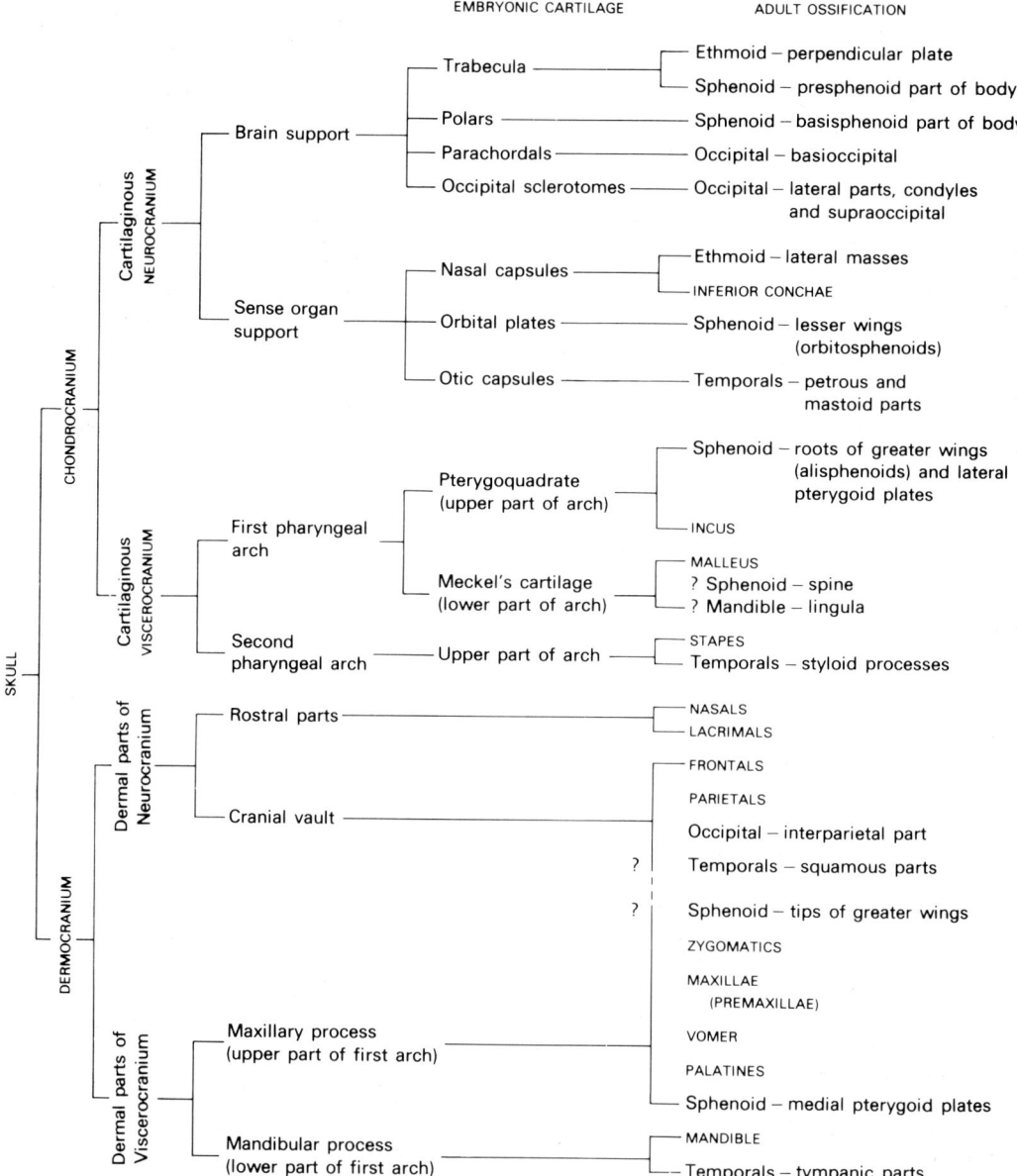

**Fig. 1.34.** Classification of embryonic primary cartilages and adult ossification in the human skull. In the right-hand column, complete individual bones are in capital letters, parts of individual bones in lower case.

Centres of ossification appear at about 6–7 weeks *in utero* within the fibrous capsule, and the sizes of the individual skull bones gradually increase, until they articulate with one another by sutures (Fig. 1.39).

By birth the increase in individual bone size is insufficient to achieve an edge-to-edge contact between all the bones of the vault of the skull. There are six resulting spaces or fontanelles between the bones which gradually close after birth (Fig. 1.40). Each fontanelle consists of a layer of tough fibrous tissue, the membrane from which the name membrane-bone is derived.

At birth the sutures are straight compared with

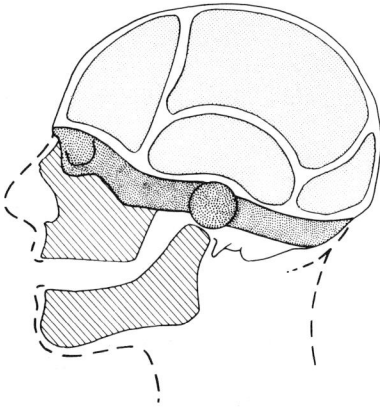

**Fig. 1.35.** The main developmental and functional divisions of the skull: cranial vault (stippled); cranial base (shaded); facial complex (hatched).

the complex interdigitations which develop later and, together with the fontanelles, they allow the bones to slide over each other when the head is compressed during birth.

FACE

The facial complex surrounds the orbit, the nasal and oral cavities, and the upper part of the pharynx. Embryonic scaffolding consists of the nasal capsule, the quadrate cartilage and Meckel's cartilage (Fig. 1.41). From these the only contributions to the bony face are the inferior turbinate bones and the ethmoid. The quadrate becomes the incus of the middle ear and the proximal end of Meckel's cartilage becomes the malleus (it is suggested that the latter cartilage and its perichondrium may also contribute the lingula of the mandible, the sphenomandibular ligament, the spine of the sphenoid and the sphenomalleolar ligament).

The majority of the face is derived from dermal bones added around the cartilaginous viscerocranium. Surrounding the nose apart from its base, these are the nasal and lacrimal bones (old dermal neurocranium), the maxillae and the vertical plates of the palatine bones. The palate, separating the oral cavity from the nose, consists of the premaxillae (see later), maxillae, vomer, and horizontal plates of the palatine bones. Outside these, the zygomatic bone buttresses the maxilla and the side of the orbit via the zygomatic arch on to the squamous part of the temporal bone. Behind the palatine bones, the medial plates of the pterygoids, attached to the sphenoid, lie on either side of the upper part of the pharynx.

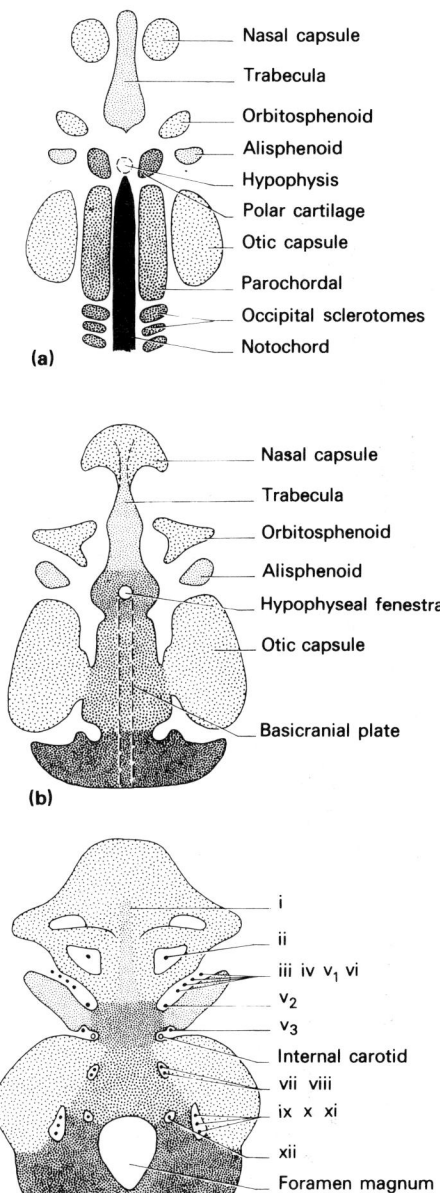

**Fig. 1.36.** Schematic dorsal view of the forming chondrocranium. (a) The primordial cartilages at about 6 weeks i.u. (b) The complete basicranial plate at 7 weeks i.u. (c) The complete chondrocranium at 12 weeks i.u., showing the relations of the internal carotid artery and cranial nerves.

The mandible (the left and right dentary), another dermal bone, contributes the whole of the lower part of the face.

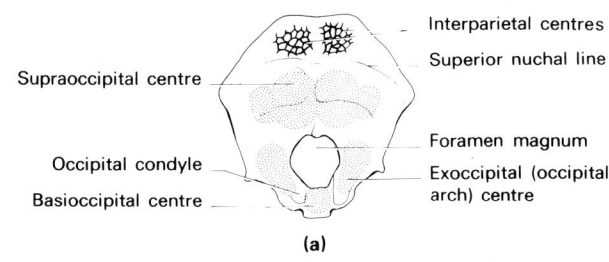
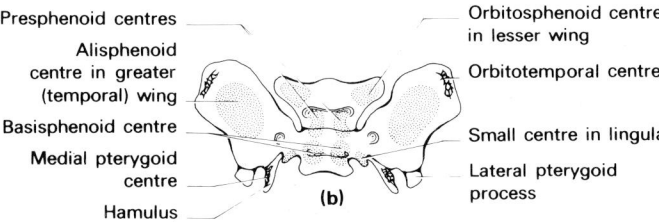
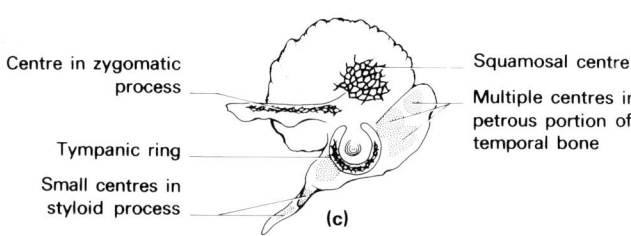

**Fig. 1.37.** Diagrams showing the location of ossification centres in three of the principle bones of the skull. Intramembranous centres are shown in black trabeculation, and endochondrial centres in stipple against an outline diagram suggesting the adult shape of the bone. (a) Occipital; (b) sphenoid; (c) left temporal.

*Nasal capsule*

The nasal capsule consists of two walls and a septum which together support the upper part of the face while the associated dermal bones are developing around it (Fig. 1.38). Later, parts of the capsule become converted into bone by endochondrial ossification.

The ossification centre for the maxilla appears at about 7 weeks *in utero* close to the lower border of the nasal capsule in the angle where the anterior superior dental nerve leaves the infraorbital nerve. From here ossification spreads out radially to form the body of the maxilla and upwards (frontal process), outwards (zygomatic process), downwards (alveolar process), and inwards (palatal process). The development of the maxilla is described in more detail later.

Centres of ossification for the premaxillae and palatine bones appear a few days after those for the maxillae. The palatine bone develops on the medial side of the wall of the nasal capsule and from here extends upwards (vertical plate) and inwards (horizontal plate). When the cartilage of the wall has atrophied the vertical plate grows forwards, overlaps the maxilla, and develops a suture with it thereby stabilizing the lateral well of the nose.

The ossification centre for the vomer appears in the mesoderm immediately beneath the cartilaginous nasal septum and from here spreads anteroposteriorly and upwards as a U-shaped gutter embracing the septum. It develops sutures below with the united palatal process of the left and right maxillae and of the palatine bones, thereby stabilizing the septum.

Anteriorly (dermal) ossification centres develop in the mesoderm lateral to the walls of the nasal capsule to form the nasal bones (9 weeks *in utero*) and the lacrimal bones (12 weeks *in utero*).

All the above are dermal bones. While they are growing, the walls of the nasal capsule atrophy. Within these walls appear ossification centres (5 months *in utero*) for the lateral masses of the ethmoid and for the inferior turbinate bones. The cartilage associated with these endochondrial bones remains and grows, and is steadily replaced by bone.

Unlike the walls of the nasal capsule which

# Embryology and Development

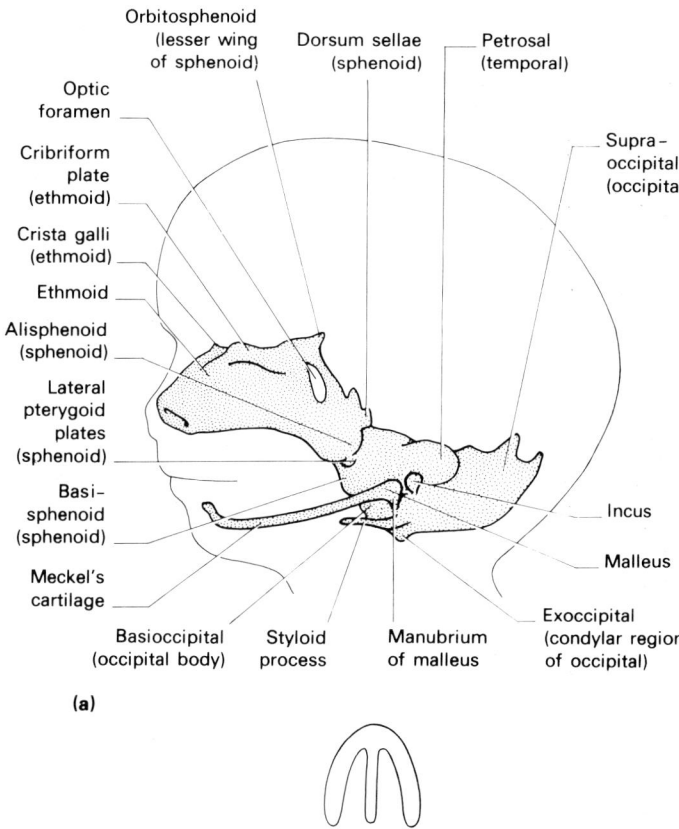

**Fig. 1.38.** (a) Diagrammatic lateral view of the chondrocranium at 12 weeks i.u. Developing intramembranous bones have been excluded. (b) Diagrammatic frontal section through the nasal capsule.

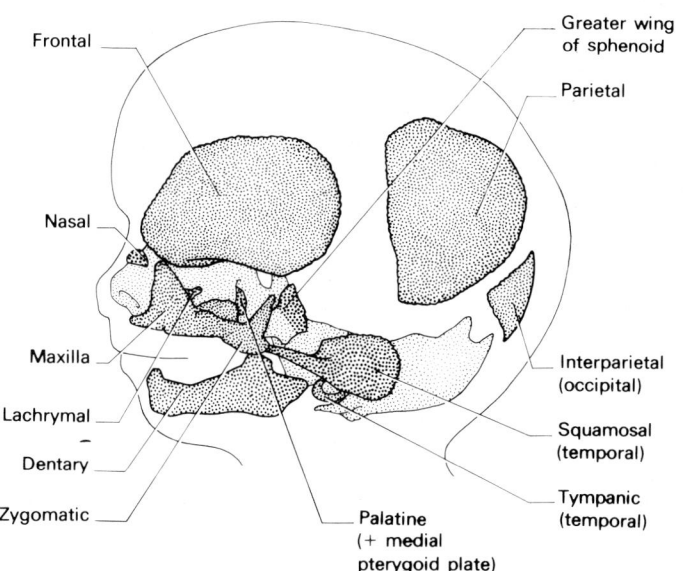

**Fig. 1.39.** The skull of a 12-week fetus showing the locations of membrane bones in relation to the chondrocranium, parts of which are undergoing endochondral ossification: cartilage (light stipple); membrane bone (heavy stipple).

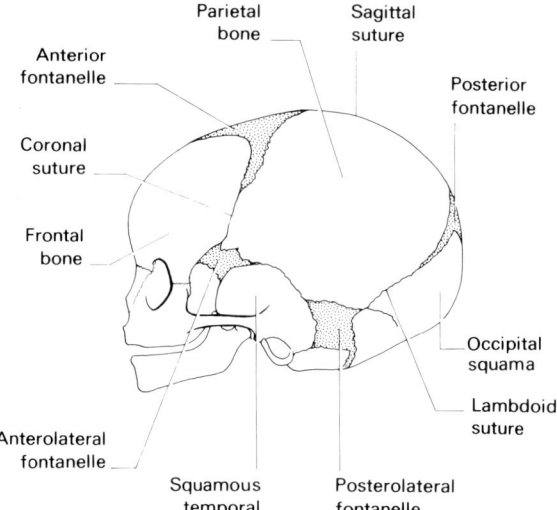

Fig. 1.40. The skull of a neonate: fontanelles (stippled) and related bones and sutures.

atrophy or are replaced by bone during fetal life, the cartilage of the septum continues growing in contact with the (dermal) vomer bone. During the first year of life an ossification centre for the vertical plate of the ethmoid appears within this cartilage. The growing cartilage is gradually replaced by bone. Ossification spreads through the septum and into the cribriform plate thus joining by bone the vertical plate of the ethmoid to its lateral masses.

*The premaxilla*

The origin of the premaxilla in the frontonasal process is controversial. In adult anthropoid apes the premaxilla is separated from the maxilla by a suture which extends over the palate and face (Fig. 1.42a). In man the premaxillary/maxillary suture never extends on to the face and is confined to the palate (Fig. 1.42b or c). One argument proposes that premaxillary centres of ossification appear a few days after the maxillary centres and that in man the maxilla grows over the facial surface of the developing premaxilla so that the latter is buried and can never be seen on the face (Fig. 1.42b). The alternative proposes that there is no separate premaxilla in man. Viewed from below (Fig. 1.42c) the ossification centre for the maxilla grows into a 'C' shape whose concavity is rapidly filled by bone and becomes an incomplete suture (the incisive fissure) which is (incorrectly) thought of as the premaxillary–maxillary suture. If the latter view (Fig. 1.42c) is correct for man, it can be visualized that the development represented by Fig. 1.42b might have been an intermediate stage between the evolution of the human condition from the ape condition (Fig. 1.42a): the pre-

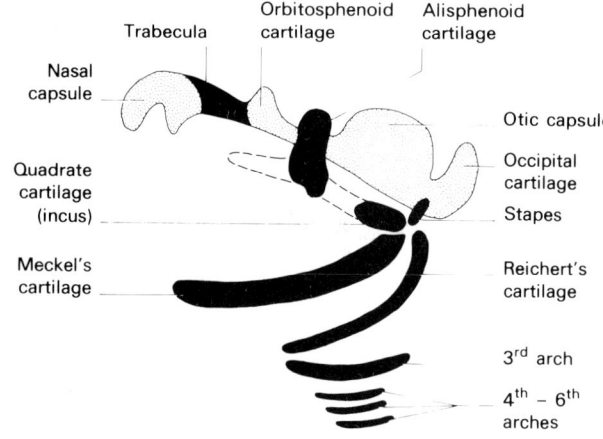

Fig. 1.41. Schematic lateral view of the cartilaginous neurocranium (stippled) and viscerocranium (black) at approximately 7–8 weeks i.u. The dotted lines indicate the incomplete chondrification of the upper part of the first branchial arch (the palatoquadrate cartilage).

# Embryology and Development

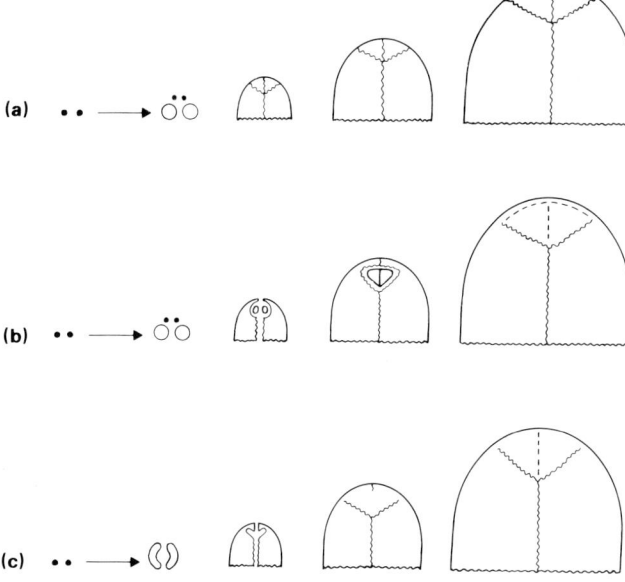

**Fig. 1.42.** (a) Ventral views of the developing palate in an ape. (b, c) The two possibilities for man (see text). Dots indicate centres of ossification.

maxillary centre of ossification became progressively reduced until the primordium finally failed to develop.

The remaining dermal bones developed in the frontonasal process are the lacrimals and nasals.

*Further support*

Two further ossification centres appear behind and lateral to each maxilla; the zygomatic bone (2 months *in utero*) and the squamous part of the temporal bone (Figs. 1.37, 1.43). The zygomatic bone forms part of the inferior and lateral margins of the orbit and buttresses the maxilla against the zygomatic process of the squamous part of the temporal bone.

*Mandible*

The lower part of the facial complex is formed by the mandible. As in the case of the upper face the mandible is a dermal bone which ossifies outside a preformed cartilage. This is Meckel's cartilage which is of viscerocranial origin and represents the lower part of the first branchial arch cartilage (Fig. 1.41). However, unlike the upper face, once the mandible begins to form, the cartilage degenerates. The development of the mandible is described in more detail later.

## DEVELOPMENT OF THE MAXILLA

The maxillary processes arise as bilateral buds

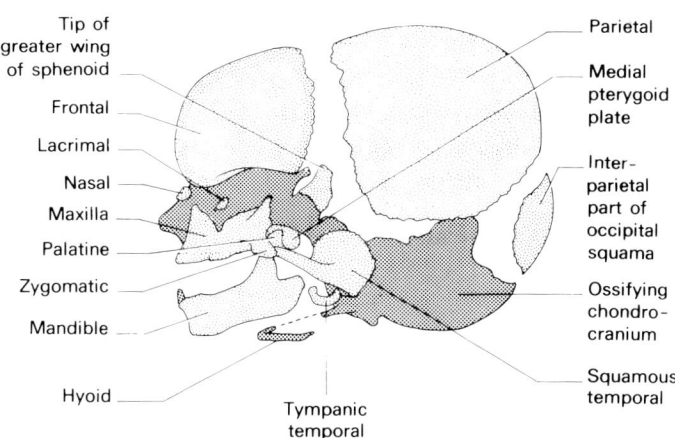

**Fig. 1.43.** Membrane bones of the fetal skull at 16 weeks i.u. (stippled).

originating from the posterior superior aspect of the mandibular processes. The two mesenchymal buds grow forward beneath the brain capsule and as the two maxillary processes approach the midline they merge with the frontonasal process to form the upper border of the mouth cavity (Fig. 1.26). As a result of the forward growth of the maxillary processes and the formation of the frontonasal processes the roof of the oral cavity becomes highly vaulted. The development of the nasal cavity and palate involves the formation of the primary palate the major part of which is derived from the embryonic frontonasal process (Fig. 1.26). The secondary palate is now developed (Fig. 1.27) and the oral cavity has been separated into an oral and a nasal cavity, continuous posteriorly at the pharynx.

In this text we have distinguished between the development and the growth of bones. The adult maxilla is described as consisting of a body and four processes, and these develop very early from the original centre of ossification. The problem of a separate origin for the premaxilla has also been mentioned.

The zygomatic process of the developing maxilla grows posterolaterally. A malar cartilage differentiates within the mesenchyme ahead of the growing edge of the process. This transient secondary cartilage is replaced by bone before birth.

The alveolar process grows from the inferior surface of the developing body of the maxilla. Buccal and lingual plates of bone grow on each side of the developing teeth which now lie in a common trough separated from the infraorbital nerve by a thin plate of bone. Septa of bone develop between adjacent teeth so that each is contained within its own crypt. However, at birth the second deciduous molar and first permanent molar share the same crypt.

The bone of the palatal process grows medially, from the region where the developing alveolar process join the body of the maxilla, and through the (soft tissue) palatal processes of the (embryonic) maxillary processes. The two palatal processes join at the midline intermaxillary suture.

Posteriorly the body of the maxilla forms a suture with the palatine bone.

At birth the maxillary sinus has not yet developed in the bone: it is merely a depression in the lateral wall of the nasal cavity.

### DEVELOPMENT OF THE MANDIBLE

The mandible is the bone of the lower region of the facial complex. It articulates on each side with the temporal bone of the skull base to form the temporomandibular joint.

The mandible ossifies directly in a mesenchymal condensation which appears on the lateral aspect of Meckel's cartilage. At this stage Meckel's cartilage consists of curved rod-like structures each arranged as bilateral 'J' shape (Fig. 1.38). Posteriorly the arches extend back to the cartilaginous otic capsules developing in the base of the skull. Anteriorly the hook of each 'J' is almost in contact with its fellow from the opposite side. An ossification centre appears for each hemimandible (dentary) at about the 6th week *in utero* in the region of the bifurcation of the inferior alveolar nerve into its mental and incisive branches.

From this centre a wave of ossification spreads anteriorly and posteriorly beneath and on each side of the inferior alveolar nerve and artery until a (dermal bone) mandible is applied to the outer surface of the cartilage framework (Fig. 1.44). The neurovascular bundle incorporated in the bone maintains openings at the mental and mandibular foramina. With further ossification the bone extends as far back as the eventual mandibular foramen. The bony structure formed up to this

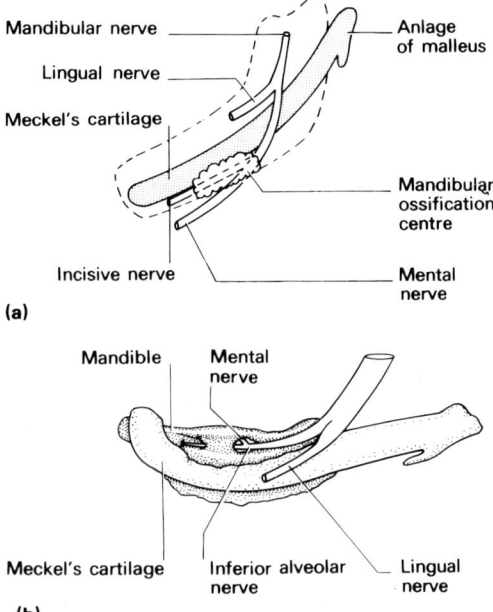

**Fig. 1.44.** (a) Scheme of centre of ossification of mandible lateral to Meckel's cartilage at the bifurcation of the inferior alveolar nerve at 6 weeks i.u. (b) Diagrammatic illustration of the development of the mandible after the bridging over of the mental and incisive nerves has commenced (8 weeks i.u.).

# Embryology and Development

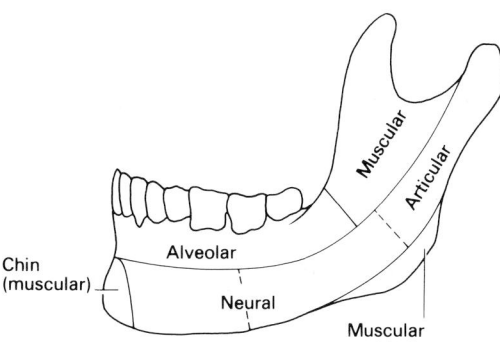

**Fig. 1.45.** The developmental segments of the mandible. The interrupted lines between neural and articular components indicate first that the original neural part of the bone is far anterior but that during development the jaw lengthens by endochondrial ossification of the developing articular part, and much of this bone finally comes to be associated with the inferior dental nerve.

point is the neural component of the mandible (Fig. 1.45) and has the appearance of a gutter or trough which lies on the outer aspect of the cartilage and contains the inferior alveolar nerve.

During the formation of the neural component of the mandible the deciduous dentition has been initiated in the overlying mucosa. However, at this stage the developing tooth germs lie somewhat above the mandible and are not contained within its structure. As the tooth germs reach the bell-stage, the bone of the mandible is extended in an upwards direction so that the teeth come to lie in a trough of bone. Each tooth is now divided from its neighbour by a bony septum. This bone surrounding the teeth is the alveolar component (Fig. 1.45) of the mandible.

Anteriorly, the growing bone partially surrounds Meckel's cartilage which now degenerates and is replaced by bone. For the remainder of its length the cartilage degenerates at some distance medial to the growing mandible.

As the bone grows backwards it develops two processes; an anterior muscular process (the coronoid process) which will give attachment to the temporal muscle and an articular process (the condylar process) which will eventually grow up to articulate with the temporal bone (Fig. 1.45).

## Secondary cartilages of the mandible

During the 10th–12th week *in utero* a condensation of mesenchymal tissue develops in the future ramal region on the superior and lateral aspect of the developing condylar process. Unlike the other stages of mandibular ossification this condensation proceeds to the formation of chondroblasts and the laying down of an area of secondary cartilage. The cartilage proliferates by differentiation of further cells from the cell rich zone in the adjacent fibrous tissue to form a cone-shaped mass whose apex extends forwards and downwards into the mandible to about the level of the mandibular foramen. The cells at the apex are replaced by bone and from here endochondral ossification (bone replacement) spreads up the cone of cartilage until by the 5th month *in utero* only the region immediately beneath the articular surface of the mandible has not been replaced. In most cases this region is not replaced by bone until the end of the second decade and it may act as a growth centre for lengthening the mandible.

Further secondary cartilages are found at two other sites in the mandible. In one a strip of cartilage forms along the anterior upper border of the coronoid process but is replaced by bone well before birth. The other site covers the anterior ends of the hemimandibles where they curl towards the mid-line. The adjacent surfaces of each bone are covered by a layer of secondary cartilage. The two layers are joined in the midline by fibrous tissue to constitute the symphysis menti. Each cartilage has a chondrogenic region, adjacent to the midline connective tissue whose growth widens the mandible. The surface of each cartilage adjacent to the bone is progressively replaced by bone. The potential for growth provided by the symphysis is lost during the first year of life when the cartilage is entirely replaced by bone and the two hemimandibles become joined across the midline transforming them into a single mandible.

The pattern of formation of the mandible shows certain similarities to that found in the maxilla. For instance the centre of ossification appears in membrane, on the outside of a preformed cartilage framework at the bifurcation of a nerve. Both bones have a neural element formed round the pathway of a nerve, and an alveolar element containing teeth. The maxilla also forms an area of secondary cartilage in its backwards extension which, like the coronoid cartilage of the mandible, does not persist into postembryonic life.

## Temporomandibular joint

When the secondary cartilage differentiates in the condylar region of the mandible its posterior edge is separated from the base of the skull by a mass of undifferentiated tissue. The condylar cartilage rapidly grows towards the developing temporal bone but the intervening region becomes organized into a layer of fibrous tissue continuous anteriorly with the future lateral pterygoid muscle.

At about 12 weeks *in utero* upper and lower clefts appear in the fibrous tissue and these form two cavities leaving between them a layer of tissue which will become the articular disc of the temporomandibular joint and which is continuous anteriorly with the developing lateral pterygoid muscle. The clefts extend their boundaries and take on the form of the upper and lower compartments of the joint. By 16 weeks *in utero* an embryonic temporomandibular joint may be recognized.

Both during development and throughout life the articular surfaces of the condyle and the temporal bone are covered with a layer of fibrous tissue consisting of sheets of collagen fibres with interspersed fibroblasts. The articular disc is composed of similar tissue.

The development of the temporomandibular joint differs in several respects from the development of synovial joints between bones of the primary cartilage skeleton (e.g. the limb bones). For instance, whereas most limb joints have completed their cavity formation by 7 weeks *in utero* the temporomandibular joint does not start forming until about the 12th week. In addition the joint develops between initially widely separated dermal bone components and, although forming synovial cavities lubricated by synovial fluid, the articular surfaces are covered by fibrous tissue and not hyaline cartilage. A further difference lies in the characteristics of the secondary growth cartilage which is found just beneath the articular surface of the condyle (Fig. 3.23).

# CHAPTER 2
# Genetics

Genetics, in the classical sense, is concerned with the contribution to biological variation made by inherited differences between individuals. On a broader scale it is also concerned with differences between populations, as well as the changes that occur in the genetic characteristics of the same population from one generation to the next. At a finer level, genetics includes the study of how gene activity is controlled within individuals to produce differences of structure and physiology between various parts of the body. Some of these aspects are dealt with in Book 1. The aim of this chapter is to give a general overall view of how inherited differences, which are fundamentally biochemical, contribute to the variation observed between individuals and populations.

## GENES, CHROMOSOMES AND GENETIC VARIATION

### Genes and chromosomes

Genes are determinants of hereditary characteristics. Each gene is an item of stored information that either specifies the structure of a particular substance or can be used to control the activity of other genes. Genes also have the capacity for accurate self replication. The information contained in them can therefore be passed unaltered from one cell generation to the next, and from a parent to its offspring. It is important to realize that the existence of genes can only be inferred from variation in the characters they produce.

The majority of known genes are located in the chromosomes. The earliest and most compelling evidence for this was the discovery that the transmission of most inherited characters from one generation to the next parallels the transmission of the chromosomes themselves. The remaining few hereditary characters do not behave in this way, and it is concluded that these are controlled by non-chromosomal genes. Non-chromosomal inheritance is not as well understood as chromosomal inheritance and is of little relevance in the present context. The following discussions are therefore concerned only with chromosomal genes.

Gene is a rather indefinite term and it is often better to be more specific. A locus is the site occupied by a gene. Loci are arranged linearly along each chromosome. An allele is one of a number of alternative forms that a gene may take and different forms of the same gene are said to be allelic. For example, the MN blood group locus in man may be occupied by either an 'M substance' producing allele or an 'N substance' producing allele. Such allelic differences provide the basis for the genetic component of variation of any character. Conversely, it is the possession of common alleles, derived from a common ancestor, that contributes to the resemblance between relatives.

In biochemical terms, an allele is a unique nucleotide sequence and its locus is the position of this sequence in the very much longer linear series of nucleotides of a chromosome's DNA. The difference between one allele and another at the same locus may be limited to only one nucleotide position in the sequence, or it may occur at more than one position.

The body is composed of two classes of cells: the somatic cells, which form the substance of the individual, and the germ cells or gametes, which are the individual's potential contribution to the next generation. The nucleus of each human somatic cell normally contains 23 pairs of chromosomes. One member of each pair is contributed by each parent so that each pair can be said to comprise a maternally derived and paternally derived chromosome. The two members of a pair are known as homologous chromosomes or homologues. One of the 23 pairs is a pair of sex chromosomes, and members of the other 22 pairs are called autosomes. Each gamete contains only one member of each chromosome pair, and its chromosome complement is known as haploid. At fertilization one gamete from each parent unite to form a single-celled zygote that subsequently develops into a new individual. As the zygote receives one member of each chromosome pair from each parent it is able to start its development with the full somatic, or diploid, complement of chromosomes.

The two members of each pair of autosomal chromosomes are potentially identical in that the same loci are present in the same sequence on both. The only differences are allelic. Each pair of autosomes is normally completely different from each of the others so that there are only two homologous autosomal loci of each type in a diploid cell, one on each member of a chromosome pair. If both alleles at a given locus are identical (it is usual to use 'locus' to refer to a pair of homologous loci) the individual is known as a homozygote (homozygous at that locus for that allele), and if the alleles are different the individual is known as a heterozygote (heterozygous at that locus).

### The sex chromosomes and X-linked genes

The sex chromosomes differ from the autosomes in that there are two quite different forms. One is the X-chromosome, which can be regarded as comparable to an autosome. Loci carried by the X-chromosome are said to be X-linked (or sex-linked) but are not necessarily directly concerned with sexual differentiation. The other is the much shorter Y-chromosome. All viable individuals possess at least one X-chromosome. The sex of an individual is dependent on whether the other member of the sex chromosome pair is another X-chromosome, associated with femaleness, or a Y-chromosome, which confers maleness. The Y-chromosome therefore carries genes essential for male sexual differentiation, but no Y-linked loci corresponding to those on the X-chromosome have been demonstrated. Females can thus be either homozygous or heterozygous for any X-linked gene, just as for an autosomal gene, but as males possess only one allele at each X-linked locus they can be neither. Males are consequently said to be hemizygous at all X-linked loci.

Over the past few years there has been increasing interest in why males, with only one copy of each X-linked gene, have similar characteristics to females, with a double dose of each X-linked gene. More specifically, heterozygotes for enzyme deficiencies controlled by autosomal genes (such as the deficiency of phenylalanine hydroxylase that causes phenylketonuria) generally have half the enzyme activity of normal homozygotes, whereas enzymes controlled by X-linked genes, such as glucose-6-phosphate dehydrogenase, usually show the same level of activity in normal males and females, despite the difference in X-linked gene dosage (Book 1). It is widely accepted that dosage compensation results from random inactivation of one or other of the X-chromosomes in each somatic cell of females at an early stage of embryonic development so that only one of the two alleles at homologous X-linked loci is able to function in any cell. This action is irreversible, and the same chromosome remains inactive in all descendants of any given cell. Therefore, in a female heterozygous at an X-linked locus, about half the somatic cells will have one allele active and the other half will have the other allele active. This means that X-linked heterozygotes are mosaics made up of patches of two different cell types. This mosaicism may or may not be detectable.

### Normal and abnormal chromosome behaviour

During growth and regeneration somatic cells give rise to more somatic cells by mitosis. Mitosis involves the replication of each chromosome so that when a parent cell divides each of its two daughter cells can receive the full somatic complement of chromosomes. The gametes are derived from somatic cells by meiosis. At the reduction division of meiosis there is cell division without chromosome replication, and, as a result, only one member of each chromosome pair passes into each gamete. For each chromosome pair it is purely a matter of chance whether a given daughter cell receives the maternally derived or the paternally derived chromosome. This chance distribution of maternal and paternal chromosomes at meiosis is known as independent assortment.

Prior to independent assortment, the members of each chromosome pair come into close contact with each other and corresponding segments may be exchanged. Therefore, the chromosomes passed into the gametes are often reconstituted, the maternally derived chromosome of each pair now containing some segments of paternal origin, and the paternally derived chromosome some segments of maternal origin. This exchange can occur anywhere along the chromosome and is known as recombination. Each chromosome segment exchanged by recombination carries many loci. Thus alleles at neighbouring loci tend to be transmitted together, whereas those at a greater distance from each other are more likely to be separated by the recombination process. The frequency with which two loci are separated by recombination can often be determined and is a measure of their physical proximity on the chromosome, known as their degree of linkage.

Occasionally something goes wrong with the assortment of chromosomes at meiosis. If members of a chromosome pair fail to become separated after recombination, one daughter cell will receive both members of the pair and the other daughter cell neither. This failure of separation is known as non-dysjunction and is responsible for producing gametes, and through them individuals, with abnormal chromosome complements. For example, if non-dysjunction of the small autosome numbered 21 occurs at the reduction division of female meiosis, one of the gametes produced will carry both of these autosomes instead of one, and the other will carry neither. If each of these cells is later fertilized by a normal sperm two different types of abnormal zygote will be formed. One will have the two autosomes 21 of maternal origin and an additional autosome 21 from the father; that is, three copies of chromosome 21 in all, a condition known as trisomy 21. The other will have only one copy of chromosome 21 (monosomy 21) which was contributed by the father. Monosomic individuals are not viable but trisomy 21, which produces Down's syndrome (mongolism), is one of the most frequently found chromosomal abnormalities. Non-dysjunction occurs sporadically and at a low frequency.

Rarely, a segment of chromosome of one pair may become attached to a member of another pair. This is known as translocation, and again chromosome 21 may be involved. Part of chromosome 21 may become attached to one of the larger autosomes so that, at the reduction division of meiosis, one of the two gametes formed receives the normal larger autosome and the other the larger autosome carrying the translocation. In addition, one of the gametes receives the normal untranslocated chromosome 21. If the normal chromosome 21 and the autosome carrying the translocation pass into the same gamete, fertilization will produce a zygote with a greater amount of chromosome 21 material than normal; two free chromosomes (one from each parent) and, in addition, the translocated portion. The result again is Down's syndrome. If the normal chromosome 21 and the autosome carrying the translocation pass into different gametes, each will have a more or less balanced haploid complement. Fertilization of the gamete containing the translocated chromosome produces a zygote with a balanced diploid complement, though such individuals will themselves produce abnormal gametes carrying both the translocation and a free chromosome 21 which, when fertilized, result in trisomy 21. Individuals carrying the translocation may therefore be unaffected but can produce more than one offspring with Down's syndrome.

### The maintenance of genetic variation

Alleles are not absolutely stable. Although they are usually transmitted unaltered from one generation to the next, rare events occur that cause changes within them. These events are called mutations, and an allele that has undergone such a change is transmitted in its new, mutant form.

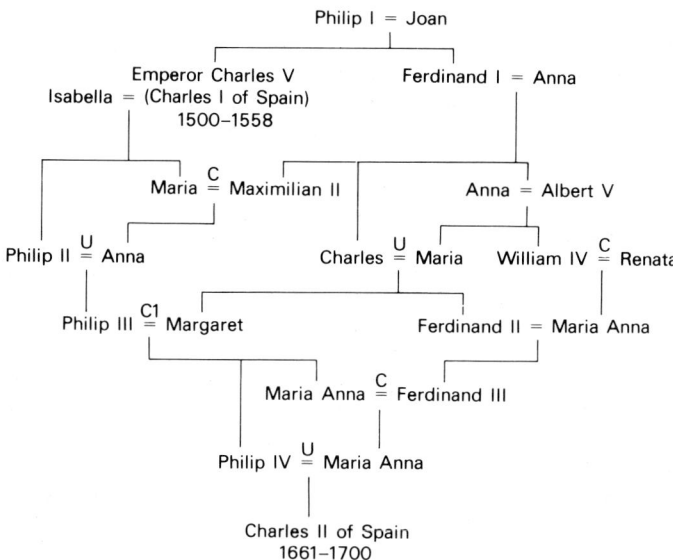

Fig. 2.1. Inbreeding among some of the Spanish Hapsburgs. In the interval between the emperor Charles V and his descendant Charles II of Spain there were three marriages between uncles and their nieces (U), three between first cousins (C) and one between first cousins once removed (C1).

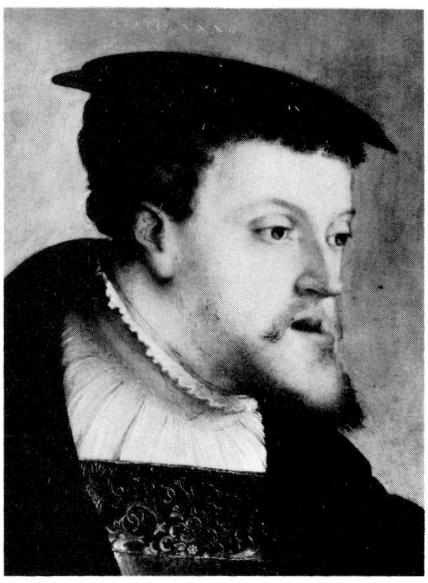 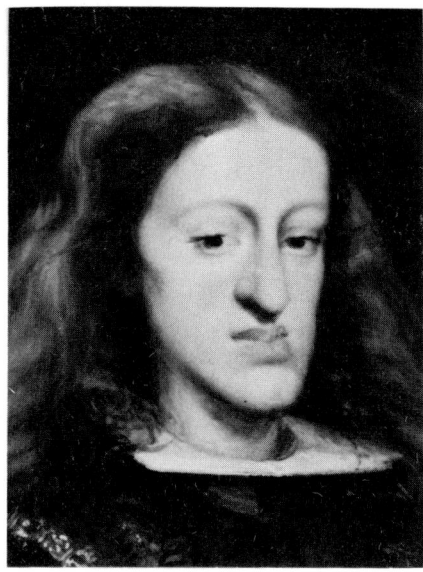

**Fig. 2.2.** The emperor Charles V (left) by Christoph Amberger [Cat. No. 556—Detail—Staatliche Museen Preussischer Kulturbesitz, Gemäldegalerie, Berlin (West)]; and his descendant Charles II of Spain (right) by Juan de Miranda Carreño (Inv. No. 1714—Detail—Kunsthistorisches Museum, Gemäldegalerie, Vienna).

Mutation increases genetic variation by introducing new genetic material. Recombination and independent assortment allow new combinations of existing genetic material to arise, but the effectiveness of these processes in creating genetic diversity depends on the mating of genetically dissimilar individuals. Mating between close relatives, known as inbreeding, therefore results in a reduction of genetic variation. This is exploited in the laboratory to produce genetically homogeneous (or nearly so) animal strains by successive generations of brother × sister mating. In man, inbreeding is never so intense, but marriage between close relatives can lead to the persistence of inherited characteristics over several generations. The protruding lower jaw of the Hapsburgs, for instance, retained a high degree of expression on the Spanish side of the family for 200 years. Persistence of extreme expression was probably contributed to by inbreeding (Figs. 2.1 and 2.2).

## GENOTYPE AND PHENOTYPE

The genetic constitution of an individual is known as his genotype. Genotype may refer to a specified locus or loci, or to all loci in general. An individual's phenotype is the final product of a combination of genetic and environmental influences. Phenotype may be used to refer to a specified character, or to all the observable properties of the individual taken together.

### Genes and characters

Different types of character can be thought of as being different distances from the fundamental level of gene activity. The further a character is removed from this fundamental genetic level the greater the likelihood that its variation is dependent on allele differences at more than one locus, and also on environmental influences. Enzymes, for instance, are products of gene expression, and in most cases it has been shown that a single locus is responsible for the structure of a single enzyme. Characters dependent on the structure of a single enzyme therefore usually show variation that is directly related to allele substitution at a single locus. For example, the most common variety of albinism results from a lack of the enzyme tyrosinase, which is necessary for the formation of pigment (Book 1). At the tyrosinase locus normal individuals possess the allele responsible for producing a normal functional enzyme, whereas tyrosinase-negative albino individuals have at this locus other alleles that are unable to produce a functional enzyme.

Morphological characters, on the other hand, such as the almost infinite number of dimensions

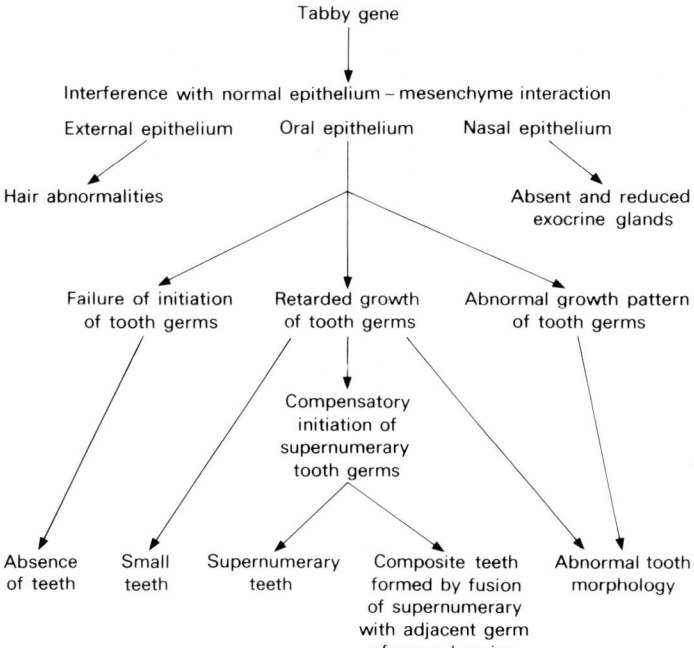

Fig. 2.3. Part of the hierarchy of developmental abnormalities caused by the mutant gene 'tabby' in the mouse.

that can be used to describe the shape of the face and jaws, are furthest removed from the fundamental genetic level and are the end results of a vast complexity of interacting developmental processes. Each gene is therefore likely to influence many morphological characters, and, since development has a basically hierarchical nature, the earlier a gene becomes active the more widespread and varied its effects are likely to be. Detectable single allele substitutions, although producing a unitary effect at the gene level, almost always result in syndromes of morphological abnormalities. When a gene is known to affect a number of different characters its action is said to be pleiotropic. For example, the most fundamental observed effect of the mutant gene 'tabby' in the mouse is an interference with the interaction between epithelium and its underlying mesenchyme that occurs during the formation of epithelial derivatives. As a consequence, these mutant mice have abnormalities of the hair, certain exocrine glands and the teeth. The teeth are generally reduced in size, of abnormal shape and sometimes absent altogether, but there may also be supernumerary teeth and composite teeth formed by fusion of two adjacent tooth germs (Fig. 2.3). The unitary action of the gene therefore has different manifestations in different developmental systems, and even within a system may have a variety of effects depending on the local conditions prevailing during development.

By contrast, the interaction that occurs between different tissues and different cell types at all stages of development allows allele substitutions at many different loci to have some effect on each morphological character. Consequently, variation in the majority of morphological characters studied cannot be shown to be due to allele substitutions at a single locus alone. Many genes and an environmental component are usually responsible. This has been demonstrated clearly for the absence of third molars in mice. Absence appears to be merely an extreme expression of small size, and is affected by many genes, diet and the lactational performance of the mother.

## Modification of gene effects

Some genes produce the same phenotype under all known conditions, but the effects of others may be modified, either by the environment, by other genes, or both. When a mutant genotype produces an abnormal phenotype in some individuals but not in others it is said to have incomplete penetrance. If, among individuals who show the abnormal phenotype, the degree of abnormality varies, the phenotype is said to have variable expressivity.

GENOTYPE AND ENVIRONMENT

The interaction between genotype and the

external environment may fall into one of a number of categories, two of which are mentioned here. First, the same genotype may produce different phenotypes in different environments. In the United Kingdom, as in many other countries, the average height for any given age group has been increasing over several years. This does not appear to be due to a change in genetic composition of the population but rather to an improvement in nutritional status and medical care. Secondly, different genotypes may react differently to the same environmental change. A normal diet causes severe mental disability in individuals with phenylketonuria but, whereas in early diagnosis a low phenylalanine diet makes all the difference between disability and mental normality to phenylketonurics, it has no comparable effect on normal individuals.

In addition to the external environment there is the internal environment of the developing individual. At any stage of development it is reasonable to assume that the same genes are active on both sides of the body, yet bilaterally represented structures regularly fail to form as exact mirror images of each other. This is partly due to differences in the local environment around the developing structures on the two sides, differences which, as far as the dentition is concerned, can lead to asymmetry of tooth size, shape and even number. The internal environment may also change as development proceeds, causing the same genotype to be expressed differently at various stages of development. The retention of a child-like voice in castrated boys, and the acquisition of a masculine voice in women who produce pathologically high levels of male sex hormones, confirm that this change in expression of the genotype is a result of an alteration in hormone production.

INTERACTION BETWEEN GENES

If an individual is homozygous (or hemizygous) at a given locus for any allele, then the observed effect must be the effect of this allele alone. When an individual is heterozygous, possessing two different alleles at the same locus, the phenotype is dependent on the relationship between the alleles. If the two alleles are symbolized by $A_1$ and $A_2$, and in heterozygotes the observed effect is entirely that of $A_2$, then $A_2$ is completely dominant over $A_1$, and $A_1$ is completely recessive to $A_2$. All levels of dominance can occur from complete dominance of one allele over its partner to a situation of no dominance where each allele is expressed unaffected by the other.

Gene interaction can also occur between loci. For example, alleles at the 'secretor' locus in man control the presence or absence in the saliva and other body fluids of ABO blood group antigens, which are specified by another locus. In homozygotes for the dominant allele, $Se$, and in heterozygotes ($Sese$) blood group antigens appear in the saliva, but in homozygotes for the recessive non-secretor allele, $se$, they do not.

A further kind of interaction occurs when a particular gene has a large effect that can be modified by several other genes, each with a small effect. It is then convenient to refer to this particular gene as the major gene and the others as minor or modifying genes. The modifying genes are collectively known as the genetic background.

In animal experiments, crossing to different inbred strains is likely to result in variation of expression of a major gene since, because of their different origins, each strain probably has a unique complement of modifiers. For instance, hemizygotes for the X-linked gene 'tabby' in the mouse have, among their dental malformations, abnormalities of the incisors. Producing the hemizygous mutant genotype in five different inbred strains by appropriate crossing, resulted in an incidence of incisor abnormalities ranging from 11% for one strain to 86% for another. The results of crossing are not predictable but depend on random differences between strains that cannot be evaluated until after the crosses have been made.

## PATTERNS OF INHERITANCE

Alleles are transmitted from one generation to the next in a predictable way. If a character is under genetic control, the distribution of the different forms of the character within families will be related to the pattern of inheritance of the alleles involved.

### Inheritance of alleles at a single locus

AUTOSOMAL INHERITANCE

The nature of meiosis is such that for any one autosomal locus each gamete contains either the maternally derived allele, $A_m$, or the paternally derived allele, $A_p$. These two types of gamete are produced in equal numbers so that half the total gamete population contains $A_m$ and the other half $A_p$. Any one gamete withdrawn at random therefore has the same chance of containing $A_m$ as it does of containing $A_p$. Such chance situations can be defined in terms of probability (symbo-

**Table 2.1.** The four possible zygotic constitutions of maternally and paternally derived alleles, $A_m$ and $A_p$, at an autosomal locus, and their probabilities of occurrence.

| | Zygotic constitutions | | Probabilities |
|---|---|---|---|
| | Allele from parent 1 | Allele from parent 2 | |
| 1 | $A_m$ | $A_m$ | $P_m \times P_m = 0.5 \times 0.5 = 0.25$ |
| 2 | $A_p$ | $A_p$ | $P_p \times P_p = 0.5 \times 0.5 = 0.25$ |
| 3 | $A_m$ | $A_p$ | $P_m \times P_p = 0.5 \times 0.5 = 0.25$ |
| 4 | $A_p$ | $A_m$ | $P_p \times P_m = 0.5 \times 0.5 = 0.25$ |
| | | Total = | 1.00 |

lized by $P$), which is measured on a scale bounded by zero and one. The value $P = 1$ denotes absolute certainty, and $P = 0$ implies complete impossibility. In any situation the sum of the probabilities of all possible alternatives is equal to one. Thus, if $P_m$ is the probability that a gamete withdrawn at random contains $A_m$, and $P_p$ is the probability that it contains $A_p$, then $P_m = P_p = 0.5$ and $P_m + P_p = 1$.

When a particular event is dependent on the previous occurrence of more than one other event, the probability of this particular event occurring is equal to the product of the probabilities of each of the events upon which it is dependent. At fertilization, which can be regarded as the random union of two gametes, the probability that a zygote will receive maternally derived alleles from both parents is equal to $P_m^2 = 0.25$. This is one of a total of four possible zygotic constitutions, illustrated in Table 2.1, based on maternal or paternal origin of the allele contributed by each gamete.

Suppose that in Table 2.1 both parents are heterozygous for the same two alleles. There would then be only three possible zygotic constitutions based on genotype: the two homozygotes, each with a probability of 0.25, and a heterozygote, with a probability of 0.5. To illustrate how this comes about suppose that the maternally derived alleles of both parents are the same, say $A_1$, and that the paternally derived alleles of both parents are also the same, say $A_2$. Constitutions 1 and 2 in Table 2.1 then represent the two homozygotes, $A_1A_1$ and $A_2A_2$ respectively, and constitutions 3 and 4 show that there are two ways in which the heterozygote, $A_1A_2$, can be formed. Each of these has a probability of 0.25, so the total probability for heterozygotes is 0.5.

Consider now the different kinds of mating that can occur with respect to an autosomal locus at which there can be either allele A or allele a. Each parent can have one of the three possible genotypes AA, Aa or aa, and for each of the three genotypes that one parent can have the same three are available for the other. Thus there is a total of $3^2 = 9$ possible parental combinations. These are illustrated in Table 2.2. However, if it is not important which parent has which genotype, these nine combinations are reduced to six possible kinds of mating by duplication. The combinations are numbered in Table 2.2 to show where the duplications arise. The six kinds of mating and their outcomes are listed in Table 2.3. If $P_A$ is the probability that a randomly withdrawn gamete contributed by a parent contains allele A, and $P_a$ is the probability that it contains a, then for heterozygous parents $P_A = P_a = 0.5$, for AA homozygotes $P_A = 1$ and $P_a = 0$, and for aa homozygotes $P_A = 0$ and $P_a = 1$. The offspring genotype probabilities in Table 2.3 are simply the products of the probabilities for alleles contributed by the two parents and are a direct indication of the relative numbers of the different genotypes that can be expected among the progeny of each kind of mating. The transmission of different alleles to different offspring is known as segregation.

### X-LINKED INHERITANCE

Gametes produced by males contain either an X-chromosome or a Y-chromosome, and these two types of gamete are produced in equal numbers. Gametes produced by females all contain an X-chromosome. The Y-chromosome of a male is therefore always inherited from his father and the

**Table 2.2.** The nine possible parental combinations with respect to a single autosomal locus with alleles A and a. The numbers in brackets show how these nine combinations are reduced to six possible kinds of mating by duplication. Pairs of cells containing the same number represent two different ways of forming the same kind of mating.

| Genotype of parent 2 | Genotype of parent 1 | | |
|---|---|---|---|
| | AA | Aa | aa |
| AA | (1) AA × AA | (2) AA × Aa | (3) AA × aa |
| Aa | (2) Aa × AA | (4) Aa × Aa | (5) Aa × aa |
| aa | (3) aa × AA | (5) aa × Aa | (6) aa × aa |

X-chromosome is always inherited from his mother. Similarly, one of the X-chromosomes of a female is always the one carried by her father and the other comes from her mother. It follows that, whereas a mother's X-linked alleles are transmitted both to her daughters and sons, a father's X-linked alleles are transmitted only to his daughters, and through them to his granddaughters and grandsons. For example, the bleeding disorder haemophilia is caused by an X-linked mutant gene. Hemizygous mutant males show the disorder, but, since the mutant allele is almost completely recessive, heterozygous females are usually unaffected and are consequently known as carriers of the gene. A haemophiliac father transmits the mutant allele to all his daughters, who as a result are carriers and who, on average, pass it on to half their sons and half their daughters. These sons are haemophiliacs and these daughters are carriers.

Consider all the possible kinds of mating that can occur with respect to an X-linked locus at which there can be either allele A or allele a. There are then three possible genotypes for the female parent, AA, Aa and aa, and for each one there are two possible genotypes for the male parent, A and a. There is thus a total of $3 \times 2 = 6$ possible parental combinations. Unlike the autosomal case there is no duplication; male and female parents can never have the same X-linked genotype. Each of the six parental combinations therefore represents a completely different kind of mating. These matings and their outcomes are listed in Table 2.4. Again, the offspring probabilities are a direct indication of the relative numbers of the genotypes that can be expected among the progeny of the different kinds of mating.

**Inheritance of characters controlled by a single locus**

A knowledge of the genetic constitution of an individual allows predictions to be made about the

**Table 2.3.** The six possible kinds of mating (see Table 2.2) with respect to a single autosomal locus with alleles A and a. The probability that a randomly withdrawn gamete from each parent will contain a given allele is shown, as are the offspring genotype probabilities.

| | Parent 1 | | | Parent 2 | | | Offspring genotype probabilities | | |
|---|---|---|---|---|---|---|---|---|---|
| | | Gamete probabilities | | | Gamete probabilities | | | | |
| Mating | Genotype | A | a | Genotype | A | a | AA | Aa | aa |
| 1 | AA | 1.0 | 0.0 | AA | 1.0 | 0.0 | 1.00 | 0.00 | 0.00 |
| 2 | AA | 1.0 | 0.0 | Aa | 0.5 | 0.5 | 0.50 | 0.50 | 0.00 |
| 3 | AA | 1.0 | 0.0 | aa | 0.0 | 1.0 | 0.00 | 1.00 | 0.00 |
| 4 | Aa | 0.5 | 0.5 | Aa | 0.5 | 0.5 | 0.25 | 0.50 | 0.25 |
| 5 | Aa | 0.5 | 0.5 | aa | 0.0 | 1.0 | 0.00 | 0.50 | 0.50 |
| 6 | aa | 0.0 | 1.0 | aa | 0.0 | 1.0 | 0.00 | 0.00 | 1.00 |

**Table 2.4.** The six possible kinds of mating with respect to an X-linked locus with alleles A and a. The probability that a randomly withdrawn gamete from each parent will contain a given allele is shown, as are the offspring genotype probabilities for the three possible genotypes of female offspring and two possible genotypes of male offspring.

|  | Female parent | | | Male parent | | | Offspring genotype probabilities | | | | |
| --- | --- | --- | --- | --- | --- | --- | --- | --- | --- | --- | --- |
|  |  | Gamete probabilities | | | Gamete probabilities | | Females | | | Males | |
| Mating | Genotype | A | a | Genotype | A | a | AA | Aa | aa | A | a |
| 1 | AA | 1.0 | 0.0 | A | 1.0 | 0.0 | 1.0 | 0.0 | 0.0 | 1.0 | 0.0 |
| 2 | Aa | 0.5 | 0.5 | A | 1.0 | 0.0 | 0.5 | 0.5 | 0.0 | 0.5 | 0.5 |
| 3 | aa | 0.0 | 1.0 | A | 1.0 | 0.0 | 0.0 | 1.0 | 0.0 | 0.0 | 1.0 |
| 4 | AA | 1.0 | 0.0 | a | 0.0 | 1.0 | 0.0 | 1.0 | 0.0 | 1.0 | 0.0 |
| 5 | Aa | 0.5 | 0.5 | a | 0.0 | 1.0 | 0.0 | 0.5 | 0.5 | 0.5 | 0.5 |
| 6 | aa | 0.0 | 1.0 | a | 0.0 | 1.0 | 0.0 | 0.0 | 1.0 | 0.0 | 1.0 |

types of offspring he produces. If there is no dominance or intermediate dominance all genotypes are phenotypically distinct, but if there is complete dominance of one allele over another it may only be possible to determine an individual's genotype through an examination of his progeny.

Table 2.5 lists the six possible kinds of mating with respect to a single autosomal locus with the alternative alleles A and a. The expected offspring segregation ratios are shown both for genotypes and also for phenotypes when A is completely dominant over a. The phenotype produced by genotypes AA and Aa is symbolized by $A$, and that produced by genotype aa is symbolized by $a$. Only three different parental combinations can be identified on the basis of phenotype alone, $A \times A$ (matings 1, 2 and 4), $A \times a$ (matings 3 and 5) and $a \times a$ (mating 6). All matings except 1 and 2 can, however, be distinguished through their offspring segregation ratios. Mating 4 has a different ratio from matings 1 and 2, and mating 3 has a different ratio from mating 5. Matings 1 and 2 can be separated by a second generation of matings of their $A$ offspring with $a$ individuals. Offspring of mating 1 are then partners in matings of type 3, whereas offspring of mating 2 contribute to some matings of type 3 and some of type 5. The transfer of dominant alleles from one generation to the next makes it possible for a dominantly controlled phenotype to occur in several successive generations of a family in the absence of inbreeding.

Table 2.6 shows a similar listing for a single X-linked locus. There are four parental combinations based on phenotype, ♀$A$ × ♂$A$ (matings 1 and 2), ♀$A$ × ♂$a$ (matings 4 and 5), ♀$a$ × ♂$A$ (mating 3) and ♀$a$ × ♂$a$ (mating 6). All matings are distinguishable on the basis of parental phenotype and offspring segregation ratio.

**Table 2.5.** The six possible kinds of mating with respect to an autosomal locus with alleles A and a. The expected ratios of the different types of offspring are shown for genotypes and for phenotypes when A is completely dominant over a.

|  | Genotypes | | Phenotypes (A completely dominant over a) | |
| --- | --- | --- | --- | --- |
| Mating | Parents | Offspring ratios AA : Aa : aa | Parents | Offspring ratios $A : a$ |
| 1 | AA × AA | 1 : 0 : 0 | $A \times A$ | 1 : 0 |
| 2 | AA × Aa | 1 : 1 : 0 | $A \times A$ | 1 : 0 |
| 3 | AA × aa | 0 : 1 : 0 | $A \times a$ | 1 : 0 |
| 4 | Aa × Aa | 1 : 2 : 1 | $A \times A$ | 3 : 1 |
| 5 | Aa × aa | 0 : 1 : 1 | $A \times a$ | 1 : 1 |
| 6 | aa × aa | 0 : 0 : 1 | $a \times a$ | 0 : 1 |

**Table 2.6.** The six possible kinds of mating with respect to an X-linked locus with alleles A and a. The expected ratios of the different types of offspring are shown for genotypes and for phenotypes when A is completely dominant over a.

| | | Genotypes | | Phenotypes (A completely dominant over a) | | |
|---|---|---|---|---|---|---|
| | | Offspring ratios | | | Offspring ratios | |
| Mating | Parents ♀ × ♂ | ♀ AA : Aa : aa | ♂ A : a | Parents ♀ × ♂ | ♀ A : a | ♂ A : a |
| 1 | AA × A | 1 : 0 : 0 | 1 : 0 | A × A | 1 : 0 | 1 : 0 |
| 2 | Aa × A | 1 : 1 : 0 | 1 : 1 | A × A | 1 : 0 | 1 : 1 |
| 3 | aa × A | 0 : 1 : 0 | 0 : 1 | a × A | 1 : 0 | 0 : 1 |
| 4 | AA × a | 0 : 1 : 0 | 1 : 0 | A × a | 1 : 0 | 1 : 0 |
| 5 | Aa × a | 0 : 1 : 1 | 1 : 1 | A × a | 1 : 1 | 1 : 1 |
| 6 | aa × a | 0 : 0 : 1 | 0 : 1 | a × a | 0 : 1 | 0 : 1 |

### More complex situations

Many characters of interest are controlled by more than one locus, possibly with more than two alleles at each locus, but the theory behind the behaviour of such characters is nevertheless based on that described for two alleles at a single locus. When considering more than one locus the probability of any genotype occurring among the progeny of a particular mating is simply the product of the probabilities for the genotypes at each of the loci taken separately, and the complexity resulting from more than two alleles at a locus can be simplified by creating a number of two allele situations in which each allele is considered in relation to all the others. As an illustration of the enormous variety of expression that can occur for a character controlled by only a small number of loci with few alleles at each locus, it has been estimated that the wide range of human skin pigmentation among individuals of mixed Caucasian and black African ancestry can be accounted for by between three and six loci with two alleles per locus.

### Demonstration of the mode of genetic control of a character

Genes are identified through variation in the characters they produce, and in particular by the distribution of different forms of each character within families. Theoretically, with unrestricted numbers of progeny from all kinds of mating, it is possible to determine the mode of genetic control of any character in great detail. However, because of restrictions of time and space in the laboratory, and because of difficulties associated with the collection of human data, it may only be practicable to make the fundamental distinction between control by a single locus and multifactorial control where many loci, or at least more than one, and an environmental component are involved. In the single locus case, analysis is based on the patterns of inheritance of the characters. The pattern of inheritance on the phenotypic level is compared with the theoretical expectations associated with different types of single locus control. The analysis of multifactorial control, on the other hand, is concerned with the size of the contributions of genetic and environmental sources to the observed variation between individuals, and rests on the degree of resemblance between relatives.

## QUANTITATIVE AND POPULATION GENETICS

Quantitative and population genetics involve extensions of the basic principles already described. They permit the analysis of, respectively, the degree of resemblance between relatives and the behaviour of genes in populations rather than families.

### Quantitative inheritance

When a character is under some degree of genetic control but no simple mode of inheritance can be demonstrated, the question of interest is: what proportion of the observed variation between individuals is due to genetic segregation and what proportion to environmental differences?

## SOURCES OF VARIATION

Variation is expressed in terms of variance and variances are additive so that the total observed or phenotypic variance, $V_P$, is composed of a genetic component, $V_G$, and an environmental component, $V_E$, so that $V_P = V_G + V_E$. The genetic variance is itself made up of three components, the additive, dominance and interaction variances. Dominance and interaction effects are dependent on particular combinations of genes at the same and different loci respectively, and are therefore not inherited in a simple manner. However, they are likely to be small and, in addition, are difficult to estimate from human data. Human genetics is therefore usually concerned only with the additive genetic component of variance, $V_A$, which is the main genetic cause of resemblance between relatives. The proportion of the phenotypic variance taken up by the additive genetic component is known as the heritability and is symbolized by $h^2$. Thus, $h^2 = V_A/V_P$. Heritability is an expression of the reliance that can be placed on an individual's phenotype as an indication of the phenotype of his relatives. If, for a particular character, there is no dominance or interaction and the observed variation is entirely additive genetic in origin (that is $V_A = V_P$ and $h^2 = 1$), then the phenotype of an individual is, on average, equal to the mean phenotype of his parents.

As heritability is a ratio of one component of the observed variation to the total, changes in any component can affect its value. Thus, the heritability of the same character in genetically similar populations could have different values under different environmental conditions. Similarly, genetically different populations are likely to show variable heritabilities for the same character in the same environment. A specific heritability estimate therefore applies only to a particular population in its own environment.

## ESTIMATION OF HERITABILITY

A common way of expressing the degree of resemblance between relatives for a continuously variable character is by a regression of offspring mean on midparent value, the mean of measurements of the character in the two parents of each family. If the two parental phenotypes are $p_1$ and $p_2$ then the midparent value is $\bar{P} = (p_1 + p_2)/2$. Suppose that $h^2 = 1$. All phenotypic variation has an additive genetic origin and the phenotype of an individual is an exact indication of his genotype. Since each individual receives, on average, half his genetic information from one parent and half from the other, the mean phenotype of offspring is $\bar{O} = (p_1/2) + (p_2/2)$. Therefore $\bar{O}$ tends to equal $\bar{P}$, and if $\bar{O}$ is plotted against $\bar{P}$ for several different families, the results average out as a straight line with a slope of one. When $h^2 = 1$, the regression of offspring on midparent value is $b_{\bar{O}\bar{P}} = 1$ and thus $h^2 = b_{\bar{O}\bar{P}}$. When $h^2 = O$, and assuming that there is no environmental reason why offspring should resemble their parents, each offspring is equivalent to a randomly selected individual from the general population, and the offspring means of all families vary around the mean of the general population. The results of plotting $\bar{O}$ against $\bar{P}$ then average out as a straight line with zero slope. When $h^2 = O$, $b_{\bar{O}\bar{P}} = O$, so that in this case also $h^2 = b_{\bar{O}\bar{P}}$ (Fig. 2.4). The equivalence of $h^2$ and $b_{\bar{O}\bar{P}}$ can in fact be shown to apply for all values of $h^2$. Different methods of analysis are available for expressing the resemblance between other sorts of relatives.

Consider a quasicontinuous variable (Fig. 2.5). Individuals are classified as either affected or non-

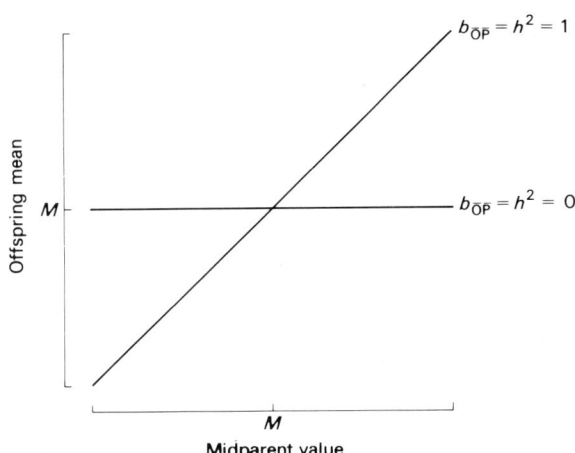

Fig. 2.4. The regression of offspring mean on midparent value. The two lines indicate the average relationships between parents and offspring for the two extremes of heritability. $M$ is the mean value of the character in the population.

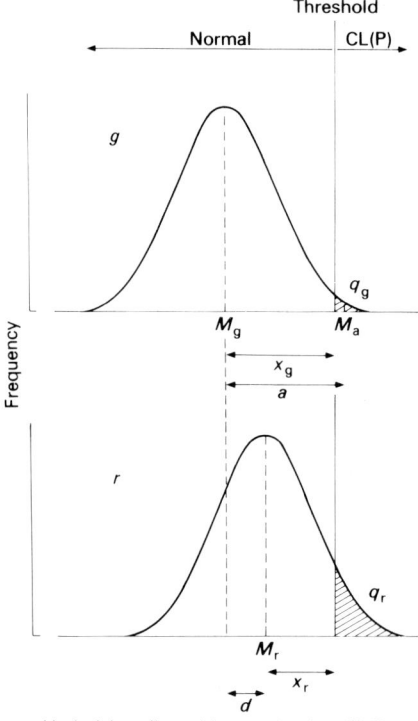

**Fig. 2.5.** Heritability estimation for a quasicontinuous or 'threshold' character, CL(P). Distributions of the general population, g, and of a group of relatives of affected individuals, r, are shown on an underlying continuous scale of disposition. The values of $x_g$ and a, and $x_r$, are derived from tables of the normal distribution given the proportions $q_g$ and $q_r$. The distance d, relative to a and the degree of relationship of the relatives used, provides the estimate of heritability.

affected. In human populations individuals affected by an abnormality or disease are usually in the minority and are the ones who attract attention. They are therefore often called index cases. As an example of a quasicontinuous variable consider cleft lip with or without a cleft of the palate, CL(P). The assumption is that for each individual a combination of genetic and environmental influences determines the level of disposition to develop the malformation. An individual whose level falls below the threshold is normal, whereas one whose level falls above it is affected. If CL(P) has no hereditary basis and is produced entirely by chance or environmental factors, then, provided all individuals are exposed to the same environment, a group of relatives of CL(P) individuals is equivalent to a random sample of the population with an incidence of the malformation approximating to that of the general population itself. On the other hand, if CL(P) is under some degree of genetic control the frequency of the malformation among relatives of index cases should be higher than among the general population. Thus, assuming that there is no environmental reason why relatives should be alike, d, the distance between $M_r$, the mean of a group of relatives of index cases, and $M_g$, the mean of the general population, is a measure of the degree to which CL(P) is a heritable condition (Fig. 2.5). This is simply the difference between $x_g$ and $x_r$ derived from applying the proportions $q_g$ and $q_r$ to tables. It must be assumed, though, that the variances of the general population and the group of relatives are the same.

The distance d must be considered in relation to a, the distance of the mean of affected individuals in the general population from the general population mean; and also to r, the degree of relationship of the relatives being used. The distance a is the maximum value that d can assume, and this can only occur if $h^2 = 1$ and if the relatives are monozygotic twins (genetically identical with their index cases, with r = 1). If the relatives used are first degree (full sibs, parents or children), second degree (aunts, uncles, nieces or nephews) or third degree relatives (first cousins) then r = 1/2, 1/4 and 1/8 respectively; these relatives have on average 1/2, 1/4 and 1/8 of their genes in common with their index case. The maximum values of d when using first, second and third degree relatives are accordingly a/2, a/4 and a/8, and these can only occur if $h^2 = 1$. The actual value of the heritability is simply the difference d expressed as a proportion of its maximum possible value. Thus $h^2 = d/ar$. Estimates of heritability for familial CL(P) from first, second and third degree relatives by this method are respectively 0.83, 0.78 and 0.81. These values suggest that the difference between familial CL(P) cases and normal individuals is probably largely (about 80%) due to the inheritance of different genes.

**Genes in populations**

Populations are described in terms of frequencies of different types of individual. Frequency, as used here, is expressed relative to the total number of individuals in the population. Used in this way, frequency is, like probability, measured on a scale bounded by zero and one, and the probability of withdrawing a particular type of individual from a population by random choice is equal to the frequency of that type in the population. Thus, in any situation, frequency and probability are numerically the same. From the genetic point of view a population can be described in terms of phenotype frequencies, genotype frequencies and 'gene' frequencies (that is allele frequencies). Starting with gene frequencies it is a simple matter to derive genotype frequencies, and therefore phenotype frequencies, if certain assumptions are made about the population. Conversely, knowing the phenotype frequencies, it is possible to determine genotype and gene frequencies. The concepts involved in these determinations are embodied in the Hardy–Weinberg law.

## THE HARDY–WEINBERG LAW

Suppose that $A_1$ and $A_2$ are two alleles at an autosomal locus, and that in a population the frequency of $A_1$ is p, the frequency of $A_2$ is q, and $p + q = 1$. From each individual taken at random the probability of withdrawing a gamete containing $A_1$ is equal to the frequency of $A_1$ ($= p$), and the probability of withdrawing a gamete containing $A_2$ is equal to the frequency of $A_2$ ($= q$). The results of random mating within the population, which is equivalent to the random union of gametes, are then as illustrated in Table 2.7. This shows that there are four possible zygotic constitutions with respect to parental origin of alleles but only three possible genotypes, as the heterozygote can be formed in two different ways. The frequencies of these genotypes, $A_1A_1$, $A_1A_2$ and $A_2A_2$, among the offspring are respectively $p^2$, $2pq$ and $q^2$.

For every $A_1A_1$ homozygote there are two $A_1$ alleles, for every $A_2A_2$ homozygote there are two $A_2$ alleles, and for every heterozygote there is one $A_1$ and one $A_2$ allele. Thus, if N offspring are produced after random mating there will be $N(2p^2 + 2pq)$ $A_1$ alleles and $N(2q^2 + 2pq)$ $A_2$ alleles. This is known as gene counting. As N individuals possess 2N alleles at an autosomal locus, and because $p + q = 1$, the frequencies of these alleles among the offspring are:

Frequency of $A_1$
$= N(2p^2 + 2pq)/2N$
$= p^2 + pq$
$= p^2 + p(1 - p) = p$

Frequency of $A_2$
$= N(2q^2 + 2pq)/2N$
$= q^2 + pq$
$= q^2 + q(1 - q) = q$

Thus the gene frequencies among the offspring of random mating are the same as in the parental generation.

Extending these principles over many generations it is clear that as long as random mating persists the gene frequencies will remain the same, and $A_1A_1$, $A_1A_2$ and $A_2A_2$ offspring will always be produced in frequencies $p^2$, $2pq$ and $q^2$ respectively. In such a situation the population is said to be in Hardy–Weinberg equilibrium. It should be stressed that the equilibrium genotype frequencies, which appear among the offspring of the first and subsequent generations of random mating, are quite independent of the genotype frequencies in the population from which the parents are drawn. They depend only on the gene frequencies.

It may also be helpful to consider the results of random mating in terms of genotypes only. Table 2.8 shows the frequencies of the nine possible parental combinations when the genotype frequencies have equilibrium values. These nine parental combinations are reduced to six kinds of mating (by duplication: they are numbered to show where the duplications arise.) The matings, their frequencies and their outcomes are listed in Table 2.9. The three genotypes of offspring, $A_1A_1$, $A_1A_2$ and $A_2A_2$, again appear in the frequencies $p^2$, $2pq$ and $q^2$ respectively.

**Table 2.7.** The four possible zygotic constitutions and three possible genotypes with respect to a single autosomal locus, and their frequencies assuming random mating. Alleles $A_1$ and $A_2$ have the frequencies p and q respectively, with $p + q = 1$.

| | Zygotic constitutions | | | | |
|---|---|---|---|---|---|
| | Allele from parent 1 | Allele from parent 2 | Frequency | Genotype | Genotype frequency |
| 1 | $A_1$ | $A_1$ | $p^2$ | $A_1A_1$ | $p^2$ |
| 2 | $A_1$ | $A_2$ | $pq$ | $A_1A_2$ | $2pq$ |
| 3 | $A_2$ | $A_1$ | $pq$ | | |
| 4 | $A_2$ | $A_2$ | $q^2$ | $A_2A_2$ | $q^2$ |

Total $= p^2 + 2pq + q^2 = 1$

**Table 2.8.** Frequencies of nine possible parental genotype combinations at an autosomal locus assuming random mating, reduced to six kinds of mating by duplication. Pairs of cells containing the same number in brackets represent two ways of producing the same kind of mating. The frequencies of the different kinds of mating, and their outcomes, are listed in Table 2.9.

|                      |           | Genotype of parent 1 |           |           |
| -------------------- | --------- | -------------------- | --------- | --------- |
|                      |           | $A_1A_1$             | $A_1A_2$  | $A_2A_2$  |
| Genotype of parent 2 | Frequency | $p^2$                | $2pq$     | $q^2$     |
| $A_1A_1$             | $p^2$     | (1) $p^4$            | (2) $2p^3q$ | (3) $p^2q^2$ |
| $A_1A_2$             | $2pq$     | (2) $2p^3q$          | (4) $4p^2q^2$ | (5) $2pq^3$ |
| $A_2A_2$             | $q^2$     | (3) $p^2q^2$         | (5) $2pq^3$ | (6) $q^4$ |

Similar theory can be applied to an X-linked locus, but account must naturally be taken of the difference in X-linked genotype between females and males.

### FACTORS TENDING TO DISTURB HARDY–WEINBERG EQUILIBRIUM

The maintenance of Hardy–Weinberg equilibrium depends on random mating within the population. Random mating means that each individual of one sex has an equal chance of mating with each individual of the opposite sex, irrespective of genotype. Random mating, as already mentioned, is therefore equivalent to random union of gametes. If particular parental genotype combinations tend to occur in matings more frequently than expected by chance, the genotype frequencies among the offspring of the parental generation will be biased in favour of those produced by the more frequent kinds of mating.

Alleles transmitted from one generation to the next can be regarded as a sample of the alleles present in the parental generation. The larger the number of alleles transmitted the more confidence there can be that the frequencies among offspring are a good indication of the frequencies in the parental generation. The Hardy–Weinberg expectations are therefore dependent on population size. In small populations allele frequencies can change markedly from one generation to the next, purely by chance.

If the locus of interest has some control over fitness, then alleles associated with poor fitness will tend to be eliminated whereas others will tend to be present at progressively increasing frequencies. Hardy-Weinberg equilibrium is therefore only established in the absence of selection. Allele frequencies are also affected by the introduction of new allelic forms through mutation, and by the introduction or loss of alleles through migration into or out of the population.

**Table 2.9.** Six possible kinds of mating with respect to an autosomal locus. The two alleles $A_1$ and $A_2$ have the frequencies p and q respectively, with $p + q = 1$. The frequency of each kind of mating (from Table 2.8) and the frequencies of the three genotypes of offspring are based on the assumption of random mating.

|   | Mating | Mating frequency | Offspring genotype frequencies | | |
|---|--------|------------------|----------|----------|----------|
|   |        |                  | $A_1A_1$ | $A_1A_2$ | $A_2A_2$ |
| 1 | $A_1A_1 \times A_1A_1$ | $p^4$    | $p^4$    | 0        | 0        |
| 2 | $A_1A_1 \times A_1A_2$ | $4p^3q$  | $2p^3q$  | $2p^3q$  | 0        |
| 3 | $A_1A_1 \times A_2A_2$ | $2p^2q^2$| 0        | $2p^2q^2$| 0        |
| 4 | $A_1A_2 \times A_1A_2$ | $4p^2q^2$| $p^2q^2$ | $2p^2q^2$| $p^2q^2$ |
| 5 | $A_1A_2 \times A_2A_2$ | $4pq^3$  | 0        | $2pq^3$  | $2pq^3$  |
| 6 | $A_2A_2 \times A_2A_2$ | $q^4$    | 0        | 0        | $q^4$    |
|   | Total  |                  | $p^2$    | $2pq$    | $q^2$    |

These factors may also tend to upset Hardy–Weinberg equilibrium.

In spite of all this, statistical tests show that in most populations of reasonable size studied the genotype frequencies are in accordance with the Hardy–Weinberg expectations. Non-random mating, random sampling variation, differential selection, mutation and migration, although they probably occur to some extent in all populations, usually do not have large enough effects to disrupt Hardy–Weinberg equilibrium to a significant extent. With this in mind, the relationships between gene frequencies and genotype frequencies described by the Hardy–Weinberg law can be used to some advantage.

## FURTHER READING

CAVALLI-SFORZA L.L. & BODMER W.F. (1971) *The Genetics of Human Populations*. San Francisco: W. H. Freeman.

EMERY A.E.H. (1979) *Elements of Medical Genetics*, 5th Edition. London: Churchill Livingstone.

FALCONER D.S. (1964) *Introduction to Quantitative Genetics*. London: Longman.

GRÜNEBERG H. (1963) *The Pathology of Development*. Oxford: Blackwell.

POOLE A.E., ed. (1975) Symposium on genetics. *Dental Clinics of North America* **19**, Number 1.

PRESCOTT G.H. & STEWART R.E., eds (1976) *Oral Facial Genetics*. St Louis: C.V. Mosby.

ROSS R.B. & JOHNSTON M.C. (1972) *Cleft Lip and Palate*. Baltimore: Williams and Wilkins.

SOFAER J.A. (1970) Dental morphologic variation and the Hardy–Weinberg law. *Journal of Dental Research* **49**, 1505.

SOFAER J.A. (1975) Genetic variation and tooth development. *British Medical Bulletin* **31**, 107.

SOFAER J.A. (1980) Single gene disorders. In *Oral Manifestations of Systemic Disease*, Chapter 2, eds. Mason D.K. & Jones H. London: W.B. Saunders.

STERN C. (1973) *Principles of Human Genetics*, 3rd Edition. San Francisco: W.H. Freeman.

WITKOP C.J. Jr., ed. (1962) *Genetics and Dental Health*. New York, Toronto and London: McGraw-Hill.

WITKOP C.J. Jr. (1965) Genetic disease of the oral cavity. In *Oral Pathology*, ed. Tieke R.W. New York, Toronto and London: McGraw-Hill.

# CHAPTER 3
# Growth and Ageing

Growth involves a series of changes and not merely the addition of material to achieve an increase in size. These changes include differentiation of various parts of the body to perform different functions and alterations in the form of the body as a whole in addition to the form of its organs and systems. For example, the thymus, which is large and prominent during childhood, gradually degenerates and is absorbed until there is little trace of it in the adult. Growth may also involve substitution, e.g. replacement of the deciduous by the permanent dentition.

Not all parts of the body grow at the same rate, nor do all parts cease growing simultaneously. Growth of one region may be influenced by that of another (e.g. endocrine system), and the degree of control depends upon the state of development reached by the controlling part.

Growth does not cease with the attainment of maturity. For instance, the lining of the oral cavity is constantly being renewed, and there may be disordered growth, as in tumours. Nevertheless, the most spectacular phase of growth occurs before birth.

**Growth processes**

There is a limit to the size that a cell can attain. This limit is set by purely physical and chemical factors. For instance, as a spherical cell grows, its volume increases with the cube of the radius, whereas its surface area increases only with the square of the radius. The volume of a cell determines its biochemical activity, since metabolism goes on all through the substance of the cell, but all the material necessary for this activity must pass in and out through the surface membrane. Therefore as the cell grows its biochemical function becomes increasingly restricted through lack of raw materials and energy, and eventually some resulting (unknown) chemical stimulus causes it to divide.

The restriction in size of individual cells can be overcome to a certain extent if a cell alters its spherical shape by flattening (epithelial cells), elongating (nerve cells) or folding up its surface membrane (interstitial cells).

The ratio between cell size and nuclear size is another factor which may play a role in determining the time at which a cell must divide. The nucleus comprises mainly chromatin, and does not increase in size with growth at the same rate as the cytoplasm. The surface area of the nucleus thus becomes inadequate to allow proper control of the cytoplasm by the nucleus. Thus it is possible that cells divide in an attempt to maintain a fairly constant ratio between the amounts of material in the nucleus and cytoplasm. Similarly, the nucleus can allow some further increase in cytoplasm by becoming flattened or lobulated, although there is a limit to the scope to which such manoeuvres are biologically possible.

The processes of growth and cell division are therefore complementary and interdependent. Growth of a cell beyond a certain size is impossible, and further growth of the tissue of which the cell is a part involves a temporary reduction in the size of the daughter cells. Similarly, cell division is normally dependent on a period of antecedent growth, without which repeated division would lead to a progressive reduction in cell size.

During this period, DNA is being synthesized, so that when the cell next divides, there is sufficient to supply each daughter cell. Cells not only divide and grow but they also tend to become 'differentiated'. This process of differentiation occurs after the early stages of embryogenesis, with the result that many tissues of the body become differentiated to perform specific functions, e.g. bone, cartilage. In general, undifferentiated cells tend to be uniform in appearance, randomly arranged, simple in structure and function, and highly adaptable to changing environmental conditions. By contrast, differentiated cells tend to be diverse and regular in appearance, to have complex structure and functions, and to be more rigid and unable to adapt. Furthermore, cellular differentiation may entail differentiation of responses to various growth-promoting stimuli, e.g. sex hormones have greater effect in certain tissues at the time of puberty than before.

The factors leading to cellular differentiation are obscure, although they appear to include the influence of other cells in the body. It is generally assumed that chemical factors control cellular differentiation, although there is little experimental data to support this supposition. Furthermore, differentiation and multiplication tend to be mutually exclusive, so that the more differentiated a cell is, the less likely it is to undergo mitosis.

Looking at the tissues of the body, three types of cell population can be recognized: those which are required to renew themselves constantly, e.g. oral mucosa; those which comprise expanding cell populations, e.g. liver; and those with static cell populations, e.g. somatic muscle and nervous tissue. Thus, when considering growth of a region of the body, many different cell populations may be involved, thereby contributing to the complexity of growth.

In the early embryo, the intercellular matrix is scanty and amorphous. Subsequently it increases in quantity and acquires viscous substances which give it a gel-like consistency and enable it to hold a large amount of fluid. Later still, the intercellular matrix may contain special compounds, e.g. collagen, whose functions are combined with those of other cells in order that specific tasks may be fulfilled, e.g. contributing to the strength of a tissue. Thus, when considering overall growth, both growth and specialization of cells and their secondary products are involved.

## Phases of growth

There are four main phases in body growth. In the early embryo, everything is subordinated to growth and there is little differentiation of function. This phase merges with a second one, where a kind of balance is achieved between growth and differentiated functional activity; the latter phase lasts until maturity. Subsequently, a third phase supervenes where the main goal is functional activity with growth repairing tissue loss due to wear and tear. This phase lasts until old age, when cells may be lost, without replacement, from various systems, with a possible result of inefficient function. In each phase, however, the balance between growth and formation can be upset by the advent of injury, which stimulates the amount of growth necessary to effect repairs.

Before birth, cell division is the main cause of growth, although other processes also occur.

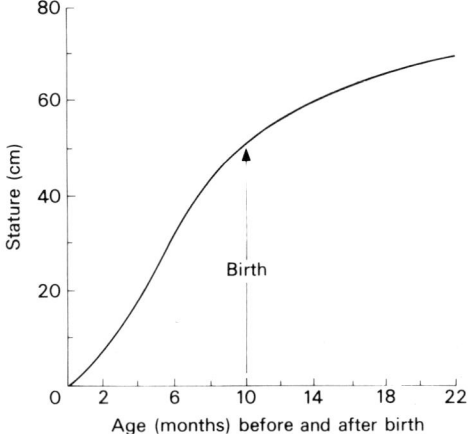

**Fig. 3.1.** Distance curve for stature before and after birth.

After birth, the emphasis shifts to the enlargement of existing cells and the laying down of intercellular matrix.

## Growth curves

The total amount of growth achieved depends upon the time for which growth proceeds, and the pace of growth per unit time. As shown in Fig. 3.1, measurements taken in a single individual at intervals when plotted against time provide a 'progress report'. This is termed a distance curve, since any point on it indicates the distance along which the body has travelled towards maturity. Alternatively, the increments of growth may be plotted against time (Fig. 3.2): this is termed a velocity curve.

In the initial stages of growth after fertilization, cell division proceeds in a geometrical pro-

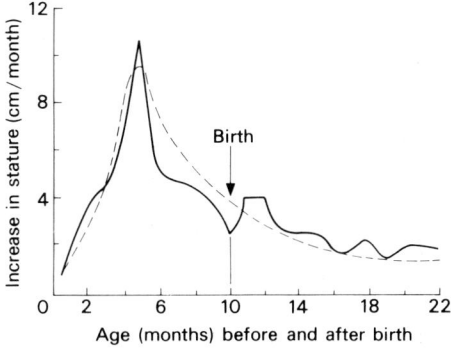

**Fig. 3.2.** Velocity curve for stature before and after birth: –, actual monthly increment; -----, smoothed curve.

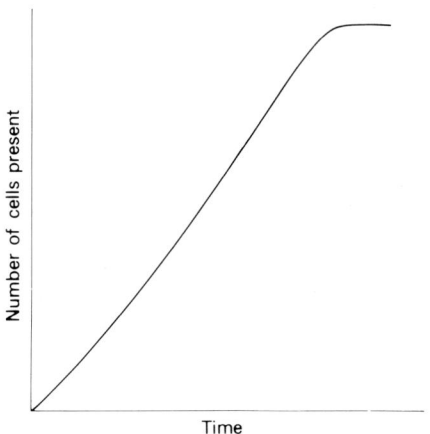

**Fig. 3.3.** Curve of logistic growth.

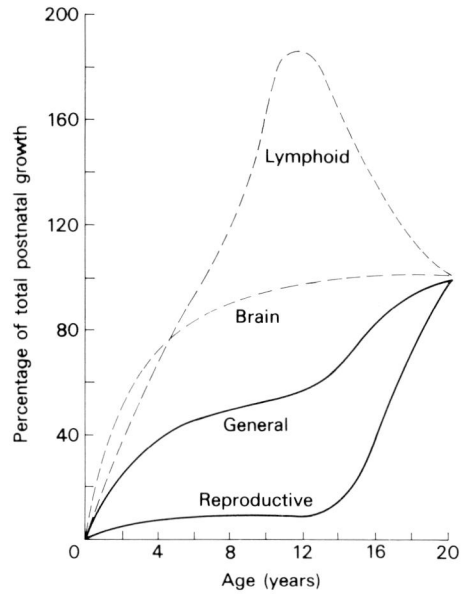

**Fig. 3.5.** Postnatal growth curve for different tissues of the body.

gression. Growth, however, slows down gradually as the adult condition is approached. Thus, growth from ovum to adult is described by a sigmoid curve (Fig. 3.3). This is termed a logistic curve and is described by:

$$W = \frac{a}{1 + be^{-kt}}$$

Where W = weight, t = time and a, b and k are constants. Alternatively, by changing the parameters of weight against time, a whole series of different growth curves may be derived (Fig. 3.4). Furthermore, the growth curves vary according to the actual tissue examined (Fig. 3.5).

## Growth in height

The human ovum measures approximately 100 $\mu$m in diameter; at birth a baby is about 50 cm long whereas an adult may be 175 cm tall. Thus, growth in height is not uniform throughout life, the maximum rate of growth occurring before birth (Fig. 3.2). Body height, however, as with many

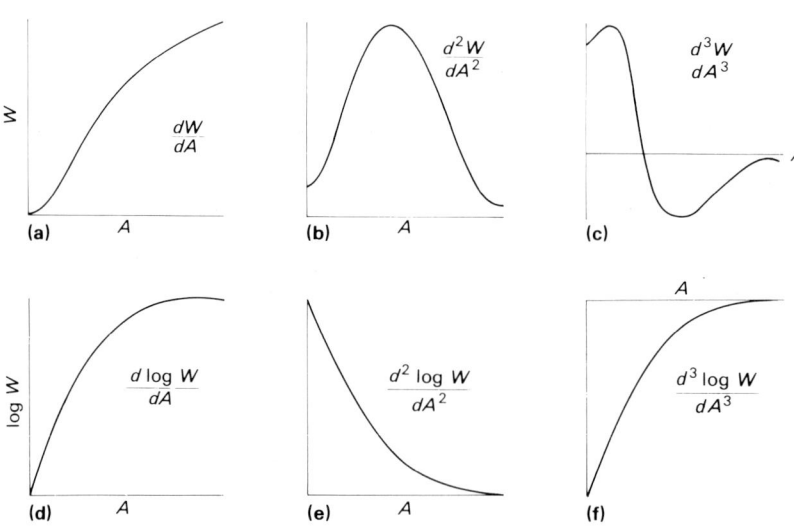

**Fig. 3.4.** Different methods of describing growth: (a) distance curve; (b) velocity curve; (c) acceleration curve; (d) curve for specific growth; (e) velocity curve for specific growth; (f) acceleration curve for specific growth. W, weight; A, time.

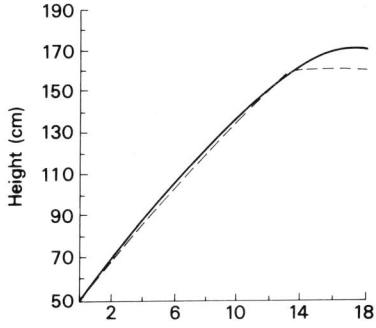
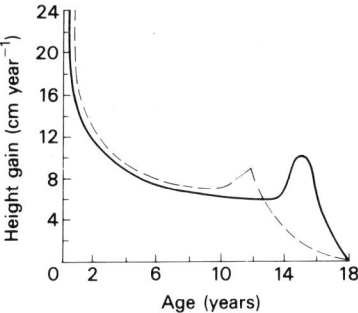

Fig. 3.6. Height and height gain per year from a cross-sectional study of Birmingham boys (solid line) and girls (broken line).

other biological parameters, is not easy to measure accurately. For instance, stature depends to a certain extent on the width of the intervertebral discs, which become compressed on standing, leading to a reduction of stature. (This compression may be up to 2 cm). Stature also depends on the degree of tension in the postural muscles, which may again vary with the time of day.

In the first year after birth, body length increases by about 50%: thereafter the annual increment decreases throughout youth, with the exception of the adolescent spurt. The adolescent spurt begins at about 10–11 years in girls and 12–13 years in boys, and in both sexes lasts approximately 2 years. (Fig. 3.6). After the conclusion of the spurt, there is a marked slowing of growth; girls reach 98% of their final height by the average of 16 years, whereas boys reach the same stage by 17 years. Up to the time of adolescence, there is little difference in the average heights of boys and girls, whereas by the age of 14 years, the 'balance' is redressed.

Even after the adolescent spurt, growth may continue in some tissues and organs. For instance, the vertebral column continues to lengthen until 30 years of age, and most skull dimensions until 60 years. These minor growth changes, however, are negligible compared with the adolescent spurt.

**Growth in weight**

At birth, a baby weighs approximately 3.4 kg, which is three thousand million times the weight of the ovum. Unlike growth in stature, the most rapid increase in weight occurs soon after birth. The rate very quickly decreases and in the ensuing 20 years, the birth weight increases by some 20 times.

Weight at birth is more variable than stature, and reflects the maternal environment more than the child's genotype. Small mothers tend to have small babies irrespective of the size of the father, and mothers of low socioeconomic groups have smaller babies than those from higher ratings. The rank of the child in the family is a factor affecting birth weight, with later children being somewhat heavier than the first born. Immediately after birth, the diminished intake of fluid leads to a transient 5% loss of birth weight, although this loss is made good within 10 days.

By the end of the first year, the birth weight has tripled, and by the end of the second it has quadrupled, subsequently settling down to a relatively steady annual increase (Fig. 3.7) until the adolescent spurt. The adolescent spurt in body weight lags behind that for height by approximately 3 months. Similarly, body weight does not achieve adult value until after stature has attained adult proportions.

**Later stages of human growth**

A special feature of human and other primate growth is the adolescent (pubertal) growth spurt, during which the rate of growth suddenly increases, later falling to zero when maturity is reached. The mechanism for timing this growth spurt is unknown: its effects may be caused by an interaction between the pituitary and hypothalamus which results from some unknown genetic trigger. Not only do individuals, but also certain organs and tissues, differ markedly in their response to the adolescent growth spurt. Consequently, for a given chronological age the organs and tissues of different individuals may show widely different degrees of maturity. For this reason, a number of other 'ages' of maturity have been devised.

SKELETAL AGE (MATURITY)

Each bone (at least the bony tissue of which it is composed) begins as a primary centre of ossifica-

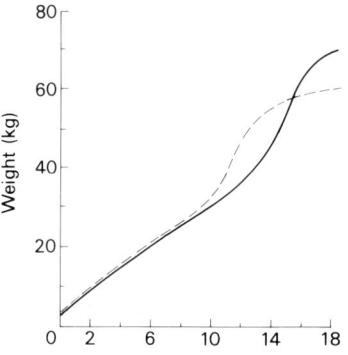

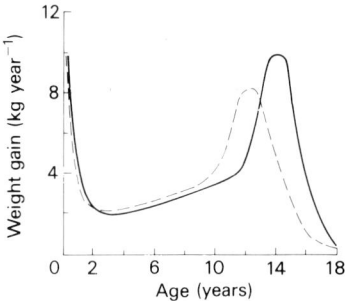

**Fig. 3.7.** Weight and weight gain per year from a cross-sectional study of Birmingham boys (solid line) and girls (broken line).

tion. It then passes through the stage of enlargement and shaping of the ossified area, acquires perhaps one or more epiphyses, and with further enlargement and shaping finally reaches its adult form with epiphyseal fusion. The sequence of events in each bone is essentially the same in all individuals, regardless of whether the stage of development of the bone (skeletal age) is advanced or retarded in relation to chronological age. Although the chronological age at which centres of ossification appear is subject to variation, skeletal age can be assessed by studying radiographs; either from the number of ossification centres present or the stage of their development.

The assessment of skeletal age is made by comparing a radiograph with a set of standards, often in the form of an atlas. In this 'atlas' method, the given radiograph is matched against skeletal standards of successive chronological ages and the standard with which the given radiograph coincides represents the skeletal age.

Whether in the form of an atlas or statistical table, different skeletal standards are provided for males and females, and for different socioeconomic and ethnic groups because different groups mature at different chronological ages. For example, during the first decade, females are more skeletally advanced than boys, possibly because genetic factors on the Y-chromosome retard skeletal development in males. Various other factors affect skeletal age, including physique (ecto-, endo-, and mesomorph, Fig. 11.29), and malnutrition. Generally environmental influences seem to have a greater effect than genetic factors.

### DENTAL AGE (MATURITY)

The eruption or noneruption of each tooth can be used to assess the dental maturity of an individual. There is controversy, however, as to whether the time when a tooth first penetrates the oral mucosa or when it achieves its occlusal location should be used as the criterion of assessment.

The deciduous dentition erupts between 6 months and $2\frac{1}{2}$ years of age. There is no evidence of significant sexual dimorphism in the eruption times of the deciduous dentition.

Surprisingly, the state of eruption of the deciduous dentition does not appear to be closely correlated with height or skeletal age nor to be affected by socioeconomic factors. Studies of twins and siblings indicate that the eruption sequence is predominantly controlled by genetic factors which differ from those controlling height and skeletal age both of which are strongly influenced by environmental effects.

The deciduous teeth tend to be lost earlier in females than males. Also, the mandibular teeth are generally exfoliated, on average, 8 to 9 months earlier than those of the maxilla.

Permanent tooth eruption provides a criterion of maturity spanning 6 to 13 years of age. Several attempts have been made to construct a scale of dental age which is based on tooth eruption times. One method is based on the average number of teeth erupted at a certain age. Tooth eruption, however, is a crude criterion for the assessment of total maturity, although it can be made more accurate in combination with radiographs of root development.

### MORPHOLOGICAL AGE (MATURITY)

Although a 'stature developmental age' (maturity) can easily be obtained by finding the age at which a given child's stature equals the height of the average child, the measure has limited application since it confounds maturity with size.

In contrast, the concept of 'shape age' is more subtle. The proportions of the body gradually change into those of the adult and this change in

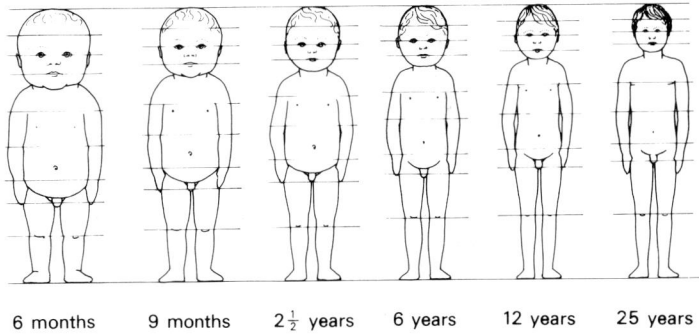

6 months  9 months  2½ years  6 years  12 years  25 years

**Fig. 3.8.** Change in body proportions during growth.

proportion provides an index of maturity (Fig. 3.8). The difficulty, however, lies in recognizing important shapes and then defining the measurements which will take into account changes in these shapes.

SECONDARY SEX CHARACTERS

This form of assessment is based on the stages of maturation in genital, pubic hair and breast development. The sequence in which secondary sex characters develop in males is much less variable than the chronological age at which such events occur. Five stages of genital, pubic hair and breast development have been outlined for boys and girls, although such stages are not discretely separated since secondary sex character development is a continuous process. Nevertheless, this form of assessment is of great value in the prediction of adult height in males and females, although it has yet to be exploited from a dental point of view (e.g. forecasting the size to which a lower jaw might later grow).

RELATIONSHIP BETWEEN DIFFERENT MEASURES OF AGE

There are a number of measures which can be used to quantify the age of an individual although only a few of the more obvious have been indicated here. During adolescence, there is a close correlation between skeletal age and the age at which the secondary sex characters appear; there is also a close correlation between the time at which secondary sex characters appear and the height spurt. By contrast, there is relatively little information for the preadolescent period. Information is particularly lacking on the degree of correlation between dental and skeletal age within any single chronological age group.

Height and skeletal age are not well correlated either with each other or with dental age. Nevertheless, people who have advanced dental development (particularly of the canines) in the immediate preadolescent years generally have an early height spurt, early menarche, early closure of the tibial epiphyses and early growth of pubic hair.

PREDICTION OF ADULT SIZE

Adult size is not necessarily predictable from an early age. The final size achieved, and the speed with which it is reached are essentially independent, although it has long been known that children with an early puberty are taller and heavier than late maturers. The rate at which a child grows is usually very regular so that it is possible to predict adult size from about 2 years of age onwards with increasing accuracy, although predictions may be inaccurate due to the variable age at which puberty may be reached. Forecasts based on the size reached for a given maturity are less accurate than those for chronological age.

In the field of dentistry, the most important prediction is that of the future facial shape, which is the resultant of growth and size in several component regions. Growth does not proceed evenly, and certain facial dimensions demonstrate marked changes in their growth rates. It is these 'spurts' that render predictions very difficult. Most predictive methods presume that the vectors of growth present at the time of prediction will remain: there is much evidence that this is untrue; for instance, mandibular growth is predominantly vertical for a time, yet inexplicably it later changes to become predominantly horizontal.

**Factors affecting growth**

The earlier the adolescent growth spurt, the more intense is its vigour, with the result that a larger adult form is produced in a shorter period of time. This relationship is not confined to stature, but also occurs in other skeletal dimensions, although whether it reflects genetic or hormonal factors, or the reactivity to hormonal factors, has yet to be elucidated.

Early maturers are not only people whose growth to maturity is usually advanced at all ages, they are also people who as adults have more weight-for-height than late maturers.

RACE AND CLIMATE

Neither climate nor race influence the timing of puberty as greatly as nutrition. However, climate seems to have a minor effect on overall growth rates.

The one racial difference that is now firmly established is the fact that skeletal maturity is more advanced in very young negroes than caucasians, and this may be associated with advancement of motor behaviour. A similar advanced maturity is apparent in the deciduous dentition and continues into the permanent dentition, despite the fact that by the time the latter erupt, the skeletal maturity of negroes has fallen behind.

HORMONES

Sexual dimorphism is only minor up to puberty, whereas during the adolescent period marked sexual differences appear in morphology, chemistry and performance due mainly to a changing pattern of hormonal secretion. The increased elongation rates of bones at puberty reflect the responses of epiphyseal cartilages to increased levels of circulating hormones. All epiphyseal plates respond to the same hormones, although they differ in the degree of their response, even within the same bone. Thus it is not only the secretion of hormones that is important in inducing pubertal changes, but also the reactivity of the target regions themselves.

The predominant hormones which influence growth are growth hormone, thyroid hormone, and androgenic and oestrogenic hormones from the ovary, testes and adrenal glands. These secretions are under the supreme control of the trophic hormones of the anterior pituitary.

Growth hormone is essential for normal childhood growth. Children with growth hormone deficiency fail to grow adequately and following the administration of growth hormone will have slightly increased growth. Excessive growth hormone production by a pituitary tumour results in gigantism if it occurs before epiphyseal fusion is completed.

Growth hormone stimulates protein synthesis.

It appears that growth hormone acts mainly through the production of a second substance. Serum for normal individuals contains a growth hormone-dependent substance (sulphation factor) which stimulates sulphate uptake by hypophysectomized rat cartilages *in vitro*, and it has been suggested that before growth hormone can exert some of its metabolic effects, it must first be converted to or initiate the formation of somatomedin, which probably occurs in the liver.

The effect of thyroid hormone on growth and maturation can be shown when it is given to infants and children with hypothyroidism. Accelerated growth and skeletal maturity often occur in the child and adolescent with hyperthyroidism.

In the normal prepubertal child, the influence of endogenous adrenocortical stimulating hormone (ACTH) and adrenal corticosteroids on growth is probably meagre: this can be deduced from the fact that in children with Addison's disease the growth patterns and skeletal age are normal before and after treatment with physiologic doses of corticosteroids. By contrast, growth is curtailed in children who receive daily pharmacologic doses of corticosteroids or their analogues. The growth retarding effect of corticosteroids appears to be related both to the suppression of growth hormone release and to the inhibition of the peripheral effects of growth hormone.

The onset of puberty is usually determined by the appearance of secondary sex characters, and is attributed to the effects of gonadal steroids. In females, the development of secondary sex characters results from both oestrogen and adrenal androgen. In both sexes, androgen produced from the adrenals is responsible for the growth of sexual hair and for the acceleration of growth and muscular development during adolescence (it is also related to the conditions of seborrhoea and acne). Children with virilizing adrenal hyperplasia, or with true sexual precocity, become exceedingly advanced in both growth and epiphyseal development. Testosterone accelerates both epiphyseal ossification and fusion.

SEASON OF THE YEAR

Growth in height is fastest in the spring and growth in weight is fastest in the autumn. These phenomena occur at all ages including adolescence.

GENETIC FACTORS

Birth measurements reflect almost entirely the action of the uterine environment, which itself depends only upon maternal factors, therefore the specific genotype of the child is largely unexpressed at this stage. At birth, only a proportion of all the genes influencing growth and development are active. Subsequently the child's genotype exerts a greater and greater effect and the resemblance to the adult status of the parents becomes increasingly marked. Obviously the height of a child results from both genetic and environmental forces interacting one with another, but it is difficult to identify the relative importance of each.

Sexual dimorphism in body size is obviously dependent upon genetic factors. There is evidence, however, that the mode of control is polygenic rather than Mendelian in nature.

Malnutrition during childhood delays growth, although man has great recuperative powers provided the adverse conditions are not carried too far or for too long. Severe malnutrition prolonged throughout a large part of the growth period, however, may cause some permanent stunting, but even under these conditions, the powers of recuperation are considerable. Furthermore, there is little evidence that malnutrition affects body shape as well as size.

ILLNESS

Most information about the effects of minor illness on the growth rate is conflicting. By contrast, both growth and maturation may slow down during major illness and stress, the degree depending upon the severity of the disease. The actual mechanisms whereby growth is slowed down probably vary from one disease to another, although a general factor in many disorders may be an increase in cortisone or a decrease in growth hormone secretion.

SOCIOECONOMIC CLASS

The growth rate of children from higher socioeconomic groups exceeds that of lower groups. Interestingly, there is also evidence that socioeconomic grouping is related to the maturity of the permanent dentition. The causes of this difference are probably multiple, although they are more closely related to home conditions than the strictly economic status of the families.

Body size is also related to social class, but whether this reflects genetic or environmental factors remains controversial. Nevertheless, variation in height and weight between different socioeconomic groups often exceeds that between different ethnic groups; an important fact to bear in mind when trying to predict future growth changes.

## SKULL AND JAWS

If a structure maintains the same proportions as it grows, the growth is said to be gnomonic (Fig. 3.9a–c). The alternative, that the growing structure changes its shape, is referred to as allometric growth (Fig. 3.9d–f). From a comparison of the shapes of a neonatal and adult human skull it is clear that allometric growth is

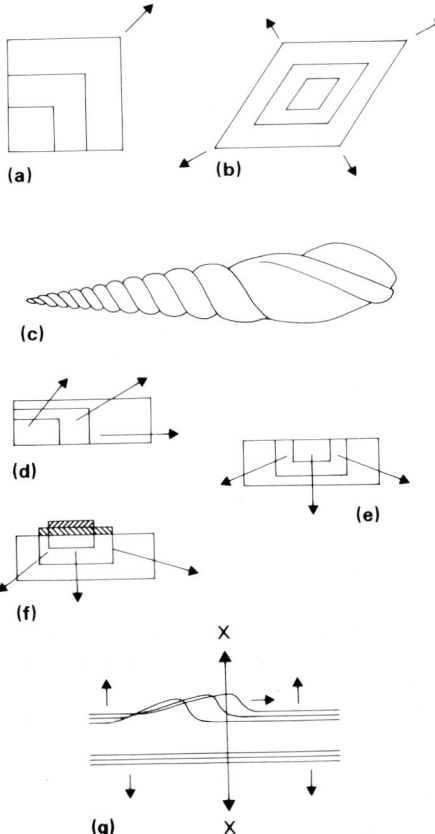

**Fig. 3.9.** (a), (b), (c) Gnomonic growth describes the fact that the shape of a structure does not change while it grows; (d), (e), (f), during allometric growth shape changes. Measurement of shape at different stages cannot help understand how a structure grows. Such measurements would be the same for (d), (e) and (f) but they grow in entirely different ways (parts of (f) are resorbed). (g): as a bone thickens, a prominence on one surface becomes relocated to the right. A section through XX would suggest that the bone is thickening on one side at three times the rate on the other side.

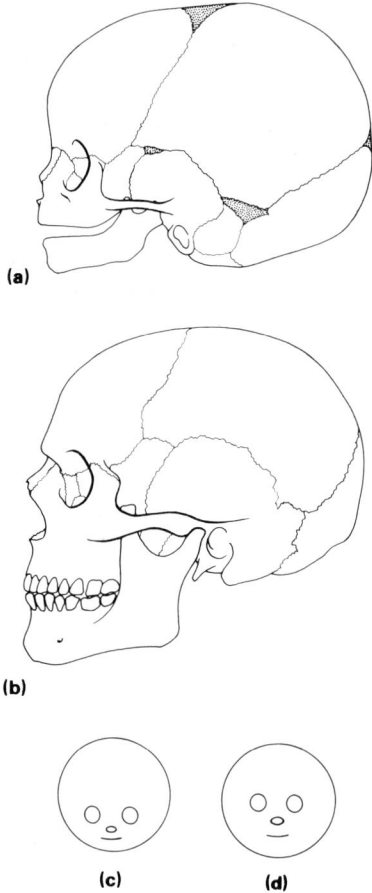

**Fig. 3.10.** Neonatal and adult skulls drawn to the same size and showing that different parts of the skull grow differently. (c), (d) Which is the child?

involved (Fig. 3.10a, b). The most glaring change in shape can be recognized by studying the cartoons in Fig. 3.10c, d. It is clear that Fig. 3.10c is the baby because subconsciously we are aware that babies have a cranium whose size is about eight times that of their face while in adults the cranio/facial volume ratio is about 1:1. This change in ratio is related to the disproportionate increase in the height of the face and suggests that the growth of the face is under a different control from the growth of the cranium.

In order to understand how growth may be controlled measurements are required and should be made with respect to a fixed reference point. For example, the shapes and sizes of the three boxes in each of Figs. 3.9d–f can be accurately measured and shown to be the same. These measurements would not be very helpful, however, because they would not indicate that each grows in an entirely different way. It is the absence of any fixed point in the growing skull which confuses all analyses: everything is moving in relation to everything else. Several techniques need to be combined in order to discover the ways in which the skull grows.

## Measuring growth

### RADIOGRAPHS

With the patient rigidly 'clamped' in a standard position, lateral skull radiographs are taken at different ages (the clamp is called a craniostat). Subsequently, tracings of the X-rays are superimposed on each other and measurements indicate growth changes. Typical reference points, planes and angles are described at the end of this section but all are arbitrarily chosen for their value in primatology, orthodontics or growth studies.

### EMBEDDED MARKERS

A. Björk pioneered the technique of embedding tiny metal markers in the jaws of growing children. These markers remained in the position and were visible on radiographs. Two radiographs of a child at different ages can be correctly superimposed using the images of the metal markers (see Fig. 3.18).

### TETRACYCLINE

Many useful antibiotics belong to the tetracycline group. These are absorbed into the bloodstream and it was accidentally discovered that they are deposited with mineralising tissues, where they become fixed. For this reason it would probably be difficult to find a tooth in any person under about 20 years of age which did not contain a tetracyline line formed during the time he was being treated with one of these very common antibiotics. The lines can only be seen if a sectioned tooth is studied under ultraviolet light, when they fluoresce brightly if the wavelength of the light is appropriate.

Tetracycline lines may be difficult to analyse unless a whole bone is reconstructed from serial sections. For example, a section in plane XX (Fig. 3.9g) would suggest that the bone is thickening on one side at three times the rate it is thickening on the other side. In fact, both surfaces are thickening at the same rate. The erroneous interpretation would have been due to the fact that a bony prominence is being progressively relocated further to the right.

HISTOLOGY

Demineralized and stained sections show evidence of bone deposition (osteoblasts) and bone resorption (osteoclasts). By reconstructing data from serial sections it is possible to deduce the overall pattern of growth (cf. tetracycline lines).

EXPERIMENTAL

Many experiments have been designed to discover how different regions contribute to growth of the skull. For example, if both condylar cartilages are removed from a growing rat there is little subsequent change in the proportions of the fully developed mandible. It can be concluded that, for growth of the rat mandible, the condylar cartilages are of minor importance.

In a different technique the condylar cartilage is removed and cultured in, for example, the brain. In this site the cartilage has very little capacity for growth. However, epiphyseal cartilage from a long bone continues to grow vigorously when transplanted. This result again suggests that, unlike epiphyseal cartilages, the condylar cartilages are not particularly important growth regions.

Any new treatment designed to correct a human facial irregularity is experimental. It must be true to say that all orthodontic procedures have originally relied on treating patients as the subjects of 'experiments'. Many treatments have been unsuccessful but there remain innumerable successful techniques filtered by the processes of trial and error. The fact that a force produced by a particular procedure effectively restores a harmonious facial contour suggests that in the abnormal condition there exists an opposite 'distorting' growth force or restraint.

**The growth of bone**

All growth is subject to restraint. For example, the weight of the body is transmitted through the epiphyseal cartilages of the leg bones and in order to increase the length of the tibia by 1 mm, the whole of the body from the femur upwards must be pushed up 1 mm. For this reason it seems clear that growing cartilage exerts a growth force. Indeed, without the existence of cartilage it is difficult to visualize how a weight-supporting bone could grow. Bone cannot grow interstitially: it can only grow at its ends. Therefore without the epiphyseal cartilages the long bones could only lengthen by means of osteoblastic activity on their articular surfaces and such fragile cells could not possibly support the weight of the body. Sometimes the forces restraining growth are minimal, such as in the skin. But even here the basal cells of the epidermis, its growing region, must push the remaining cell layers outwards.

In summary, to understand the growth of the skull it is necessary to visualize the forces which produce growth and the restraints which must be overcome. The rate of growth is proportional to the difference between growth force and restraint. In order to produce growth the genes can only operate through an intermediate creation which generates force.

METHODS OF BONE GROWTH

*Cartilage*
The growth of endochondral bones is described elsewhere (Book 1). Two varieties of cartilage exist; primary and secondary (Book 1). At birth the spheno-occipital synchondrosis (Figs. 3.11a, 3.13) and the nasal septum are almost all that remain of the primary cartilaginous skeleton of the skull. Secondary cartilages are growing in the mandibular condyle and at the mandibular symphysis (Fig. 3.11b). When transplanted and cultured in a different region none of these cartilages grow well, which suggests that none produces a growth force comparable to that of epiphyseal cartilages (which grow vigorously in culture).

*Subperiosteal deposition*
Apart from their articular surfaces, the outer surfaces of all bones are covered by periosteum which is a two-layered structure. The outer surface of fibrous tissue covers an inner osteogenic layer from which osteoblasts are derived (Fig. 3.11c). Although subperiosteal bone deposition is obviously important to skull growth the fact that many regions, such as the facial surface of the maxilla, are constantly being resorbed indicates that other growth forces are necessary.

*Sutures*
The many sutures present in the skull seem to indicate their importance in skull growth. In terms of histological structure, where two bones meet at a suture the two periosteal layers continue round the edge of each bone, in the skull the osteogenic layer being called the cambial layer and the fibrous layer being called the capsular layer (Fig. 3.11d). The two capsular layers are joined by a uniting layer.

If a suture, together with the bone on either side,

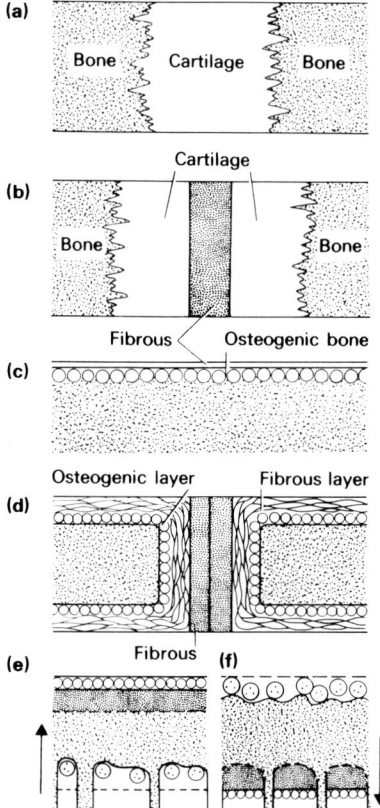

**Fig. 3.11.** Diagrammatic representation of (a) synchondrosis; (b) symphysis; (c) periosteum; (d) suture. (e) Bone deposited under the periosteum is compensated by removal of bone from the endosteum (and vice versa, f).

is dissected from a growing skull and cultured in a different site it shows very little capacity for growth. This particular experiment suggests that sutures are not sites of primary growth. That is, sutures do not provide a growth force but are themselves subjected to a growth force from elsewhere. For example, it is now widely believed that the growing brain pushes the calvarial bones outwards thereby tensing and potentially widening the associated sutures which respond by depositing bone. Sutural growth is a response to the expansion of a growing internal organ or region: the sutures provide a force which resists but allows the brain to grow.

*Functional matrices*
It is easy to visualize that the growing eye and brain are probably responsible for causing growth at the sutures between the bones which surround them. The concept of functional matrices extends this idea to account for the growth of other bones.

The head contains regions responsible in part or in whole for the functions of digestion, respiration, vision, neural integration and so on. The part of the skull responsible for each function is known as a functional cranial component. Each functional cranial component consists of the soft tissues and spaces which undertake the function, the functional matrix; the skeletal tissues which support and/or protect the soft tissues are together known as the skeletal unit. The size and shape of the skeletal unit are the result of scleroblast (osteoblast, chondroblast) and osteoclast activity but the coordination of this cellular activity is not under direct genetic control. The growth of the skeletal unit is controlled by its associated functional matrix which itself grows in response to the requirements of the function it undertakes.

There are two types of functional matrix: periosteal and capsular. Periosteal matrices are exemplified by muscle attachments to bone, and capsular matrices by their contained functional spaces, such as the mouth, or functional organs, such as the eye.

The only contentious part of this hypothesis seems to relate to the implication that a functional space such as the nasal cavity, mouth or pharynx can, merely by functioning as a space, in some way induce its capsular matrix to force bones apart. Unfortunately it is the growth of the bones surrounding these cavities, the facial bones, which are the most difficult to analyze and understand.

*Remodelling*
The shapes of all the skull bones are changed as they grow but these changes are not solely due to growth. Equally radical changes in shape are produced by resorption. The combination of growth in some regions and resorption in others is known as remodelling (e.g. Fig. 3.9g). Remodelling describes how the shape of a bony contour may be changed but it is not an explanation of the change.

It might seem that the subperiosteal deposition of (compact) bone would thicken the cortex of the bone. However, where bone is deposited subperiosteally it is removed from the endosteum by osteoclasts and vice versa (Fig. 3.11e, f).

The internal arrangement of trabeculae in bone is said to be organized in response to the forces which need to be withstood. The trabeculae are constantly being remodelled in response to small changes in these forces.

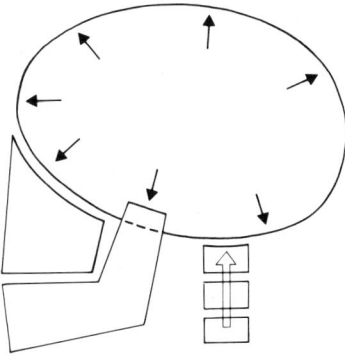

Fig. 3.12. The neurocranium is supported on the vertebral column. The maxilla is carried on the anterior end of the neurocranium, the mandible on the middle of the neurocranium. Growth of the neurocranium carries them apart.

## The influence of the brain and eye

The neurocranium is articulated with the remainder of the body by means of the atlanto-occipital joints and the face is joined to the neurocranium at the anterior half of the cranial base (Fig. 3.12). In order to understand the growth of the face it is first necessary to describe the growth of the bony neurocranium because the upper face and the mandible are each attached to different parts of the shifting, sliding, cranial base.

### GROWTH OF THE NEUROCRANIUM

At birth the spheno-occipital synchondrosis, a remnant of the primary cartilaginous base of the skull, separates the sphenoid and occipital bones (Fig. 3.13). The only other remaining cartilage lies in the midline floor of the anterior cranial fossa and will ultimately be ossified to become the cribriform plate of the ethmoid during the 3rd year of life (Fig. 3.14). The spheno-occipital synchondrosis is obliterated in about the 15th year. Experimental data (see above) suggest that neither of these cartilages provides a significant growth force. Together with the sutures between the frontal, sphenoid, petrous temporal and occipital bones, they may form new bone in response to tensional forces generated by the growing brain. In the same way the calvaria is induced to grow at the sutures between the frontal, parietal, sphenoid, temporal, and occipital bones. Sutural growth continues up until about the end of the first decade by which time the cranium is almost its adult size. Subsequently the bones are thickened

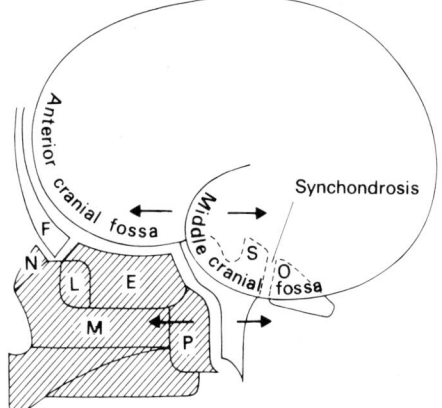

Fig. 3.13. Most of the upper face is carried by the floor of the anterior cranial fossa. Only the back of the vomer and the pterygoid plates are supported by the sphenoid bone in the floor of the middle cranial fossa. (F, frontal; S, sphenoid; O, occipital; L, lacrimal; E, ethmoid; M, maxilla; P, palatine). Shaded region is the upper face. Due to growth of the frontal lobes of the brain the middle cranial fossa (and pterygoid plates) is carried back with respect to the anterior cranial fossa.

on both surfaces indicating that the cranial cavity, but not necessarily the brain, is reduced in size.

The upper face (Fig. 3.13) is almost entirely carried by the floor of the anterior cranial fossa (the frontals, cribriform plate of the ethmoid, and lesser wings of the sphenoid). Only a very small part consisting of the back of the midline vomer and the pterygoid plates surrounding the upper part of the pharynx are carried by the body of the sphenoid which forms the mid-line base of the middle cranial fossa. Therefore, growth of the frontal lobes, expanding the cranial base, carries the upper face forwards and potentially separates the maxilla (lying below the anterior cranial fossa)

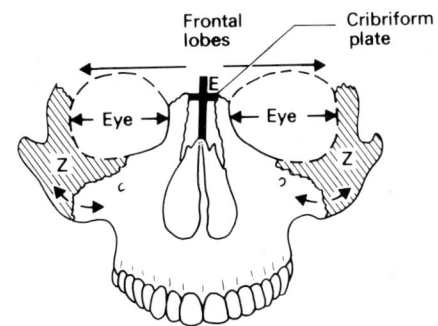

Fig. 3.14. Growth of the frontal lobes and eyes pushes the zygomatic bones apart thereby widening the upper face. The ethmoid (and frontal) bone acts as a strut.

from the pterygoid plates (lying below the middle cranial fossa). This potential separation is compensated by a continuous growth at the back of the maxilla, the region in which the permanent molar teeth are developing, growing and erupting in sequence.

The mandible is carried on the temporal bone which forms part of the floor of the middle cranial fossa (Fig. 3.12). Therefore the maxilla is being carried forward in relation to the mandible. The middle cranial fossa is also widening, in response to the growing brain, with the result that the mandibular condyles are carried apart.

GROWTH OF THE EYE

Not only is the brain lengthening but it is also widening. Furthermore, the eyes are growing but are prevented from expanding medially by struts, the frontal and ethmoid bones, with the result that the zygomatic bone is carried outwards, the zygomatico-maxillary suture is tensioned, bone is developed, and the zygomatic and maxillary bones widen (Fig. 3.14). The maxilla is largely separated from the anterior cranial fossa by the ethmoid and lacrimal bones although it does articulate by its frontal process with the frontal bone. Growth of the eye pushes the maxilla downwards away from the cranial base with the

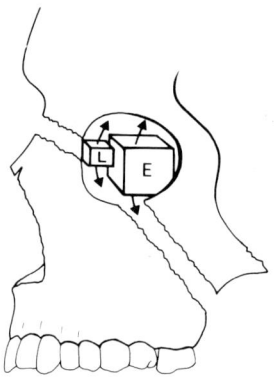

**Fig. 3.15.** Growth of the eye thrusts the maxilla downwards and forwards thereby tensioning the sutures around the lacrimal (L) and ethmoid (E) bones.

result that the ethmoid and lacrimal bones medially, and the zygomatic bone laterally grow vertically in response to tension at their sutural surfaces (Fig. 3.15). This sutural growth is most rapid during the first few years of life and it ceases by about 17 years of age.

**Growth of the maxilla**

The above growth forces displace the maxilla downwards and forwards and the maxilla grows partly due to the tensions developed at sutures in response to these forces. Other growth forces are less easy to visualize. Of these, the growing dentition is probably very important. Just as the growing brain causes the calvaria to expand, so the growing dentition could cause the maxilla to expand: resorption on the endosteal surface of the alveolar bone induces deposition on the periosteal surface.

It has often been proposed that growth of the (midline) nasal septum thrusts the maxilla downwards and forwards. However, although experimental data indicate that it may be an important growth centre in some animals, it does not seem to be true of man. Congenital absence of the septum produces very little facial deformity in children and suggests that the septum grows in response to lengthening of the face rather than that it causing the lengthening.

It is convenient to describe the growth of the maxilla in three planes.

VERTICAL

The frontal process of the maxilla lengthens by sutural growth (frontomaxillary suture) in response to tension developed due to growth of the eye (Fig. 3.16). The infraorbital nerve, just beneath the eye, is also pushed down with the result that its foramen moves little in relation to the inferior margin of the orbit but separates markedly from the frontomaxillary suture.

Beneath the orbit lies the body of the maxilla and its alveolar process. The depth of this region increases rapidly at times which correspond with the eruption of the deciduous teeth and later the permanent teeth. As each tooth erupts it 'carries with it' developing alveolar bone (Fig. 3.16).

*Palate*

The vertical growth of alveolar bone in response to tooth eruption would deepen the palate enormously were it not for the fact that bone is correspondingly deposited over the whole of the palatal surfaces of the maxilla and palatine bones. The palate deepens during growth because more bone is deposited on the alveolar margins than on the palate (Fig. 3.17). The potential thickening of the palate is compensated by resorption over the whole of its nasal surface with the result that the vertical dimension of the nasal cavity increases.

# Growth and Ageing 75

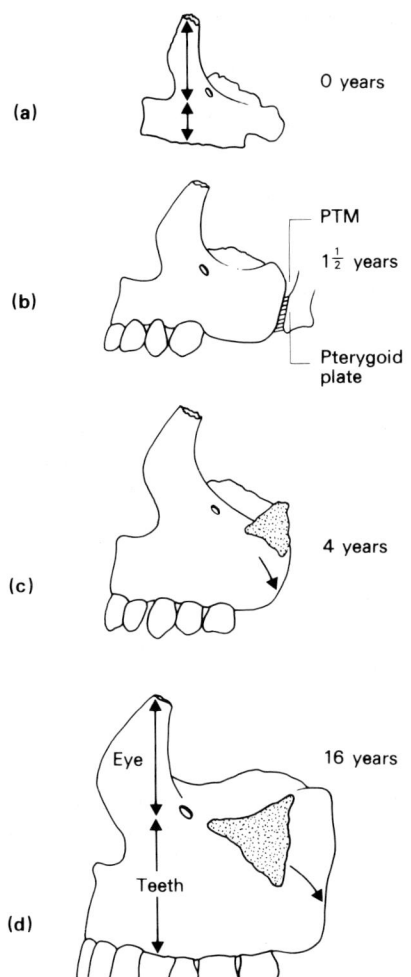

Fig. 3.16. Outlines of the maxilla at various ages (after Sicher and du Brul). PTM = pterygomaxillary fissure.

## ANTEROPOSTERIOR

The maxilla is carried forward on the floor of the anterior cranial fossa against the restraint of the muscles of facial expression; in particular, the buccinator muscle. This restraint could account for the observation that much of the facial surface of the maxilla is generally being slowly resorbed throughout the growth period. The maxilla grows or is thrust forward at a greater rate than the bone is resorbed with the result that its anterior surface appears to grow forward. Because bone cannot grow interstitially, the maxilla can only lengthen by bone formed at its posterior surface (Fig. 3.18). The maxilla has sutural connections with the horizontal plate of the palatine bone and with the part of the palatine bone which intervenes between the maxilla and the pterygoid plates (Fig. 3.13). About half the posterior surface of the maxilla is covered by soft tissue at $1\frac{1}{2}$ years (Fig. 3.16): above is the pterygomaxillary fissure and below is the tuberosity of the maxilla which contains the developing molar teeth. What is the origin of

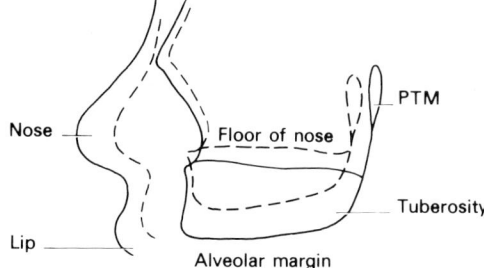

Fig. 3.18. Metal implants are used correctly to locate tracings of the upper face made from a child at two different ages. PTM = pterygomaxillary fissure (after Björk).

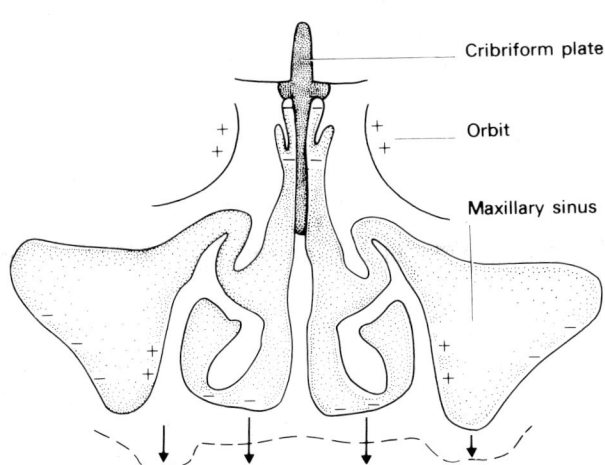

Fig. 3.17. A coronal section of the maxilla illustrating growth of the palate, nose and antrum.

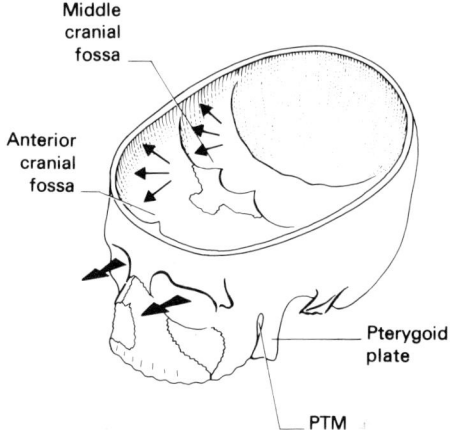

**Fig. 3.19.** Growth of the anterior cranial fossa leads to tensioning of the sutures which separate the pterygoid plates and the maxilla (after Enlow).

the force which causes the maxilla to lengthen in this region?

The maxilla is being carried forward by growth of the frontal lobe of the brain. In addition the anterior surface of the temporal lobe grows against the greater wing of the sphenoid (anterior wall of the middle cranial fossa) which carries the pterygoid plates (Fig. 3.19). Therefore the growing temporal lobe of the brain might seem to contribute to the forward thrust of the maxilla via the pterygoid plates. If this is true the sutures between the pterygoid plates and the maxilla would be compressed and there would be no sutural growth here.

In partial answer to this problem, the eye grows within the orbit and thrusts back against the greater wing of the sphenoid. This growth could separate the maxilla from the pterygoid plates, thereby tensioning the relevant sutures leading to bone formation and lengthening of the maxilla. It is also true that during growth the anterior surface of the anterior cranial fossa moves progressively further in front of the anterior surface of the middle cranial fossa. Therefore the maxilla is carried further forward than the pterygoid plates with the result that the sutures between them are tensed and the maxilla is lengthened.

The growing dentition may also provide a force leading to growth of the free surface of the tuberosity of the maxilla (Fig. 3.16, 4 years) but it seems unlikely that it could induce growth at the posteriorly adjacent sutures.

A functional matrix, in this case the oropharynx, could produce a force which tensions the relevant sutures.

WIDTH

The upper face is widening due to growth of the eye and the frontal lobes of the brain. This growth widens the upper surface of the maxilla by the development of bone in the tensioned zygomatic/maxillary suture at the inferior margin of the orbit (Fig. 3.14). The maxilla is widening posteriorly, perhaps in response to the growth and development of the molar teeth it contains. The mid-palatal suture is widening up to about 7 years of age, possibly in response to tensioning due to the growing eyes. Muscular activity and growth of the tongue may also exert a lateral thrust. Finally, resorption of the anterior surface of the maxilla also leads to an apparent widening because the narrower anterior few millimetres are being removed.

### Growth of mandible

The mandible is cradled in space by the medial pterygoid and masseter muscles (Fig. 3.20). The condyle is attached to the temporal bone by the capsular and temporomandibular ligaments. In this account it is assumed that the condylar cartilage does not normally produce a growth force but rather that as the mandible is carried away from the temporal bone the potential space is filled by new cartilage. If this view is correct, what forces carry the mandible away from the temporal bone?

The most obvious, but not necessarily correct, answer is that the mandible is firmly attached via muscles and ligaments to the hyoid bone, larynx and trachea. As the upper cervical vertebrae

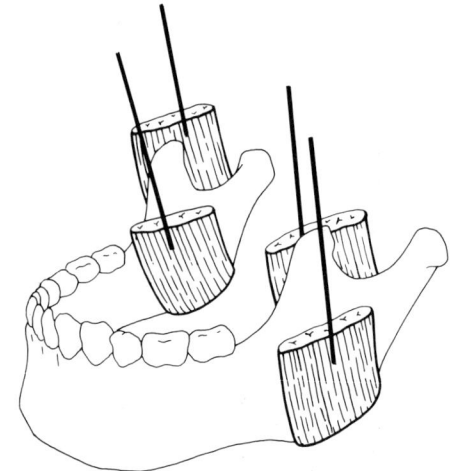

**Fig. 3.20.** The mandible is cradled by the medial pterygoid and masseter muscles.

lengthen they carry the cranium and upper face away from the mandible (Fig. 3.12). The potential space is filled by the maxilla and body of the mandible in front, and by condylar growth behind. In other words, the cranium is carried away from the mandible.

Unlike the remainder of the skull no bony restraints, with the exception of the glenoid fossa, prevent the mandible growing. It therefore seems that the shape of the mandible is partly moulded by the surrounding soft tissues restraining its growth. Because the amount and action of these restraints are impossible to predict it is easier to describe the growth of the mandible and to deduce the restraints from the pattern of growth.

CONDYLAR CARTILAGE

The pattern of mandibular growth is ideally studied by reference to the metal implant technique devised by Björk (Fig. 3.21). Such a study

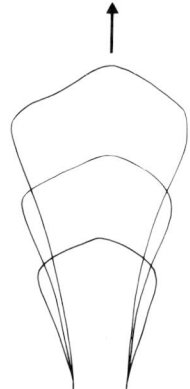

Fig. 3.22. The coronoid process grows back and is resorbed anteriorly (after Enlow).

*Histology*

The structure of the growing condylar region is shown in Fig. 3.23. Four or five cells down from the fibrous tissue covering the articular surface lies a zone of cell division, the chondrogenic layer. A few of the daughter cells contribute to the rather inactive layer of flattened cells adjacent to the fibrous tissue. Following cell division the new chondroblasts secrete the precursors of cartilage, including collagen and glycosaminoglycans, and become separated. It is notable that the chondroblasts inside the cartilage matrix do not divide nor do they become arranged in regular columns (cf. epiphyseal cartilage). Following matrix secretion, just as in epiphyseal cartilage, the chondroblasts become hypertrophied as they draw back the matrix they secreted 1 or 2 days earlier. Some of the cartilage remains and is mineralized but the majority is lost as the cartilage lacunae are broken open and the encapsulated chondrocytes are freed into the tissue spaces. The wide open spaces at the

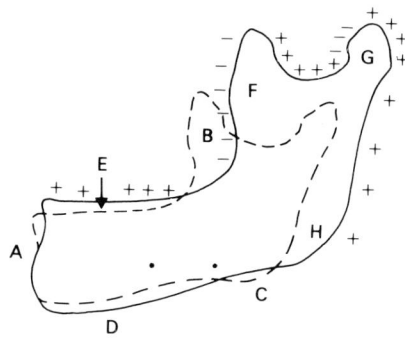

Fig. 3.21. Tracings of a mandible made from radiographs of a child at different ages and superimposed by reference to two metal implants (after Björk).

demonstrates that the condylar cartilage grows upwards and backwards. The way in which space may be created for this new tissue is described above. It is also possible that the growing tongue may thrust the mandible forwards.

It can be seen (Figs. 3.21 and 3.22) that during its backward growth bone is removed from the periosteal surfaces of the condyle which face anteriorly. In compensation, bone is laid down on the adjacent endosteal surfaces. This is an example of growth in conical regions (V-shaped) (Fig. 3.16) which is most commonly seen in the metaphysis of long bones. By endosteal deposition and periosteal resorption the cone enlarges and moves towards its wider end.

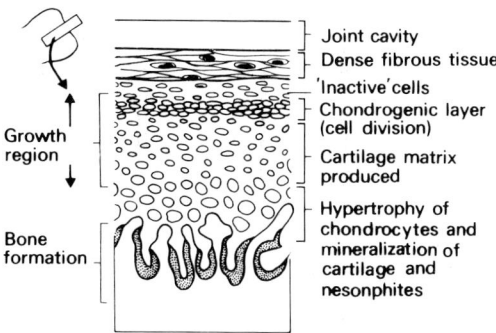

Fig. 3.23. The histology of the growing condyle of the mandible (inset shows orientation).

bony end of the cartilage contain numerous budding capillaries which bring potential osteoblasts into the region. These cells lay down bone on the surface of the mineralized cartilage. Away from this activity the mineralized cartilage and newly formed, woven bone are resorbed and replaced by fine-fibred bone.

Studies in which the newly formed cartilage cells in the chondrogenic layer are labelled indicate that it takes 5 or 6 days before the surviving chondrocytes are shed into the developing bony canals. The fate of these chondrocytes is not known.

ANTEROPOSTERIOR AND VERTICAL GROWTH (FIG. 3.21)

The ramus of the mandible lengthens by growth of the condylar cartilage and by periosteal bone formed at its posterior border. In compensation, bone is removed from the anterior surface of the condylar and coronoid processes. It can be seen that the lower anterior half of the ramus steadily becomes incorporated in the body of the mandible and is the means by which the body lengthens. The mandible is carried or thrust forwards against the lips. This restraint may account for the small amount of resorption anteriorly adjacent to the incisors.

The ramus of the mandible increases in height by growth of the condylar cartilage and by bone deposited in the base of the sigmoid notch and at the posterior border and tip of the coronoid process. A little bone is removed at the depth of the concavity beneath the lower border of the ramus. The growth of bone at the angle of the jaw leads to change in the mandibular angle from about 135° in the newborn to about 100° in the adult although the angle is very variable (Fig. 3.24).

The main increase in the depth of the body is due to the development of alveolar bone. There is little lower border growth.

WIDTH

During the 1st year of life the mandible widens anteriorly due to the formation of cartilage on each side of the mandibular symphysis (Fig. 3.11b); this cartilage is later replaced by bone. When the chondrogenic layers cease growing the remaining cartilage is replaced by bone and the two halves of the mandible are united.

The ramus of the mandible widens above due to growth of the condylar cartilages. These are following the adjacent glenoid fossae which are themselves separated by the effect of the widening brain on the bone of the middle cranial fossa.

Areas of bone formation and resorption are shown in Fig. 3.25. In histological sections

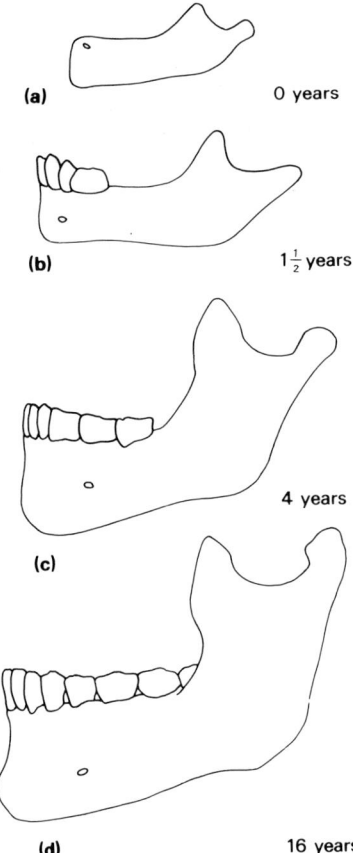

Fig. 3.24. Outlines of the growing mandible at different ages (after Sicher and du Brul).

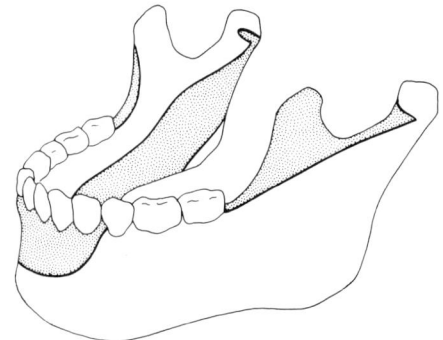

Fig. 3.25. The surfaces of the mandible are shaded to show regions where bone is resorbed. Bone is deposited in the remaining regions (but at very different rates) (after Enlow).

# Growth and Ageing

periosteal deposition is normally related to adjacent endosteal resorption and vice versa (Fig. 3.11e, f).

## ROOM FOR THE LOWER THIRD MOLARS

A radiograph of a 16-year-old adolescent may seem to indicate that there will be insufficient space to accommodate the developing third molars. Such space is created in three ways. First, mesial drift is carrying the molar teeth forwards. Second, the anterior border of the coronoid process is resorbed. Third, the alveolar bone rises up the sloping border of the coronoid process (Fig. 3.26).

## THE MENTAL FORAMEN

In the neonatal jaw the mental foramen is close to the lower border: in the adult it lies midway between upper and lower borders: in the aged and edentulous it is close to the upper border. The movement is accounted for in the following way (Fig. 3.27).

The mental nerve is angled backwards and upwards as it emerges from the mental foramen. It then passes further back before turning upwards and forwards into the lips. As bone is deposited on the buccal surface of the jaw, the foramen rises. When the teeth are lost, the alveolar bone is resorbed with the result that the mental foramen approaches the upper border.

## Nose and antrum

The height of the nose is increased in two ways. First, the growing eye tensions the frontomaxillary suture thereby deepening the upper half of the nose (Fig. 3.15). Second, with the downgrowth of the palate, the nasal surface of the palate is resorbed thereby deepening the lower half of the nose (Fig. 3.17).

The length of the nose is increased by the bone deposited behind the maxilla, at the suture be-

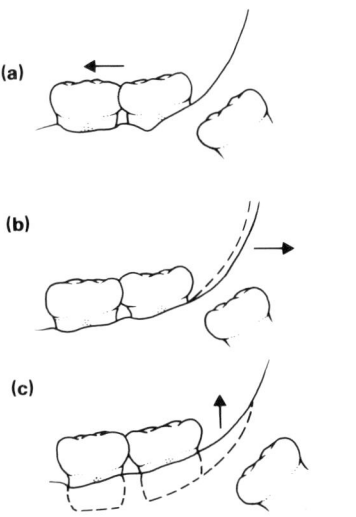

**Fig. 3.26.** Mechanisms by which space may be made available for a developing lower third molar.

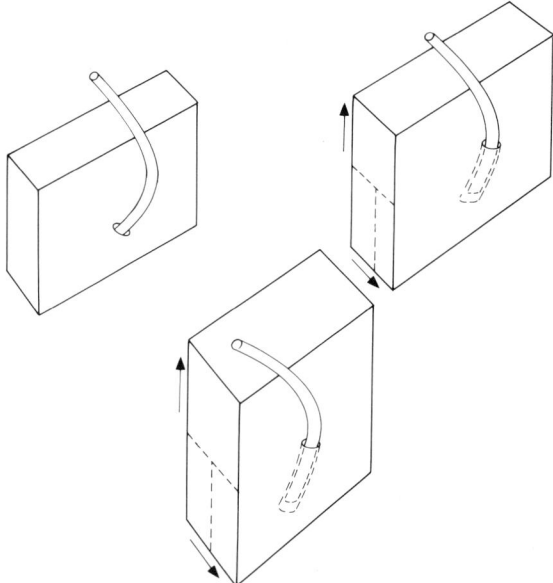

**Fig. 3.27.** The mental foramen rises up the mandible as bone is deposited on the buccal surface.

tween the horizontal plate of the palatine bone and the maxilla, and at the posterior free border of the palatine bone (Fig. 3.18). The width of the nose is increased by the growth of the eyes (Fig. 3.14).

At birth the antrum is merely a slight depression in the lateral well of the nose. By 7 years of age it has reached about half its adult size by resorbing the body of the maxilla (Fig. 3.17). The function of the antrum and the forces which control this resorption are unknown. The following unlikely suggestions have been made: the space lightens the bone; it adds resonance to the voice; the warm air inside the antrum is added to inspired air thereby raising its temperature. It is possible that the bone which would lie inside the antrum is resorbed because it does not support any load.

## Palate

The growth of the palate is described with growth of the maxilla.

## Zygomatic arch (Fig. 3.28)

The zygomatic arch is displaced backwards and outwards by remodelling as room is created for the growing temporal muscle and more support is provided for the masseter muscle. The amount of resorption beneath the anterior surface of the zygomatic bone determines the prominence of the 'cheek bone'.

## Some cephalometric markers

Some reference points used in studies of growth and of primates are shown in Fig. 3.29. They are selected either because they are usually clearly seen on lateral skull radiographs or because they facilitate analyses of development.

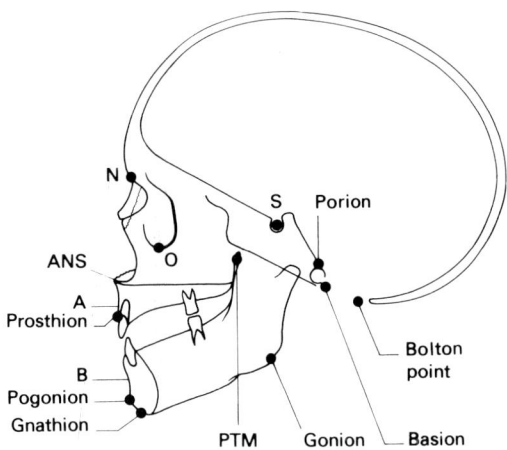

**Fig. 3.29.** Some reference points on the skull.

Some reference planes are shown in Fig. 3.30.
N (Nasion); the end of the frontonasal suture in the midline.
O (Orbitale); the most inferior point on the lower border of the left orbit.
ANS (Anterior nasal spine); the most anterior point on the floor of the nasal cavity.

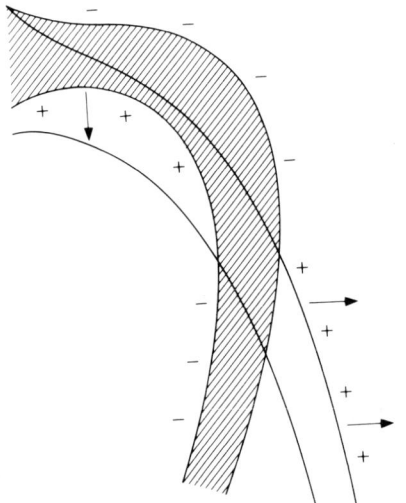

**Fig. 3.28.** Remodelling of the growing zygomatic arch of the right side seen from above.

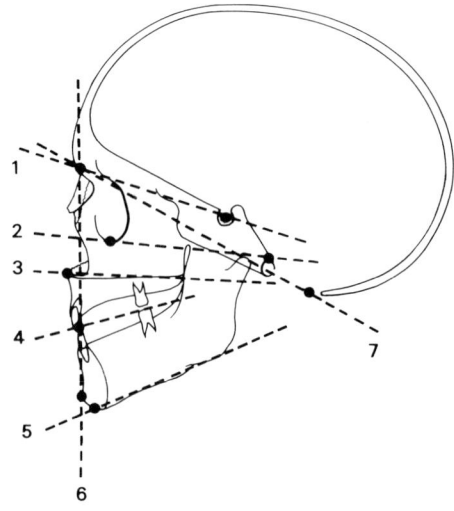

**Fig. 3.30.** Some reference planes on the skull.

A (Supraspinale); the deepest point in the concavity between ANS and prosthion.
Prosthion; the most anterior bony point between the upper incisor teeth.
B (Supramentale); the deepest point in the concavity between pogonion and the most anterior bony point between the lower incisor teeth.
Pogonion; the most anterior point on the chin.
Gnathion; the point where the anterior border of the mandible meets the lower border.
Gonion; the mandibular plane (see below) and a line tangent to the posterior border of the mandible are drawn. The angle joining these lines is bisected. Gonion is the point where this line cuts the angle of the mandible.
PTM (Pterygomaxillary fissure)
Basion; the lowest point on the anterior margin of the foramen magnum.
Bolton point; the deepest point on the notch behind the occipital condyle.
Porion; the midpoint on the upper margin of the external acoustic meatus.
S; the midpoint of sella turcica.

The following planes are drawn in Fig. 3.30.
1   Sella-nasion.
2   Frankfort plane (orbitale-porion).
3   Palatal plane: upper surface of hard palate.
4   Occlusion plane: incisive edge of the upper central incisor to the contacting surfaces of the upper and lower first molars.
5   Mandibular plane: tangent to the lower border of the mandible and passing through gnathion.
6   Facial plane: nasion to pogonion.
7   Bolton plane: Bolton point to nasion.

## AGEING

Whilst ageing can mean many things to different people it can be defined formally as the progressive loss of homeostatic efficiency that occurs at the latter end of the lifespan. Senescence is the term employed for the state reached when the loss of efficiency is fully evident; in man this is usually after the age of 65 years.

The processes of ageing and the problems they pose have only received concentrated attention, comparable to that accorded to development and growth, over the past 2 or 3 decades. Consequently many of the facts have yet to be established and answers to the questions that arise remain controversial.

Living tissues have powers of repair and, at a cellular or subcellular level, most if not all parts are gradually being replaced all the time. By impairing

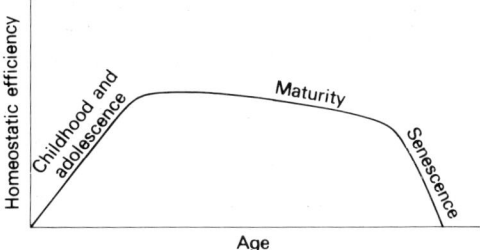

Fig. 3.31. Curve to show human life span.

these processes, disease and injury may play a part in the changes that occur in the organism with the passage of time. Nevertheless a great deal of evidence suggests that senescence is not simply due to the cumulative effect of partial recovery from environmental injury. Intrinsic age change is the term employed for the concept of change attributable to the passage of time *per se* however well the organism may be protected from its environment.

The human life span is depicted in a simple way in Fig. 3.31. Body efficiency gradually develops in childhood and adolescence until maturity is reached. After a period of little change, there is a gradual decline in powers. The time at which ageing becomes evident varies but many changes associated with, or possibly the cause of, the decline occur earlier than is generally supposed. Deteriorative changes begin in joints as early as 25–30 years and minor vascular changes similar to those of old age can be detected almost as soon. Other changes begin much later.

The view that life is finite and, apart from accident and disease, is determined by some kind of genetic clock has received support in recent years from the work of Hayflick which suggests that there is a limit to the number of times cells can mitose and that this number is related to the life span of the particular species. He found that whereas cell cultures of fibroblasts from human embryos died out after about 50 population doublings (roughly equivalent to mitoses), those from young adults seemed to be limited to about 30 doublings. Embryonic fibroblasts from short-lived species, such as chicks and mice, survived only for about 15 doublings. If cells do continue to divide after these finite periods, they do so as mutated cells which are often neoplastic if transplanted back into host animals.

Previously, attitudes towards ageing had been very much influenced by the accounts of continuous culture of cells for periods of 30 years or more. There is reason to believe that this is accounted for by the crude extracts of embryos which were part of the frequently changed media in which the cells were grown. These extracts probably contained living cells which were thus continually being added to the culture.

Some important experiments appear to be out of accord with the concept of a finite life for cells. By serial transplantation from old to young rats, skin has been kept alive for 6–7 years which is longer than twice the normal life span of the rat. This can be partially explained by the activity of chalones, hormone-like substances produced by cells which inhibit mitosis in cells of their own type. In organized tissues these substances act on the tissue population locally, but in a cell culture they would diffuse into the culture medium and be too diluted to affect the cells. It may well be that, through the activity of chalones, individual somatic cells *in vivo* never reach the limit of their capacity for cell division. In any case, *in vivo* only a few members of a cell population mitose at any one time.

Factors affecting ageing may be grouped under a number of headings:

HEREDITY

Ageing is governed to a major extent by genetic factors; human longevity can be predicted with a fair degree of accuracy from the average of the ages at death of both parents and the four grandparents of the subject. The age at death was much closer for a large number of pairs of identical twins than for a comparable group of non-identical twins and a number of dramatic examples have been reported of identical twins, living apart in widely different environments, dying within a month of each other.

DIET

Some of the earliest and most clear-cut experiments on ageing showed that, in rats raised on diets calorie-deficient but adequate in all other respects, sexual maturity was delayed but life expectancy was greatly increased. Comparable evidence in man is not available but there is evidence that an excess of calories has the reverse effect; obesity shortens life sufficiently for insurance companies to take account of it in calculating premiums.

IONIZING RADIATION

Whole body exposure of experimental animals to ionizing radiation produces changes, such as greying of hair, cataracts, chromosomal aberrations and tissue fibrosis, which mimic ageing, but the changes are not identical; for instance, although the fibrosis would lead to secondary parenchymatous changes, and therefore would produce widespread functional disorder, the fibrosis is periarteriolar and pericapillary and does not match the more diffuse connective tissue changes of senescence. Nevertheless, it has been suggested that cosmic radiation, to which all living things are exposed, might be the primary cause of ageing.

Whether the long-term survivors of atom bombs show an abnormal pattern of ageing is disputed. On the whole, although radiation in various ways may shorten life, as can many things including smoking, radiation does not seem to do so by simulating or speeding up natural ageing.

The following section gives an account of known systematic changes in the ageing process. In many ways, the tissues of the elderly differ in structure and behaviour from those of the young and, with the vastly increased proportion of the elderly, it is important to be aware of these differences so that they can be taken into account in assessing disease processes.

## Changes associated with advanced age

ORGAN ATROPHY

There is a general reduction in the weights of various organs with advancing age after maturity is reached. This applies to the brain, liver, kidney, endocrine glands and various secretory glands, including probably the salivary glands, and is associated with a decline in the numbers of parenchymatous cells or units; for example kidneys in advanced age may have lost about half their nephrons. Heart and skeletal muscle tend not to be involved in this general organ involution until a late senile stage.

VASCULAR CHANGES

The characteristic change in large arteries, usually commencing in the aorta and often as early as the end of the second decade, is atherosclerosis. The lesions consist essentially of patches of fibrosis in the intima with deposition of lipid substances, including free and esterified cholesterol. The affected areas are at first small but gradually, with advancing age, become larger, confluent and more widespread, involving the coronary and cerebral arteries and other major arteries especially those of the lower limb. The changes in the vessel walls, combined with the formation of thrombus on the luminal surfaces, may obstruct the lumen in the coronary and cerebral vessels, leading to myocardial and cerebral ischaemia or infarct. Atherosclerosis is much more common in materially prosperous, and probably overfed, societies than in simple agrarian ones or in the chronically undernourished.

Changes in the smaller arteries and in arterioles tend to begin later in life, in the 4th and 5th decades, and are different from those in the large arteries. The vessels become tortuous, less elastic and histologically the tunica media is affected. There may be an increase in elastin and calcium content in this layer.

Changes in the capillary network are very marked, probably more widespread and more closely connected with the ageing process *per se* than the foregoing. Manifestations of them can be seen in living skin and mucosa with the naked eye and, for example, in the retina with the ophthalmoscope.

On the arterial side of the capillary network, the vessels tend to become angularly tortuous in association with an increase in the density of the adventitia. In skin and mucosa, localized dilatations of the capillary bed may give rise to the spider naevi of the elderly. The venules develop saccular dilations which can be large enough to be seen with the naked eye in skin and mucosa. The sublingual varicosities which are almost universal over the age of 65 years are gross examples of these changes and of ones which occur in the capillary bed throughout the body.

NUCLEAR CHANGES

There is said to be a steady decrease in the nucleocytoplasmic ratio with advancing age. Chromosome studies in both experimental animals and man show that chromosomal aberrations tend to occur in liver cells with increasing frequency and in leukocytes, which also lose their sex chromatin.

Evidence for any general reduction of nuclear activity with advancing age, for example of cell replacement in epidermis, is inconclusive.

LIPOFUSCIN, AGEING PIGMENT

There is a small amount of evidence that catabolic products may accumulate in ageing cells, perhaps impairing their efficiency, and of changes in their enzyme activity. Most notable is the accumulation of a yellowish solution-resistant pigment, known as lipofuscin, contained within the lysosomes of the cytoplasm. Such pigment is particularly common in neurons, both of the central nervous system and of autonomic ganglia, tending to increase after the age of about 30 years in man, but it also occurs in other species. Heart muscle is another tissue in which a similar pigment accumulates with age, leading to what is known as brown atrophy. Lipofuscin, which has been called ageing pigment and does appear to represent the accumulation of unwanted products in the cell, is a complex substance. Fundamentally it is a lipoprotein and is rich in heavy metals.

The only cells in which lipofuscin has been described are fixed postmitotic cells; that is ones which, having differentiated, never mitose. Neurones, cardiac and skeletal muscle cells, and the rod and cone cells of the eye belong to this category, and so do odontoblasts.

Lipofuscin is not encountered in tissues in which cells are regularly replaced by mitosis, such as epidermis, gut epithelium and lymphoid tissue. Lipofuscin, or a similar pigment, does, however, tend to accumulate in liver cells which normally do not divide. Liver can be regenerated, under certain conditions such as chemical damage or trauma, and it is said that the regenerated liver cells are devoid of pigment. This is part of the evidence that mitosis has a rejuvenating effect on cells.

HEALING

It is generally believed that healing of both tissue and bone is retarded in the aged. Some experimental evidence supports the belief.

THE SKELETON

After the 5th decade, there is an overall reduction in the weight of the skeleton, by loss of trabecular bone and thinning of the cortical bone. Only in advanced age is this osteoporosis associated with reduction in the outer dimensions of the bones; a feature of such change is a stepwise loss of stature due to collapse of the vertebrae, one by one (Garn 1975). Osteoporosis is a predisposing cause of fractures in the elderly; for example, fracture of the femoral neck.

These changes appear to be comparable to the disuse atrophy that occurs in bones immobilized for long periods, such as splinted fractures and paralysed limbs, and indeed senile osteoporosis may be secondary to the diminished muscle power and general inactivity of old age. On the other hand, dietary deficiency may play a part and the fact that post-menopausal women are particularly liable to osteoporosis and that senile osteoporosis often responds to steroid therapy suggests that an endocrine disturbance, particularly of the adrenogenital complex, plays a part.

JOINTS

Quite early in life, even by 30 years of age, most joints, but particularly heavily stressed joints like the knee, show minor degrees of degenerative changes or failure to combat the wear and tear to which they are subjected. These changes appear to be the first stages of a process which in certain instances results in osteoarthritis. In the early stages of these changes, articular cartilage and in the mandibular joint, articular fibrous tissue, lose their smooth character and slits appear, leading to fraying of the surface.

Changes in joints and the skeleton as a whole are sufficiently related to advancing age to be the main means of determining age for forensic purposes; for example, changes at the pubic symphyseal surfaces and thinning of the scapula.

SKIN

Wrinkling of the skin is one of the most easily visible signs of advanced age and loss of skin elasticity one of the most easily demonstrated changes. If the skin of an aged person is picked up and pinched between the fingers, a few seconds elapse before it returns to flatness, whereas in the young it returns immediately. The loss of elasticity is due to changes in the dermis which are not fully understood but are worthy of detailed consideration because it is probable that similar changes occur in connective tissue throughout the body, including the stromal tissue of parenchymatous organs. They are perhaps as close to being changes due to the passage of time *per se* as any we know about.

Dermis is a connective tissue in which the intercellular elements, collagen, reticulin and ground substance, predominate. The ground substance is probably not homogeneous in either chemical composition or physical properties. Its structural and physicochemical organization is difficult to study and is therefore not fully understood. Parts are likely to be in a gel or semi-solid state while other parts are more fluid. In fact it is possible that the ground substance is essentially a gel with spaces or channels which contain a more fluid phase which carries electrolytes and water-soluble substances at a near molecular level between blood capillaries and the tissue drainage system of lymphatics. The rheological and hydrodynamic properties of the substance in which the collagen and elastin fibre networks lie contribute to the elasticity of skin; for instance the deformity of its gel phase and the flow of its semi-solid or fluid components from place to place must play a part in the skin-pinching phenomenon referred to above. Changes in the ground substance, such as increased cross-linking between the complex molecules of which the ground substance is composed, or increased polymerization, could affect its fluid–gel state, its viscosity or flow properties and thereby change the skin-pinching reaction. Changes of this sort would be difficult to detect.

Collagen and elastin have only a very slow turnover rate in adult life but some evidence suggests that there is a gradual increase in the collagen content of dermis and other connective tissues with advancing age. There is considerably more evidence that the characteristics of both collagen and elastin are changed with age. Collagen becomes less water-soluble, more resistant to enzyme digestion and undergoes certain physical changes; for instance, its thermal contraction is increased. These chemical and physical changes are explained by an increase in the molecular bonds or crosslinks between its units.

Chemical analysis and histological sections stained conventionally for elastin suggest an increase in the amount of elastin in the dermis. However, this appears to be due to the conversion of collagen into an elastin-like substance which has been called collastin or pseudoelastin and which does not have elastic physical properties. There may be an actual loss of true elastin. These changes in the fibres of connective tissue, particularly the loss of true elastin, could account for the loss of elasticity of skin in advanced age.

ENDOCRINE SYSTEM

Atrophic changes occur in all parts of the endocrine system in advancing age and a decline in the activity of the system undoubtedly mediates some of the changes of senescence; for example a lowering of the basal metabolic rate, an age-associated reduction in glucose tolerance which is explained in terms of a decrease in the efficiency of pituitary–pancreatic mechanisms, and a decline in the output of the adrenogonadal 17-ketosteroids.

IMMUNITY SYSTEM

Circulating levels of gamma globulin increase with age, probably as the cumulative effect of immune responses to past infections. There is some evidence of the deposition of denatured gamma globulin in the tissues; for example, as a component of amyloid, a complex glycoprotein which is sometimes found in the tissues of the elderly though it is more commonly secondary to chronic sepsis or neoplastic disease.

The ability to form antibodies in response to exogenous antigens decreases with age; this would explain why the elderly tend to succumb to infectious disease. However, the levels of auto-antibodies increase in old, otherwise healthy, people and there is a corresponding rise in the incidence of various autoimmune diseases.

CENTRAL NERVOUS SYSTEM

Neurones are fixed post-mitotic cells; hence the statement that we are as old as our neurones. They are one of the types of cell in which lipofuscin tends to accumulate with advancing age; however, lipofuscin has been found in the neurones of quite young children.

There is some evidence of a gradual loss of brain neurones throughout life but much-quoted dramatic estimates of a loss of the order of 100 000 neurones every day are unreliable and not meaningful unless expressed as percentages of the total number of brain cells. Certainly, however, in really advanced age there is about a 20% loss of brain weight and the degenerative changes which tend to be found in the brainstem nuclei would account for the shakiness and loss of locomotor coordination seen in old age.

One of the deteriorations of brain function of old age is loss of memory, at least of memory for recent events because that for remote events tends to remain much longer and may even appear to be enhanced. There tends also to be a loss of the ability to concentrate thought: this is related to loss of memory and could indeed account for it. The loss of the ability to concentrate thought and attention explains also the difficulty experienced by the elderly in learning new skills and in accepting new ideas.

Large complex psychological adjustments are needed to meet the changes associated with retirement from the activities and habits of working life and an increasing awareness of the ensuing loss of physical and mental ability. These adjustments are not always made successfully without help.

## General theories of ageing

The foregoing concerns the changes and possible parts of the mechanisms concerned in ageing rather than the ultimate causes. These ultimate causes are still the subject of speculation and controversy, though several hypotheses worthy of discussion have been advanced. The principal hypotheses summarized here are not mutually exclusive; the causes of ageing, as well as its effects, are likely to be multifactorial.

PROGRAMMED AGEING

All cells contain information in the DNA upon which their behaviour throughout life depends. It has been suggested that ageing occurs because cells eventually run out of programme. A more meaningful suggestion is that cells contain information for their death at a certain time, a sort of built-in obsolescence, perhaps after a certain number of replications of DNA or transcriptions of RNA. Hayflick's observations clearly fit this concept. Some mechanism of this sort presumably is involved in the female menopause. Further, programmed, precisely timed cell death is involved in a number of embryonic processes such as the degeneration of many branchial arch arteries (Fig. 1.19) and part of the mesonephric duct. Deciduous trees carry programmes for cell death and annual plants for total organismal senescence.

SOMATIC MUTATION THROUGH
CHANCE ERRORS OF REPLICATION

Another hypothesis is that ageing is due to a deterioration in replication, not as the result of inborn information carried in the genes, but by the accumulation of chance (stochastic) errors in the replication of DNA or in the transcription of RNA, in particular that related to the enzyme systems whereby cells operate. There is no reason to suppose that these replication processes are invariably perfect. Every fault in replication or transcription would be transmitted to the descendants of the cells and the accumulation of occasional errors in the course of many generations would obviously lead to irreversible deterioration in the efficiency with which the cells operate.

It is easiest to understand this in the case of cells which, like surface epithelia, are continuously mitosing, but the effect would be even greater on fixed post-mitotic cells because, in a population of dividing cells, the accumulation of past errors would to some extent be eliminated by natural selection; the worst affected cells would tend to die and the least affected would have correspondingly more descendants.

## AUTOAGGRESSION

Autoimmunity, perhaps better called autoaggression, has been postulated as the predominant mechanism in ageing. A somatic mutation could arise in a stem cell of the lymphoid system which would cause the cell to respond immunologically to the antigens of the body's own tissues. A descendant population, or 'forbidden clone', of the stem cell, or the humoral products of such a population, could wage a 'warfare' against target cells which they were tolerant towards before the mutation. Alternatively, target cells might undergo an error of replication whereby they produced molecules antigenic to the body's own immune system. Such abnormal immune reactions, especially if multiplied in respect of many organ tissues, could produce the widely diverse changes of ageing.

An important objection to the autoimmune hypothesis of ageing is that it is out of accord with the well-established fact that females are more susceptible to recognized autoimmune disease and yet their life spans tend to be longer.

## CROSS-LINKING HYPOTHESIS

The cross-linking of collagen as a feature of ageing has been referred to above. Similar cross-linking of various multiple-chained proteins, including DNA and RNA, has been suggested as the ultimate cause of ageing. A comparison has been made with the cumulative cross-linking that ages a number of polymers such as rubber. Gradual inactivation of DNA by irreversible histone binding is another possible but hypothetical deteriorative change.

## CUMULATIVE EFFECT OF CELL DAMAGE

There are a number of ways in which, theoretically, damage could occur within cells and which might be cumulative. For instance, it is conceivable that the chemical reactions within cells, especially if aberrant, could produce enough heat to denature cell proteins or DNA. The possibility exists that cosmic, ultraviolet and other forms of atmospheric radiation to which all life forms are exposed could produce slowly cumulative cell damage.

A number of examples of relatively innocuous permanent colonization of cells by viruses are recorded and it is possible that more exist than have yet been discovered. The accumulation of these viruses could lead to a widespread deterioration of cell function.

## FREE RADICAL HYPOTHESIS

Free radicals are molecules possessing an unpaired electron and thus are strong oxidizers. They occur transiently in oxidation–reduction in cells and could theoretically cause cell damage especially if they accumulated. There has been a little success in extending the life span of experimental animals with a variety of antioxidant substances added to food.

## POTENTIAL AGE-LENGTHENING SUBSTANCES

Many of the hypotheses concerning ageing are susceptible to tests by the use of recently produced pharmacological preparations; for example, immunosuppressant substances, radioprotectants, including high atmospheric oxygen tension, antioxidant substances, ones which increase lysozome stability or inhibit protein cross-linking, enzyme activators and substances which can inhibit the formation of lipofuscin in neurones and even remove it. However, although research on these lines is proceeding, no strong leads have emerged.

# FURTHER READING

AMBROSE A. (1969) *Stimulation in Early Infancy.* London: Academic Press.
BJÖRK A. (1963) Variations in growth pattern of the human mandible. *Journal of dental Research* **42**, 400.
CHEEK D.B. (1968) *Human Growth. Body Composition, Cell Growth, Energy and Intelligence.* Philadelphia: Lea and Febiger.
COMFORT A. (1974) The position of aging studies. *Mechanisms of Ageing and Development* **3**, 1.
D'ARCY THOMPSON W. (1942) *On Growth and Form.* Cambridge: University Press.
ENLOW D.H. (1973) Growth and the problem of the local control mechanism. *American Journal of Anatomy* **136**, 403.
ENLOW D.H. (1975) *Handbook of facial growth.* Philadelphia: W.B. Saunders.
FILIPSSON R. (1975) A new method for assessment of dental maturity using the individual curve of number of erupted permanent teeth. *Annals of Human Biology* **2**, 13.
GOLDMAN R. & ROCKSTEIN M. (1975) *The Physiology and Pathology of Human Aging.* New York: Academic Press.
HALL D.A. (1976) *The Ageing of Connective Tissue.* New York: Academic Press.
KOSKI K. (1971) Some characteristics of cranio-facial growth cartilages. In *Cranio-facial growth in man* (eds. Meyers R.E. & Krogman W.M.) Oxford: Pergamon Press.

LOWREY G.H. (1973) *Growth and Development of Children*. Chicago: Year Book Medical Publishers.

MEDAWAR P.B. (1960) *The Future of Man*. London: Methuen.

MOORE W.J. (1975) Bone growth and remodelling. In *Applied physiology of the mouth* p. 73, ed. Lavelle C.L.B.. Bristol: John Wright.

ROCKSTEIN M., SUSSMAN M.L. & CHESKY J. (1974) *Theoretical Aspects of Aging*. New York: Academic Press.

SINCLAIR D. (1973) *Human Growth after Birth*. London: Oxford University Press.

TANNER J.M. (1962) *Growth at Adolescence*. Oxford: Blackwell Scientific Publications.

TIMIRAS P.S. (1972) *Developmental Physiology and Aging*. New York: Macmillan.

YOUNG J.Z. (1971) *An Introduction to the Study of Man*. London: Oxford University Press.

# CHAPTER 4

# Evolution and Adaptation of the Vertebrate Mouth

Nearly all forms of classification have their drawbacks. For example; viruses seem to have properties by which they could be classified as either living or non-living; some unicellular organisms can be classified either as plants or as animals. In an attempt to reduce the number of uncertainties, new criteria may be formulated to distinguish between what should be recognised as living or non-living, plant or animal and so on. No matter how carefully they are formulated there are always problems, and the vertebrates are no exception.

Vertebrates belong to a larger group of animals, the phylum Chordata. The chordates are defined as those animals having a notochord (Fig. 1.13f) at least at some stage in their life history. For the last 500 million years the huge majority of chordates have developed, around their notochord, a cartilaginous or bony vertebral column consisting of articulated segmental elements. But some chordates (e.g. lampreys) which do not have true vertebrae are far more like 'vertebrates' than are other members of the chordate subphyla. Such animals share with the 'vertebrates' a dorsal hollow nerve cord which terminates in an expanded brain and associated paired sense organs. These features, rather than the vertebral column itself, are used to identify animals belonging to the subphylum Vertebrata of the phylum Chordata.

The vertebrates can be subdivided in several different ways (Table 4.1). The Agnatha are unique in having no jaws; the rest of the vertebrates (Gnathostomata) have jaws. The Agnatha, Chondrichthyes (having a purely cartilaginous skeleton) and Osteichthyes (a bony skeleton) constitute the Pisces (fish). All the rest are Tetrapods (have four limbs) although some, such as snakes, have lost these limbs during evolution. The Pisces together with Amphibia produce eggs which develop without forming an amnion (Fig. 1.11c). All the remainder develop an amnion. Only the birds (Aves) and mammals are endothermic. This last classification may have to be revised if it is shown, as has recently been suggested, that dinosaurs were endothermic. One way out of this problem is to take the dinosaurs out of the Class Reptilia and to create a new Class Dinosauria which could include their only descendents, the birds. Man constructs classifications for his own convenience (Table 4.2 and Fig. 4.1).

## AGNATHA: JAWLESS FISHES

Living jawless vertebrates, the lamprey and the hagfish (subclass Cyclostomata), are present-day survivors of the first level or grade of vertebrate evolution (Fig. 4.1). They should not necessarily be regarded as 'primitive' because, apart from the basic characteristics which define the Class Agnatha, they have little in common with their lower Palaeozoic ancestors. Their highly specialized structure and biology has enabled the agnathans to survive over 400 million years in the presence of potential competition from more 'advanced' forms. In cyclostomes the notochord remains prominent in the adult as the primary axial skeleton; vertebrae are poorly developed and never ossified, being at best irregular, cartilaginous growths. The skull consists of a series of cartilaginous boxes developed in association with areas of the brain and the sense organs, joined to form a composite neurocranium. The other skull component, the viscerocranium, which in gnathostomes includes the upper and lower jaws, is constructed from a series of cartilaginous rods developed in support of the pharynx and gills.

### Cyclostomes

Lampreys are both marine and freshwater: most species are obligate parasites of other fishes. They attach themselves firmly to a host by their muscular suctorial mouth (Fig. 4.2a) and rasp a hole through its skin with a powerful tongue-like organ

**Table 4.1.** Division of the subphylum Vertebrata.

| | | | | |
|---|---|---|---|---|
| Agnatha | Agnatha | | | |
| Placodermi | Gnathostomata | Pisces | Anamniotes | Ectothermic |
| Chondrichthyes | | | | |
| Osteichthyes | | | | |
| Amphibia | | Tetrapoda | | |
| Reptilia | | | | ? ? |
| Aves | | | Amniotes | Endothermic |
| Mammalia | | | | |

**Table 4.2.** Nature, origin, and classification of vertebrates.

Class **Agnatha**: jawless vertebrates
 *Subclass **Ostracodermi**: ostracoderms, including cephalaspids, anaspids and pteraspids
  Subclass **Cyclostomata**: cyclostomes, including lampreys and hagfishes

*Class **Placodermi**: placoderms, including arthrodires, antiarchs, and acanthodians

Class **Chondrichthyes**: cartilaginous fishes
  Subclass **Elasmobranchii**: elasmobranchs, including *pleuracanths, *cladodonts and sharks and rays
  Subclass **Holocephali**: chimaeras

Class **Osteichthyes**: bony fishes
  Subclass **Actinopterygii**: ray-finned fishes
   Infraclass **Chondrostei**: chondrosteans, including sturgeons and paddlefishes
   Infraclass **Holostei**: holosteans, including gars and the bowfin
   Infraclass **Teleostei**: teleosts
  Subclass **Sarcopterygii**: fleshy-finned fishes
   Infraclass **Dipnoi**: dipnoans or lungfishes
   Infraclass **Crossopterygii**: crossopterygians or lobe-finned fishes

Class **Amphibia**: amphibians
 *Subclass **Labyrinthodontia**: labyrinthodonts
  Subclass **Lissamphibia**: salamanders, frogs and toads and apoda

Class **Reptilia**: reptiles
  Subclass **Anapsida**: *stem reptiles and turtles
  Subclass **Lepidosauria**: lizards, snakes and *Sphenodon*
  Subclass **Archosauria**: crocodilians, *dinosaurs and *flying reptiles
 *Subclass **Euryapsida**: euryapsids, including plesiosaurs and ichthyosaurs
 *Subclass **Synapsida**: mammal-like reptiles

Class **Aves**: birds
 *Subclass **Archaeornithes**: ancestral birds
  Subclass **Neornithes**: familiar birds

Class **Mammalia**: mammals
  Subclass **Prototheria**: monotremes or egg-laying mammals
  Subclass **Theria**: mammals bearing 'live' young
   Infraclass **Metatheria**: marsupials or pouched mammals
   Infraclass **Eutheria**: higher or 'placental' mammals, including nearly all mammals not native to Australia

*Indicates an extinct group.

armed with several small teeth. Each tooth is a thickened keratinization of the oral ectoderm sometimes supported by a cartilaginous base (Fig. 4.2b). They are referred to as horny or 'false' teeth since they are developmentally unrelated to the (mesodermal) dentine teeth of gnathostomes. Because the mouth is continuously blocked during feeding, the animal breathes by pumping water through the gill apertures in both directions; for this reason the gill chambers themselves are of a very different design to those of gnathostome fishes.

The hagfish and slimehags are non-parasitic but are extensively adapted for a saprophagic life. They burrow into and eat the soft gill region of dead or moribund fishes. Although they have no jaws, hagfish can use their muscular mouth and enlarged tongue (which is armed with recurved horny teeth) to bite in a way similar to gnathostomes. Hagfish secrete large amounts of mucus through lateral body glands as a defence against predators.

The larval stage of the lamprey is important because it has a structure which is probably closer to that of an ancestral vertebrate than is the adult. In this larva the skin is the predominating surface for respiratory exchange of gases while the primary function of the gills seems to be an aid to feeding. A pharyngeal current draws water in through the mouth over a mucus-secreting sub-pharyngeal gland and out through the gills. The thick viscid mucus traps food particles and, when laden, is drawn back into the oesophagus. In this animal the mouth is an inlet and the gills are an outlet for the stream of water which is sweeping food over the sub-pharyngeal gland. This gland has the property of concentrating iodine and when

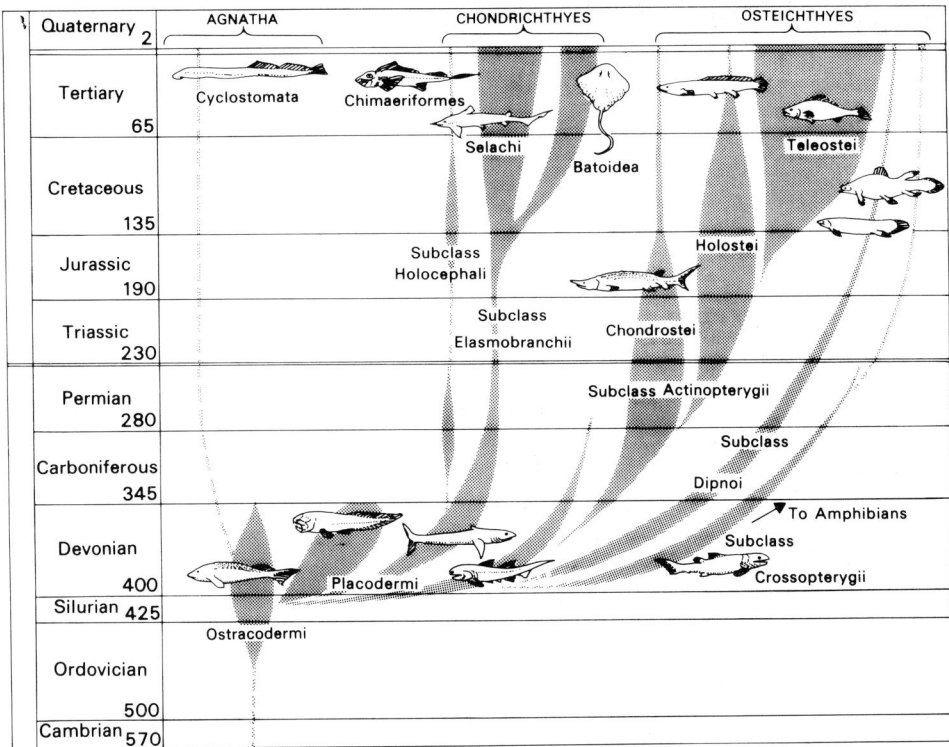

**Fig. 4.1.** A phylogeny of fishes showing their radiation and relative abundances in time. Figures in left-hand column are millions of years before present.

a critical concentration has been reached it directs metamorphosis: it becomes the thyroid gland.

### Ostracoderms

The earliest appearance of recognizable vertebrates in the fossil record was made during the Ordovician period by the ostracoderms (Fig. 4.2c), jawless ancestors of the cyclostomes, which in contrast to the living soft-bodied forms possessed an exoskeleton of calcified (fossilizable) tissues. Their locomotion must have been clumsy since, in the majority of cases, they lacked any form of lateral stabilizing appendage. Paired fins evolved in a later ostracoderm group. The carapace of the head region was formed by fusion of the numerous dermal plates which covered the body. These polygonal plates or tessarae each comprised a surface layer of tubular dentine underlain and supported by layers of spongy and lamellar acellular bone (Fig. 4.2d). Dentine was therefore among the first vertebrate hard tissues to appear in the fossil record.

How did the ostracoderms gain a selective advantage by developing a layer of dentine on their outer surfaces? The answer may possibly lie in the fact that dentine is avascular yet extremely sensitive. It is unlikely that touch or pressure reception alone would be an adequate reason to evolve dentine, as well as bone, in the dermal armour since receptors could easily have been placed in the soft tissues which probably filled the spaces between the dentine nodules. Sensitivity to temperature change also was probably not of much importance to an animal of this level of organization. The following argument suggests that the monitoring of osmotic changes in the environment was a likely function of primitively formed dentine.

The earliest vertebrate remains come from what was clearly a marine environment, the Harding Sandstone of the Ordovician period. Subsequently the ostracoderms are found in what was evidently a freshwater environment, the Old Red Sandstone from the Devonian in Wales. This suggests that the vertebrate organization first arose in the sea and that coincident with the spread of vegetation into fresh waters, the evolution of

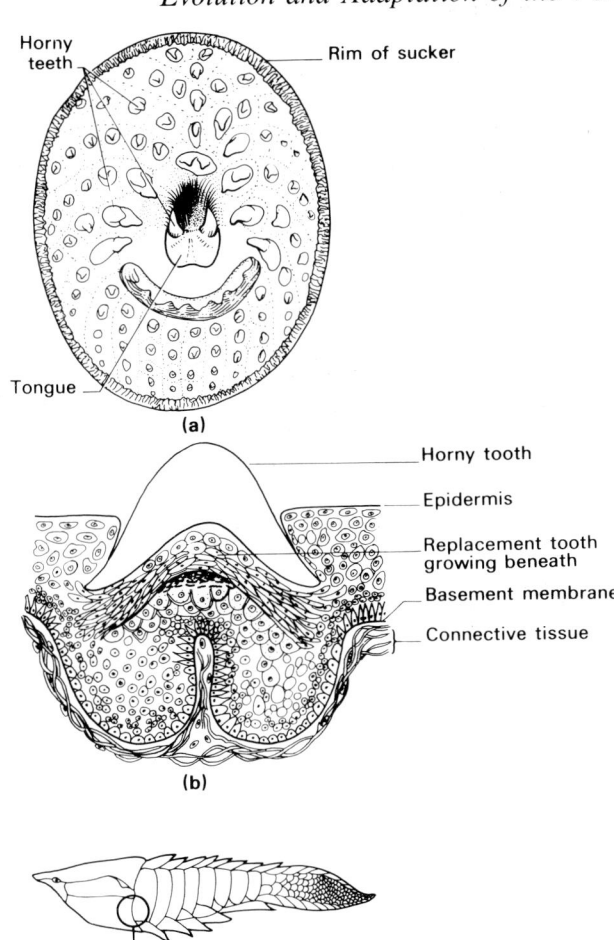

Fig. 4.2. (a) Mouth of lamprey (inner aspect). (b) Horny (epidermal) tooth of lamprey (vertical section). (c) An early jawless fish (ostracoderm). (d) The body armour was made up of tessarae—bony plates which supported dentine nodules; these were fused together over the head region to form a carapace.

vertebrates during the Ordovician and Silurian periods was marked by the gradual excursion into waters of reduced salinity. For this environmental change, the formation of dentine on the surface layer of the dermal armour might have provided cautionary information to the organism while its kidneys had yet to elaborate their water-excreting salt-conserving functions sufficiently to cope with the freshwater habitat.

Although the above argument suggests a selective advantage for the evolution of dentine, the selective advantage for laying down bone in the skin is less obvious. The possibilities are; as a store of phosphate, as a protection against predation and as a support for the dentine nodules.

## PLACODERMI—EARLY JAWED FISHES

The ostracoderm mouth was toothless and, being bordered by plates of dermal armour, was probably rigidly open (unlike the mouth of the cyclostomes). Respiration and feeding were carried out by a 'vacuum-cleaner' pharynx capable of pumping water and mud in through the mouth and out through the gills. From this stream the gills would have filtered such organic material and minute organisms as the sea or river beds contained. The ostracoderm radiation was therefore confined to environments in which a supply of small particulate food was available. The first

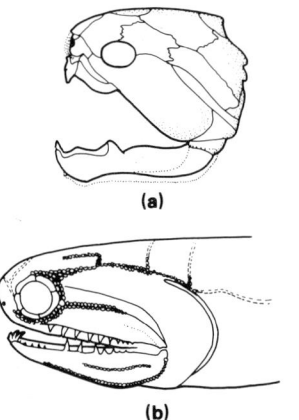

**Fig. 4.3.** Placoderms. (a) *Dinichthys* (with jaws bearing bony projections and blades). (b) *Ischnacanthus* (Acanthodii; true dentine teeth).

appearance of jawed vertebrates, the placoderms (Fig. 4.3), during the Silurian period coincided with a decline in both the numbers and the variety of ostracoderm types. Placoderms were structurally further advanced in possessing mobile paired fins and jaws which, although clearly experimental and quite unlike anything living today, must have placed their possessors firmly at the top of the food chain. The simultaneous appearance of jaws and teeth, capable of capturing and killing other animals as a source of food, heralded an entirely new vertebrate type, the predator. This set the main course for subsequent vertebrate evolution, towards increased mobility and rapacity, and further allowed the vertebrate organization to adapt to and exploit a vast array of habitats during succeeding geological periods.

In placoderms, thick dermal armour was formed only over the anterior part of the body while the tail was covered by thin bony scales, or, in later Devonian forms, was completely naked. The jaws were not only of value in the new predatory role but also became, in other groups, a better means of defence than cumbersome body armour. The reduction in body armour continued in the several lines of placoderm descendants (leading to cartilaginous and bony fish) as selection put increasing advantage on speed and manoeuvrability.

With their new role as predators, the placoderms evolved internal bones by ossifying their cartilaginous endoskeleton; amongst these were the jaw bones. Two different attempts were made to increase the efficiency of the jaws. In one attempt the jaw bone was extended into sharp blades which were exposed and acted as teeth (Fig. 4.3a). Some of these animals achieved enormous sizes (up to 5 m long). Another group, the acanthodians, evolved true teeth (Fig. 4.3b). The internal bony skeleton of the acanthodians was further developed in the Osteichthyes that first appeared in the rivers and lakes of the middle Devonian continent.

## CHONDRICHTHYES

The entirely cartilaginous skeleton of sharks and rays was at one time held as evidence that these forms are survivors of the earliest gnathostome radiation and that they are more primitive than the bony fishes.

With increased knowledge of the fossil record and of the relationships between different groups, it now appears that the absence of bone in cartilaginous fish was a result of reduction. In fact cartilaginous and bony fishes appeared at about the same time in the fossil record. (Fig. 4.1).

The head skeleton of Chondrichthyes consists of two primary components; a neural part, or neurocranium, formed by a central cartilaginous box surrounding the brain to which are fused six additional boxes enclosing or supporting the three paired special sense organs; the nasal, orbital and otic capsules; a visceral part, or viscerocranium, which consists of a series of paired cartilaginous rods (the branchial arches) containing and supporting the underlying pharynx. The neurocranium and part of the viscerocranium develop together and become joined during embryogenesis to form a composite structure—the chondrocranium. These structures are recognisable in all vertebrates, including man, although in Chondrichthyes the chondrocranium reaches its fullest development.

### Segmentation of the head

Although the original pattern in which the vertebrate head developed has become largely obscured in all recent vertebrates, there are sufficient data to recognize an archaic symmetry. Just as in the remainder of the body, so in the head region of an ancestral gnathostome, a series of dorsal somites developed on each side of the neural tube (Fig. 4.4a). As the neural tube closed, neural crest cells were 'pinched out' and migrated down the flanks of the head between the dorsal somites and then around the ventrally situated pharynx. Contact with the endoderm of the pharynx induced each stream of neural crest cells to develop a bar of cartilage. Between each cartilage

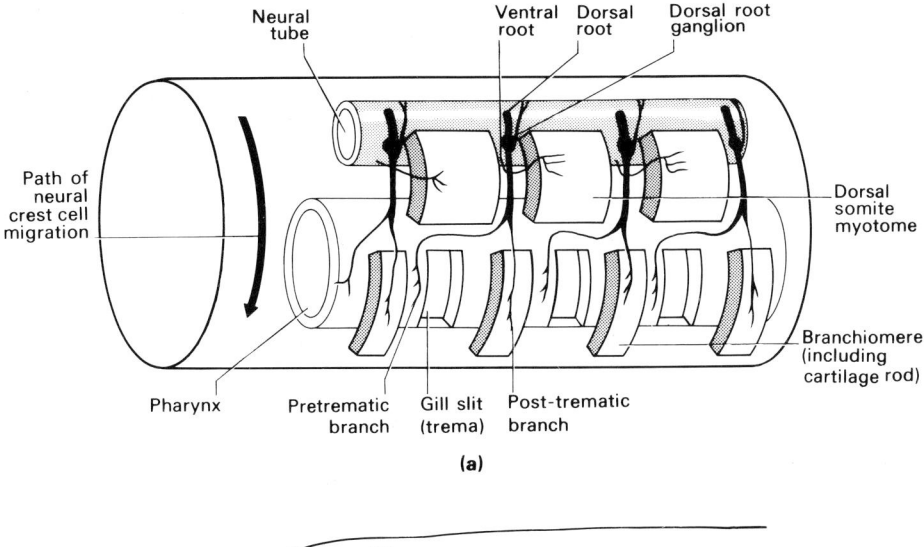

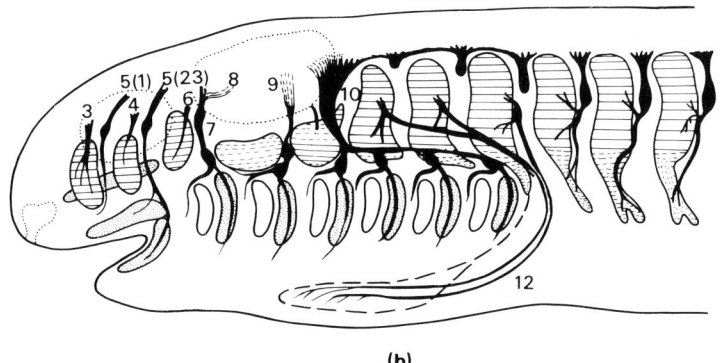

**Fig. 4.4.** Segmentation. (a) Diagrammatic view of the vertebrate pharynx. (b) Dogfish embryo: development and courses of cranial dorsal and ventral root nerves (numbered).

developed a gill slit which therefore corresponded in position with a dorsal somite. Some of the neural crest cells also induced the ectoderm between each somite to thicken into a placode from which, together with the neural crest cells themselves, developed a ganglion of nerve cells. This dorsal root ganglion lay in the spaces between each somite and therefore above each gill cartilage and its associated muscle, together known as a branchiomere.

Each dorsal root nerve supplied visceral sensory and motor branches to its branchiomere behind a gill slit (post-trematic branch) and a small visceral sensory branch to the skin in front of this gill slit (pretrematic branch). It also had a small somatic sensory twig to the dorsal skin. The dorsal muscle (myotome) received its motor supply from the equivalent ventral root nerve.

The above simple pattern is still recognizable in the recent Chondricthyes (Fig. 4.4b). For example, the 3rd, 4th and 6th (ventral root) cranial nerves go to the first, second or third myotomes (which have become extrinsic muscles of the eye in modern vertebrates); the 7th nerve still has pre- and post-trematic branches; the pre- and post-trematic branches of the 5th nerve are maxillary and mandibular divisions of the trigeminal supplying the visceral branchiomere associated with the jaws.

NEUROCRANIUM

The notochord, the primary axial skeleton of the body, lies under the nerve cord and extends as far forwards as the pituitary. As the midbrain grows it is supported below by a pair of parachordal

94                                   *Chapter 4*

cartilages, one on each side of the notochord, developing in the mesoderm (Fig. 4.5a,b). In front of this the forebrain is supported by two further cartilages, the trabeculae cranii; behind the parachordals the brain stem is supported by occipital cartilages which develop from occipital somites. These three axial sets of cartilages are joined laterally by three further pairs, the nasal, optic and otic capsules surrounding or supporting the nose, eye and ear respectively. All these cartilaginous elements grow and fuse to become the neurocranium. With such a skull the brain extends forward between the optic capsules. In the skull of amniotes (Table 4.1) the paired trabeculae cranii are fused to form a single median trabecula and the brain now lies behind, and not between, the orbits (Fig. 4.5c). In man, the trabecula is probably represented partly by the vertical plate of the ethmoid (mesethmoid) and partly by the anterior part of the sphenoid body (presphenoid).

VISCEROCRANIUM

The viscerocranium (pharyngeal skeleton) is composed of a series of jointed cartilaginous arches which surround the pharynx. Muscles acting on the rods in each arch squeeze and relax the enclosed pharyngeal tube thereby sucking water into the pharynx and driving it out through the gill slits. It is assumed that in the archaic condition all the cartilaginous arches were alike (Fig. 4.4a). During the early evolution of Agnatha the most anterior pair, which can be called arch 0, tilted upwards to support the lengthening forebrain (Figs. 4.6a and b); these are the trabeculae cranii of Fig. 4.5. The next two arches are the mandibular and hyoid, arches 1 and 2 respectively. To understand the evolution of these arches it is necessary to describe an unmodified arch in a recent cartilaginous fish (Fig. 4.7). Each cartilaginous rod consists of four elements, a small dorsal pharyngobranchial, a larger epibranchial and ceratobranchial, and a small hypobranchial. The hypobranchials of each side are jointed across the midline ventral to the pharynx by a basibranchial plate which also connects successive arches together.

The upper jaw was derived from the epibranchial and the lower jaw from the ceratobranchial of the first arch (Figs. 4.6b, c): in Chondrichthyes they are known as the palatopterygo-quadrate bar and Meckel's cartilage respectively. The fibrous connection between these cartilages became the jaw joint. The branchial adductor muscle has been retained and enlarged to close the mouth (Fig. 4.7). The second, hyoid, arch

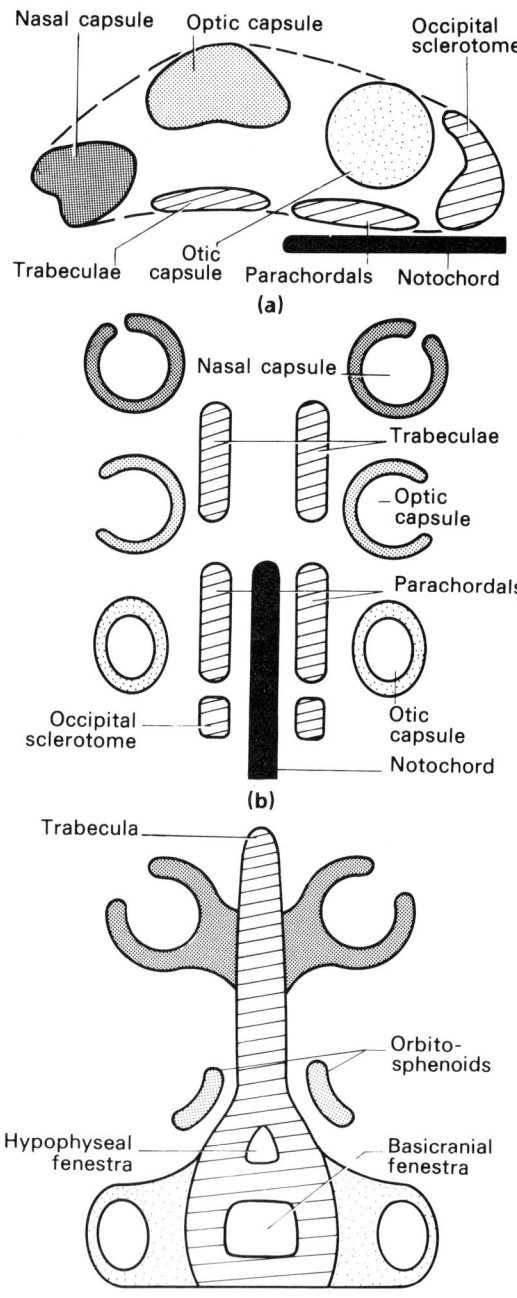

**Fig. 4.5.** Development of the vertebrate neurocranium (diagrammatic): (a) lateral view; (b) dorsal view (dogfish); (c) dorsal view (mammal).

has become modified to support the altered elements of the first arch (Figs. 4.6c, d) while the cleft between first and second arch became the spiracle (p. 104).

# Evolution and Adaptation of the Vertebrate Mouth

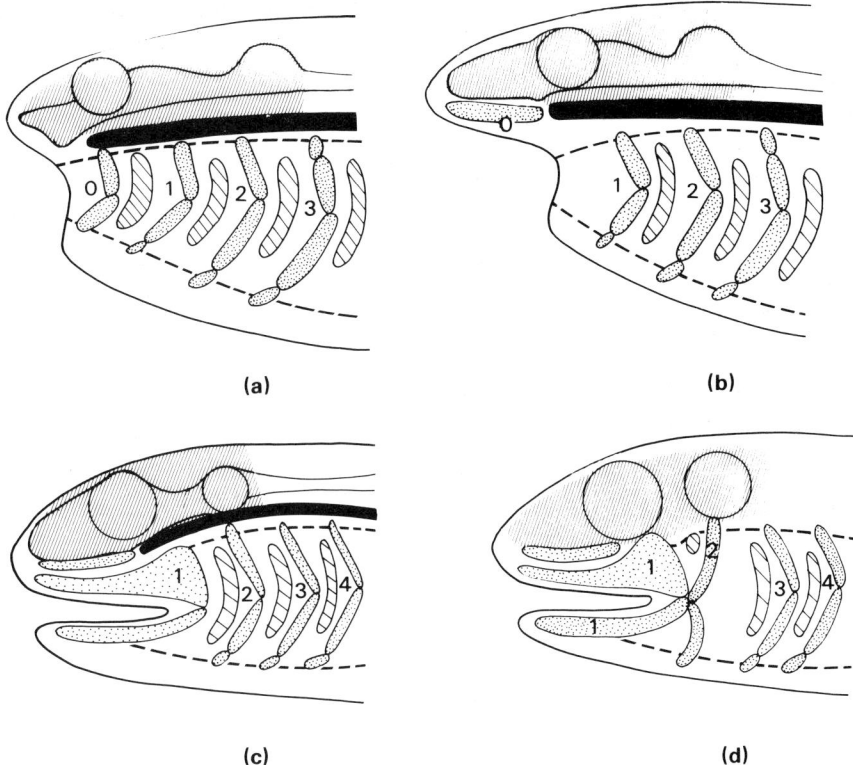

**Fig. 4.6.** Evolutionary modification of the branchial arches. (a) Earliest stage; all arches unmodified, notochord almost terminal. (b) Agnathan stage: arch 0 supports forebrain; arch 1 (mandibular) supports the mouth. (c) Early gnathostome stage: arch 1 supports the mouth and forms upper and lower jaws; arch 2 is unmodified. (d) Later gnathostome stage (compare with Fig. 4.4b): arch 2 modified as an accessory support for the jaws; gill slit 2 reduced in size (spiracle).

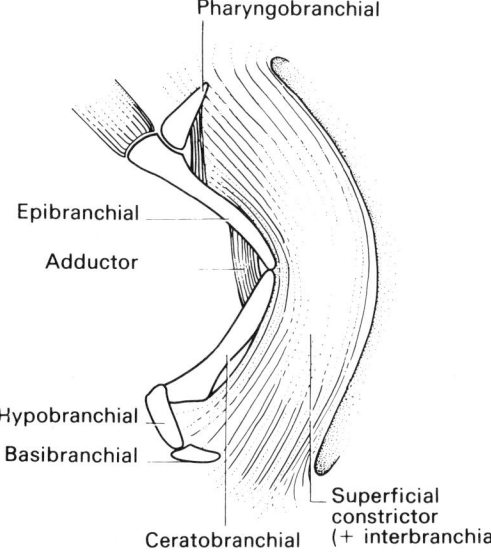

**Fig. 4.7.** A single gill arch of a dogfish and its musculature.

In Chondrichthyes, the mandibular arch cartilages actually form the upper and lower jaws of the adult fish. In the jaws of all other gnathostomes, the mandibular arch cartilages are reduced in importance by the addition (during development) of dermal bones which perform the functions of tooth support and muscle attachment (Fig. 4.28); these include the premaxilla and maxilla of the upper jaw; the dentary and most of the post-dentary bones of the lower jaw. However, the 'primary' embryonic jaws serve the all-important function of providing a structural framework for the soft tissues of the embryo in which the dermal bones are formed. Additionally, parts of the mandibular arch cartilage persist into the adult stage, endochondrally ossified, as elements of the jaw joint—the (upper jaw) quadrate and the (lower jaw) articular bones of amphibians, reptiles and birds and their homologues in mammals—the incus and malleus of the middle ear (Fig. 10.3). A further part of the primary upper jaw persists in mammals as the

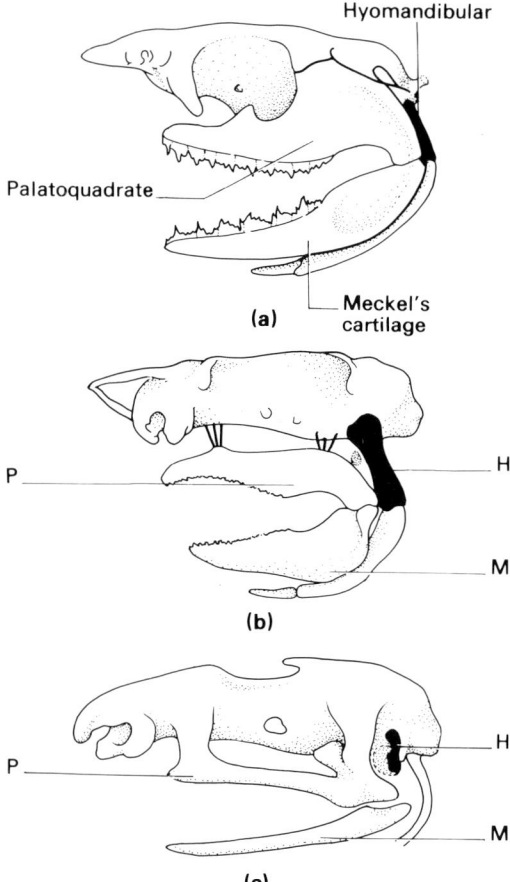

Fig. 4.8. Jaw attachments to the neurocranium in vertebrates: (a) amphistylic; (b) hyostylic; (c) autostylic.

recent species of sharks (e.g. *Chlamydoselache*, *Heterodontus*), the upper jaw is attached directly to the otic region of the cranium and is additionally supported by the hyomandibular cartilage, which attaches dorsally to the otic capsule and ventrally to the jaw joint region. The hyomandibular is derived from the dorsal (epibranchial) element of the second (hyoid) arch: the remainder of the arch (ceratohyal and basihyal) comes to lie below and behind Meckel's cartilage. This manner of jaw suspension, with the upper jaw quite firmly attached to the cranium, is known as amphistylic (Fig. 4.8a).

In the most modern sharks (Fig. 4.8b) attachment of the upper jaw to the cranium is reduced to ligaments and its principal support comes from the hyomandibular. This flexible attachment is known as hyostylic. By not having the upper jaw firmly attached to the skull, it becomes possible to protrude the jaws into a wider gape giving these fishes a clear advantage as predators.

In the line of evolution from placoderms which resulted in land vertebrates (tetrapods) just the opposite occurred. The connection between palato-pterygo-quadrate and cranium was reinforced and the hyomandibular connection to the upper jaw was broken; an attachment type known as autostylic (Fig. 4.8c). This option freed the hyomandibular for another, more remarkable, transformation into the sound transmitting stapes of the tetrapod middle ear (Fig. 4.20).

alisphenoid cartilage (=epipterygoid) which ossifies as part of the sphenoid greater wing in man.

### Jaw attachment of the neurocranium

In most early fishes (Placodermi, early Chondrichthyes and Osteichthyes), and some

### Teeth of Chondrichthyes

Teeth evolved from the body armour of the ancestral agnathans (Fig. 4.9a). The armour was reduced so increasing the mobility of the animal (Fig. 4.9b), ultimately becoming a placoid scale with a dentine-like body and a bony base embedded in, and attached to, the dermis (Fig. 4.9c). In the region of the jaw opening these scales spread over the lips onto the jaw bones (Fig. 4.9d) becoming, by definition, teeth.

As its jaws increase in size an animal requires

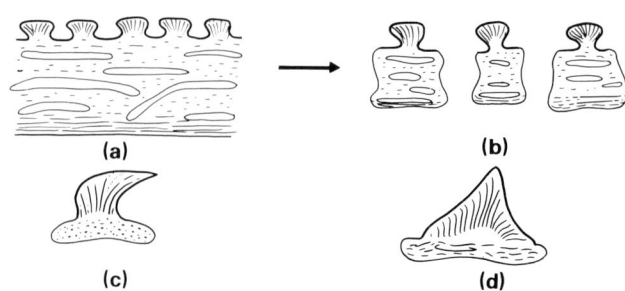

Fig. 4.9. Evolution of teeth and placoid scales by reduction of primitive dermal armour.

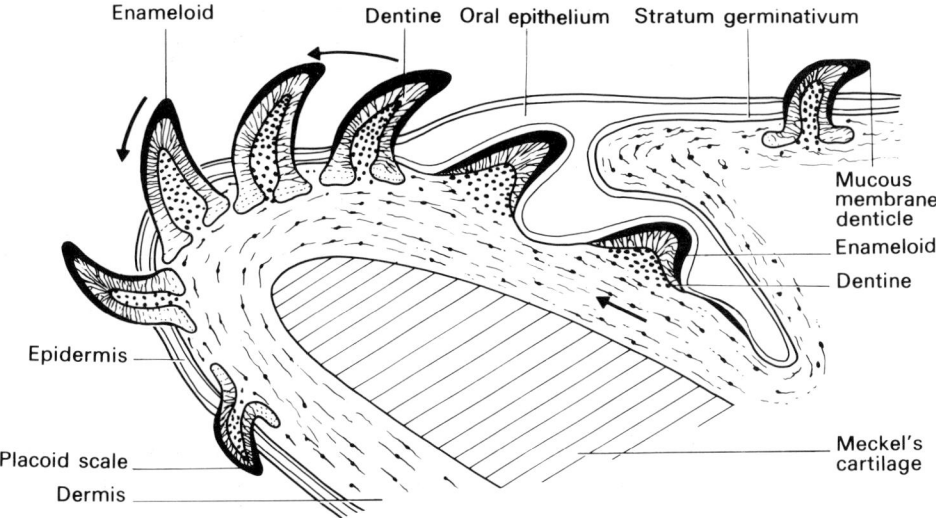

**Fig. 4.10.** Tooth succession in a dogfish (for explanation see text).

increasingly large teeth. To meet this requirement most vertebrates, apart from mammals, continue to replace their teeth throughout life. The following mechanisms exist in Chondrichthyes (Fig. 4.10). Each tooth develops at the end of a deep invagination of the oral epithelium which lines the oral aspect of a jaw cartilage. Between the epithelium and the cartilage is a thick layer of fibrous tissue which seems to act as a conveyor belt. As the new tooth grows it develops a bone-like base of osteodentine (Fig. 6.5) within and attached to the fibrous tissue which conveys the

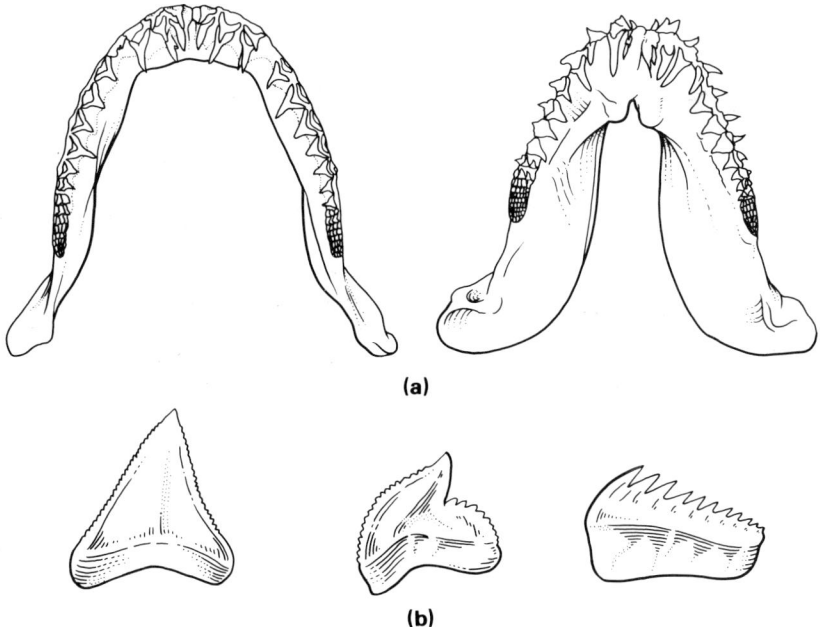

**Fig. 4.11.** (a) Dentition of shark (*Carcharias*): left, upper jaw; right, lower jaw. (b) Shark teeth—variations of form: left to right; Great white, Tiger, Comb-toothed shark.

tooth towards its functioning position at the edge of the jaws. After a short time the functioning tooth is rolled over the jaw, becomes loosened, and is shed, falling to the ocean floor.

The subclass Elasmobranchii contains almost all the surviving members of the class Chondrichthyes (Fig. 4.1). The subclass consists of two orders the Selachii (sharks) and the Batoidea (rays and skates).

Most of the sharks are agile predators with fearsomely sharp batteries of pointed teeth (Fig. 4.11a). Most are piscivorous and a few of the larger species eat seals and sealions. The great white shark (*Carcharodon*), known to be a man-eater, is among the largest living species reaching a length of some 10 m.

Nearly all shark teeth are flattened buccolingually producing a sharp serrated cutting edge (Fig. 4.11b). They serve not only as offensive weapons, capable of inflicting disabling wounds on the largest of prey, but also as a means of snatching and piercing small prey that is to be swallowed whole.

The rays and skates are predominantly bottom-living invertebrate eaters. For this function their morphology has departed strikingly from that of sharks. The tail is no longer the main propulsive organ and has become reduced and whip-like. The body is flattened dorso-ventrally with greatly enlarged pectoral fins which are used in bird-like flapping locomotion. Their ventral mouth is ideally situated for feeding off the bottom of the ocean but poorly situated for inspiration, a function which is taken over by the greatly enlarged, dorsally placed, spiracle.

The dentitions of rays are characteristically tooth pavements made up of flat-surfaced rhombic, hexagonal or polygonal teeth (Fig. 4.12a). *Pristis*, the sawfish, has an elongated rostrum armed with enlarged placoid scales which is possibly used, by side-to-side thrusts of the head, to strike out and kill among shoals of fish.

The egregious *Pristis* is an example of a shark-like ray. There are also examples of ray-like sharks, for example the genus *Heterodontus*, which feed on hard-shelled molluscs and echinoderms, have pointed, prehensile teeth anteriorly and crushing teeth posteriorly. The angel shark (*Rhina*: Fig. 4.12b) is most unusual in that a precise occlusion develops between upper and lower dentitions. Finally, the basking shark (*Cetorhinus*) is one of a disparate group, including some mammals and bony fish, which feed on the plankton. In *Cetorhinus*, the plankton is sieved by greatly elongated mucous membrane denticles which bridge the gill clefts.

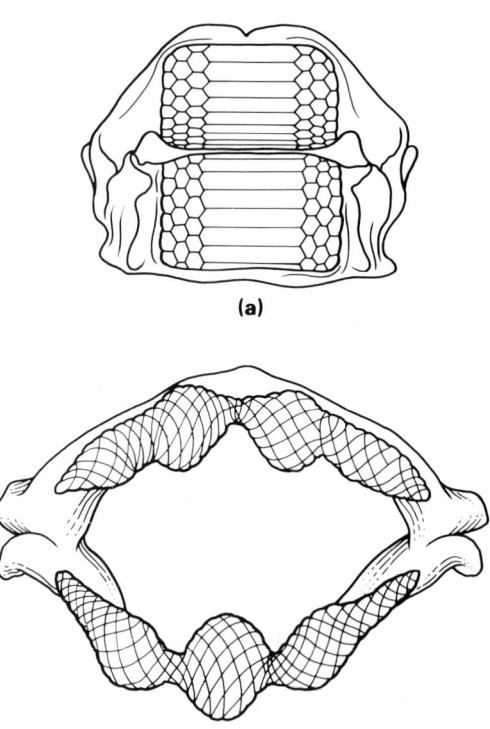

**Fig. 4.12.** (a) Dentition of a ray (*Myliobatis*). (b) Dentition of the angel shark (*Rhina*).

## OSTEICHTHYES

Bony fish fall into three naturally distinct subcategories which have evolved independently from placoderm ancestors (Fig. 4.1). The Actinopterygii ('ray-finned') include, together with various fossil types, the teleosts, the most advanced and abundant extant group of fishes. The Dipnoi ('double breathing') include the modern lung fishes and their abundant ancestors. The Crossopterygii ('tassle-finned') are, from an evolutionary point of view, the most important group since they gave rise, in late Devonian times, to land tetrapods. Only one species, the coelacanth, is known to survive today. The Dipnoi and Crossopterygii are often grouped together in a subclass (Sarcopterygii) since both groups have fleshy, amphibian-like, lobed fins.

Lungs were present (in addition to gills) in many of the Devonian bony fishes; probably because the freshwater habitats of those times, being restricted, murky and often ephemeral, had placed a premium on the ability to breathe air directly.

Although this muddy environment was clearly advantageous for filter feeders (e.g. ostracoderms) it must have made life difficult for the recently evolved predators. By late Devonian times the freshwater predators had secured a greater survival advantage by extending their adaptation to new habitats: the actinopterygians moved downstream into the seas; the crossopterygians evolved a land form, the amphibians; the Dipnoi stayed to survive the rigours of the original environment by more extensive physiological changes—for example, they were able to withstand long periods of summer drought by digging burrows in the mud and suspending their metabolism—a phenomenon analogous to hibernation. By taking the most conservative of the three options, the Dipnoi secured survival in an unfavourable habitat but had to forego the explosive evolutionary expansion which characterized the colonization of new adaptive zones by the other types. Being bound to one specific environment has resulted in a slow decline of the group since Devonian times so that there are only three extant genera.

## Actinopterygii

The ray-finned fishes became the dominant group from Carboniferous times both in the seas and, with the return of more equable climatic conditions, in fresh water. Today there are about 20 000 known species of which some are extremely numerous, e.g. the atlantic herring population is estimated at about $10^{12}$ individuals. Of these 20 000 species all but a handful are members of the infraclass Teleostei. This handful of survivors includes; the sturgeons (Chondrostei), and the bowfins and garpikes (Holostei) from the Mississippi river.

Much of the superiority of actinopterygians over their elasmobranch competitors can be traced to the fact that bone has wider possibilities as a structural material than cartilage. With the advantage of this high strength, low bulk material actinopterygians achieved greater speed and manoeuverability (rayed fins), more efficient respiration, and a bewildering array of skull adaptations (Fig. 4.13a) far beyond the engineering potential of cartilage.

Many of the advanced actinopterygians have developed the thin bones of the face into a complex system of levers incorporating a jointed premaxilla (Fig. 4.13b) which can be projected forwards quickly to seize prey. The same system was subsequently adapted as the basis for feeding on vegetation thereby broadening horizons for what was previously a strictly carnivorous group.

## TEETH OF TELEOST FISHES

Although a great variety of skull shapes and feeding mechanisms exists, teleost teeth have departed little from the simple conical or button-shaped form. Very few have elaborated crown forms that could parallel the enormous variety of occluding shapes evolved by mammals. However, both the number of teeth and the total area of the mouth and pharynx to which teeth are attached are not equalled by any other vertebrates; teeth may be formed not only on the premaxilla, maxilla and dentary but also on the palatine, pterygoid, vomer, splenial and bones of the pharyngeal skeleton. In the majority of predacious forms there are two upper arcades; a marginal set of strong recurved teeth on the premaxillae and sometimes the maxillae (edentulous in most forms) and an inner set on the primary upper jaws (palatopterygoids). In the lower jaw, teeth are generally confined to the dentaries but in moray eels large teeth are formed on the ceratohyals (second branchial arch) which, lying medial to the dentaries, function as a second pair of lower jaws. Additionally, there is often a whole array of fine hair-like teeth covering the roof of the mouth and insides of the throat whose function is to secure a slippery prey for swallowing. Some have a uniquely teleost refinement in which the large marginal teeth are hinged to facilitate the entry of prey into the mouth but prevent its escape (Fig. 7.3).

In most species the teeth are used for catching, retaining and swallowing prey (e.g. pike, Fig. 4.14a); in a few species (e.g. piranha: Fig. 4.14b) they are used for biting and cutting large prey, or (e.g. sheep's head fish: Fig. 4.14c) for scraping up and crushing shelled invertebrates. Some of the more advanced teleosts (e.g. wrasses, carp and perch), which have specialized as vegetarians or small invertebrate feeders, have largely abandoned the marginal dentition in favour of pharyngeal teeth which develop in the mucous membrane of the throat in connection with the bones of the branchial skeleton. In the carp, teeth are confined to the lower pharyngeal bones and bite against a keratinized pad on the pharynx roof—a system reminiscent of some ungulate mammals. The shapes of pharyngeal teeth have become modified for various requirements, being rounded, conical, hooked or spoon-shaped in different carp species. The extremely protrusible premaxillae of carps is used to 'gulp' large quantities of mud or water with its contained food.

The herring (*Clupea*) lives on microscopic plankton and has developed a filtering system analogous to whalebone whales, whereby the

100   *Chapter 4*

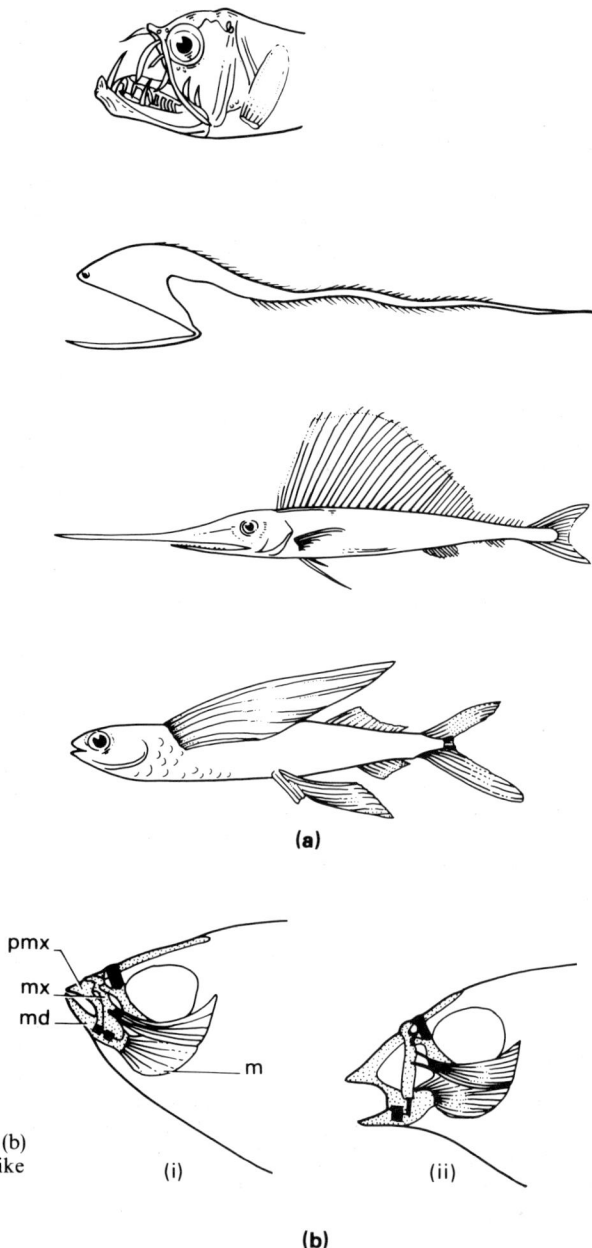

**Fig. 4.13.** (a) Structural diversity of teleost fishes. (b) The protrusile premaxilla of an advanced perch-like teleost: (i) mouth closed; (ii) mouth opened with premaxilla (pmx) drawn forward (m, jaw muscle; ligaments in black).

'exhaled' respiratory current is sieved by the gills: the dentition is reduced and the jaws feeble.

### Dipnoi

Because they share many structural features with amphibians (including lungs and the partial separation of pulmonary and systemic circulations) the Dipnoi were once regarded as their ancestors. Not long ago they were deposed from this exalted position because they lack true internal nostrils (choanae) and the well-defined skull architecture shared by the Devonian crossopterygians and the first amphibians (Fig. 4.1). Also their highly specialized mode of life, especially their feeding and dentition, makes them an unlikely ancestor for anything except more lungfish. Since they were faced with similar environmental problems the

# Evolution and Adaptation of the Vertebrate Mouth

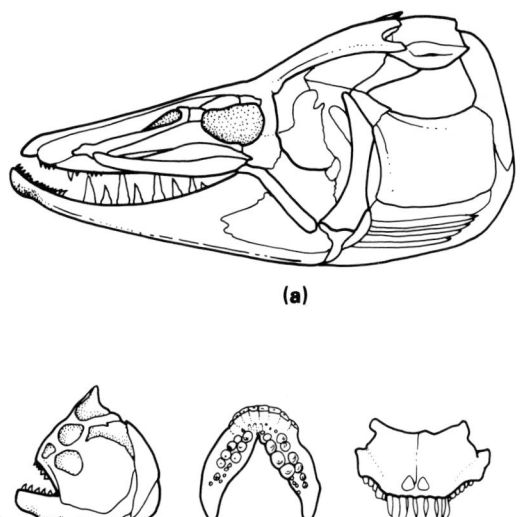

**Fig. 4.14.** Teeth of teleosts: (a) Pike (*Esox*); (b) Piranha (*Serrasalmus*); (c) Sheep's Head (*Sargus*).

amphibious characteristics of lungfishes clearly evolved in parallel with those of the crossopterygians.

There are three surviving genera of lungfish distributed in the rivers of the southern hemisphere. There is no maxilla or premaxilla in the skull and no marginal dentition on either jaw. Toothplates developed on the palate and on the insides of the lower jaw occlude precisely and are used for crushing shellfish, although their diet also includes vegetable material.

## Crossopterygii

The great majority of this group of fishes belong to the fossil order Rhipidistia which includes the intermediates between the placoderms and amphibians. The remainder are the coelacanths.

The Rhipidistia flourished in Devonian and Carboniferous freshwater environments becoming rare and disappearing in the early Permian. The remaining line of descent, the coelacanths, became adapted to a marine life through the Mesozoic, making their last appearance in the fossil record during the late Cretaceous. The discovery in 1938 of the single surviving genus of coelacanth, *Latimeria*, off the South African coast was an event unparalleled in the history of zoology; not only is it a very different kind of fish than anything else living but it is a descendant of an early stage of our own ancestry which has survived unknown for more than 60 million years! What it can tell us about our ancestry, however, is a little less spectacular because the coelacanths opted for a marine existence which brought about considerable modification of the appendicular skeleton away from the almost pentadactyl limbs of devonian rhipidistians. As in the ray-finned fishes, there has been a reversion to obligate gill breathing, the lungs being reduced to a single dorsal swim-bladder. Nonetheless, *Latimeria* has retained some characteristics which help us to understand the anatomy of fossil crossopterygians. *Latimeria* is a large predator with abundant teeth both along the margins of the jaws and on the palate. The majority of these are small conical pegs but along the jaw margins are groups of much larger single-pointed tusks similar to those in the Rhipidistia.

The Rhipidistia are a very important group of 'main line' vertebrates because they are transitional between placoderms and amphibians. They first appear in Lower Devonian strata, becoming the dominant freshwater predators of their time. Their relationship with the placoderms is obscure: it can only be presumed that they evolved during the late Silurian from an acanthodian-type ancestor (Fig. 4.3b).

Many of the dermal bones of the head can be recognized in mammals and have been named accordingly (Fig. 4.15). Each major stage in subsequent evolution, amphibian to reptile to mammal, involved a sequential 'loss' of dermal bones.

The bodies of rhipidistians were covered by 'cosmoid' scales, each having a thin outer layer of ganoin (=enameloid, Fig. 6.7) and a much thicker layer of cosmine (=vasodentine, Fig. 6.6b) supported by layers of lamellated bone. Layers of enameloid and vasodentine also covered the dermal bones of the head so that the whole body was encased in a type of dentine.

The dentition consists of single or double rows of small sharp conical (haplodont) teeth on the marginal bones while on the bones of the palate (vomer, palatine and ectopterygoid) and on an inner bone (coronoid) of the lower jaw there are much larger fangs arranged in pairs (Fig. 4.15). Fangs were replaced alternately so that there was always a functioning tooth in each pair. All the teeth have a pronounced superficial grooving which in section appears as a labyrinthine infolding of the dentine (=plicidentine, Fig. 6.6a). The term labyrinthodont is applied to this type of tooth and to the almost identical type found in the first amphibia (Fig. 4.16).

The demise of Rhipidistia during the early

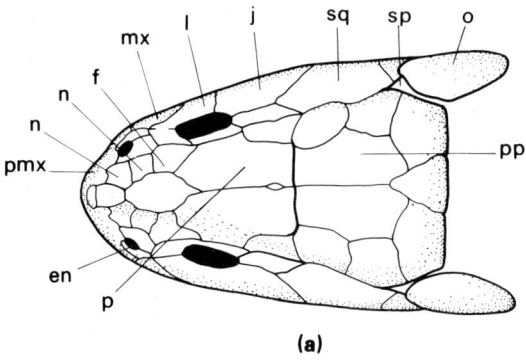

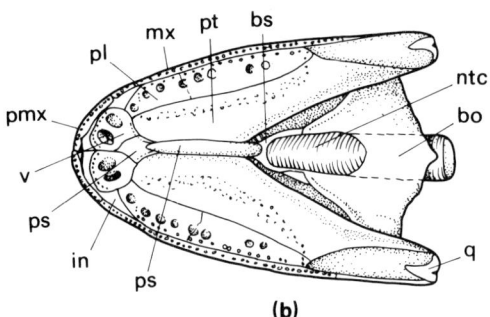

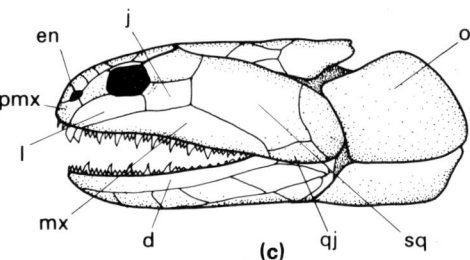

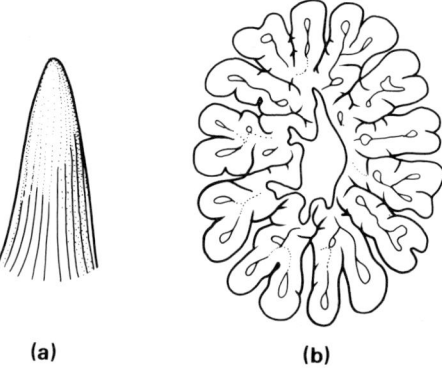

Fig. 4.16. Labyrinthodont teeth of Rhipidistia and Carboniferous Amphibia. (a) Whole tooth showing superficial grooving. (b) Transverse section showing infolded and 'nipped-off' pulp chambers.

Fig. 4.15. The skull of a Devonian rhipidistian fish: (a) dorsal, (b) ventral and (c) lateral views. Key (human homologues in parentheses): bo, basioccipital; bs, basisphenoid; d, dentary (mandible); en, external naris; f, frontal; in, internal naris; j, jugal (zygomatic); l, lacrimal; mx, maxilla; n, nasal; ntc, notochord; o, occipital; p, parietal; pl, palatine; pmx, premaxilla; pp, postparietal (supraoccipital); ps, presphenoid; pt, pterygoid; q, quadrate (incus); qj, quadratojugal; sq, squamosal (temporal); v, vomer; sp, spiracle. After Romer (1971).

Permian can be linked with the drying out of many of the stagnant waters that had earlier given them a survival advantage due to their ability to breathe air. The possibility also exists that they failed in direct competition with their own descendants, the amphibia, which replaced them ecologically during Permo-Triassic times.

## AMPHIBIANS

The class Amphibia contains two subclasses (Fig. 4.17); the Labyrinthodontia is an extinct group (U. Devonian–Triassic) of large, heavily armoured animals which included forms transitional between Rhipidistia and Reptilia. The subclass Lissamphibia contains all the modern forms (frogs, salamanders etc.).

Although amphibians are tetrapods, they cannot be regarded as true land animals; with few exceptions they are dependent on an aquatic medium, at least for fertilization, embryogenesis, and the larval stage of their life history. Adult amphibians, not being able to resist desiccation as well as higher tetrapods, can never move very far from open water or a humid environment. Some have evolved mechanisms which enable them to vacate the communal pond, with its heavy predation of eggs and larvae by substituting a 'private' pond in which external fertilization and larval survival are more successful. For example, a tree frog species rolls up a leaf around its body to make a small cup in which the eggs and albumen are deposited. As the tadpoles develop, the decreasing pH of the water in the cup dissolves the gum which was used to stick the leaf together. The leaf then springs open and showers the young into the water beneath. Other species have made more thorough attempts at emancipation from open water by becoming ovoviviparous. In *Pipa dorsigera*, for example, the eggs develop inside deep-lidded pouches on the back of an adult; the tadpole develops an expanded vascularized tail as a placenta for gas exchange and its entire larval life is passed within the pouch.

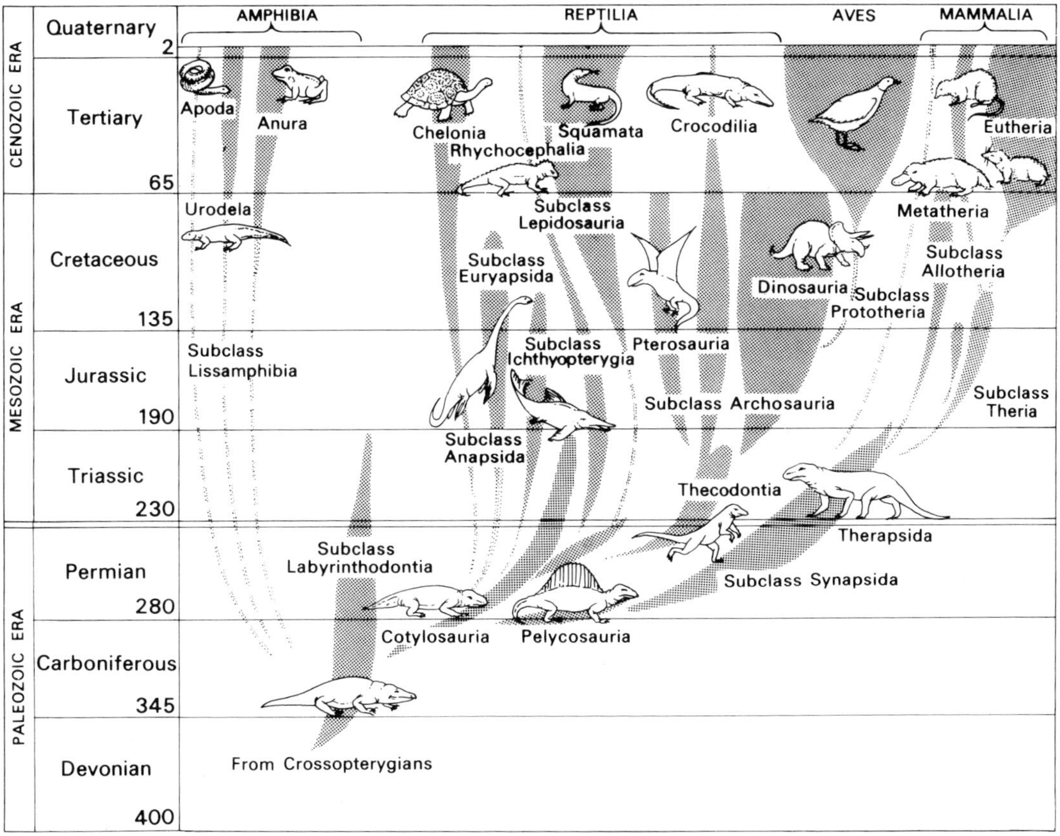

# Evolution and Adaptation of the Vertebrate Mouth

**Fig. 4.17.** A phylogeny of tetrapods. Figures in left-hand column are times in millions of years before present for the start of the period.

Adult amphibians breathe air and by using their limbs as holdfasts, they can convert their fish-like body flexure into forward locomotion over a solid medium (Fig. 4.18). These two adaptations (lungs and pentadactyl limbs) were already present or latent in rhipidistians. Other important, but less obvious, differences between the fish and amphibian structures must have developed during the change of medium. These include the adaptation of the sense organs to aerial stimuli.

### Adaptation of sense organs

NOSE (Fig. 4.19)

In elasmobranchs, the nose is a blind-ended cavity, lined by olfactory epithelium, which is evacuated and refilled by flexure of the cranium (Fig. 4.19a). In bony fishes respiration produces less flexure of the cranium so water is moved into and out of the nasal cavity largely by cilia. The

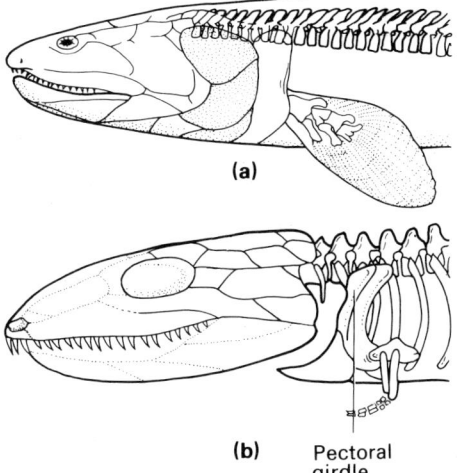

**Fig. 4.18.** Diagram of the relationship of pectoral girdle and forelimb to the skull in (a) a rhipidistian fish and (b) an early amphibian. Loss of the gills and opercular bones (stippled) freed the girdle from the skull.

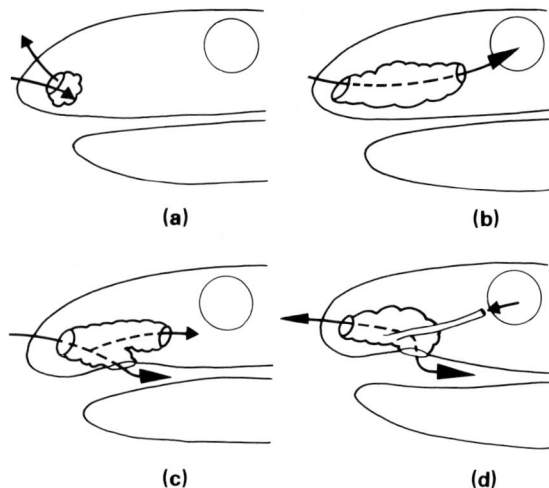

**Fig. 4.19.** The nasal passages in vertebrates: (a) elasmobranchs; (b) bony fish; (c) rhipidistian; (d) amphibian.

cavity is lengthened and its orifice divided so as to enlarge the sensory area and create a one-way passage for the olfactory current (Fig. 4.19b). In rhipidistians a new channel joined the nasal 'tube' to the oral cavity creating an internal nostril (Fig. 4.19c). Contractions of the visceral muscles, instead of cilia, now produced the olfactory current. This mechanism was perfectly adapted for aerial olfaction; since air is much less viscous than water cilia cannot induce it to flow in anything approaching the volume that can be moved by lungs or a buccal pump. The sniffing of smells involves the action of visceral muscles in all tetrapods. In the evolution of amphibians from rhipidistians the nasal passage was lengthened and became mucus-secreting so that air-borne molecules could still be dissolved in water before being sensed. The mucus also protects the delicate olfactory epithelium from desiccation.

EYE

The eye became protected from desiccation and abrasion by the development of eyelids, oil-producing glands and lacrimal glands producing a watery secretion. A lacrimal duct connecting the eye with the nasal cavity (Fig. 4.19d) serves to drain away secretions.

EAR

A fish is able to perceive pressure vibrations because they are conducted through the jaw as pressure waves to the otic capsule via the hyomandibular (Fig. 4.20a). Within the otic capsule is the sacculus, a region of the inner ear where the pressure waves are transduced to neural signals. In amphibians the pressure waves of air-borne sound cause a specialized region of the skin (tympanum) to vibrate together with a bony rod, the stapes, which is attached to the inside of the tympanum. The other end of the vibrating stapes is attached to a membrane closing the fenestra ovalis in the inner ear. Vibrations of this membrane cause pressure waves to develop in the perilymphatic fluid filling the inner ear cavity (Fig. 4.20c, d). This tympanic apparatus concentrates sound energy from a large tympanic membrane to a small stapedial footplate. The evolution of the middle ear with its stapes can now be considered.

In rhipidistians the hyomandibular is a strut which attaches the upper jaw to the otic capsule of the neurocranium (amphistylic attachment; Figs. 4.6d and 4.20a). The spiracle, the pharyngeal cleft of the hyoid arch, is a cleft in front of the hyomandibular connecting the pharynx with the outside (Fig. 4.20b). Behind the hyomandibular and attached to it by an opercular process (Fig. 4.20b) is the large opercular bone (Fig. 4.18a), a flap which covers, protects and assists operation of the underlying gills.

The (air-breathing) amphibians lose gills and the bones behind the spiracle (Fig. 4.18b). They also need to detect sound vibrations in the air. The pharyngeal cleft of the hyoid arch is expanded medially and laterally (becoming the tympanic cavity of the middle ear) to surround the hyomandibular ( = stapes). The opercular process of the hyomandibular is attached to a new structure, the tympanum, which is a sheet of tissue walling off the old spiracular cleft: the medial end of the hyomandibular attaches to a similar sheet of tissue developed in the wall of the otic capsule: the

# Evolution and Adaptation of the Vertebrate Mouth

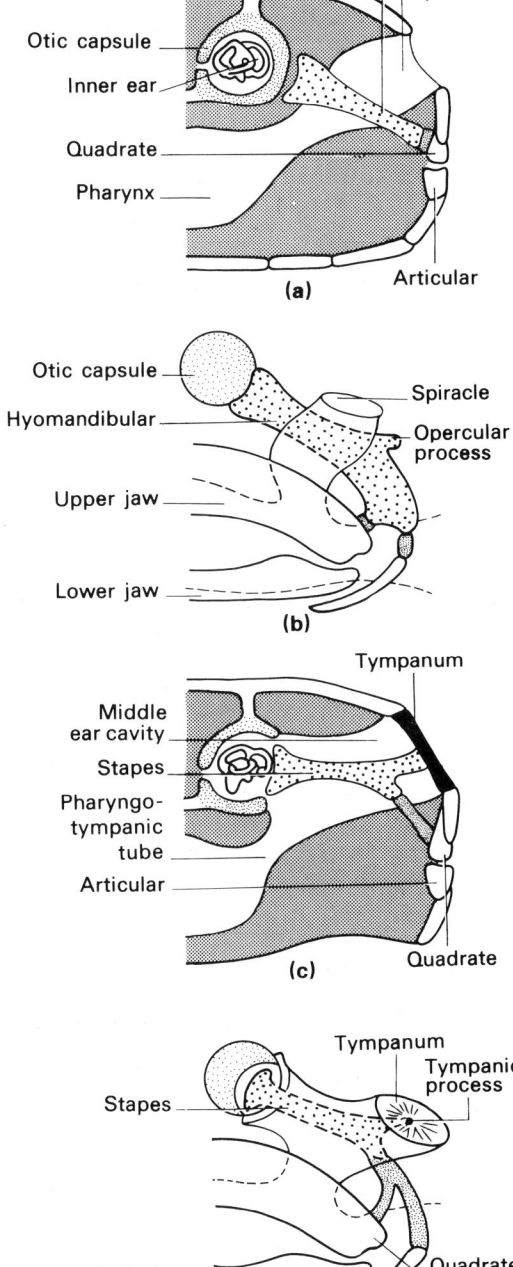

Fig. 4.20. Evolution of the amphibian middle ear. Diagrammatic rhipidistian fish: (a) in transverse section; (b) in lateral view, dermal bone not shown. Amphibian: (c) in transverse section; (d) in lateral view, dermal bone not shown.

attachment to the quadrate is retained. It can be seen that the middle ear cavity retains the same communication with the pharynx as did the spiracle. In tetrapods this is the pharyngotympanic tube.

Further changes were associated with the loss of gills. These included the incorporation of redundant parts of the branchial arch skeleton into support of the trachea and construction of a larynx.

### Dentitions of labyrinthodont amphibians

Labyrinthodonts were large (up to 10 ft) lumbering predators—the dominant animals of Carboniferous swamps. It is ironic that with this first appearance of a dense lush land vegetation (to which we owe most of our coal formations) there were no herbivorous vertebrates around to exploit it: at this time the food chain between large vertebrates and vegetation was still indirect, with fish, insects and other invertebrates as intermediates. It was not until the close of the Carboniferous that herbivorous vertebrates (some of the early reptiles) first evolved.

The labyrinthodonts inherited the simple conical teeth and alternately replaced tusks of the rhipidistians. The jaw muscles were unable to move the jaws laterally: only straight up and down movement was possible.

### Modern amphibians

ANURANS (TAILLESS AMPHIBIANS); FROGS AND TOADS (Fig. 4.17)

The many differences between larval and adult forms of both frogs and toads include those between the dentitions. Tadpoles, though not averse to feeding on a piece of raw meat in a jam jar, are naturally vegetarian. Their sucker-like mouths are equipped with numerous small keratinized teeth. During the rearrangement of the mouth and branchial arches at metamorphosis, the horny teeth are replaced by true dentine teeth on the margins of the premaxilla and maxilla and on the vomer bone in the palate. In the frog the teeth are bicuspid and are confined to the upper jaw. The lower jaw develops keratinized pads on its inner surface. Adult toads are toothless. Characteristic of tetrapods is the development of a protrusible tongue (absent in most fishes) in the floor of the pharynx from musculature of the occipital somites. The tongue is kept sticky by glandular secretions and is used by most terrestrial amphibians to catch insects which are retained by the dentition and swallowed whole.

URODELES

Tailed amphibians may be completely aquatic (mud puppies), semiterrestrial (newts), or more fully terrestrial (salamanders). Unlike the Anura, true teeth are present in both the larval and adult forms and are usually present on both the upper and lower jaws.

## REPTILES

Reptiles became the first fully terrestrial vertebrates being emancipated from water by developing the amniotic egg. The egg is fertilized internally and the zygote develops in a bath of watery fluid contained by an extraembryonic membrane—the amnion. In reptiles and birds, the large egg yolk contains sufficient food reserves for complete embryogenesis together with a further water supply, the egg white. An intermediate larval form, with its own special requirements such as a feeding apparatus is not required. The amniote embryo is protected from damage and desiccation by further membranes and a leathery or calcareous shell. In mammals, the egg is not self-supporting and has such a small yolk that the embryo must be fed by the mother via the tissues of her reproductive tract (viviparity). Since they are difficult to define by any other single characteristic, it can be said that reptiles are those amniotes which are neither birds nor mammals.

Armed with this new egg which protects the delicate embryo both from desiccation and, to some degree, from predation, the reptiles radiated rapidly into the terrestrial environment of the Permian period (Fig. 4.17) subdividing it through the Mesozoic era into finer and finer niches; they were so successful that they dominated the land for over 200 million years. Some lines of descent (pterosaurs and, later, birds) entered a new adaptive zone, the air, whilst others (e.g. turtles and ichthyosaurs) returned to the sea where their advanced specification gave them a measure of success over the established inhabitants.

Both the evolution and classification of reptiles are marked by differences in the pattern of skull fenestration (the 'windows' in dermal roofing bones of the skull (Fig. 4.21) through which emerge the jaw adductor muscles allowing them to be attached to both inner and outer surfaces of the skull bones). Initially, these modifications provided an increased area for the attachment of the

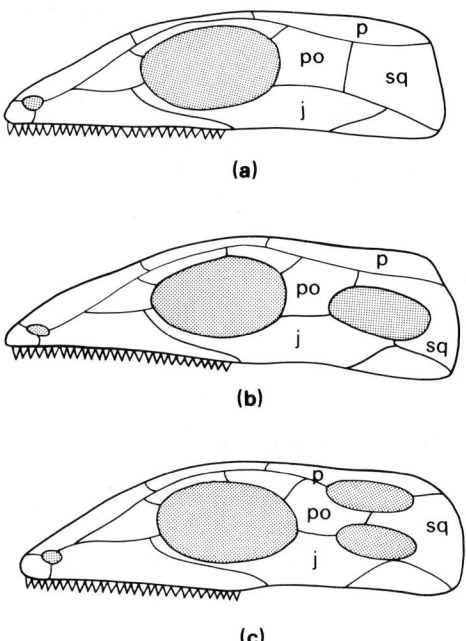

Fig. 4.21. Diagram to illustrate the patterns of skull fenestration in reptiles: (a) anapsid type (stem reptiles, chelonians); (b) synapsid type (mammal-like reptiles); (c) diapsid type (archosaurs and lepidosaurs).

muscle fibres. In one group (the mammal-like reptiles or synapsids) the skull opening enlarged to such an extent that the muscle mass was almost entirely attached on the outside surfaces of the skull bones. In this position they were able to differentiate into components with very different sites of attachment and directions of pull (Figs. 4.21b and c, and 4.22).

**Anapsid reptiles (skull roof lacking fenestration) (Fig. 4.21a)**

The first reptiles (from upper Carboniferous deposits) had a complete skull roof inherited with little modification from their labyrinthodont ancestors. These stem reptiles had an inextensive radiation before being largely replaced by their more efficient descendants, the order Synapsida. Perhaps the most significant feature of their short-lived radiation was the first evolution of herbivorous land vertebrates. These had laterally expanded, multicuspid cheek teeth capable of dealing with vegetation. Carnivorous members of this group were smaller and usually possessed a marginal dentition of conical teeth. In some forms, the appearance of one or more larger killing teeth towards the anterior end of the jaw can be viewed

# Evolution and Adaptation of the Vertebrate Mouth

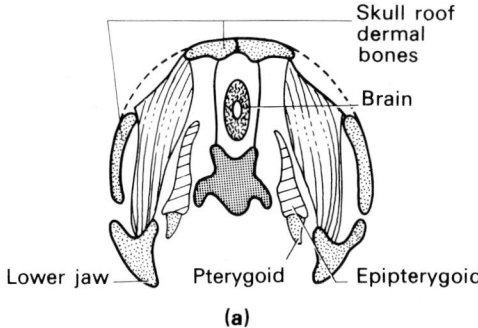

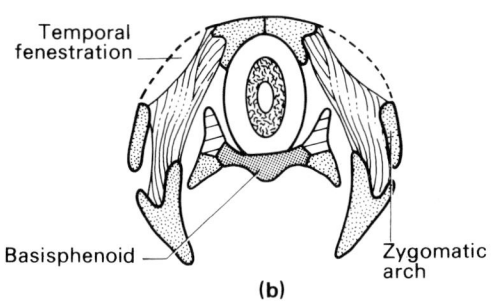

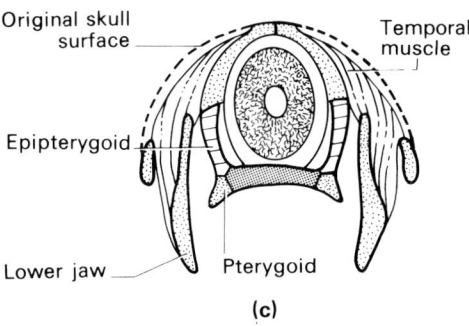

**Fig. 4.22.** Diagrammatic transverse sections of the skull and jaws of (a) a primitive synapsid reptile (pelycosaur), (b) an advanced synapsid reptile (therapsid) and (c) a mammal. Part of the lateral walls of the cranium were originally membraneous (a). The expanding brain later became protected by a downgrowth of the roofing bones and incorporation of a spur (epipterygoid) from the palate to form a complete bony box for the brain. In mammals the epipterygoid is known as the alisphenoid and in man as the greater wing of the sphenoid (b, c). By this process the lower jaw adductors, originally inside the cranial roof (a), come to lie outside it in the zygomatic arch (jugal = zygomatic and squamosal bones). The primary upper jaw (epipterygoid, pterygoid) was originally separate from the cranium (a) but became immovably attached to it (b). (See Romer.)

as one of the first steps towards heterodonty; i.e. differentiation between the sizes and shapes of teeth along the row in relation to different functions.

Present-day survivors of the anapsid reptile stock are the tortoises and turtles (Chelonia). With the passage of 300 million years, chelonians have departed widely from their anapsid ancestors. They are edentulous: the jaw bones support a sharp-edged horny beak which has become an efficient functional equivalent of teeth in several animals (e.g. birds).

**Diapsid reptiles** (Fig. 4.21c)

With the exception of the Chelonia all modern reptiles (lizards, snakes and crocodiles) have, or have had in their evolutionary history, two skull roof fenestrations. The crocodile is the closest living reptilian relative of the Dinosaurs and, together with a few other mesozoic reptile types, they are placed in the subclass Archosauria (ruling reptiles). The remaining diapsids form the subclass Lepidosauria (scaly reptiles).

LEPIDOSAURS

The most primitive living lepidosaurs, and incidentally, the only one to retain a complete diapsid skull with two arches (Fig. 4.23a) is the New Zealand *Sphenodon*. In other respects also the sphenodon retains a very early level of lepidosaur structure especially the skeleton, joints and musculature.

The dentition of *Sphenodon* is specialized. The hook-shaped premaxilla supports large conical tusks; the dentary bears a single row of small conical teeth which, by anteroposterior jaw movements, slice between two rows of upper teeth, one on the maxilla, one on the palatine; an advanced jaw mechanism for an otherwise primitive reptile.

In Squamata (lizards and snakes) the continuity of the lower temporal arch of the primitive diapsid skull has been broken (Fig. 4.23b). The quadrate bones, robust pillars which support the posterolateral corners of the skull are the dorsal components of the jaw joint and have become more extensively movable following loss of the quadratojugal and support from the jugal. The hinged joints (quadrate, pterygoid, maxilla, etc., Fig. 4.24a) constituting a streptostylic skull are found in many lizards. When a protractor muscle contracts the quadrate swings forwards and the muzzle is raised. This greatly increases the gape. In many lizards the streptostylic quadrate forms the

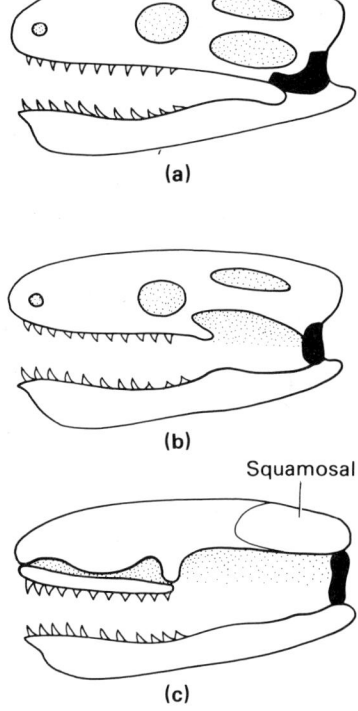

**Fig. 4.23.** Diagram to show the progressive loss of the temporal arches and increase in freedom of the quadrate in diapsid reptiles: (a) *Sphenodon*; (b) a lizard; (c) a snake. (Quadrate in black.)

basis of a kinetic chain (Fig. 4.24a), by means of which the upper jaw can be raised in relation to the braincase.

In an extinct group of marine lizards, the mosasaurs, the gape was even further increased by the development of a fibrous joint midway along the lower jaw.

Lizards usually have homodont dentitions consisting of conical teeth but some unusual variations exist. For example, *Iguana* has serrated teeth which are used to slice vegetation into swallowable chunks. *Heloderma* (the Ghila monster of Central America) has specialized venom teeth whose labial walls are infolded to make a canal for injecting venom. Several forms, such as *Callopistes*, have pointed anterior teeth and rounded posterior teeth; a simple form of heterodonty. The dentitions are usually polyphyodont although many species with acrodont dentitions (Fig. 7.4b) do not replace their teeth after the adult stage is reached, (e.g. agamids, chameleons).

Snakes have taken streptostylic kinetism a stage further than lizards. Both lower and upper tem-

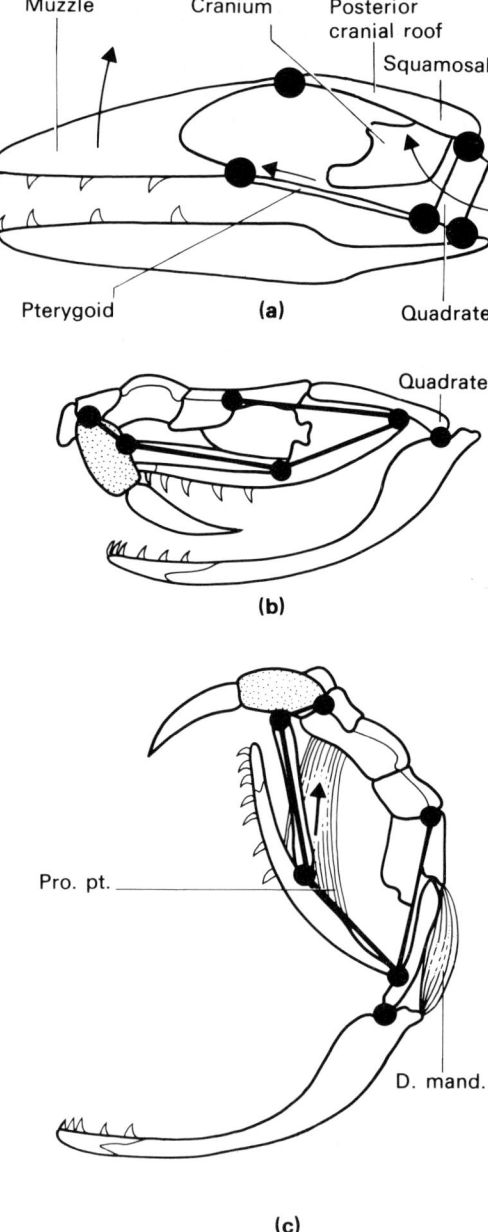

**Fig. 4.24.** Diagram to show mechanism of streptostylic skulls. (a) Simple streptostylic skull of a lizard. Rotation of the quadrate about its hinge joint with the squamosal (arrowed) pushing the pterygoid strut forward in relation to the cranium which in turn causes the muzzle to hinge up in relation to the posterior cranial roof and cranium. The position of the hinge joints are shown by black dots.
(b) Specialized streptostyly of venomous snakes. The skull elements form a kinetic chain whereby opening the jaws causes the maxillae to be rotated and their attached fangs erected into the strike position (c).

poral arches are lost, leaving the quadrate only loosely attached to the rest of the skull by its dorsal joint with the squamosal (Fig. 4.23c). The greatly increased mobility of the quadrate allows the mouth to be considerably broadened in the region of the jaw joints so that large prey can be swallowed whole. A distensible mental 'symphysis', which consists only of ligaments, allows the two lower jaw halves to be pulled apart as the mouth cavity expands. Venomous snakes (e.g. vipers and cobras) catch and immobilize their prey, prior to swallowing, by injecting a haemolytic or neurotoxic venom secreted by a specialized maxillary gland. The long maxillary teeth or fangs are erectile in most species and lie folded back along the roof of the mouth when not in use (Fig. 4.24b). The marginal bones of the skull (pterygoid, palatine and ectopterygoid) are only loosely attached to the cranial bones and act as push-pull levers to rotate the maxilla. Simultaneous contraction of the protractor, pterygoid and depressor mandibulae muscles causes the mouth to be opened and the fangs erected (Fig. 4.24c). Venom is injected into the prey through a mesial groove in each fang: in vipers, this groove is very deep and the free edges fuse across to form an enclosed tube whose opening is subterminal, as in a hypodermic needle (Fig. 4.25).

Additional specializations of venomous snakes include the extremely sensitive infrared detectors of pit-vipers, by which they locate the warm bodies of mammal and birds.

Non-poisonous snakes are generally egg-eating or constricting. The fangless dentition (e.g. *Python*, Fig. 10.2) consists of many very sharp recurved teeth attached to nearly all the bones in the mouth. The skull is extensively kinetic allowing the upper and lower jaws to 'climb' around large prey objects. *Dasypeltis* feeds exclusively on birds' eggs and has a reduced dentition. The egg is swallowed entire, greatly distending the oesophagus; the latter is contracted, pushing the egg against a much enlarged process of a neck vertebra which extends through the gut wall. This cracks the shell, the egg contents are swallowed and the shell is regurgitated.

In snakes the ear is degenerate with the tympanic membrane, middle ear cavity and eustachian tube failing to develop. However, the stapes remains articulated between the inner ear and quadrate. Snakes hear by bone conduction through the head and also through the body via the vertebrae and lungs which act as an amplifier.

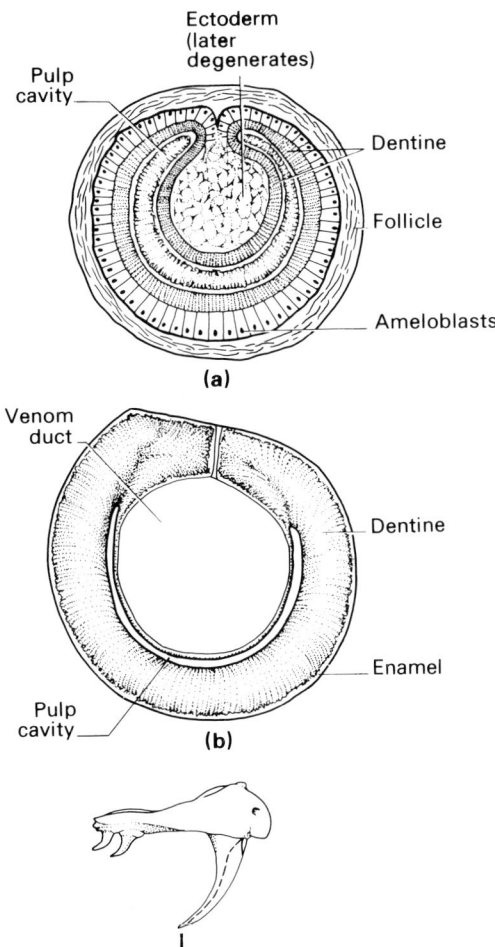

Fig. 4.25. Venom fangs of snakes. (a) Development of the viper fang; transverse section prior to closure of tube. (b) Transverse section of fully developed fang of a rattlesnake (c) Lateral view of fang and venom duct of a cobra (note the sub-terminal opening of the duct).

ARCHOSAURS (Fig. 4.17)

The great reptilian radiation which replaced the synapsid (mammal-like) reptiles as dominant land vertebrates and suppressed the mammals into an insignificant ecological position, took place during the Triassic period with the evolution of various diapsid types (Fig. 4.21c). Thecodonts, crocodiles, pterosaurs and dinosaurs flourished through the Mesozoic era—the 'Age of Dinosaurs'. Of these many forms only the crocodiles are still extant.

The earliest archosaurs were fast-running bipeds (probably the key to their success over the slower quadrupedal mammal-like reptiles) but the crocodiles specialized for a semi-aquatic existence which returned them to a short-limbed quadrupedal body form. The very strong flattened tail, dorsal positioning of the eyes, and closeable nostrils are all aquatic modifications. The nasal cavity is separated from the mouth cavity by ingrown and fused palatal folds (of premaxilla, maxilla and palatine bones) which form a hard palate extending right to the back of the mouth. The development of a secondary palate in crocodiles is an example of convergent adaptation; both the crocodiles and the mammals have evolved the same structure independently after their divergence from the common ancestor (in this case a Carboniferous Anapsid). The selective advantage of a structure need not be, and indeed often is not, the same in two groups, except in the most general terms: the palate in crocodiles and mammals separates the air-way and food-way. In crocodiles it seems to be a directly aquatic adaptation allowing the mouth to be opened under water.

In mammals, the secondary palate originally evolved in association with mastication. First, it protected the sensitive nasal mucosa and delicate turbinate bones from ingested food. Second, by completing a 'box' section through the snout it greatly strengthened the support of the upper cheek teeth. Finally, it later enabled the animal to breathe through the now isolated nasal passages while it chewed or suckled. For this last function it can be viewed as a 'pre-adaptation'; the secondary palate developed before suckling evolved.

Teeth of crocodiles (and most archosaurs) differ from lepidosaurs in having a gomphosis (thecodont attachment). Since they do not occlude their teeth, the significance of this flexible 'independent tooth suspension' in crocodiles is obscure. The teeth are invariably conical with replacement teeth developing in small niches at the base of the alveoli. *Alligator* is an American crocodilian which is distinguishable from other crocodiles because the upper teeth overlap the lowers. In *Crocodylus* the upper and lower teeth interlock.

DINOSAURS

The dinosaurs were extraordinarily successful creatures, who dominated the earth for over 130 million years (the whole of the Jurassic and Cretaceous periods), radiating and adapting to ecological niches whose diversity has been equalled only by the mammals. Since all we know of dinosaurs is their apparently reptile-like bones and teeth, palaeontologists have customarily dressed them in reptilian clothing; that is to say they are conventionally reconstructed as lumbering cold-blooded creatures with sprawling posture, low metabolic rate and all the slow, heavy, and unmanageable characteristics that have come to be associated with their name. In truth, however, not all dinosaurs were giants. Some were small, lightly built, agile creatures not unlike flightless birds. Indeed the ancestry of the birds has been found among some small dinosaurs of the Jurassic (Fig. 4.17). Furthermore an often overlooked, but indisputable, fact is that the dinosaurs as a group totally eclipsed the mammals during the whole of their long history. Some modern palaeontologists have questioned the 'reptilian prejudice' underlying the more conventional dinosaur reconstructions and have started to look more closely at the evidence presented by the bones and teeth and the formative environments of the sedimentary rocks in which they are found. Researchers have been able to demonstrate that the limbs of even the largest dinosaurs were in fact constructed for an erect (not sprawling) posture and gait. Furthermore, some suppose that the dinosaurs were endothermic and maintained a high constant body temperature. The evolution of bird characteristics (e.g. insulation, increased brain size, care of the young, separation of pulmonary and systemic circulations) is thought to have preceded the origin of birds, and to have been the common property of many small carnivorous dinosaurs of the Jurassic. While these (and the birds) remained oviparous, a number of other forms had probably evolved viviparity as a means of overcoming the limitations, especially of size, imposed by egg laying.

It seems possible that the dinosaurs had evolved far from what we understand as a reptilian physiology: perhaps as far as have the mammals and birds. Some workers emphasize that dinosaurs differ so much from modern reptiles that they warrant a separate class status (Dinosauria) just as much as do Aves and Mammalia.

Accepting current classification, the informal name 'dinosaur' describes two diapsid reptile orders; the Saurischia and Ornithischia.

*Saurischian dinosaurs*
The predatory nature of *Tyrannosaurus* is clearly expressed by its powerful jaws and formidable dentition of recurved dagger-like teeth. It was the last of a long evolutionary line of bipedal carnivores; the ultimate both in size (30 ft long) and specialization, i.e. structures such as the jaws and teeth were accentuated whereas others were reduced, e.g. the apparently functionless forelimb (Fig. 4.26a). The dentition was adapted for killing and seizing prey but not for chewing.

# Evolution and Adaptation of the Vertebrate Mouth

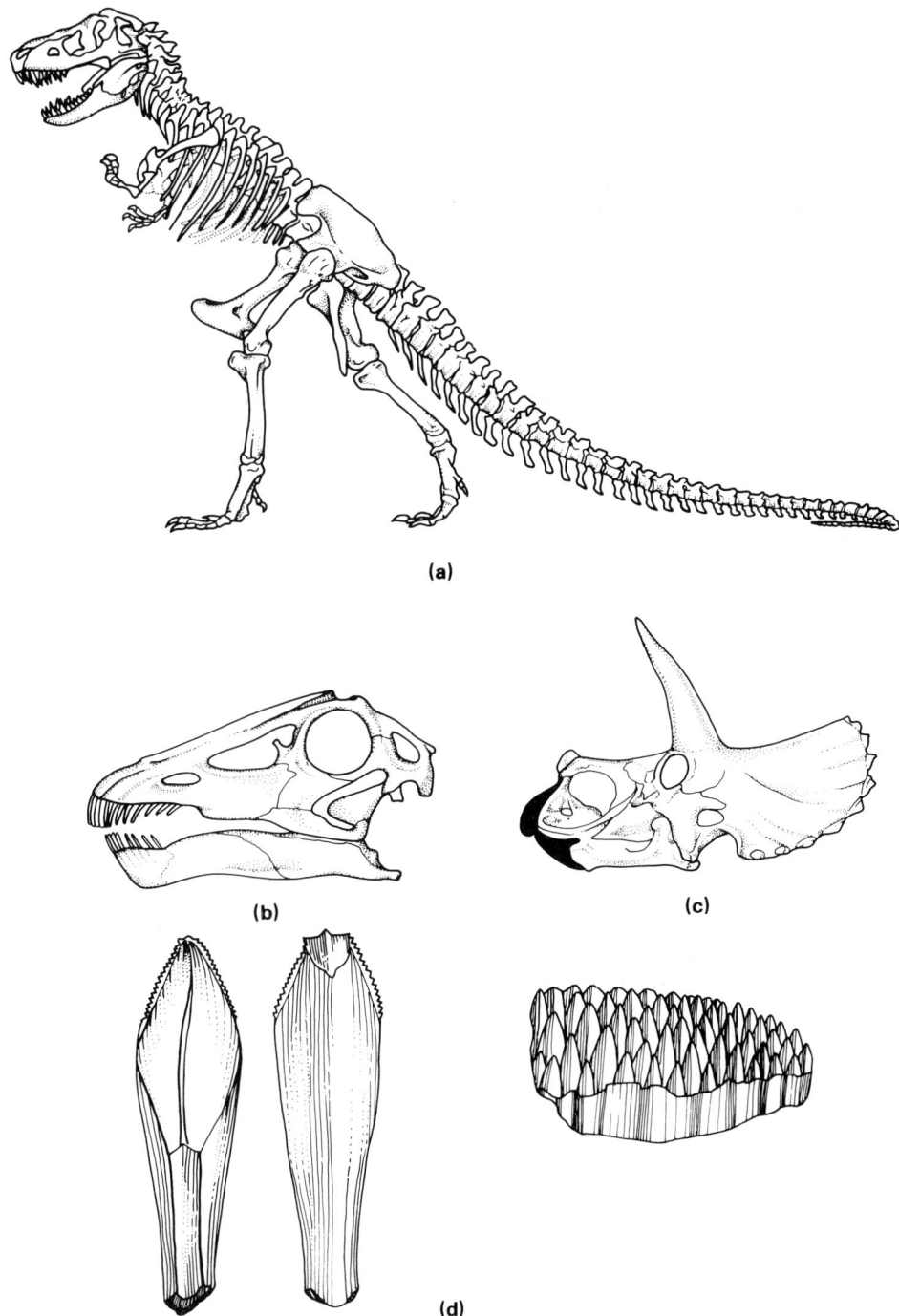

**Fig. 4.26.** Dinosaurs. (a) *Tyrannosaurus*, a large Saurischian carnivore. (b) Skull of *Brontosaurus*, a giant quadrupedal, herbivorous saurischian. (c) Skull of a quadrupedal, ornithischian (*Triceratops*). The rostral and predentary bones (black) were probably covered by a horny beak. (d) Isolated teeth (left) and tooth battery (right) of the ornithischian dinosaur, *Anatosaurus*.

Herbivorous saurischians were the largest ever land animals, reaching lengths of up to 90 ft. Although characterized as sluggish semiaquatic creatures who could not carry their own weight on land, it is possible that they were the adaptive equivalent of elephants; not only fully terrestrial but also able to move about at a fair speed. A more appropriate description might be 'elephantine giraffe' since their long necks would have allowed them to eat tree-top foliage. Their dentitions were very weak, their skulls and jaw musculature small (Fig. 4.26b). Usually there were only a few slender teeth in each quadrant situated at the front of the jaw in the position of 'cropping' incisors. With this feeble equipment it is hard to understand how *Brontosaurus* could process sufficient food to develop, or even maintain, its enormous bulk. One answer may be the stones (gastroliths) that are sometimes found within the ribcages of the fossils; these could have been used for 'ball-mill mastication' as in the gizzard of birds. Another animal which swallows stones is the crocodile; here the gastroliths seem to have the additional function of ballast, keeping the approximately cylindrical body submerged on an even keel in the water.

*Ornithischian dinosaurs*
The entirely herbivorous Ornithischia differ from the Saurischia not only in the bird-like structure of the pelvis (from which their name derives) but also in the presence of a median predentary bone in the lower jaw. The predentary was often serrated and cropped against a toothless premaxilla; both were presumably covered by a horny beak (Fig. 4.26c). Behind these, on the maxilla and dentary, were rows of crenulated cheek teeth which, in some advanced forms, developed a very efficient grinding occlusion. In the hadrosaurs of the Upper Cretaceous, for example, the cheek teeth were arranged in parallel banks, several rows deep, so that as many as 700 could have been functional at any one time (Fig. 4.26d). The functions of the elaborate cusps and crests in a single mammalian tooth are undertaken here by a close-packed multiplicity of single-cusped teeth. Other ornithiscians, the ceratopsians (e.g. *Triceratops*, an adaptive equivalent of *Rhinoceros*), had only one or a few parallel rows of cheek teeth but in these a very high replacement rate compensated for wear. The dinosaurs became extinct towards the end of the Cretaceous, for reasons that are as yet unknown, leaving only the birds as their direct descendants.

**Marine reptiles** (Fig. 4.17)
Several groups of early reptiles, directly descended from land-living forms, had a successful evolution in the seas of the Mesozoic era. These include the diapsid mosasaurs and two groups possessing a single high temporal fenestration—ichthyosaurs and plesiosaurs. The ichthyosaurs are particularly interesting because they achieved an extreme aquatic specialization; reducing their pentadactyl limbs to stabilizing fins and developing a dorsal fin and a strong, vertically fluked, caudal fin. In brief they evolved a totally piscine appearance and capability. Dolphins have specialized in a similar way (convergent evolution); their similarities extend to the shape of the skull and form of the dentition.

## BIRDS

The earliest bird species is *Archaeopteryx* from the Upper Jurassic. *Archaeopteryx* was a lightweight carnivorous dinosaur with feathered arms; however, it had diverged markedly from its terrestrial or arboreal forebears by evolving a larger brain with an expanded cranium and a consequent reduction of the temporal bars. The long narrow jaws bore single rows of conical teeth. In modern birds, all that remains of the ancestral reptilian dermal roof is the lower temporal bar (jugal and quadratojugal). Above this, a single large fossa (the upper bar is lost) communicates with the orbit. In many modern birds the skull is highly kinetic (Fig. 4.27); the anterior part is joined to the brain case by a flexible lamina of bone in the naso-frontal region. The upper jaw is rotated upwards on the cranium when the lower jaw is depressed, since rotation of the quadrate transmits forward thrust to the maxilla through the pterygoids and the quadratojugal-jugal bar. However, unlike the lizard, the upper and lower jaws are linked by an inextensible postorbital ligament between the cranium and lower jaw; this allows the mouth to be kept shut with little muscular exertion—since the lower jaw cannot fall without the upper jaw being raised. The jaw muscles are large only in birds of prey. Birds have no teeth (except the caruncle, or hatching tooth which is a horny false tooth used to break open the egg); some of their functions are taken over by a horny beak, ensheathing upper and lower jaws, whose size and shape varies with different feeding habits. Some birds use tools, such as a cactus-spine to extract insects from beneath the bark of a tree; others crack hard-shelled food by beating it against a stone. Food is predigested by maceration in the crop followed by 'ball-mill' crushing in the muscular grit-containing gizzard. These structures, particularly well-developed in

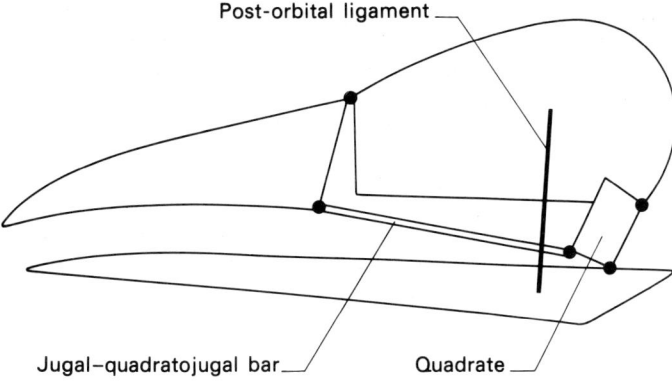

Fig. 4.27. The kinetic skull of a bird. (For explanation see text.)

grain-feeders, are poorly developed in carnivores whose sharp beaks can adequately prepare their food.

## SYNAPSID REPTILES (MAMMAL-LIKE REPTILES)

During the Permian and Triassic periods, before the emergence of dinosaurs, synapsid reptiles were the major vertebrate land fauna (Fig. 4.17). In the various synapsid types are seen gradual and 'progressive' adaptations in parallel 'towards' the mammalian level. The dentary bone of the lower jaw increased in size and took over the attachment areas of the jaw adductor muscles while the postdentary bones became correspondingly reduced in size as they assumed an increasingly important role in hearing as well as jaw articulation. These developments (together with a reduction in the numbers of generations of teeth, an increase in heterodonty and many other characteristics that can be taken as evidence of improved mastication) evolved in those several lines of descent which, at the close of the Triassic, crossed the boundary which distinguishes reptile from mammal. Mammals are somewhat arbitrarily defined as that group of vertebrates having a squamosal-dentary (=temporomandibular) jaw joint (cf. quadrate-articular of reptiles) and a three-bone middle ear (cf. one bone of reptiles). By this definition, the fossil record shows that the class Mammalia includes descendants of more than one evolutionary line. Mammals must therefore constitute a class of multiple (polyphyletic) origin.

### Jaw articulation and middle ear apparatus of mammals and reptiles

In all mammals the lower jaw consists of a single element, the dentary. Anteriorly it bears the teeth, posteriorly it develops an ascending ramus with a coronoid, angular and articular process (the mandibular condyle). These three processes of the dentary have the same names as the separate individual bones which occupied the equivalent positions in the reptile jaw (Fig. 4.28). Of the reptile postdentary bones, the splenial, coronoid and surangular have disappeared (they have no homologue in mammals); while the positions and functions of the articular (plus prearticular) and angular have been changed, just like those of the quadrate of the upper jaw.

In non-mammals the lower jaw articulates with the upper jaw by the quadrate–articular joint, the concave surface of the articular bone fitting around a convexity of the quadrate. The quadrate lies at the posterior corner of the skull at the end of a series of bones (premaxilla, maxilla, pterygoid jugal, quadratojugal, quadrate) along the upper jaw. A single auditory ossicle, the stapes (known as the columella auris in reptiles), has two outwardly directed processes; one braced against the quadrate, the other being attached to the tympanum (Fig. 4.20). The inner end of the stapes fits into the fenestra ovalis of the otic capsule.

In mammals the condyle of the lower jaw articulates with a fossa in the squamosal bone (= squamous temporal of man). The stapes has a single outwardly directed process articulating with the incus (quadrate) which in turn articulates with the malleus (= articular). The malleus is attached to the tympanum by a lever arm, the manubrium mallei. The incus and malleus are separate from the jaw and skull but remain articulated with each other, being intercalated between the stapes and the tympanic membrane as a part of the vibration–transmission mechanism of the middle ear. A third bone, the angular bone of a reptile, has also lost its connection with the lower jaw and is instead fused with the skull in mammals. It supports the membranous tym-

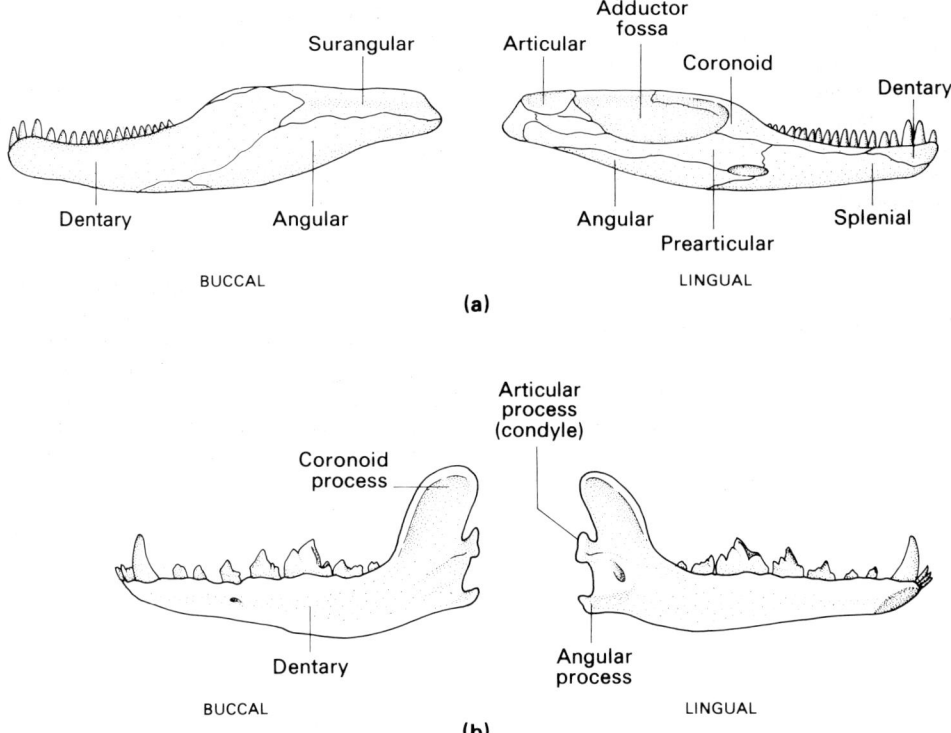

**Fig. 4.28.** Lower jaw of (a) a primitive reptile and (b) a recent mammal.

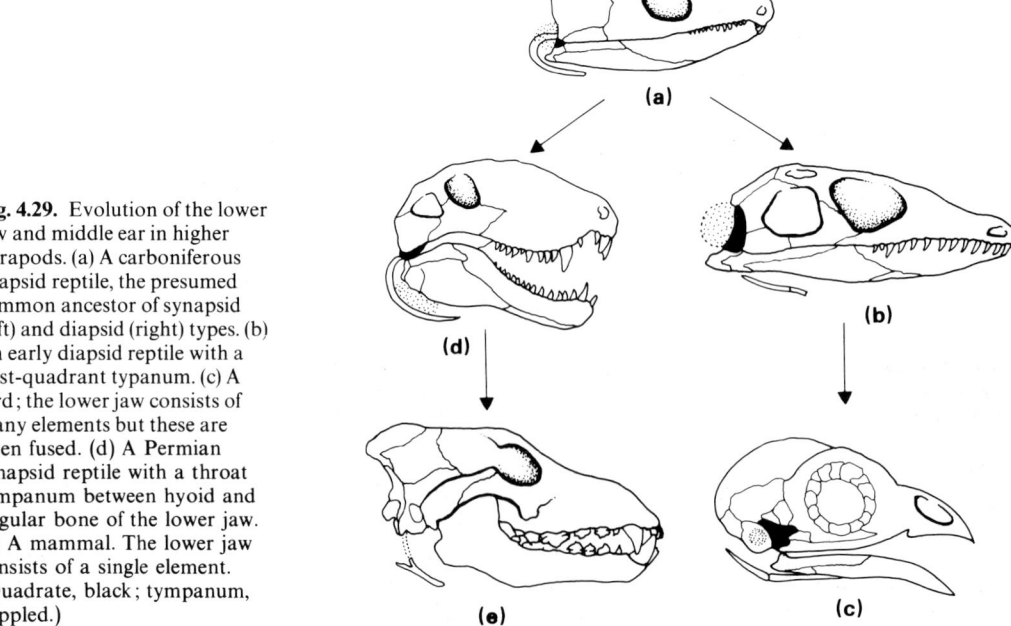

**Fig. 4.29.** Evolution of the lower jaw and middle ear in higher tetrapods. (a) A carboniferous anapsid reptile, the presumed common ancestor of synapsid (left) and diapsid (right) types. (b) An early diapsid reptile with a post-quadrant typanum. (c) A bird; the lower jaw consists of many elements but these are often fused. (d) A Permian synapsid reptile with a throat tympanum between hyoid and angular bone of the lower jaw. (e) A mammal. The lower jaw consists of a single element. (Quadrate, black; tympanum, stippled.)

panum and in most mammals it is known as the tympanic bone. In man it has become a part of the (composite) temporal bone although it still develops from separate dermal ossification centres.

The articulating chain consisting of three bones, stapes–incus–malleus, is present in both recent reptiles and mammals but the function is entirely different. In the former it is a jaw joint, in the latter a 'hearing aid'.

## Evolution of the mammalian jaw joint and middle ear

To understand the evolution of the mammalian middle ear it is important to note that the tympani of recent amphibians, reptiles and mammals are not homologous. Each type has evolved independently and in a different position in each line. In other words the common ancestor of diapsid reptiles (the basal stock of modern reptiles) and synapsid reptiles (the basal stock of mammals) either had no tympanum at all or had developed a simple middle ear apparatus which subsequently became improved in two quite different ways. (Fig. 4.29)

In diapsid reptiles (Fig. 4.29b) and their descendants, the birds (Fig. 4.29c), the tympanum developed behind (and was supported by) the quadrate. In mammal-like reptiles, the tympanum formed on the lower jaw, lateral to the articular, and was supported in this position by the angular and hyoid bones. (Fig. 4.29d) The reasons for this difference of strategy was probably to do with the relative sizes and postures of the two types of reptiles; the mammal-like reptiles evidently found an advantage in keeping an 'ear to the ground'. Initially, in the earlier mammal-like reptiles (Fig. 4.30a) the hyoid bone would have transmitted tympanic vibrations directly to the stapes and inner ear, but in later forms of mammal-like reptile (Fig. 4.30b, c) the hyoid bone transmission route decreased in importance as tympanic vibrations were transmitted through the jaw joint bones to the stapes. The small quadrate was streptostylic (attached moveably to the skull) and the

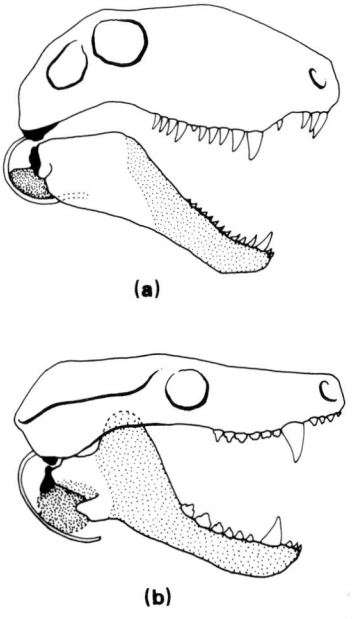

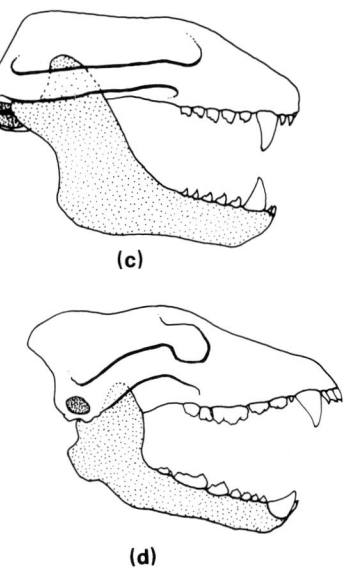

Fig. 4.30. Jaw and ear evolution in mammals. (a) *Dimetrodon*, a Lower Permian mammal-like reptile; a tympanum (heavy stipple) is situated on the posteroinferior border of the mandible. Vibrations were transmitted to the stapes by the articular-quadrate jaw joint (black) and by the hyoid. (b) *Thrinaxodon*, a Lower Triassic mammal-like reptile; the tympanum is supported additionally by a reflected lamina of the angular (=tympanic) bone. The dentary is enlarged and the post-dentary bones are reduced in size. (c) Late Triassic mammal-like reptile; two jaw joints operate side by side, the medial one (quadrate-articular) also transmitting vibrations from the tympanum which is still attached to the lower jaw by the angular (=tympanic). The hyoid is no longer a vibration transmitter. (d) Mammal; one jaw joint (squamosal-dentary) and the tympanic bone together with the tympanum is fused to the skull rather than to the lower jaw. The quadrate (=incus) and articular (=malleus) have no jaw joint function in the adult. The lower jaw consists of a single bone (dentary).

articular–angular complex was only loosely attached to the adjacent postdentary bones; quadrate and articular could both articulate the jaw and transmit vibrations of the tympanum to the inner ear The evolutionary advantage of subsequently separating the quadrate, articular and angular ossicles from the jaws was the reduction in ligamentous and muscular impedance which previously limited the sensitivity or frequency response of the middle ear. The progressive diminution of the postdentary bones in mammal-like reptiles, was an essential prerequisite of this separation. The selective advantage for each increment of size reduction must have been the improved hearing which resulted from decreased mass and inertia of the transmission elements. As the postdentary bones decreased in size and loosened their attachment to the tooth-bearing dentary bone (stippled in Fig. 4.30), the jaw joint became increasingly weakened. However, the dentary had increased in size proportional to the diminution of the postdentary bones and had taken over the attachment areas of the jaw musculature: also, the temporal fenestration had increased to such an extent that the dorsal attachment of the jaw musculature now spread over a much larger area. (Fig. 4.22)

Differentiation of the single reptilian adductor muscle into separate units (temporalis, masseters and pterygoids) with different directions of pull effectively reduced the masticatory loading of this weakened jaw joint (Fig. 10.3).

The most remarkable aspect of the change in which the bones of the old jaw joint moved with the ear is not that it occurred at all but that it evolved without interrupting either jaw movement or hearing. Although the quadrate and articular became separated from the skull there was never a time when the lower jaw had no articulation with the upper; before this separation took place, the dentary had already established contact with the squamosal close to the pre-existing jaw joint. Advanced mammal-like reptiles with four jaw articulations (two on each side) are well known from the fossil record of the Upper Triassic (Fig. 4.30c).

Although clearly the result of selection for improved hearing, further advantages were gained from the reorganization of the musculature: there was a great increase in bite force across the postcanine teeth and, more important still, the varied musculature could produce side to side movements of the lower jaw. Chewing was finally possible.

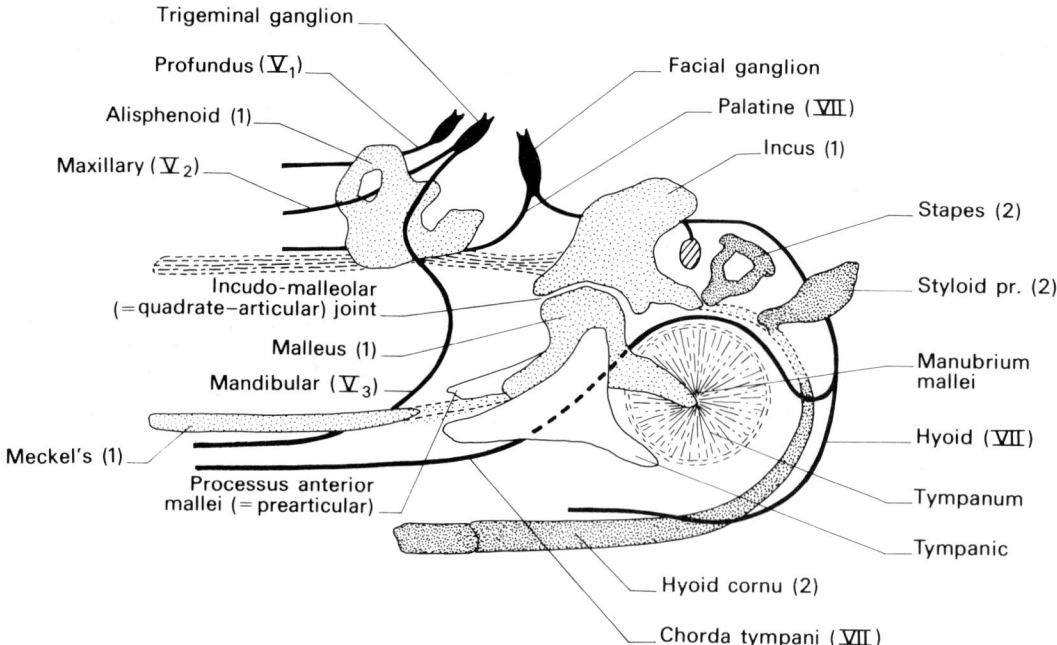

Fig. 4.31. Diagram of the disposition in lateral view of first and second arch cartilages and their relationship to the dorsal root cranial nerves (black) in a mammal embryo. Cartilage, degenerating cartilage or non-chondrifying arch mesenchyme, stippled. The alisphenoid (=greater wing of sphenoid) and incus cartilages are all that remain in a mammal of the primary upper jaw (palato-pterygo-quadrate bar).

# Evolution and Adaptation of the Vertebrate Mouth

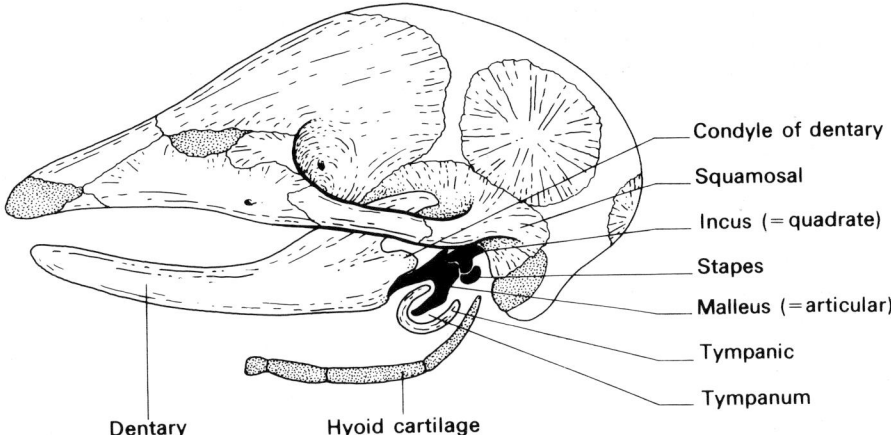

**Fig. 4.32.** Skull of an embryo mammal at a stage when the jaws are articulated by the primary (incudomalleolar) jaw joint. Presumptive auditory ossicle cartilage, black; other cartilage, stippled; dermal bones, lined.

## Ontogeny of the mammalian jaw apparatus
(Figs. 4.31 and 4.32)

Although the sequence of changes which occur in embryological development does not exactly repeat their sequence of evolutionary appearance, the ontogeny of the mammalian jaw apparatus broadly confirms the findings of palaeontology. Namely that, early in development, Meckel's cartilage and the quadrate cartilage form the posterior ends of the developing upper and lower jaws; their articulation together constitutes the first or primary joint between the jaws. As development proceeds the posterior end of Meckel's cartilage ossifies as the malleus, parts of its fibrous sheath persist as the anterior ligament of the malleus and the sphenomandibular ligament, and the remainder is almost completely removed. The dentary (a dermal bone whose growth is supplemented in modern mammals by a secondary growth cartilage) grows back and develops an articular process (condyle). A similar sequence of events is seen in the upper jaw, involving the quadrate cartilage (incus) and a dermal ossification (the squamosal).

Finally a joint forms between the dentary and squamosal bones. For a brief period there are two jaw joints on either side, incudomalleolar and squamodentary. Thereafter the former bones became isolated within the middle ear cavity just posterior to the squamodentary jaw joint. Meanwhile the tympanic bone, which first appears in the mesenchyme of the mandibular process just lateral to the posterior end of Meckel's cartilage, becomes attached to the skull.

## FURTHER READING

ALLIN E.F. (1975) Evolution of the mammalian middle ear. *Journal of Morphology* **147**, 403.
GOODRICH E.S. (1930) *Studies on the Structure and Development of Vertebrates.* London: Macmillan.
ROMER A.S. (1971) *The Vertebrate Body*, 4th Edition. Philadelphia: W. B. Saunders.
ROMER A.S. (1966) *Vertebrate Palaeontology*, 3rd Edition. Chicago: Chicago University Press.
STAHL B.J. (1974) *Vertebrate History: Problems in evolution.* New York: McGraw-Hill.

# CHAPTER 5

# Tooth Morphology

Although it is easy to understand what a tooth is, it is difficult to construct a strict definition. This is due to a great diversity in the structure and function of teeth found in vertebrates. For a human tooth, a suitable definition might be—a hard body in the mouth, attached to, but not forming part of the jaws, which is primarily concerned with the comminution of food.

The basic form and constituent tissues of a human tooth are shown in Fig. 5.1. The human tooth, like most mammalian teeth, is composed of three quite different types of hard tissue, enamel, dentine and cement. It is the dentine which forms the bulk of the tooth. The anatomical crown of the tooth is covered by enamel. The junction between enamel and dentine is the amelodentinal (enamel/dentine) junction. The anatomical root of the tooth is covered by cement, the junction between dentine and cement being the cementodentinal junction. The junction between the enamel and cement (i.e. the crown and root) is the cervical margin or cervix of the tooth.

The fundamental structural unit of dentine is the tubule. Dentinal tubules run from the inner, pulpal, surface towards the amelodentinal and cementodentinal junctions. The tubules are occupied, at least in part, by cellular processes of the dentine-forming cells, the odontoblasts, whose cell bodies line the pulpal surface of the dentine. This differs significantly from cement and bone where the tissue-forming cells, the cementocytes and osteocytes, and their processes, become completely embedded in the matrix. Because dentine contains odontoblast processes which give it the capacity to react to physiological and pathological stimuli, it is considered a living tissue. The colour of the dentine can be seen through the relatively translucent enamel and gives colour to the crown. Although dentine is less hard than enamel, it is more resilient and acts as support for the brittle enamel.

Most important, and unlike dentine and cement, enamel contains no cellular inclusions. The basic morphological unit of enamel is the prism or rod. In longitudinally sectioned teeth, the prisms extend roughly perpendicularly from the amelodentinal junction to the surface (Fig. 6.21). Each prism consists largely of submicroscopic crystals of hydroxyapatite and it is the arrangement of these crystals which gives a prism its structural identity and strength. The hard enamel protects the softer underlying dentine as well as providing a unique masticatory surface for crushing, grinding and chewing nutrient particles.

Cement is a hard, 'bone-like' tissue arranged in thin layers around the tooth root. It is the least hard of the three dental tissues, its properties being very similar to those of bone. However, whilst bone is vascularized and innervated, cement is avascular and has no innervation.

All the dental hard tissues are calcified tissues, most of the calcium being in the form of (crystalline) hydroxyapatite, $Ca_{10}(PO_4)_6(OH)_2$. The hydroxyapatite crystals in enamel are far larger than those of the other hard tissues. The organic matrix of dentine and cement is collagenous and differs significantly from that of enamel which contains proteins unique to this tissue. By (wet) weight enamel, dentine and cement contain 96, 70 and 65% inorganic material respectively.

Like dentine, the inner core of loose connective tissue, the dental pulp, is derived from mesenchyme of the dental papilla. Indeed, because of the close relationship between the dentine and pulp in terms of development, structure, function and reactions, the collective term pulpodentinal complex is sometimes used to indicate the two tissues. The dental pulp is the nutritive portion of the tooth and is protected from external noxious stimuli by the overlying hard tissues. The pulp cavity consists of a pulp chamber in the crown and a number of root canals, the number depending upon the particular tooth. The pulp chamber is a single cavity varying in shape according to the outline of the crown. Where the crown has well-developed cusps, the pulp chamber may project as pulp horns (pulp cornua). Generally each root has

# Tooth Morphology

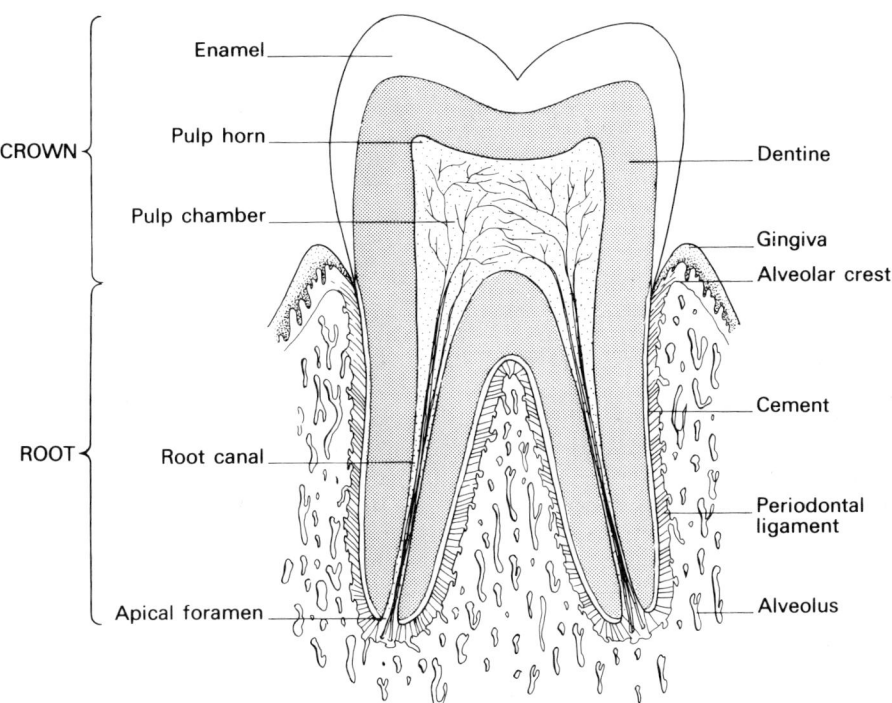

**Fig. 5.1.** Buccolingual section through an upper molar showing the distribution of the dental and supportive tissues.

a single root canal which tends to be oval in cross section. Each root canal opens by a foramen or foramina at the apex of the root. The apical foramen rarely opens at the exact anatomical apex of the tooth, but about 0.5–1 mm from it. The pulp is continuous with the connective tissues of the periodontal ligament through the apex of each root. Accessory root canals are generally found in the apical third of the root and are branches of the main root canal. They end in accessory foramina and are more commonly seen in young patients because they become obliterated by cement and dentine as the patient ages. Accessory canals which open approximately at right angles to the main pulp cavity are termed lateral canals and are most commonly found at the root bifurcation of posterior teeth. The components of the pulp are common to all loose connective tissue; cells, fibres, ground substance, blood vessels and nerves. It is composed of approximately 25% organic material and 75% water by weight.

The tissues which support the teeth in the jaws are collectively termed the periodontium and comprise: the alveolar bone which houses the sockets for the roots of the teeth; the periodontal ligament, a connective tissue which attaches the cement to the alveolar bone; the gingiva (gums); the cement.

The periodontal ligament is the dense, fibrous connective tissue occupying the space between the root of the tooth and the alveolus. Above the alveolar crest, the ligament is continuous with the connective tissues of the gingiva whilst at the apical foramen it is continuous with that of the dental pulp. The average width of the periodontal space is 0.2 mm, though there is considerable variation between and within individual teeth. Like other connective tissues, the periodontal ligament consists of a stroma of fibres in a gel of ground substance containing cells, blood vessels and nerves.

Alveolar bone is that part of the mandible and maxilla in which the teeth are located. Alveolar bone is sufficiently 'plastic' to remodel according to the functional demands placed upon it. Consequently, it readily adapts to the movements of teeth during their developmental, eruptive and functional periods. Morphologically, no distinct boundary exists between the body of the mandible (and maxilla) and its alveolar process. Two parts of the alveolar bone can be described; first, the thin lamina of compact bone which lines the tooth

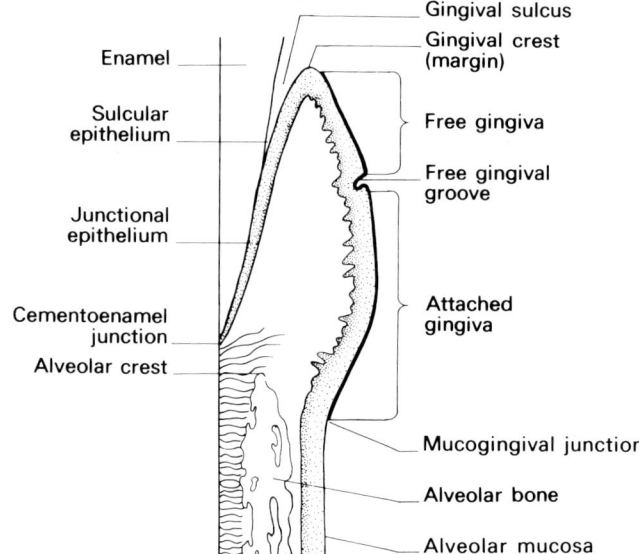

**Fig. 5.2.** Buccolingual section showing the gingiva.

sockets and which gives attachment to the fibres of the periodontal ligament, the lamina dura; second, the bone which surrounds and gives support to the socket. Alveolar bone has the same physical and chemical properties as bone found elsewhere in the body. Its chemical composition is similar to that of cement.

The gingiva (Fig. 5.2) is firmly attached to the periosteum of the alveolus and to the teeth. It may be subdivided into free and attached gingiva. The interdental papilla is that part of the gingiva which fills the space between teeth. The free gingiva is separated from the tooth by a fluid-filled gutter, the gingival sulcus, which is lined by sulcular epithelium. The gingiva adheres to the tooth by means of the junctional epithelium. In health, the gingival sulcus may be between 0.1 and 1 mm deep.

Finally, it must be emphasized that the appearance of the dental tissues is dependent upon the method used to prepare the specimen. Thus, in ground sections the delicate connective tissues of the pulp, periodontal ligament and gingiva are removed by the act of grinding the tissues to obtain a thin section. In decalcified material the soft connective tissues and organic matrix of the calcified tissues are retained but, unless the decalcifying procedure is carried out with exceptional care, the highly mineralized enamel is lost.

## HUMAN TOOTH FORM

Man has two generations of teeth (diphyodonty); the deciduous and the permanent dentitions. The first of the deciduous teeth appear in the mouth at about 6 months after birth, the deciduous dentition is complete at about 2–3 years, and the last deciduous tooth is replaced at about 12 years. The first of the permanent teeth enters the mouth at about 6 years and the permanent dentition is complete at about 18 years. The dentitions are mixed between 6 and 12 years.

The teeth are set in upper and lower arches shaped like a catenary (i.e. like a chain suspended at its two ends). For descriptive purposes the dentition is subdivided into four quadrants and the teeth are identified according to quadrant (right or left, upper or lower).

In common with all other mammals, any tooth developing in the premaxilla is called an incisor regardless of its form or its function. The most anterior tooth on the maxilla is called a canine, again regardless of form or function. Since only one tooth in the quadrant can be the most anterior tooth there can only be one upper canine in each quadrant, by definition. Any tooth behind the canine is a molar; if it is replaced it is called a deciduous molar; if it is not replaced it is called a permanent molar; if it replaces a deciduous molar it is called a premolar.

In a normal lower jaw, the tooth occluding immediately in front of the upper canine is called a lower canine, regardless of form or function. Any tooth in front of the lower canine is called a lower incisor. The teeth behind the lower canine are defined in the same way as those behind the upper canine.

Despite the apparently arbitrary method used

for defining teeth, it so happens that in most mammals, including man, the teeth within a class (incisor, canine or molar) generally have similar shapes and are different from those in other classes. But there are many exceptions. For example, by definition an elephant tusk is an incisor and a walrus tusk is a canine. The caniniform tooth in the permanent lower dentition of a mole lies behind the upper canine: therefore it is a premolar.

Human incisors are named according to their relationship to the midline. Thus, the incisor nearest the midline is the central or first incisor, the incisor which is more laterally positioned being named the lateral or second incisor (Fig. 5.3). All human incisors have blade-like crowns and are used to incise food.

Human canines have a stout cone-shaped crown. They are the longest rooted and probably the most stable teeth in the dental arches, acting as 'anchor teeth'.

The canines and incisors together are often referred to as anterior teeth. Apart from their function in mastication, they have considerable aesthetic importance and play a role in the formulation of many speech sounds.

The premolars are essentially bicuspid (two cusps) teeth peculiar to the permanent dentition (by definition). Structurally and functionally they are intermediate between the canine and molars. In the complete permanent dentition there are two premolars in each jaw quadrant. The most anterior premolar is called the first premolar and the premolar behind it is the second premolar (Fig. 5.3).

The molars have large chewing surfaces and usually two or more roots. Their position, close to the powerful jaw closing muscles, and shape make them suitable grinding teeth. In the deciduous dentition there are two molars in each quadrant; in the permanent dentition there are three molars in each quadrant. Like the premolars, the molars are distinguished according to their antero-posterior position. Thus, there are first and second deciduous molars (Fig. 5.4) and first, second and third permanent molars (Fig. 5.3). The molars and premolars are sometimes collectively referred to as posterior or check teeth.

In summary, there are 20 teeth in the complete deciduous dentition ten in each jaw; in the complete permanent dentition there are 32 teeth, sixteen in each jaw. The dental formula for the deciduous dentition of man is

$$DI\frac{2}{2} DC\frac{1}{1} DM\frac{2}{2} = 10$$

and for the permanent dentition

$$I\frac{2}{2} C\frac{1}{1} P\frac{2}{2} M\frac{3}{3} = 16.$$

To simplify tooth identification a dental shorthand is often used in clinical situations. As you look at a patient, imagine a cross with the horizontal bar place between upper and lower jaws and the vertical bar running between the upper central incisors and lower central incisors. The symbol used to describe each quadrant is derived from this cross—

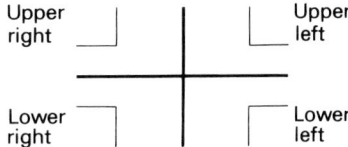

The permanent teeth in each quadrant are numbered 1–8 (Fig. 5.3) and the equivalent deciduous teeth are lettered A–E (Fig. 5.4). Thus, the upper right second permanent molar is allocated the 7⌋ and the lower left deciduous canine, ⌈C. This system of dental shorthand is termed the Zsigmondy System. An alternative scheme has been devised by the Federation Dentaire Internationale in which the quadrant is represented by a number, i.e.

1 = upper right quadrant  
2 = upper left quadrant  
3 = lower left quadrant  } Permanent  
4 = lower right quadrant  
5 = upper right quadrant  
6 = upper left quadrant  
7 = lower left quadrant  } Deciduous  
8 = lower right quadrant  

The deciduous or permanent number prefixes a tooth number. According to this system, the upper right second permanent molar is symbolized as 1,7 and the lower left deciduous canine as 7,3 (not C).

SURFACES AND RIDGES OF THE
TEETH (Figs. 5.3 and 5.5)

The outer surfaces of the anterior teeth face forwards towards the lips and are consequently termed labial surfaces. The corresponding surfaces of the posterior teeth face the cheeks (buccinator muscle) and are termed buccal surfaces. The inner surfaces of all the teeth in the lower jaw face the tongue and are called lingual surfaces. The corresponding surfaces in the upper jaw are called palatal surfaces. The anterior teeth have medial and lateral neighbours; the posterior

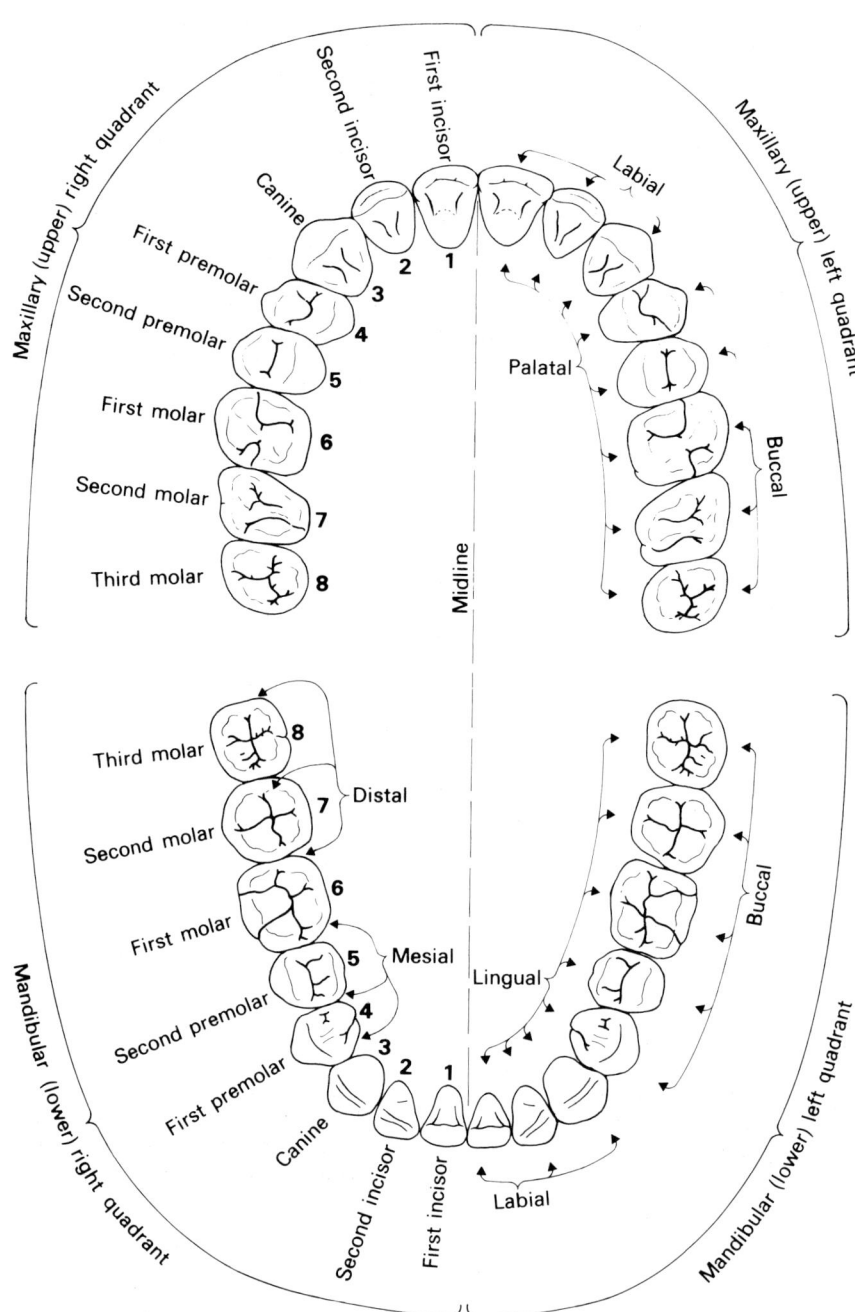

**Fig. 5.3.** Occlusal view of the upper and lower permanent teeth.

teeth have anterior and posterior neighbours. The vertical surfaces of two adjacent teeth that face one another are called contact surfaces or proximal surfaces. Dentists usually call the contact surface of a tooth which faces the next tooth forward in the arch the mesial surface; the contact surface which faces the next tooth behind is known as the distal surface. The cutting edge of anterior teeth is termed the incisal edge. The chewing or occlusal surfaces of posterior teeth are those surfaces that come into contact with antagonists.

For descriptive purposes, the junctions of the

# Tooth Morphology

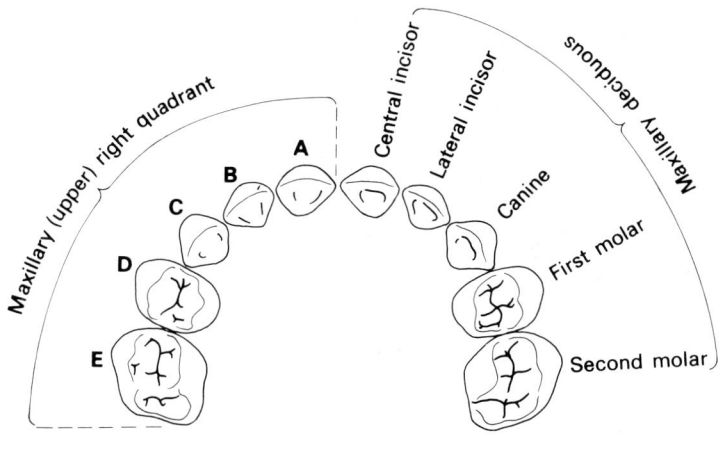

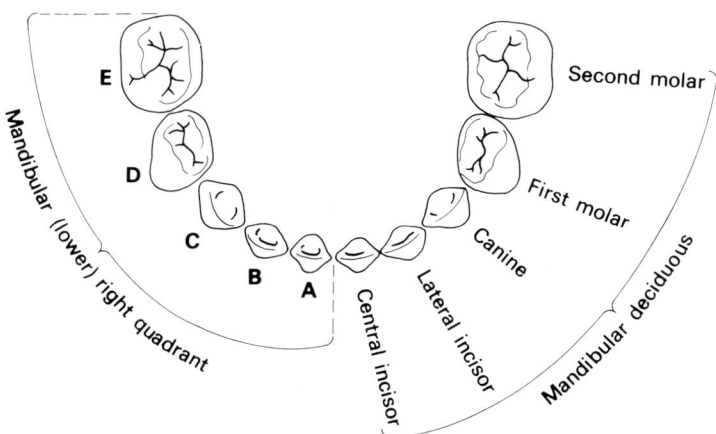

**Fig. 5.4.** Occlusal view of the upper and lower deciduous teeth.

crown surfaces are referred to as line angles and point angles (Fig. 5.6). A line angle is formed by the junction of two surfaces, for example the mesiolabial angle of anterior teeth; a point angle is formed by the junction of three surfaces, for example the mesiolabioincisal point angle of anterior teeth.

The crowns of teeth may show a number of elevations or ridges (Fig. 5.5):

A cusp is a pronounced elevation on the occlusal surface of a posterior tooth.

A tubercle is a small elevation on the crown which may or may not be typical.

A cingulum is a bulbous convexity near the cervical region of a tooth.

A ridge is any linear elevation on the surface of a tooth.

Marginal ridges are ridges at the mesial and distal edges of the occlusal surfaces of posterior teeth. Some anterior teeth have equivalent ridges.

A fissure is a long cleft between cusps or ridges.

A fossa is a rounded depression.

*Cusp nomenclature*

Cusps can be identified according to zoological terminology (Fig. 10.15) but dentists normally indicate them according to the surfaces of the crown (e.g. mesiobuccal cusp).

## The permanent dentition

THE UPPER FIRST (CENTRAL) PERMANENT INCISOR

*Average dimensions*

Crown height, 10.5 mm; root length, 13.0 mm; mesiodistal crown diameter, 8.7 mm; labiopalatal crown diameter, 7.0 mm.

*General description* (Fig. 5.7)

Like all incisors this tooth is characterized by its rather sharp and narrow incisal edge. Here it is centrally positioned over the root. Two grooves

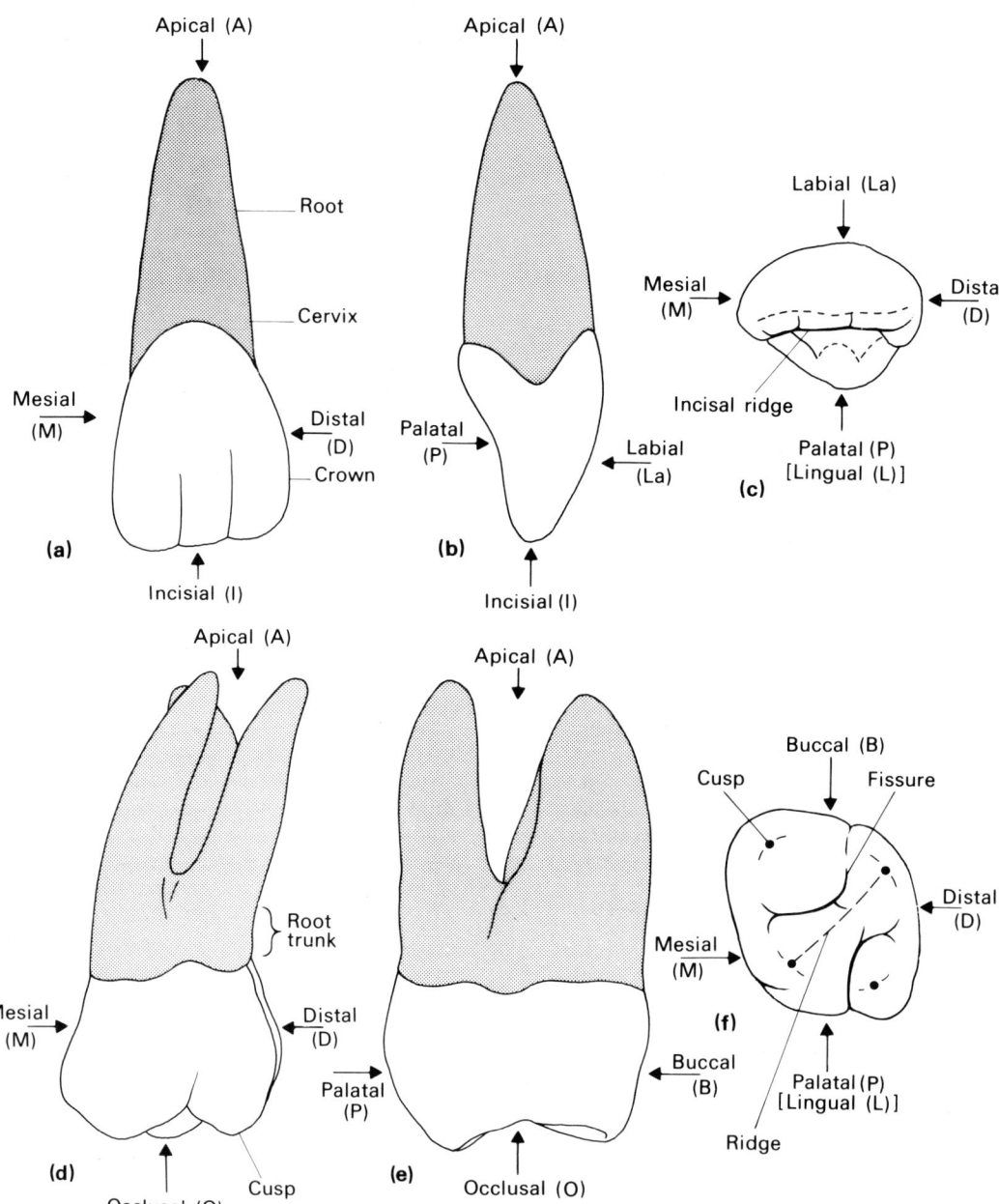

**Fig. 5.5.** Views of individual upper permanent teeth showing the various tooth surfaces. (a) Labial view of left central incisor; (b) mesial view of the left central incisor; (c) incisal view of left central incisor; (d) buccal view of left first molar; (e) mesial view of left first molar; (f) occlusal view of left first molar. (The abbreviations on Fig. 5.5 are used in subsequent descriptions of the individual teeth.)

which may run on to the labial surface correspond to the divisions between three tubercles (mammelons) seen on the incisal margins of newly erupted incisors. The mammelons are usually worn flat soon after eruption. The smoothly convex labial surface of the crown is roughly trapezoidal. From a labial view the mesial surface appears straight and approximately at right angles to the incisal edge. The distoincisal angle is more rounded and the distal outline more convex. Viewed palatally the middle and incisal regions of the crown are concave, giving a slightly shovel-

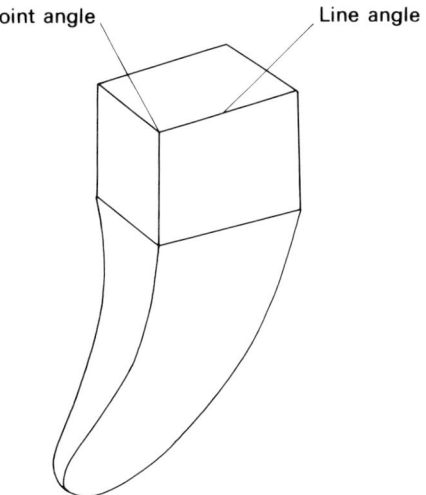

**Fig. 5.6.** Schematic diagram of a tooth illustrating the difference between the terms line angle and point angle.

shaped appearance to the incisor. The cingulum is a smooth, prominent convexity against which the lower incisors bite. The palatal surface is bordered by mesial and distal marginal ridges, often poorly developed, which merge with the cingulum and pass towards the incisal angles. The mesial and distal views of the crown illustrate the fundamental wedge-shape of all incisors. The outline of the labial surface is convex whilst the outline of the palatal surface is concavo-convex.

The sinuous cervical margin is concave towards the crown on the palatal and labial surfaces and convex towards the crown on the mesial and distal surfaces, the curvature on the mesial surface being the most pronounced of any tooth in the dentition.

The single stout root of this incisor tapers towards the apex. The root is roughly circular in cross-section.

*Pulp morphology*

Viewed from the labial surface the pulp chamber follows the general outline of the crown and is usually widest incisally. In a young tooth the pulp chamber has three pulp horns which correspond to the mammelons: viewed distally, the pulp tapers towards the incisal ridge edge, and widens cervically. Following a constriction, the (usually) single and centrally placed root canal tapers towards the apical foramen where it occasionally bends distally or labially. In cross-section the root canal tends to be roughly circular but tapering palatally. With age, the dimensions of the pulp cavity diminish as secondary dentine is laid down. The tip of the pulp chamber recedes until it may come to lie almost at the cervical level and the root canal narrows especially in the mesiodistal plane.

*Variations* (Fig. 5.8)

The shapes of the crowns of upper central incisors are very variable. Three basic types may be seen; tapering, square and ovoid, with varying combinations. For example the incisor illustrated in Fig. 5.7 may be classified as square-tapered.

The shape of the cingulum is variable. It may be single, divided, or replaced by prominent portions of the marginal ridges. Where the marginal ridges are exaggerated the tooth has a distinct 'shovel-shape' (Fig. 5.33). Occasionally, a slight ridge of enamel may run towards the incisal edge, dividing the palatal surface into two shallow depressions.

UPPER SECOND (LATERAL) PERMANENT INCISOR

*Average dimensions*

Crown height, 9.0 mm; root length, 13.0 mm; mesiodistal crown diameter, 6.5 mm; labiopalatal crown diameter, 6.0 mm.

*General description* (Fig. 5.9)

The shape of the lateral incisor is very variable, although generally it is like a slightly modified, small upper central incisor. From the incisal aspect it has a more rounded outline. Viewed labially, the mesioincisal and particularly the distoincisal angle are more rounded than those of the central incisor. The palatal aspect of the crown is also similar to that of the central incisor, though the marginal ridges and cingulum are often more pronounced. Consequently, the palatal concavity appears deeper. Lying in front of the cingulum is a pit, the foramen cacumen. The mesial and distal aspects of the lateral incisor differ little from those of the central incisor.

The course of the cervical margin and the shape of the root are each similar to those of the central incisor.

*Pulp morphology*

The pulp cavity of the upper lateral incisor is similar to, but smaller than, that of the upper central incisor.

*Variations* (Fig. 5.10)

The lateral incisor is commonly missing from the dental arch (about 1–2% of individuals). It is not uncommon for it to be a rudimentary cone termed a 'peg' lateral incisor (a further 1–2% of indiv-

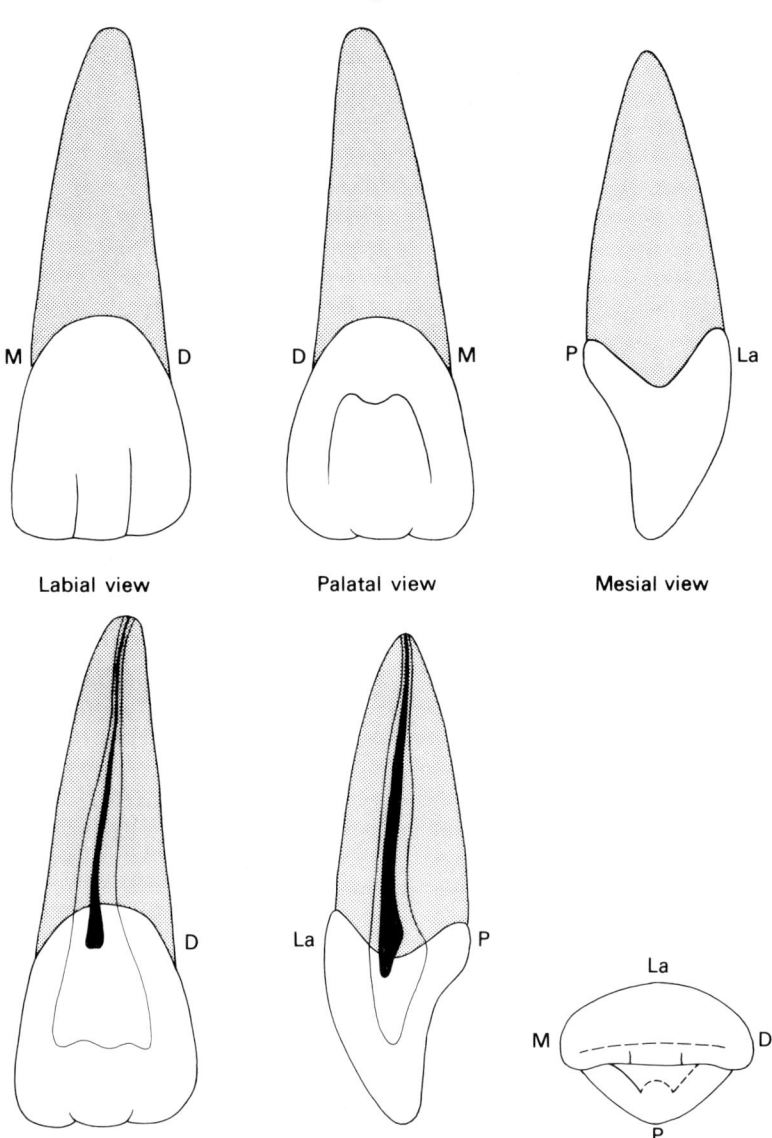

**Fig. 5.7.** The left upper first (central) permanent incisor. The pulp cavity has been superimposed on two diagrams. The outline represents the shape in a young tooth; the solid region is the shape in a very old tooth.

iduals). The distal curvature may be increased to produce a prominent bulge. Like the central incisor, the cingulum occasionally has a number of additional tubercles, some of which may become very prominent. A groove of variable depth may cross the cingulum and extend down to the root surface. Occasionally, the foramen cacumen extends deeply into the substance of the tooth.

In an extremely important variation the apical part of the root has a sharp distal bend. If such a tooth is rotated during extraction the root apex breaks off.

THE LOWER FIRST (CENTRAL) PERMANENT INCISOR
*Average dimensions*
Crown height, 9.0 mm; root length, 12.5 mm; mesiodistal crown diameter, 5.3 mm; labiolingual crown diameter, 6.0 mm.

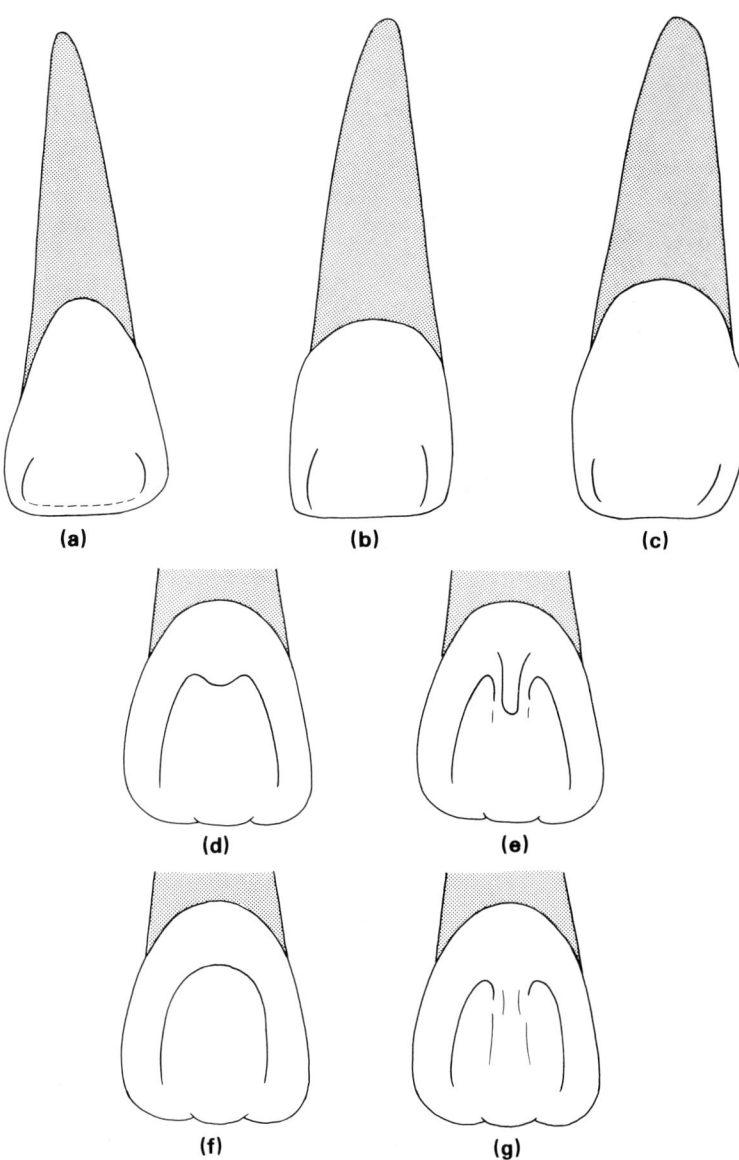

**Fig. 5.8.** Morphological variations of the upper first permanent incisor. (a) Tapering crown form; (b) square crown form; (c) ovoid crown form; (d) single cingulum; (e) divided cingulum of marginal ridges; (f) cingulum replaced by convergence; (g) cingulum and longitudinal ridge.

*General description* (Fig. 5.11)

The lower incisors are the narrowest teeth in the permanent dentition, the first being smaller than the second. They have similar shapes and can be distinguished from the upper incisors not only by their size but also by their mesiodistally flattened roots and the poor development of their marginal ridges and cingula. Viewed incisally, the lower first permanent incisor has a bilaterally symmetrical triangular shape. In the newly erupted tooth, three mammelons are usually present on the incisal edge. Viewed labially the crown of the incisor is almost twice as long as it is broad. The incisal edge is straight and is normally worn approximately at right angles to the long axis of the tooth. The mesial and distal incisal angles are generally sharp. Lingually, the marginal ridges and cingulum are far less pronounced than those of the upper

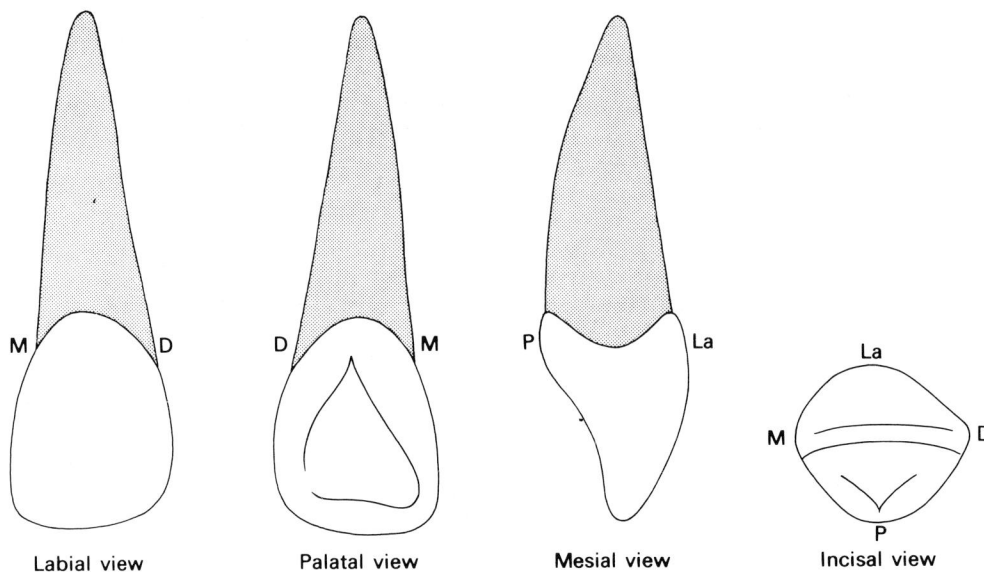

**Fig. 5.9.** The left upper second (lateral) permanent incisor.

incisors, the lingual surface being smooth and slightly concave.

The single root is very flattened mesiodistally and frequently grooved on the mesial and distal surfaces. Because they are symmetrical it is not possible to distinguish between extracted left and right lower central incisors.

*Pulp morphology*
The pulp chamber is similar to that described for the upper central incisor, being broadest incisally with three pulp horns, although the pulp horns are less well-developed. The pulp chamber is oval in cross-section, being wider labiolingually than mesiodistally, and is constricted at the cervical margin. In distal view the root canal in the young only narrows in the middle third of the root. The root canal is oval in cross-section, being compressed mesiodistally. With age, the pulp cavity becomes considerably constricted and ultimately its roof lies at the level of the cervical margin. However, the root canal remains rather wide in its labiolingual dimension except near the apex of the tooth.

*Variations*
Lower incisors have fairly constant shapes. Sometimes the crown is markedly tilted towards the lingual side of the tooth. Occasionally the root canal may bifurcate.

THE LOWER SECOND (LATERAL) PERMANENT INCISOR

*Average dimensions*
Crown height, 9.5 mm; root length, 14.0 mm; mesiodistal crown diameter, 5.8 mm; labiolingual crown diameter, 6.5 mm.

*General description* (Fig. 5.12)
This tooth is very like its neighbouring central incisor although it can usually be distinguished due to its asymmetry. First, the distal surface diverges at a greater angle from the long axis of the tooth giving it a fan-shaped appearance and the distoincisal angle is more acute and rounded. Second, when viewed incisally, the incisal ridge deviates distally in a lingual direction.

*Pulp morphology*
This differs little from the lower central incisor. However, the root canal often divides in the mid-third of the root to give a labial and lingual branch.

*Variations*
Like the mandibular central incisor, morphological variations are uncommon.

THE UPPER PERMANENT CANINE

*Average dimensions*
Crown height, 10.0 mm; root length, 17.0 mm;

# Tooth Morphology

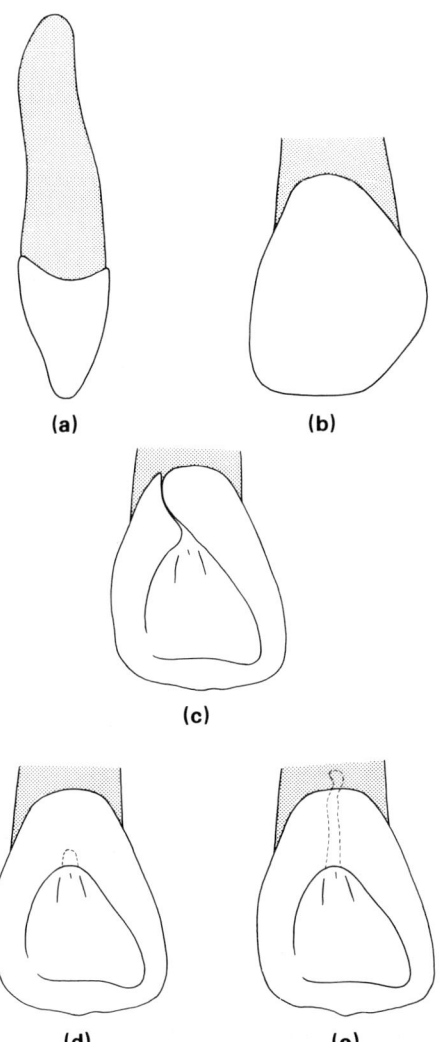

**Fig. 5.10.** Morphological variations of the upper second permanent incisor. (a) Peg-shaped lateral incisor; (b) distal lobe on distal surface of crown; (c) groove on palatal surface arising from the cingulum; (d) usual depth of foramen cacumen; (e) extended foramen cacumen.

in size of a central mammelon at the expense of mesial and distal mammelons. Prominent longitudinal ridges often pass from the cusp tip down both the labial and palatal surfaces. The labial surface of the canine may be marked by the longitudinal ridge which extends from the cusp towards the cervical margin. The cusp occupies at least one third of the crown height. The tooth expands as a distal bulge, the distal surface meeting the root at more of an angle than the mesial surface. The palatal surface has distinct mesial and distal marginal ridges and a well-defined cingulum. The longitudinal ridge from the tip of the cusp meets the cingulum and is separated from the marginal ridges on either side by distinct depressions. Viewed mesially or distally, the distinctive feature of this tooth is its stout cingulum, the labiopalatal dimension being greater than any other anterior tooth.

The cervical margin follows a similar course to the incisors though the curves are less pronounced. The curvature of the cervical margin on the distal surface is less marked than that on the mesial surface.

The root is the largest and stoutest in the dentition. Because its labial surface is wider than its palatal surface it has a somewhat triangular cross-section. The mesial and distal surfaces of the root are often grooved longitudinally.

*Pulp morphology*
The pulp chamber is narrow with one pulp horn which points cuspally. Both the pulp chamber and the single root canal are wider labiopalatally than they are in the mesiodistal plane. The root canal does not constrict markedly until the apical third of the root is reached. The root canal is oval or triangular in cross-section except in its apical third, where it is circular.

*Variations* (Fig. 5.14)
Variations in the shape of this tooth are common, though rarely sufficient to make the tooth appear deformed or atypical. The tip of the cusp may vary from a blunt apex to a sharp nipple-shaped point. The slopes of the cusp may be steep or slight and sometimes there are accessory cusplets, especially on the distal side. The occurrence of a well-developed palatal cingulum is not uncommon and it is present as a small cusp. Frequently the tip of the root bends mesially or distally.

## THE LOWER PERMANENT CANINE

*Average dimensions*
Crown height, 11 mm; root length, 15.5 mm; mesiodistal crown diameter, 7.6 mm; labiopalatal crown diameter, 8.0 mm.

*General description* (Fig. 5.13)
This is a stout tooth with a well-developed cingulum and the longest root in the dentition. Viewed cuspally it is asymmetrical. A plane passing through the tip of the cusp and the middle of the cingulum has more of the tooth on its distal than its mesial side. It is thought that the pointed shape of the canine tooth is related to an increase

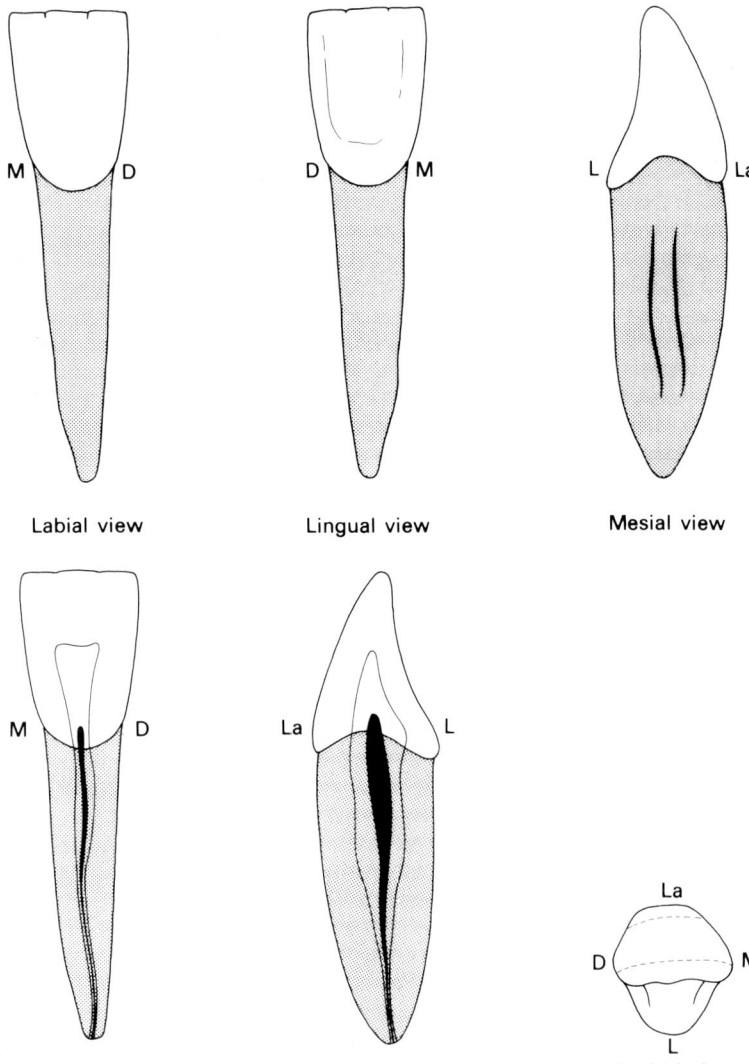

**Fig. 5.11.** The left lower first (central) permanent incisor and the shape of its pulp.

mesiodistal crown diameter, 6.8 mm; labiolingual crown diameter, 7.5 mm.

*General description* (Fig. 5.15)
This tooth is similar to the maxillary canine but is smaller, more slender and more symmetrical. The cusp is generally less prominent. Indeed, with attrition, its cusp may be lost, with the result that the tooth resembles an upper lateral permanent incisor. No distinct longitudinal ridges run from the tip of the cusp on to the labial and lingual surfaces. Viewed labially, the blunt cusp occupies one fifth of the crown height. The crown is narrower mesiodistally than the upper canine so that it appears longer, narrower and more slender.

The mesial and distal profiles converge only slightly towards the cervix. On the lingual surface the cingulum, marginal ridges and fossae are indistinct. The lingual surface is much flatter than the palatal surface of the upper canine, and is like the lingual surface of the mandibular incisors. Viewed mesially and distally, the wedge-shaped appearance of the canine can be seen clearly. These proximal surfaces are longer than those of the maxillary canine. The labiolingual diameter of the crown near the cervix is less than the corresponding labiopalatal diameter of the maxillary canine.

The single root is compressed mesiodistally with well-marked developmental grooves on both sides.

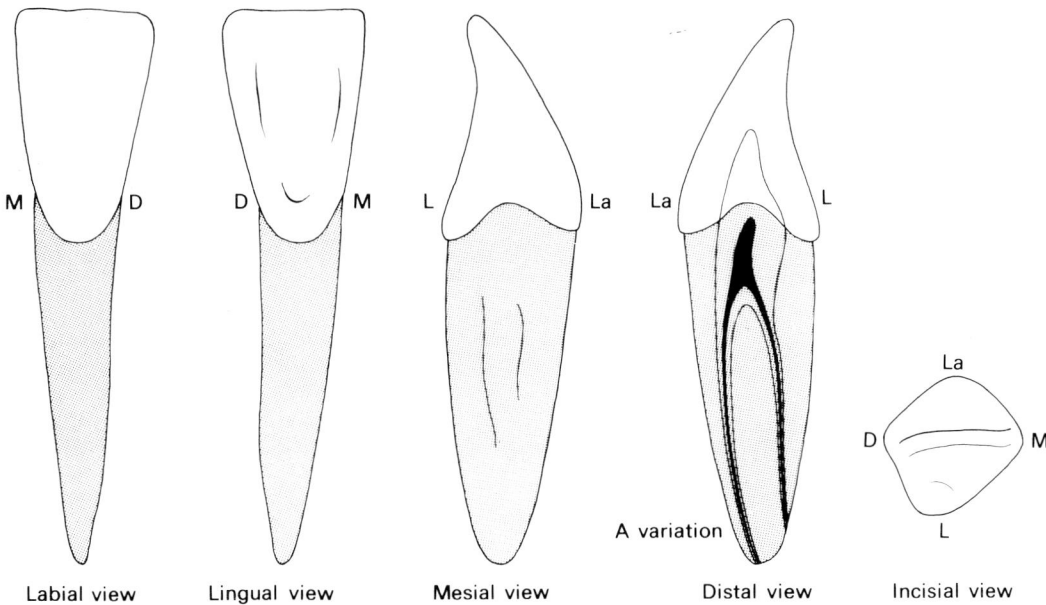

**Fig. 5.12.** The left lower second (lateral) permanent incisor and a variant in the shape of its pulp.

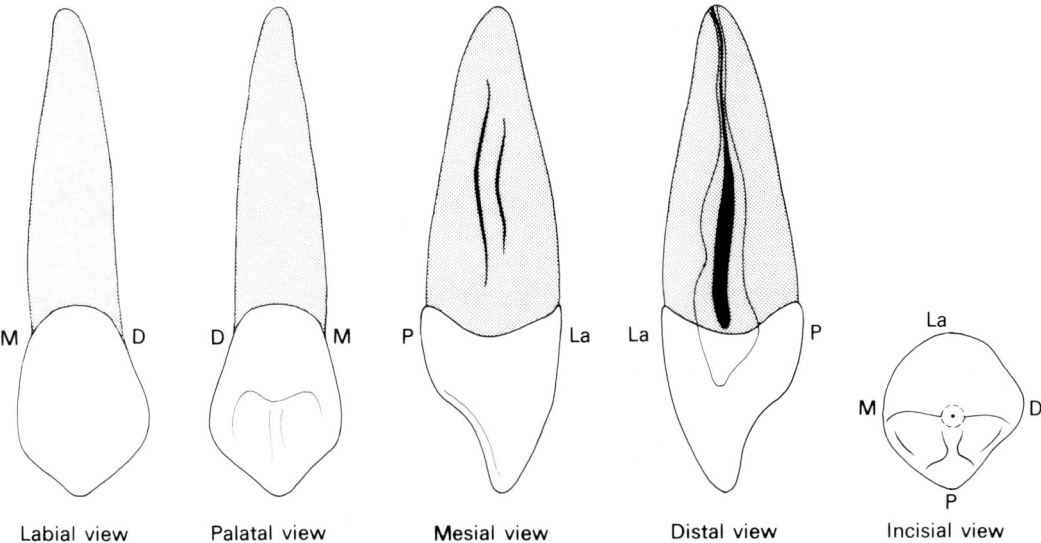

**Fig. 5.13.** The left upper permanent canine and the shape of its pulp.

*Pulp morphology*

The pulp cavity of this tooth resembles that of the maxillary permanent canine, though it tends to be slightly smaller in all dimensions. As with the lower incisors (Fig. 5.12) the root canal may divide into two branches towards the apex of the tooth.

*Variations* (Fig. 5.16)

The most important variation is the bifurcation of the root into labial and lingual roots. There are varying degrees of bifurcation ranging from deep grooving of a single root to clearly separated roots. Variations similar to those described for the

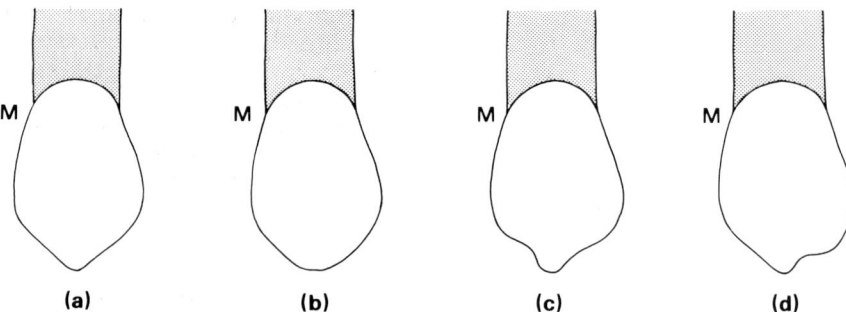

**Fig. 5.14.** Morphological variations of the upper permanent canine. (a) normal cusp tip; (b) blunt cusp tip; (c) nippled cusp tip; (d) accessory cusplet on distal slope of main cusp.

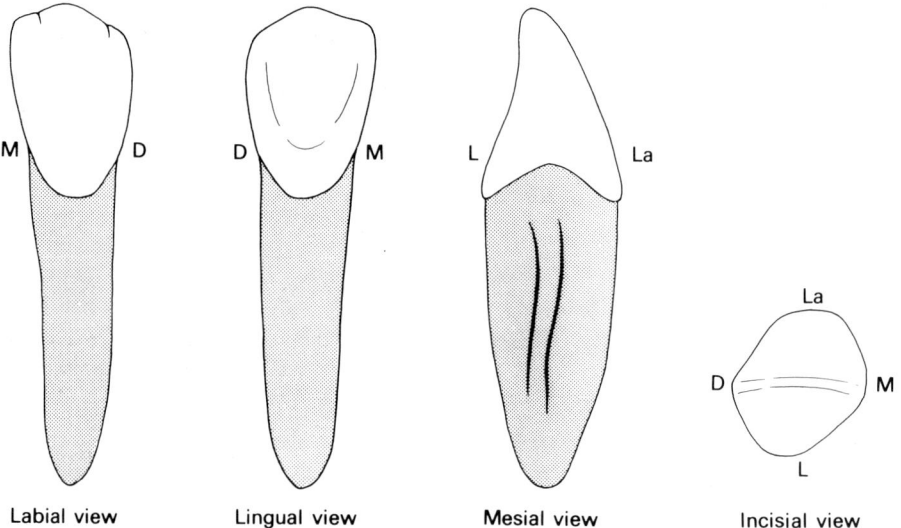

**Fig. 5.15.** The left lower permanent canine.

upper permanent canine may be seen in the shape of the cusp, its slopes and accessory cusplets, and in the prominence of the ridges on the lingual surface.

THE UPPER FIRST (PERMANENT) PREMOLAR

*Average dimensions*
Crown height, 8.5 mm; root length, 14.5 mm; mesiodistal crown diameter, 7.0 mm; buccopalatal crown diameter, 9.0 mm.

*General description* (Fig. 5.17)
Premolars are transitional between canines and molars. Like all premolars this tooth has two main cusps, buccal and palatal. From the occlusal aspect, the crown is roughly oval with the long axis buccopalatally. The mesiobuccal and distobuccal corners are less rounded than the mesiopalatal and distopalatal corners. The mesial and distal borders of the occlusal surface are marked by distinct mesial and distal marginal ridges. The occlusal fissure usually crosses the mesial marginal ridge on to the mesial surface. Viewed buccally, the first premolar resembles the adjoining canine. A longitudinal ridge passes down the buccal cusp. Viewed palatally, the buccal part of the crown is larger in all dimensions than the palatal part. The palatal cusp deviates mesially. From the mesial aspect, the unequal height of the unworn cusps is seen clearly. The fissure usually extends across the mesial

# Tooth Morphology

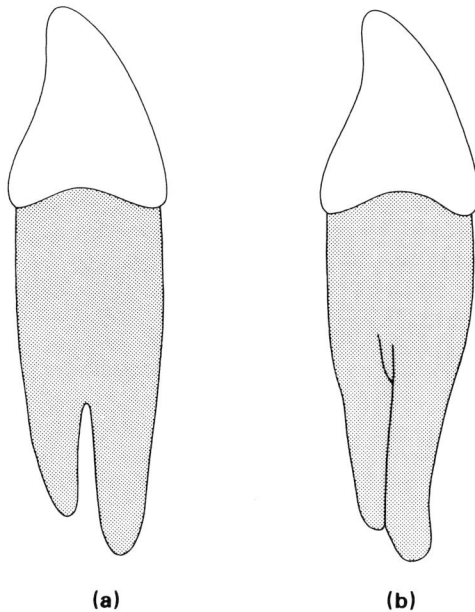

**Fig. 5.16.** Morphological variations of the lower permanent canine. (a) Bifurcated root in apical third of root. (b) Root bifurcation extending towards cervix.

the orifices are funnel-shaped. The root canals are usually straight and taper evenly from their origin to the apical foramina. In cross-section, the root canals are generally round. With age, the general shape of the pulp cavity remains the same but its dimensions, particularly the height of the pulp chamber, are reduced.

*Variations*
From its occlusal aspect the crown varies from squarish oval to triangular oval always with the greatest width buccally. The occlusal fissure may not extend onto the mesial surface of the tooth. Sometimes there is a single root and rarely there may be three (two buccal and one palatal, the condition in anthropoid apes).

THE UPPER SECOND PREMOLAR

*Average dimensions*
Crown height, 8.5 mm; root length, 14.0 mm; mediodistal crown diameter, 6.8 mm; buccopalatal crown diameter, 9.0 mm.

*General description* (Fig. 5.18)
The tooth looks like the adjacent first premolar except for the following features. Its occlusal surface is more rounded. The central fissure appears shorter and does not cross the mesial marginal ridge. From the buccal aspect the crown is slightly smaller and more rounded. The two cusps are smaller and more equal in size than those of the first premolar. Mesially and distally, the tooth appears similar to the adjacent first premolar but there is no canine fossa or fissure on the mesial surface. The cusps are more equal in size. The root is usually single.

*Pulp morphology*
The second premolar has a single root with a single root canal and its pulp chamber extends apically well below the cervical margin. Variations are frequent. Sometimes the root canal branches in its apical third to form two apical foramina. Frequently, the tooth has two root canals which join to form a common apical foramen. The appearance of the pulp cavity viewed from the buccal aspect is similar to that in the adjacent first premolar. In cross-section the root canal is oval.

*Variations*
Occasionally, the central fissure is replaced by a single deep pit. From this central pit supplemental grooves radiate in the form of an 'X'. Rarely the tooth has two roots.

marginal ridge from the occlusal surface. The cervical third of the mesial surface is marked by a distinct concavity, the canine fossa. Unlike the mesial aspect, the distal aspect of the crown lacks a fissure and canine fossa.

The cervical margin follows a fairly level course around the crown, deviating slightly towards the root on the buccal and palatal surfaces and away from the root on the mesial and distal surfaces.

There are usually two roots, a buccal and palatal root, though sometimes there may be only one. Where there are two roots the bifurcation generally occupies half their length. However, even a single root is deeply grooved on its mesial and distal surfaces.

*Pulp morphology*
Whether the tooth has one or two roots, it has two root canals leaving a single pulp chamber. If the tooth is single-rooted the two root canals may merge to form a common apical foramen. The pulp chamber is wide buccopalatally with two distinct pulp horns pointing towards the cusps. From the buccal view the pulp chamber is much narrower. The floor of the pulp chamber is rounded with the highest point in the centre. It usually lies within the root just apical to the cervix. Where the root canals arise from the pulp chamber

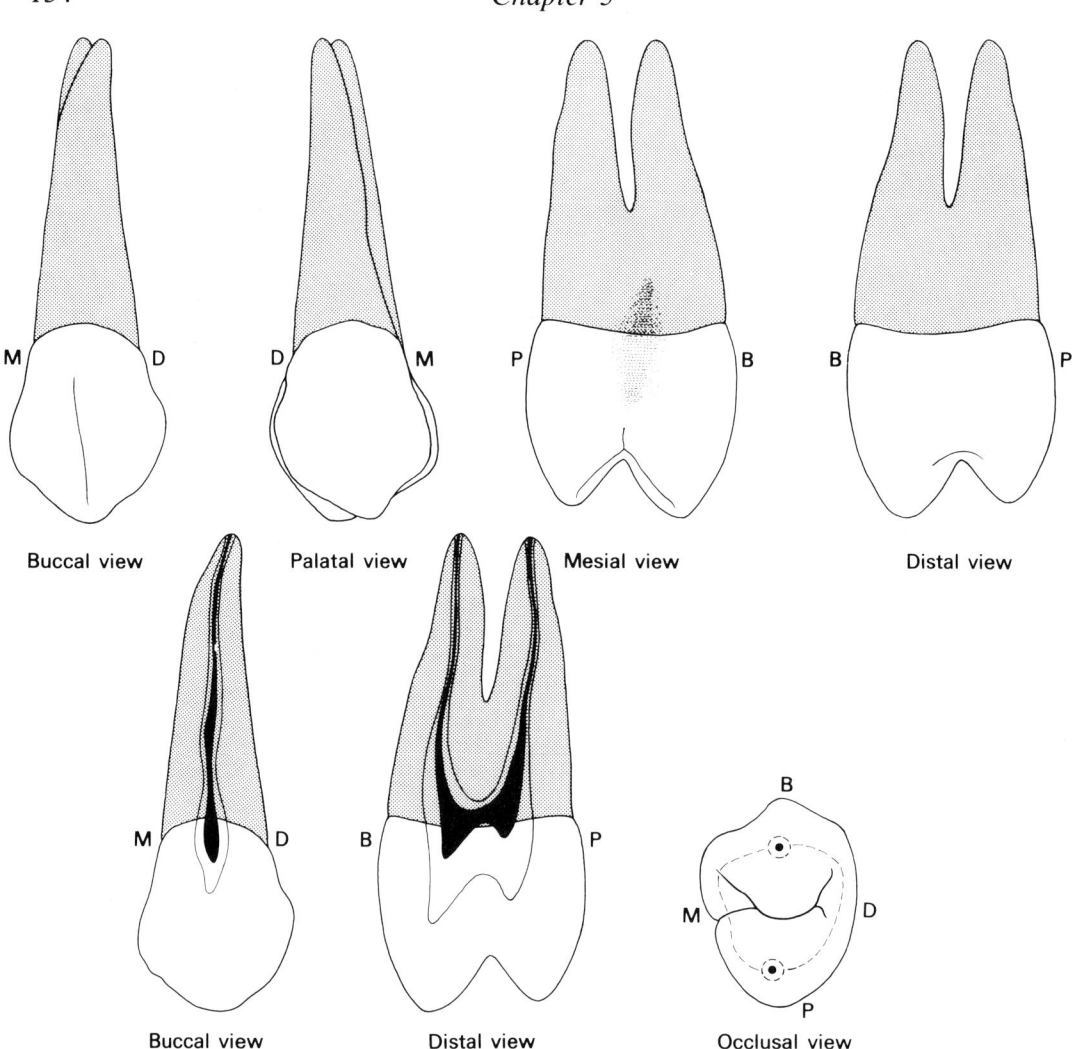

Fig. 5.17. The left upper first permanent premolar and the shape of its pulp.

THE LOWER FIRST PREMOLAR

*Average dimensions*
Crown height, 8.5 mm; root length, 14.0 mm; mesiodistal crown diameter, 7.0 mm; buccolingual crown diameter, 7.5 mm.

*General description* (Fig. 5.19)
This is the smallest premolar. Since it has a dominant buccal cusp and a very small lingual cusp which is similar to a cingulum, some consider it to be a modified canine. Unlike the upper premolars, from the occlusal aspect the crown appears to have a semicircular buccal cusp and triangular lingual cusp which is displaced mesially. The buccal and lingual cusps are connected by a blunt, transverse ridge which divides the occlusal surface into mesial and distal pits. The mesial pit is smaller than the distal pit. A fissure often extends from the mesial pit on to the mesiolingual surface of the crown. Viewed buccally, the crown is nearly symmetrical. From the lingual aspect, the entire buccal profile and the occlusal surface are visible. Thus, the lower first premolar differs from other premolars in that its occlusal plane does not lie perpendicular to the long axis of the tooth. The tilt of the occlusal plane can also be appreciated from the mesial and distal aspects: the lingual cusp is less than half the size of the buccal cusp.

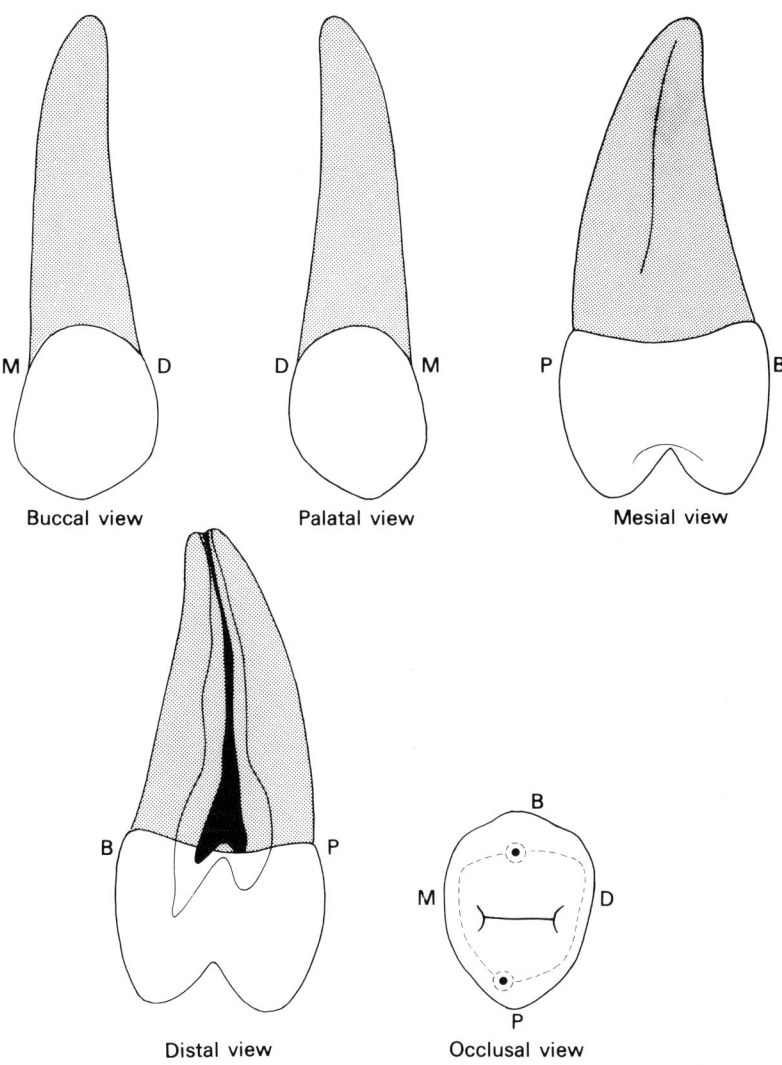

**Fig. 5.18.** The left upper second permanent premolar and the shape of its pulp.

The cervical margin follows an almost level course around the tooth. The root is single, conical and oval to round in cross-section.

*Pulp morphology*
The pulp chamber in this tooth, like the upper premolars, is wider buccolingually than it is mesiodistally. Unlike the pulp chamber of the upper premolars, there is usually only one pulp horn which extends into the buccal cusp. Occasionally, a small pulp horn may pass to the lingual cusp. There is a single root canal which becomes constricted towards the middle third of the root. The canal may temporarily branch in the middle third to form two separate root canals which rejoin near the apical foramen. In cross-section the root canal is round.

*Variations*
Although there is generally a single lingual cusp, there may be as many as four or it may be absent altogether. The position of the lingual cusp relative to the buccal cusp is variable. The transverse ridge between the buccal and lingual cusps may run uninterruptedly or it may be divided into buccal and lingual parts by a deep central groove from the mesial and distal fossae. The size and prominence of the transverse ridge

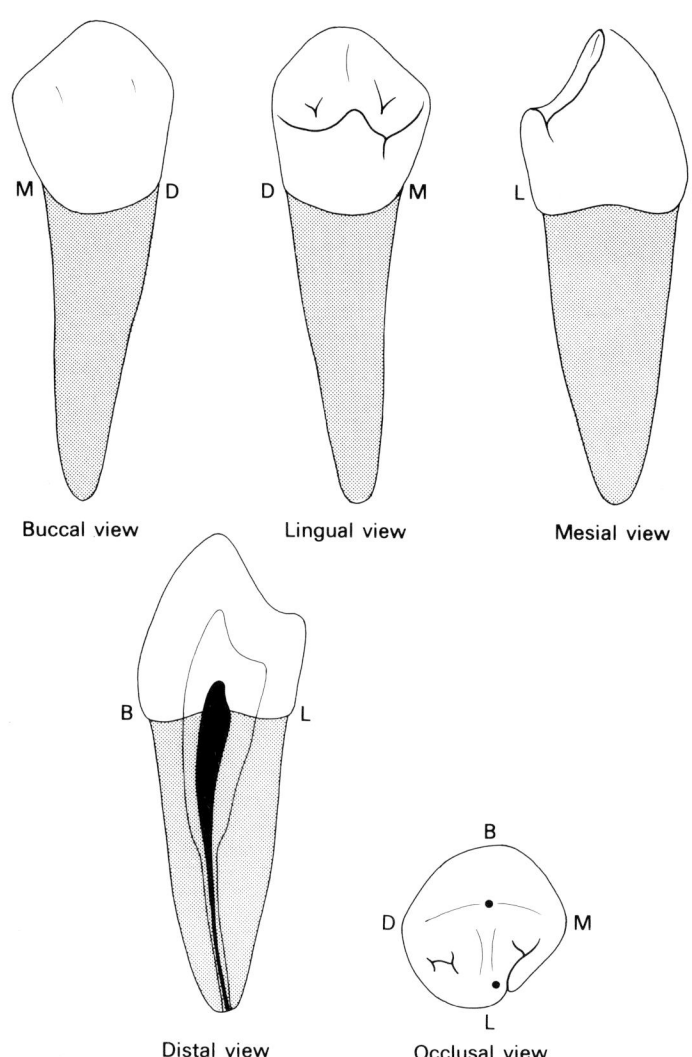

**Fig. 5.19.** The left lower first permanent premolar and the shape of its pulp.

varies greatly and it may be accompanied by several accessory transverse ridges. A further fissure may extend from the distal pit to the distolingual surface. The size and prominence of the marginal ridges vary considerably. A style or lobe may be seen on the buccal cusp margin and where it is prominent may form a cusplet. Occasionally, there are two roots, buccal and lingual.

THE LOWER SECOND PREMOLAR

*Average dimensions*
Crown height, 8.0 mm; root length, 14.5 mm; mesiodistal crown diameter, 7.1 mm; buccolingual crown diameter, 8.0 mm.

*General description* (Fig. 5.20)
This tooth resembles the neighbouring lower first premolar, though several significant differences enable one to distinguish between them. The crown of the second premolar is generally larger than that of the first premolar. Its lingual cusp is better developed although it is not quite as large as the buccal cusp, which appears correspondingly reduced in size. From the occlusal aspect, the buccal outline is semicircular and the lingual outline is rectangular. The cusps are separated by a well-defined mesiodistal occlusal fissure. Unlike the first premolar, the apices of the cusps are not usually joined by a transverse ridge. The lingual cusp is subdivided into mesiolingual and distolingual cusps, the mesiolingual cusp being wider and

# Tooth Morphology

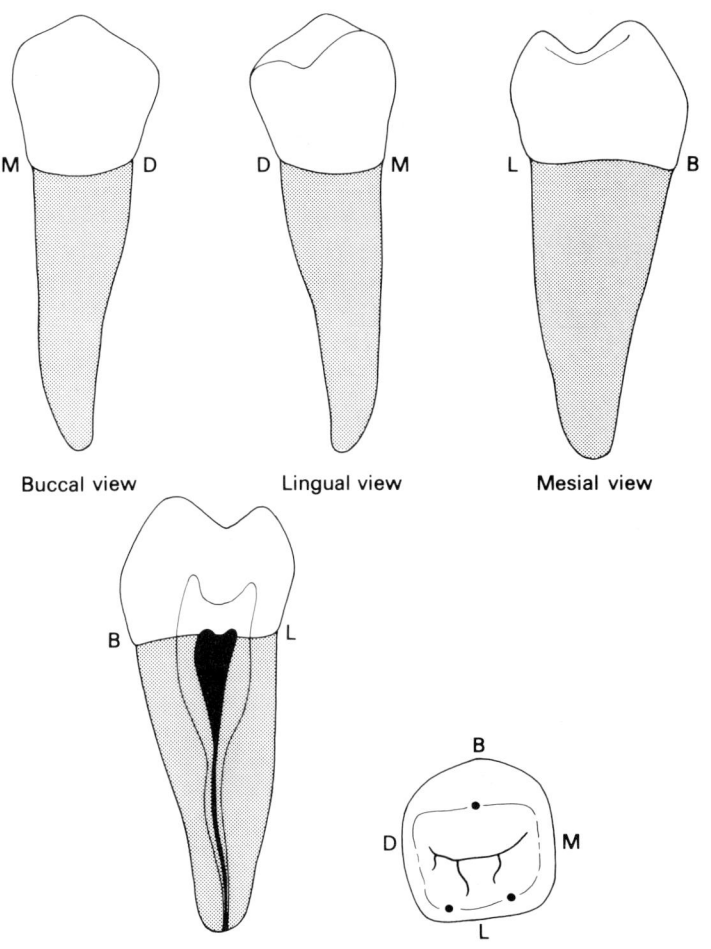

Fig. 5.20. The left lower second permanent premolar and the shape of its pulp.

higher than the distolingual cusp. From the buccal aspect the buccal cusp appears shorter and more rounded than that of the first premolar. Lingually, the mesiolingual cusp is larger than the distolingual cusp. From the mesial and distal aspects, the occlusal surface is roughly horizontal. The crown appears wider buccolingually than that of the first premolar and the buccal cusp does not incline far over the root.

The cervical margin follows an almost level course around the tooth. The root is single, conical and nearly round in cross-section. Generally, the root is thicker than that of the first premolar.

*Pulp morphology* (Fig. 5.20)
This differs little from that described for the mandibular first premolar. However, the pulp chamber of this tooth usually has two well-developed pulp horns projecting towards its cusps.

*Morphological variations* (Fig. 5.21)
The most common variations relate to the number of lingual cusps, the variants being one or three. The pit-groove pattern on the occlusal surface is variable. In rare instances, the root (and therefore the root canal) may bifurcate near its apex. In about 1% of individuals this tooth is absent.

### THE UPPER FIRST PERMANENT MOLAR

*Average dimensions*
Crown height, 7.5 mm; root length, 12.5 mm; mesiodistal crown diameter, 10.5 mm; bucco-palatal crown diameter, 11.0 mm.

*General description* (Fig. 5.22)
The upper first permanent molar is usually the largest molar. Viewed occlusally, the crown, like

138    Chapter 5

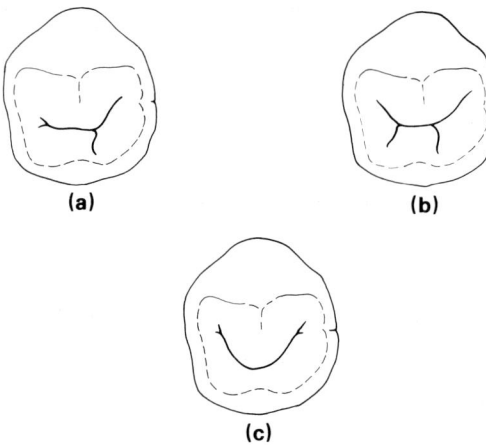

Fig. 5.21. Morphological variations of the lower second permanent premolar. (a) Y-shaped fissure pattern; (b) H-shaped fissure pattern; (c) U-shaped fissure pattern.

all upper molars, is rhombic in outline, the mesiopalatal and distobuccal angles being obtuse and the longest diameter of the crown running from the mesiobuccal to the distopalatal corners. It has four cusps separated by an incomplete H-shaped fissure. The cusps are named according to their positions i.e. mesiobuccal, mesiopalatal, distobuccal and distopalatal. An oblique ridge crosses the occlusal table diagonally from the mesiopalatal to the distobuccal cusp through the bar of the 'H'. An accessory cusplet of variable size is often seen on the palatal surface of the large mesiopalatal cusp. This cusplet is termed the tubercle of Carabelli and is found on about 60% of upper first permanent molars. Mesial and distal marginal ridges connect the pairs of mesial and distal cusps respectively. On either side of the oblique ridge lies a fossa, the mesial fossa being U-shaped and larger than the distal. From the distal fossa a fissure runs parallel to the oblique ridge on

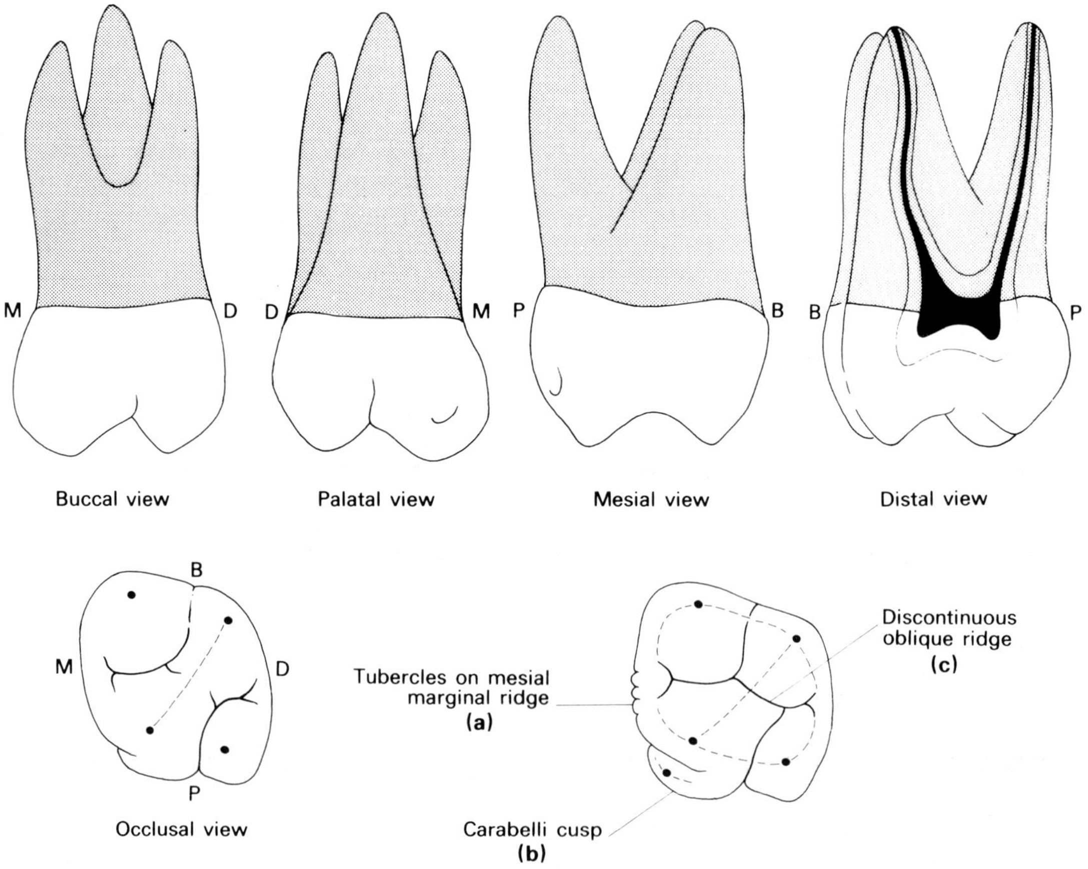

Buccal view     Palatal view     Mesial view     Distal view

Occlusal view

Tubercles on mesial marginal ridge
(a)

Carabelli cusp
(b)

Discontinuous oblique ridge
(c)

Fig. 5.22. The left upper first permanent molar, its pulp and variants of its occlusal surface. (a) Large cusp of Carabelli, (b) tubercles on the mesial marginal ridge, (d) discontinuous oblique ridge.

to the palatal surface and separates the palatal cusps.

From the buccal aspect, the buccal cusps are about equal in height though the mesiobuccal cusp is wider than the distobuccal cusp. A buccal groove is present. Viewed palatally, the disproportion in size between the mesiopalatal and distopalatal cusps is most evident. The mesiopalatal cusp is blunt and occupies approximately three-fifths of the mesiodistal width of the palatal surface. The distopalatal is the smallest cusp on the crown. The palatal fissure terminates approximately halfway up the palatal surface, from the proximal views; because of the convexity of the palatal surface the palatal cusps appear nearer the centre of the tooth.

The cervical line follows a fairly even contour around the tooth.

There are three roots (two buccal and one palatal) arising from a common root base. The palatal root is the longest and strongest, and is circular in cross-section. The buccal roots are more slender and are flattened mesiodistally; the mesiobuccal root is usually the larger and wider of the two.

*Pulp morphology* (Fig. 5.22)
The pulp chamber of this tooth is quadrilateral in shape, wider buccopalatally than mesiodistally. From the roof four pulp horns arise, one to each of the major cusps. The pulp horn to the mesiobuccal cusp is the longest. The pulp horns to the palatal cusps are the least distinct. The floor of the pulp chamber generally lies below the cervical margin. From the floor, three root canals arise, their orifices being funnel-shaped. A root canal lies in the middle of each root. The more divergent the roots, the closer together lie the orifices of the root canals. The root canal of the mesiobuccal root leaves the pulp chamber in a mesial direction. In cross-section, it appears as a narrow slit, being wider buccopalatally. Its anatomy may be complicated by irregular branching or bifurcation near the apical foramen. The palatal root canal is the widest and longest of the three root canals. For most of its course it is round in cross-section. With age, the canals become much finer and their orifices more difficult to find.

*Variations* (Fig. 5.22)
One of the most common variations relates to the tubercle of Carabelli on the mesiopalatal cusp. Such variations range from complete absence to pit, groove, tubercle, cusplet or cusp (Fig. 5.33). A transverse ridge ('anterior transverse ridge') extends diagonally from the mesiobuccal corner between the mesial marginal ridge and the mesiobuccal cusp towards the centre of the occlusal surface. The oblique ridge is very variable. Where it is discontinuous, a fissure joins the distal and mesial fossae. Supplemental grooves from the main fissure are common but highly variable. The buccal and palatal grooves sometimes terminate as pits on the buccal and palatal surfaces. A common variation is the appearance of tubercles on the mesial marginal ridge; the distal marginal ridge rarely shows such tubercles. The degree to which the roots diverge is variable. Occasionally, the buccal roots may be abnormally short. The distobuccal root shows a particular tendency to curve irregularly. Rarely, the distobuccal and palatal roots may be fused.

THE UPPER SECOND PERMANENT MOLAR

*Average dimensions*
Crown height, 7.0 mm; root length, 11.5 mm; mesiodistal crown diameter, 9.8 mm; buccopalatal crown diameter, 11 mm.

*General description* (Fig. 5.23)
This tooth closely resembles, but is smaller than, the adjacent first molar. Occlusally the rhomboid form is more pronounced. The occlusal fissure pattern is similar to the first molar but is more variable and supplemental grooves are more numerous. Palatally, the distopalatal cusp is reduced in size. A tubercle of Carabelli is not usually found on the mesiopalatal cusp.

Like the first molar, the second molar has three roots (two buccal and one palatal). However, they are shorter and less divergent than those of the first molar and may be partly fused. The apex of the mesiobuccal root is generally in line with the centre of the crown, unlike that of the first molar which generally lies in line with the tip of the mesiobuccal cusp.

*Pulp morphology*
The pulp cavity of the upper second molar may be regarded essentially as a smaller replica of that of the neighbouring first molar. The differences are due to the more convergent roots of the second molar.

*Morphological variations*
Variations in morphology of the upper second permanent molar are quite common. The most common relate to the size of the distopalatal cusp. Total reduction of this cusp is common, giving the

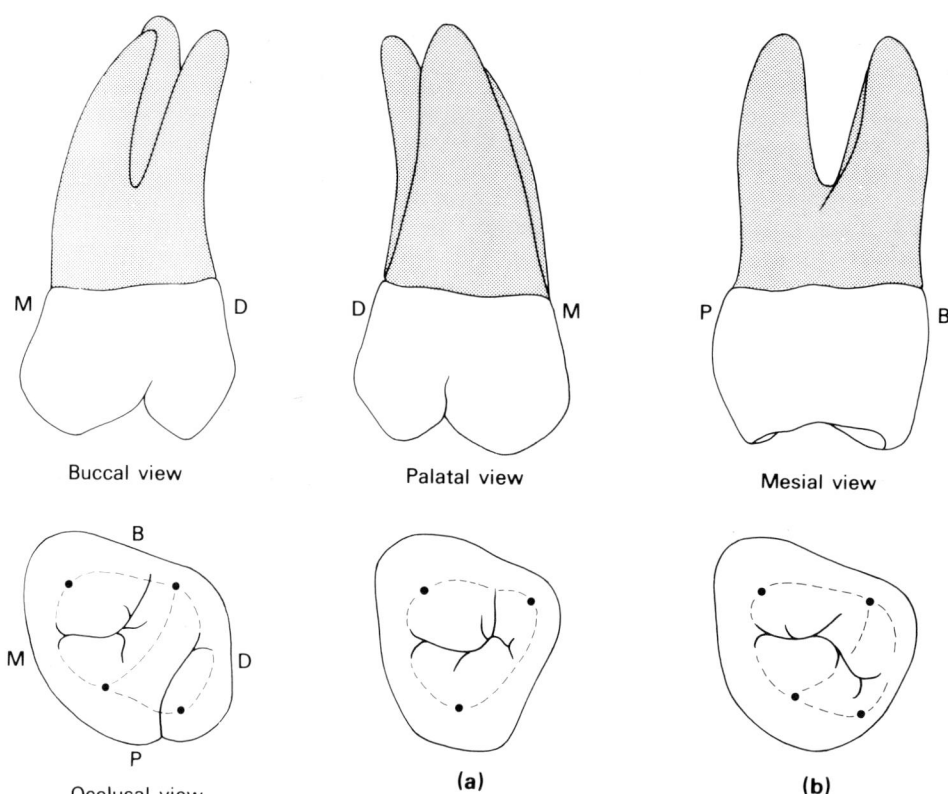

**Fig. 5.23.** The left upper second permanent molar and variations in its occlusal surface. (a) Absence of distopalatal cusp; (b) very small distopalatal cusp and fissure crossing oblique ridge.

occlusal table a triangular outline. The fissure pattern is highly variable as is the morphology of the roots. The mesiobuccal and palatal roots, or even all three roots, may be completely or partially fused.

THE UPPER THIRD PERMANENT MOLAR

*Average dimensions*
Crown height, 6.5 mm; root length, 11.0 mm; mesiodistal crown diameter, 8.6 mm; buccopalatal crown diameter, 10.0 mm.

*General description* (Fig. 5.24)
This tooth is the most variable in the dentition. Its shape may range from that characteristic of the adjacent upper molars to a peg-like tooth. The crown is usually triangular with three cusps. The roots are often fused and irregular in form. The shape of the pulp cavity is very variable. Unlike the lower third molar, with which it might be confused, it never has a rectangular occlusal surface. It is the most common tooth to be absent from the dentition.

THE LOWER FIRST PERMANENT MOLAR

*Average dimensions*
Crown height, 7.5 mm; root length, 14.0 mm; mesiodistal crown diameter, 11.0 mm; buccolingual crown diameter, 10.0 mm.

*General description* (Fig. 5.25)
Viewed occlusally the crown of this tooth has a roughly rectangular outline, being broader mesiodistally than buccolingually. This shape is characteristic of lower molars; upper molars are rhomboid. The occlusal surface is divided into buccal and lingual parts by a mesiodistal fissure which arises from a deep central fossa. The buccal side of the

# Tooth Morphology

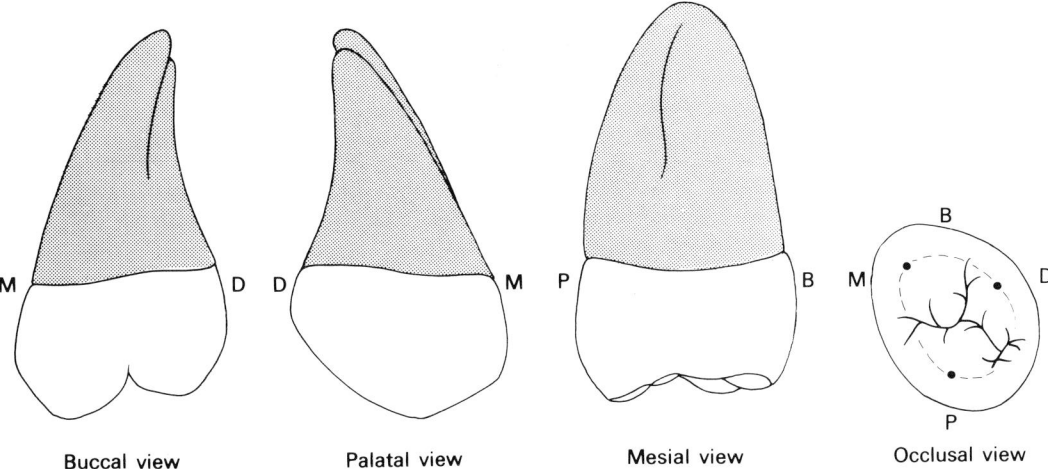

**Fig. 5.24.** The left upper third permanent molar.

occlusal table has three distinct cusps; mesiobuccal, distobuccal and distal. Each cusp is separated by a groove which joins the mesiodistal fissure. On the lingual side the two cusps are mesiolingual and distolingual. The fissure separating the lingual cusps joins the mesiodistal fissure in the region of the central fossa. The lingual cusps tend to be more pointed and prominent though they are not disproportionately larger than the mesiobuccal and distobuccal cusps. The tips of the buccal cusps are displaced lingually, rounded and lower than the lingual cusps. Because of the lingual displacement of the tips of the buccal cusps most of the buccal surface is visible from the occlusal view and this provides a further distinction between upper and lower molars. The smallest cusp is the distal one which is displaced towards the buccal surface. In most cases, the mesiolingual cusp runs into the distobuccal cusp across the floor of the central fossa. From the buccal aspect the relative sizes of the three cusps can be appreciated; the mesiobuccal cusp is the largest and the distal the smallest. The fissure separating the mesiobuccal and distobuccal cusps arises from the central fossa on the occlusal surface and terminates halfway down the buccal surface in a buccal pit. From the lingual aspect the mesiolingual is the larger of the two cusps. The fissure between the lingual cusps does not extend far down the lingual surface. Viewed mesially the buccal surface appears markedly convex especially at the cervical third of the crown. This convexity produces the characteristic lingual inclination of the buccal cusps.

The cervical margin follows a uniform contour around the tooth. Unlike the upper molars, lower molars have only two roots (mesial and distal). The two roots arise from a common base. Both roots are flattened mesiodistally and the mesial root is usually deeply grooved. Both roots curve distally.

*Pulp morphology* (Fig. 5.25)
The pulp chamber of this tooth is wider mesiodistally than it is buccolingually. It is also wider mesially than distally. There are five pulp horns projecting to the cusps, the lingual pulp horns being longer and more pointed. The floor of the pulp chamber lies at or just below the level of the cervical margin. The root canals leave the pulp chamber through funnel-shaped orifices of which the mesial are finer than the distal. The mesial root has two root canals, mesiobuccal and mesiolingual. Generally, the mesiobuccal root canal follows a tortuous path. The mesiolingual canal is straighter and slightly larger in cross-section than the mesiobuccal root canal, though both are circular in cross-section. Occasionally, the two canals may join in the apical fifth of the root. The distal root has a single root canal. This is considerably larger and more oval in cross-section than the mesial root canals. It generally follows a straight course. Rarely, the distal root has two root canals. With age the pulp cavity becomes constricted, particularly the roof of the pulp chamber.

*Variations*
These are described in the section on racial differences at the end of this Chapter (see Fig. 11.11).

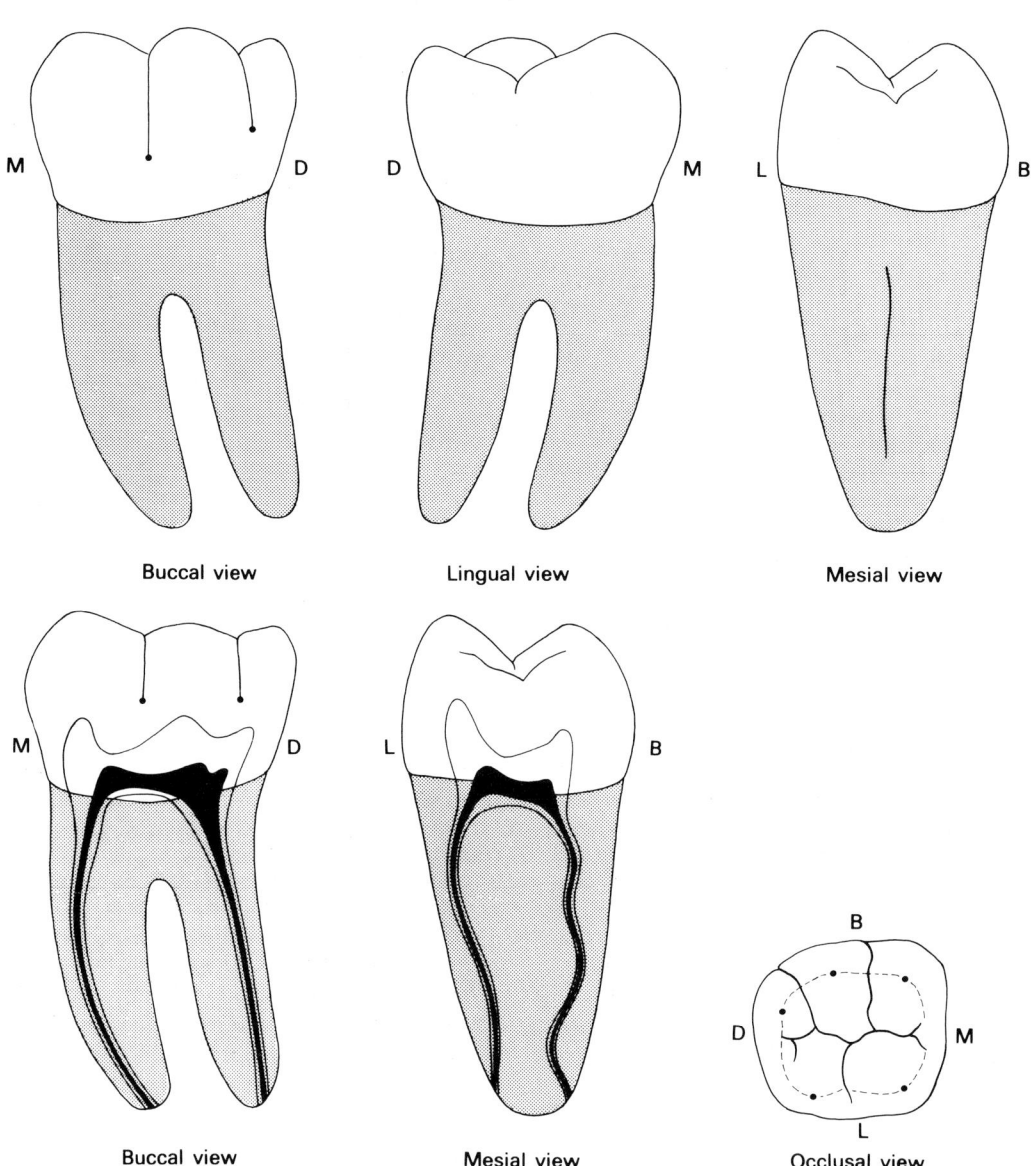

**Fig. 5.25.** The left lower first permanent molar and the shape of its pulp.

THE LOWER SECOND PERMANENT MOLAR

*Average dimensions*
Crown height, 7.0 mm; root length, 12.0 mm; mesiodistal crown diameter, 10.6 mm; buccolingual crown diameter, 9.8 mm.

*General description* (Fig. 5.26)
Viewed occlusally the crown usually has a regular rectangular shape. There are four cusps, the mesiobuccal and the mesiolingual cusps being slightly larger than the distobuccal and distolingual cusps. The cusps are separated by a cross-shaped occlusal fissure though it may be complicated by supplemental grooves. From the buccal aspect, the crown appears smaller than that of the first molar. A fissure extends between the buccal cusps from the occlusal surface to terminate approximately halfway up the buccal surface. Like the adjacent first molar, the buccal surface is markedly convex. Lingually the crown is

# Tooth Morphology

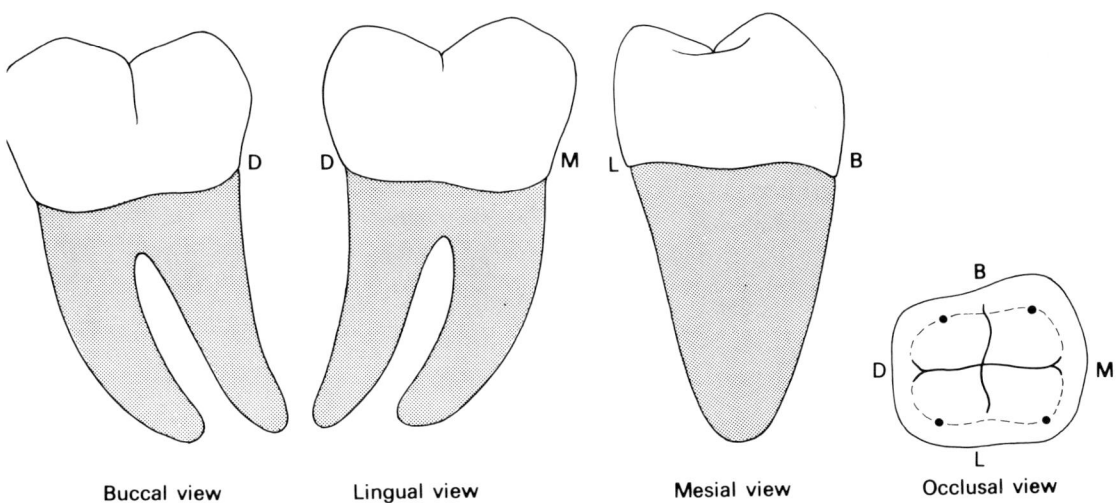

**Fig. 5.26.** The left lower second permanent molar.

noticeably shorter occlusocervically than the first molar. The mesial and distal aspects of the second molar resemble those of the first molar though, because there is no distal cusp, the proximal surfaces are more equal in terms of their convexity.

The mesial and distal roots are flattened mesiodistally and are smaller and less divergent than those of the first molar. Indeed, they may be partly fused. The distal inclination of the roots is usually more marked.

*Pulp morphology*
This closely resembles that of the adjacent first molar, though there are only four pulp horns.

*Morphological variations* (Fig. 5.33).

## THE LOWER THIRD PERMANENT MOLAR

*Average dimensions*
Crown height, 7.0 mm; root length, 11.0 mm; mesiodistal crown diameter, 10.3 mm; buccolingual crown diameter, 9.5 mm.

*General description* (Fig. 5.27)
Although its shape is variable, it is not as variable as that of the upper third permanent molar and it is generally possible to recognize the rectangular outline typical of lower molars. The crown is the smallest of the lower molars though occasionally it may be as large as the first molar. It has four or five cusps. Its occlusal fissure pattern is irregular. As a

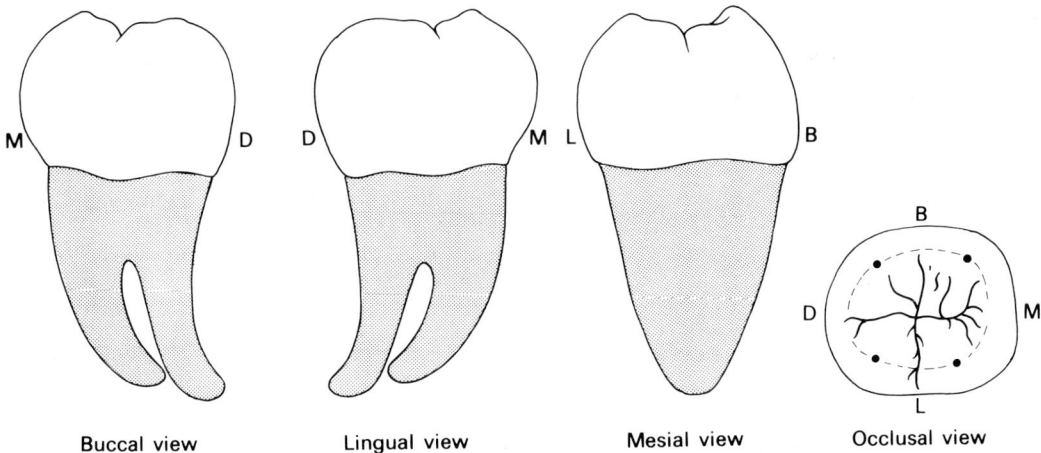

**Fig. 5.27.** The left lower third permanent molar.

rule, the roots are greatly reduced and are fused. They show a marked distal inclination. The tooth is commonly absent from the dentition and pulp morphology is extremely variable.

**The deciduous dentition**

Like the permanent dentition the deciduous dentition has two incisors and one canine in each quadrant but has no premolars (by definition) and only two molars. The deciduous teeth differ from the permanent teeth in the following respects:

1 The deciduous teeth are smaller than their corresponding permanent successors (Fig. 5.28) though the mesiodistal dimensions of the premolars are generally less than those for the equivalent deciduous molars.
2 Deciduous teeth have more consistent shapes.
3 The crowns of deciduous teeth appear bulbous, often having pronounced labial or buccal cingula.
4 The cusps of newly erupted deciduous teeth are more pointed.

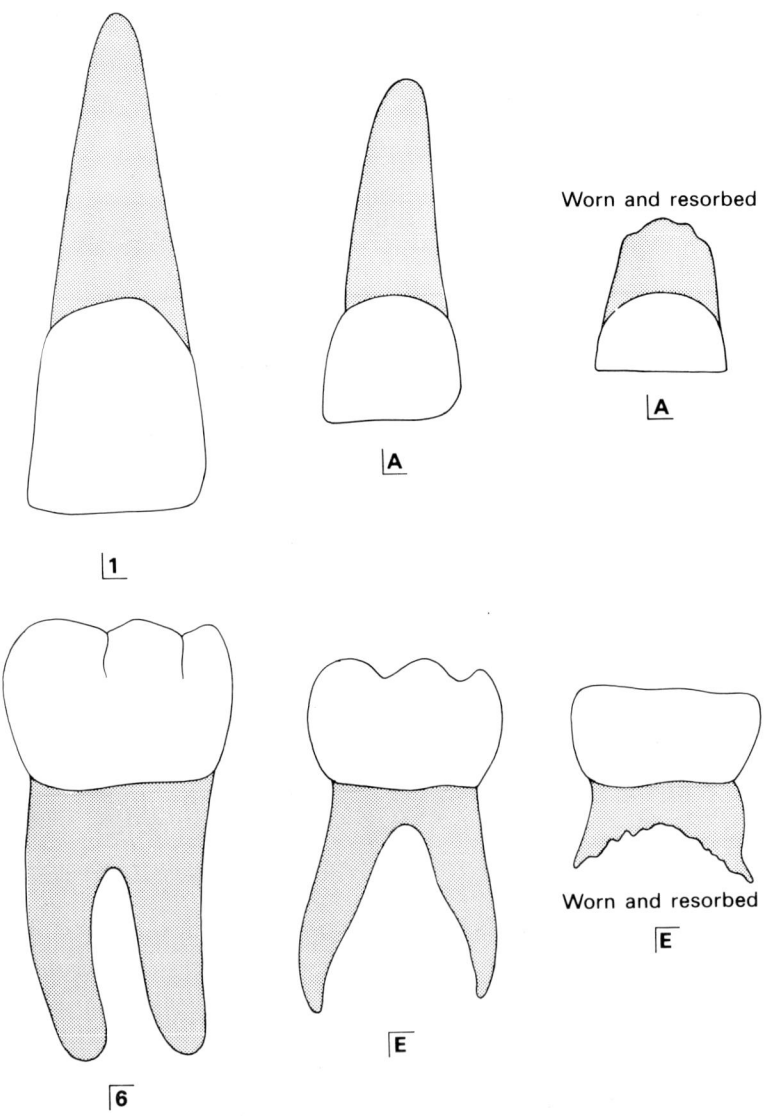

**Fig. 5.28.** Comparison between the sizes of permanent and deciduous teeth and the appearance of resorbed and worn teeth: central incisors and molars.

5 The crowns of deciduous teeth are whiter, less mineralized and become very worn.

6 The cervical margins of deciduous teeth are more sharply demarcated and pronounced than those of the permanent teeth; the enamel bulging at the cervical margins rather than gently tapering.

7 The roots of deciduous teeth are shorter and less robust than those of the permanent teeth (see 1).

8 The roots of the deciduous incisors and canines are longer in proportion to the crown than those of their permanent counterparts.

9 The roots of the deciduous molars are widely divergent, extending beyond the dimensions of the crown.

10 The pulp cavities of deciduous teeth are proportionally larger than those of the permanent teeth.

THE UPPER FIRST (CENTRAL) DECIDUOUS INCISOR

*Average dimensions*
Crown height, 6 mm; root length, 10.0 mm; mesiodistal crown diameter, 6.5 mm; labiopalatal crown diameter, 5.0 mm.

*General description* (Fig. 5.29)
This tooth has a similar shape to the corresponding permanent tooth. However, since the breadth of its crown nearly equals its height it appears plumper than its permanent successor. From the incisal view the straight incisal edge is centred over the bulk of the crown. Unlike the permanent tooth, no mammelons are developed on the incisal edge. The labial surface is slightly convex in all planes and unmarked by grooves, lobes or depressions. The mesioincisal angle is sharp and acute, whilst the distoincisal angle is more rounded and obtuse. On the palatal surface the cingulum is a very prominent bulge which extends for some distance up the crown. Unlike its permanent successor, the marginal ridges are ill-defined and the concavity of the palatal surface shallow. Mesial and distal views show the typical shovel-shaped appearance of the crown. From this view, the low, rounded cingulum can be seen at the margin of the labial surface.

As with all deciduous teeth, the cervical margins are more pronounced but less sinuous than their permanent successors.

The fully formed root is conical, tapering to a rather blunt apex. Compared with the corresponding permanent tooth, the root is longer in proportion to the crown. Most specimens have severely worn incisal edges.

*Pulp morphology* (Fig. 5.30)
The pulp chamber follows closely the outline of the tooth. The pulp tissue is closer to the surface of the tooth than for the permanent successor. The pulp canals are wide and there is no clear distinction between pulp chamber and root canal.

THE UPPER SECOND (LATERAL) DECIDUOUS INCISOR

*Average dimensions*
Crown height, 5.6 mm; root length, 10.2 mm; mesiodistal crown diameter, 5.2 mm; labiopalatal crown diameter, 4 mm.

*General description* (Fig. 5.29)
This tooth is similar in shape, though smaller, than the maxillary first deciduous incisor. However the mesioincisal angle is more acute and the distoincisal angle is more rounded. The palatal surface is more concave and the marginal ridges are more pronounced. Viewed incisally the crown appears almost circular in contrast to the central incisor which appears diamond-shaped. Like the first deciduous incisor, there is a rounded, labial cingulum cervically. The palatal cingulum is generally lower than that of the central incisor.

The course of the cervical margin and the shape of the root are similar to the first deciduous incisor.

*Pulp morphology*
This differs little from that described for the upper first deciduous incisor.

THE LOWER FIRST (CENTRAL) DECIDUOUS INCISOR

*Average dimensions*
Crown height, 5.0 mm; root length, 9.0 mm; mesiodistal crown diameter, 4.0 mm; labiolingual crown diameter, 4.0 mm.

*General description* (Fig. 5.29)
This tooth has a similar shape to its permanent successor, though it is much shorter and has a low labial cingulum.

The single root is more rounded than the corresponding permanent tooth.

*Pulp morphology*
Like the deciduous upper incisors, the pulp cavity is wide and follows closely the crown outline. Occasionally, the root canal may bifurcate into labial and lingual branches.

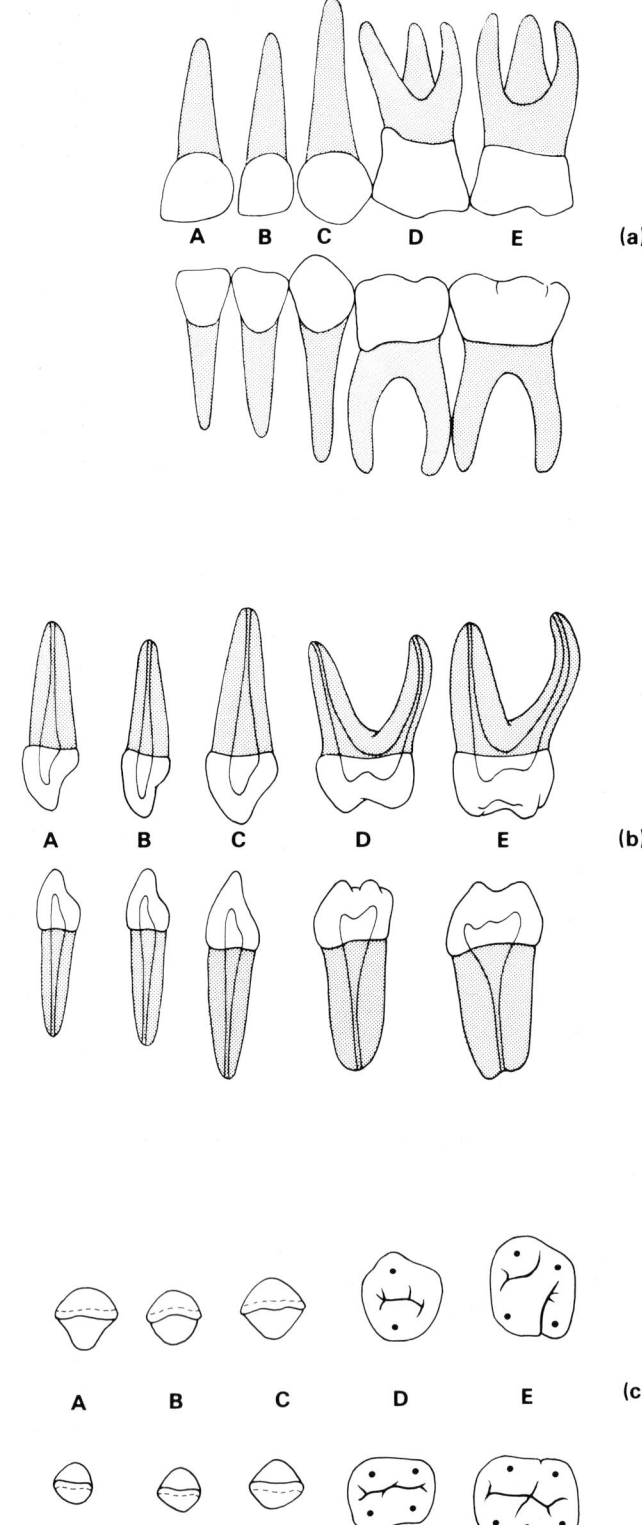

**Fig. 5.29.** Morphology of the deciduous dentition (left side). (a) Buccal view; (b) view with superimposed pulp outlines; (c) occlusal view.

## Tooth Morphology

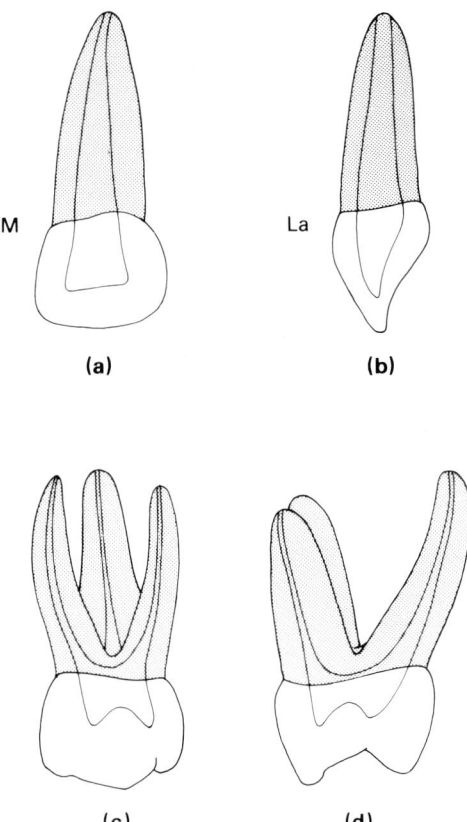

**Fig. 5.30.** Pulp shapes: (a) Labial view of upper deciduous incisor; (b) distal view of upper deciduous incisor; (c) buccal view of upper deciduous molar; (d) distal view of upper deciduous molar.

THE LOWER SECOND (LATERAL) DECIDUOUS INCISOR

*Average dimensions*
Crown height, 5.2 mm; root length, 9.8 mm; mesiodistal crown diameter, 4.5 mm; labiolingual crown diameter, 4.0 mm.

*General description* (Fig. 5.29)
Like the other deciduous incisors, the lower second deciduous incisor resembles its permanent successor. It is wider than the lower first deciduous incisor and is asymmetrical.

THE UPPER DECIDUOUS CANINE

*Average dimensions*
Crown height, 6.5 mm; root length, 13.0 mm; mesiodistal crown diameter, 6.8 mm; labiopalatal crown diameter, 7.0 mm.

*General description* (Fig. 5.29)
This generally symmetrical tooth has a fang-like appearance, being similar to, though more bulbous than, its permanent successor. When viewed labially or palatally its bulge gives the crown a diamond-shaped appearance with the crown margins overhanging the root profiles. The mesiodistal width of the crown is greater than its height.

The root is long compared with the crown height and is triangular in cross-section.

*Pulp morphology*
The pulp cavity follows the outline of the tooth and has a single pulp horn pointing towards the cusp. Like that of the deciduous incisors, the root canal is wide and there is no clear distinction between it and the pulp chamber.

THE LOWER DECIDUOUS CANINE

*Average dimensions*
Crown height, 6.0 mm; root length, 11.2 mm; mesiodistal crown diameter, 5.5 mm; labiolingual crown diameter, 4.9 mm.

*General description* (Fig. 5.29)
This tooth is more slender than the upper deciduous canine. The crown is asymmetrical with the cusp tip displaced mesially. On the lingual surface the cingulum and marginal ridges are less pronounced than the corresponding structures on the palatal surface of the upper deciduous canine. The mesiodistal width is less than the height.

The root is single and slightly triangular in cross-section.

*Pulp morphology*
This is similar to that described for the upper deciduous canine.

THE UPPER FIRST DECIDUOUS MOLAR

*Average dimensions*
Crown height, 5.1 mm; root length, 10.0 mm; mesiodistal crown diameter, 7.1 mm; buccopalatal crown diameter, 8.5 mm.

*General description* (Fig. 5.29)
This tooth, which is the most atypical of all molars, both deciduous and permanent, appears to be intermediate between a premolar and a molar. It is the smallest molar. Viewed occlusally, the crown is an irregular quadrilateral. However, the

mesiobuccal corner is extended to produce a prominent buccal bulge. The buccal and palatal cusps are separated by a mesiodistally running occlusal fissure. The buccal cusp is the most prominent. A shallow buccal fissure may extend from the central mesiodistal fissure to divide the buccal cusp into two, the mesial part being the larger. The palatal cusp may also be subdivided into two. Viewed from the buccal aspect, the crown appears squat, its height being less than its width. Marginal ridges linking the buccal and palatal cusps are not crossed by fissures.

The tooth has three roots (two buccal and one palatal) which arise from a common base. The mesiobuccal root is flattened mesiodistally. The distobuccal root is smaller and more curved. The palatal root is the largest and is round in cross-section. The distobuccal and palatal roots may be partially fused.

*Pulp morphology* (Fig. 5.30)
The pulp chamber in this tooth is large in relation to the tooth size. Pulp horns to the two main cusps are well-developed. Additional cusps may have additional pulp horns. Each root has a root canal but the root canal system is more complicated than that of permanent molars, often branching.

THE UPPER SECOND DECIDUOUS MOLAR

*Average dimensions*
Crown height, 5.7 mm; root length, 11.7 mm; mesiodistal crown diameter, 8.4 mm; buccopalatal crown diameter, 10.0 mm.

*General description* (Fig. 5.29)
This tooth closely resembles the upper first permanent molar, though its size, whiteness, widely diverging roots and low buccal cingulum help to distinguish it. A tubercle of Carabelli on the mesiopalatal cusp is often well-developed.

*Pulp morphology*
The pulp cavity is large in relation to tooth size. The pulp chamber gives off pulp horns to each of the main cusps.

THE LOWER FIRST DECIDUOUS MOLAR

*Average dimensions*
Crown height, 6.0 mm; root length, 9.8 mm; mesiodistal crown diameter, 7.7 mm; buccolingual crown diameter, 7.0 mm.

*General description* (Fig. 5.29)
From the occlusal aspect the crown appears elongated mesiodistally and is an irregular rectangle, the buccal and lingual surfaces being parallel. Like the upper first deciduous molar, the mesiobuccal corner is extended to form a buccal bulge. The occlusal table is usually divided into buccal and lingual parts by a mesiodistal fissure. The buccal part consists of two ill-defined cusps, the mesiobuccal being larger than the distobuccal. The lingual part of the tooth is narrower than the buccal part and also has two cusps, the mesial being the larger. The mesial cusps are larger than the distal cusps. A transverse ridge may connect the mesial cusps, dividing the mesiodistal fissure into a distal fissure and a mesial pit. Often a distal pit may be found just mesial to the distal marginal ridge. A supplemental groove from the mesial pit may extend over the mesial marginal ridge. The lower first deciduous molar has two divergent roots, mesial and distal, which are flattened mesiodistally. The mesial root is often grooved.

*Pulp morphology*
The pulp cavity is large in relation to the size of the tooth. Pulp horns project from the pulp chamber into each of the four main cusps. Like the permanent molars, the mesial root generally has two root canals, the distal root one.

THE LOWER SECOND DECIDUOUS MOLAR

*Average dimensions*
Crown height, 5.5 mm; root length, 12.5 mm; mesiodistal crown diameter, 9.7 mm; buccolingual crown diameter, 8.7 mm.

*General description* (Figs. 5.28, 5.29)
This tooth is similar to the lower first permanent molar. However, it is smaller, narrower, whiter, has widely diverging roots and has more convex mesial and distal surfaces.

*Pulp morphology*
The pulp cavity resembles that seen in the lower first permanent molar, though the pulp chamber is relatively wider and the root canals relatively narrower. There are two root canals in the mesial root and one in the distal root.

**General remarks**

From the above descriptions it should be possible to locate the original position of an isolated tooth and to decide whether it is a permanent or deciduous tooth. But a tooth betrays much more than this.

AGE

*Root development*
Each tooth begins to mineralize, has its crown formed, erupts and has its roots completed at times which are, within limits, typical for that tooth (p. 323). By studying the degree to which a particular tooth has developed, the age of its owner at the time of extraction can be assessed with some accuracy. For example, the crown of the lower first permanent molar is complete at 3 years of age. When it erupts at 6 years, about half of its root is formed. The root is complete at 9 years, therefore requiring about 3 years to form the remaining half. A rough calculation suggests that a first permanent molar whose roots are about three-quarters complete came from an individual between 7 and 8 years old.

*Attrition*
The longer a tooth has functioned the more heavily worn it appears. But the amount of wear depends on the roughness of the diet: most Europeans wear down their teeth far less than Eskimos and Aborigines. Therefore, in the absence of knowledge of the diet, attrition provides only a poor indication of tooth age. Nevertheless, a 14-year-old will not have a very heavily worn second permanent molar.

*Gingival attachment*
The gingivae, which are firmly attached to the neck of the tooth, gradually recede down the root with age: the process of getting 'long in the tooth'. Although the rate of this recession is very variable, the older a person the further from the enamel is the gingival attachment. The position of this attachment can almost always be recognized on an isolated tooth. On many teeth a fine dark line separates a smooth coronal part of the root from a roughened apical part. On other teeth, calculus (tartar) has collected on that part of the root coronal to the gingival attachment: calculus can only develop on surfaces in contact with saliva.

*Cement*
The thickness of cement increases with age: the thicker the cement, the older the tooth.

*Colour*
Old teeth are much darker than young teeth but the assessment of age from colour requires considerable experience. However, many extracted teeth have been whitened in bleaching solutions making a correct assessment impossible.

RACE

There are many distinguishing features between the teeth of different races (p. 151) but most of these can only be recognized from statistical analysis and are of little or no value in the recognition of isolated teeth.

DEVELOPMENTAL DEFECTS

Unlike bone, fully developed enamel and dentine are almost totally unaffected by general disease (caries is a localized disease). However, every transient injury during its development leaves a permanent record in the tooth. If the disease is sufficiently serious the developing enamel is permanently marked by a ridge or a white line. The position of the defect on a particular tooth is determined by the extent to which that tooth is developed at the time of the disease.

ANOMALIES

The shapes of teeth within a species are astonishingly constant. For this reason it can be interesting to collect teeth whose shapes are anomalous. The student is easily 'tricked' by upper molars with two roots; by lower molars with three roots; by upper molars with one buccal and two palatal roots; by lower premolars with two roots, etc. It is important to remember that the shapes of crowns are more constant than the shapes of roots. Crowns can be oddly shaped, particularly those of the third molars. Paramolar tubercles, accessory cusps on the buccal sides of cheek teeth, can be very confusing.

**Protective features**

Several features common to all the cheek teeth seem to be important because they protect the adjacent gingiva. It is usually essential that the shapes of these features are restored when they are replaced by a filling material.

CONTACT POINTS (Fig. 5.31a)

The mesial surface of a tooth normally abuts firmly against the distal surface of an adjacent tooth. This contact is maintained by the process of mesial drift (p. 326) despite the constant abrasion of contact areas. If a contact area is not adequately restored food easily gets wedged between the teeth, which is a common irritation. If the space between teeth is wide enough food can easily wedge between them but it is as easily removed.

MARGINAL RIDGES (Fig. 5.31a)

All the cheek teeth, and to a lesser extent the anterior teeth, have marginal ridges. These ridges deflect most of the food, potentially driven between adjacent teeth by their opponents, on to the occlusal surfaces. If the marginal ridge is not restored by filling material food rapidly compacts between the teeth leading to inflammation of the gingiva.

CURVATURES OF CHEEK TEETH (Fig. 5.31b)

The buccal cusps of lower cheek teeth bite between the buccal and lingual cusps of upper cheek teeth (Fig. 9.1) with the result that food trapped between them is forced up over the palatal sides of upper teeth and down over the buccal sides of lower teeth. Adjacent to each of the upper cheek teeth the palatal gingiva is protected by a strongly curved tooth surface: it is the buccal surfaces of lower cheek teeth which are more curved.

**Development, resorption, fracture**

An unduly short root may be due to the fact that it is not yet fully developed, or that it has been resorbed or fractured.

**1** A fully developed root has an almost invisible apical foramen. If the exposed part of the pulp canal in a root is large, the tooth was almost certainly still developing when it was extracted. The edges of a developing root are smooth, thin and sharp, and funnel into a narrowing hollow (Fig. 5.32a).

**2** Only deciduous teeth are normally (as opposed to pathologically) resorbed. The resorbed surface is rough and is usually on the lingual side of anterior teeth and between the roots of

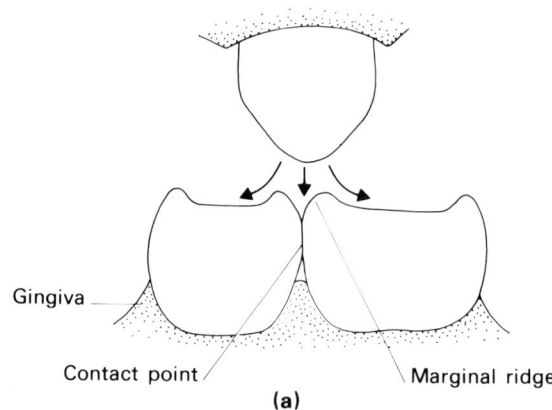

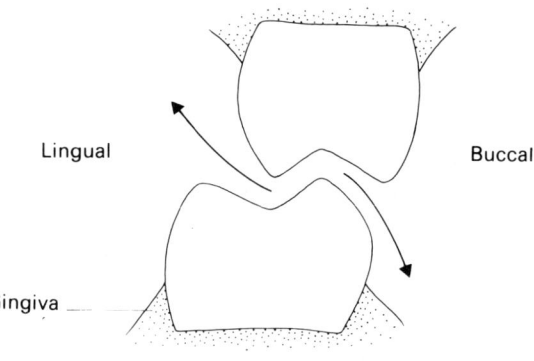

**Fig. 5.31** Morphology of teeth in relation to the displacement of food (arrow). (a) Buccal view; (b) lateral view.

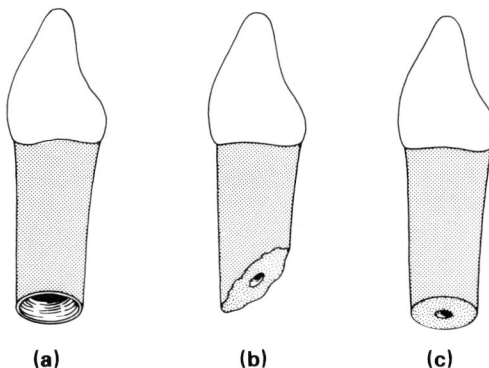

**Fig. 5.32.** Variations in the appearance of the root apex. (a) Developing root; (b) resorbing root; (c) fractured root.

molars. If the resorption is confined to the root, the exposed pulp canal is very small (Fig. 5.32b).
3 Fractured roots have a straight, smooth surface usually with a narrow exposed root canal (Fig. 5.32c).

## RACIAL DIFFERENCES OF TOOTH MORPHOLOGY

A race is usually defined as a subdivision of a species formed by individuals who share common biological characteristics. Races can however be distinguished not only biologically but also from the cultural point of view, though the cultural differences are probably largely secondary to the biological ones and to differences of environment. The biological characteristics that have been used traditionally to distinguish the races of man are skin pigmentation, facial form and body build; characteristics that have been shown to be highly heritable. These have been chosen simply because they are conspicuous but heritable differences between races undoubtedly exist for a wide variety of less noticeable characteristics. The highly heritable nature of the biological characteristics distinguishing one race from another indicates that differences between races are fundamentally of genetic origin. Nevertheless, only a small proportion of all known human genetic variation appears to be responsible for racial differences. It has been estimated that, of the worldwide total of human genetic variation, about 80% occurs within races and only about 20% accounts for the biological differences between races.

It has long been known that minor morphological variation is superimposed on the basic shapes of human teeth. In common with the variation shown by other biological characteristics, much of this minor dental variation is found within races; different individuals of the same race often show different manifestations of each morphological variable. However, a proportion also occurs between races, so that individuals from a particular race tend to have a particular constellation of morphological features, with different constellations being typical of different races. In fact, minor differences of tooth shape have contributed to the characterization of the races of man and have been used to provide an indication of racial affinity between human populations. Both contemporary and past populations can be compared. The study of contemporary populations requires intraoral examination or, preferably, plaster casts of the teeth; that of past populations requires adequate skeletal or fossil remains. Nevertheless, it must be remembered that the use of a particular variant for the biological characterization of races is only valid if the variant is known to be largely under genetic control. This condition is probably fulfilled for most minor variants of tooth shape; in other words, individuals probably have particular dental morphological characteristics because they have inherited particular genes and not simply through chance or for some environmental reason. Direct evidence for the genetic control of a character comes from studies of resemblance between relatives, and for tooth morphology such studies are few and far between.

Even so, it is justifiable to use tooth morphology for studying racial affinity, provided it is borne in mind that the underlying basis for the observed variation is not yet fully understood. Affinity is measured by comparing the frequencies of different morphological variants in different groups. A similar percentage frequency of the same highly heritable variant form in two groups implies a high degree of affinity, whereas the greater the difference in frequency the lower the affinity and the greater the biological distance between the groups. Data for more than one variable can be combined to provide a single estimate of biological distance between two groups, and the larger the number of variables used the more reliable the estimate. A comparison of the pattern of racial affinities derived from a study of tooth morphology with the pattern based on other, better understood, biological criteria can provide a clue to the underlying basis of dental morphological variation. If the patterns are similar it is reasonable to infer that dental morphological variation is likely to have a high degree of genetic deter-

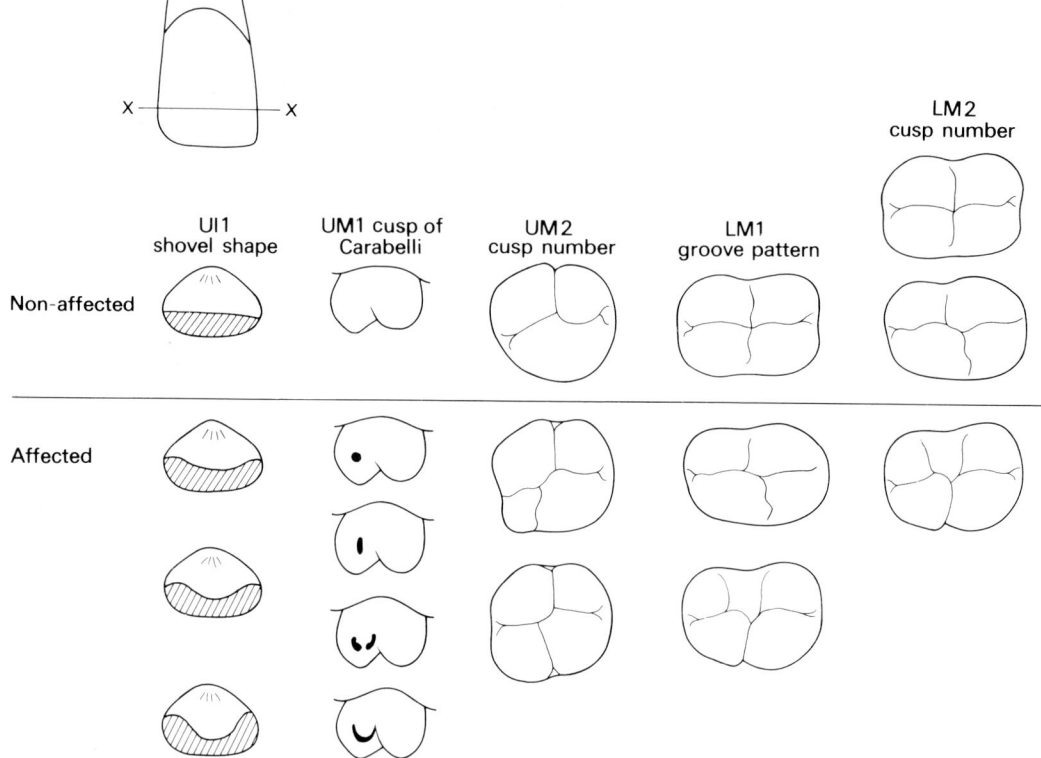

**Fig. 5.33.** Morphological variables on the upper central incisor (UI1), upper first and second molars (UM1 and UM2), and lower first and second molars (LM1 and LM2); and division of the range of variation of each into two categories, nonaffected and affected. Diagrams are modified from Lee G. T. R. and Goose D. H. (1972). The inheritance of dental traits in a Chinese population in the United Kingdom. *Journal of Medical Genetics* **9**, 336.

mination and can therefore make a useful contribution to the biological characterization of human populations.

There have been many studies of the frequency of variant forms for dental morphological characters in different populations. Five of the more commonly studied characters are illustrated in Fig. 5.33. They all appear to behave as quasi-continuous variables; that is, the variant form is either present or absent, but when present it can show different levels of expression from the lowest to the most extreme. For example, the upper second molar may have three cusps or four cusps but the fourth cusp, when present, varies in size. Some indication of the range of expression of the different characters is given in Fig. 5.33 but for the present purpose all the variables are regarded as all-or-none characters; in other words, a tooth is considered to be either non-affected or affected. The relevant characteristic of a population is the proportion of teeth affected.

The frequencies of the variant forms reported for different populations of the same racial group sometimes differ considerably. This must be partly because of real differences between samples taken from the different populations, but undoubtedly is also due to differences between the scoring criteria of different investigators. The most reliable estimate of the frequency of a variant in a given race is therefore the frequency of affected teeth in a group composed of as many samples as possible pooled together. Table 5.1 lists the lowest and highest frequency values found in the literature, each calculated from a single sample, and the pooled frequency estimate, calculated for teeth from several samples, for each of the five dental morphological characters in seven racial groups. The low and high values indicate the considerable range of variation in frequency reported for some of the characters in some racial groups. The pooled frequency estimates can be used to derive the most reliable pattern of affinities between different racial groups.

Many different statistical procedures, some very complex, have been used to combine observations on several characters to express biolog-

**Table 5.1.** The percentage frequency of affected teeth (%A) for five dental morphological characters in seven racial groups. For each character and each group the 'low' and 'high' values are the lowest and highest reported in the literature by different investigators, and the 'pooled' value is the frequency of affected teeth over several separately reported samples combined. N is the number of individuals on which each frequency is based. Sources of the data are given in SOFAER J.A., et al. (1972) Population studies on south-western Indian tribes. V. Tooth morphology as an indicator of biological distance. *American Journal of Physical Anthropology*, **37**, 357.

| Racial group: | | CAU Caucasian | | SEM Semitic | | NEG Negro | |
|---|---|---|---|---|---|---|---|
| Character | Estimate of %A | N | %A | N | %A | N | %A |
| UI1 Shovel shape | Low | 100 | 17.0 | 137 | 41.5 | 264 | 16.6 |
| | High | 212 | 91.0 | 60 | 47.0 | 807 | 44.4 |
| | Pooled | 1833 | 40.5 | 197 | 43.2 | 1193 | 37.2 |
| UM1 Cusp of Carabelli | Low | 91 | 41.0 | 30 | 62.0 | 389 | 2.0 |
| | High | 140 | 85.7 | 30 | 93.0 | 274 | 57.7 |
| | Pooled | 3789 | 59.5 | 197 | 73.9 | 663 | 25.0 |
| UM2 Cusp number | Low | 53 | 58.0 | 137 | 30.5 | 78 | 100.0 |
| | High | 50 | 87.5 | 30 | 73.0 | 78 | 100.0 |
| | Pooled | 103 | 72.3 | 197 | 42.1 | 78 | 100.0 |
| LM1 Groove pattern | Low | 85 | 86.0 | 30 | 53.0 | 133 | 86.9 |
| | High | 75 | 96.0 | 137 | 70.4 | 49 | 100.0 |
| | Pooled | 221 | 91.6 | 197 | 65.7 | 182 | 90.4 |
| LM2 Cusp number | Low | 61 | 1.0 | 60 | 0 | 167 | 18.6 |
| | High | 356 | 14.0 | 137 | 7.0 | 69 | 53.7 |
| | Pooled | 611 | 11.0 | 197 | 4.9 | 285 | 28.2 |

| Racial group: | | PAC Pacific and Australia | | ASI Asia | | ESK Aleut and Eskimo | | AMI American Indian | |
|---|---|---|---|---|---|---|---|---|---|
| Character | Estimate of %A | N | %A | N | %A | N | %A | N | %A |
| UI1 Shovel shape | Low | 167 | 41.0 | 269 | 85.0 | 499 | 99.2 | 342 | 100.0 |
| | High | 59 | 88.1 | 259 | 97.7 | 267 | 100.0 | 342 | 100.0 |
| | Pooled | 1045 | 56.8 | 1817 | 92.8 | 766 | 99.5 | 342 | 100.0 |
| UM1 Cusp of Carabelli | Low | 67 | 19.4 | 339 | 31.9 | 60 | 13.3 | 41 | 12.0 |
| | High | 30 | 33.0 | 339 | 31.9 | 61 | 78.3 | 200 | 83.5 |
| | Pooled | 97 | 23.6 | 339 | 31.9 | 384 | 66.3 | 844 | 60.2 |
| UM2 Cusp number | Low | 53 | 69.8 | 887 | 84.6 | 91 | 65.7 | 53 | 66.2 |
| | High | 104 | 100.0 | 887 | 84.6 | 118 | 72.9 | 97 | 91.8 |
| | Pooled | 256 | 88.7 | 887 | 84.6 | 264 | 69.6 | 241 | 82.1 |
| LM1 Groove pattern | Low | 57 | 54.9 | 40 | 100.0 | 29 | 41.4 | 53 | 76.9 |
| | High | 20 | 100.0 | 40 | 100.0 | 30 | 97.0 | 55 | 100.0 |
| | Pooled | 77 | 66.6 | 40 | 100.0 | 202 | 88.2 | 270 | 95.1 |
| LM2 Cusp number | Low | 97 | 12.5 | 19 | 19.0 | 30 | 43.0 | 55 | 32.0 |
| | High | 20 | 48.0 | 21 | 31.0 | 58 | 66.1 | 53 | 72.0 |
| | Pooled | 232 | 24.6 | 40 | 25.3 | 124 | 57.4 | 197 | 60.4 |

ical distance between populations. Each has its own application. Probably the simplest that is suitable for the present purpose is the square root of the sum of squared differences of percentage frequency over all characters studied; that is, $\sqrt{\sum (P_1 - P_2)^2}$, where $P_1$ and $P_2$ are percentage frequencies of a particular variant in the two populations being compared. Distances calculated in this way, based on the five dental morphological variables illustrated in Fig. 5.33,

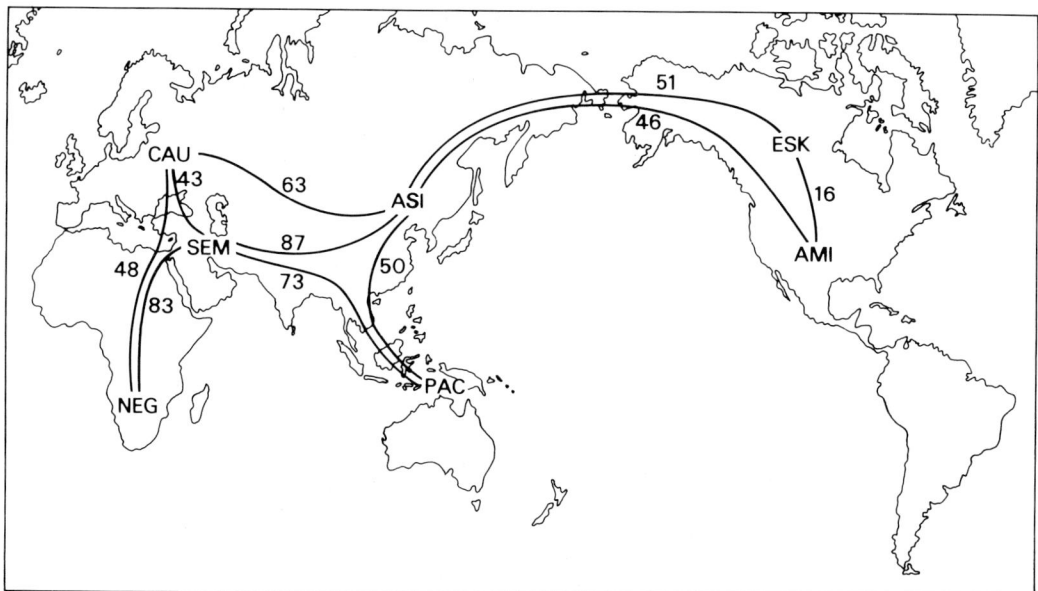

**Fig. 5.34.** A comparison between geographical distances along possible routes of migration and 'dental morphology distances' (given in figures against corresponding routes) separating neighbouring racial groups. The dental morphology distances are calculated from the frequencies of affected teeth for five dental morphological characters in several samples pooled for each racial group (see Table 5.1). (CAU = Caucasian: SEM = Semitic: ASI = Asian: ESK = Aleut and Eskimo: AMI = American Indian: PAC = Pacific and Australia: NEG = Negroid)

are shown on a world map in Fig. 5.34. The position of each racial group is marked at approximately the geometric centre of the area from which samples contributing to the pooled frequency value were drawn. The geographical distances between racial groups, along possible routes of migration, are indications of the ease of admixture and consequently of genetic similarity. Provided there are no extreme geographical or cultural barriers between particular races, the shorter the geographical distance the shorter the biological distance.

Four 'triangular' relationships between neighbouring racial groups are shown on the map: CAU–SEM–NEG, CAU–ASI–SEM, SEM–ASI–PAC and ASI–ESK–AMI. For each of these the 'dental morphology distance' is least between the two geographically closest groups. For example, the dental morphology distance between the Caucasian and Semitic groups is less than that between either of these groups and the Asians. The dental morphology distances therefore show some degree of correspondence with the geographical distances, and so, assuming that biological distance is closely associated with geographical distance, the dental morphological variables considered here seem to be of some use for indicating biological relationships between populations.

It can be argued that racial differences of tooth morphology do reflect fundamental biological differences between races. However, there is still a need for family studies of tooth morphology to provide direct and more detailed information about the genetic control of human dental morphological variation. Until this information becomes available the precise value of dental morphological differences as indicators of biological distance, and the relative usefulness of different morphological variables for biological characterization, will be a matter for speculation.

# FURTHER READING

DOWNER G.C. (1975) *Dental Morphology*. Bristol: Wright.

HARTY F.J. (1976) *Endodontics in Clinical Practice*. Bristol: Wright.

KRAUS B.S. & JORDAN R.E. (1965) *The Human Dentition before Birth*. Philadelphia: Lea & Febiger.

KRAUS B.S., JORDAN R.E. & ABRAMS L. (1969) *Dental Anatomy and Occlusion*. Baltimore: Williams and Wilkins.

SCOTT J.H. & SYMONS N.B.B. (1974) *Introduction to Dental Anatomy*, 7th Edition, Edinburgh: Livingstone.

WHEELER R.C. (1974) *A Textbook of Dental Anatomy and Physiology*, 5th Edition. London: Saunders.

# CHAPTER 6
# Dental Tissues

## EVOLUTION

The teeth of vertebrates have a common basic structure. The body of the tooth always consists of dentine, which is a moderately hard tissue. The functional surface is generally covered by a layer of a much harder, more highly mineralized tissue, of which there are two forms, enamel and enameloid. This chapter is devoted to the evolutionary history of these three tissues. One major group of vertebrates, the birds, lack teeth altogether. The lampreys, hagfishes, frog larvae (tadpoles), turtles and the platypus lack true teeth but have evolved horny structures which take their place (see Fig. 4.2). These horny tissues are derived from the oral epithelium by keratinization and will not be considered further. Dental tissues associated with tooth attachment are dealt with in a later chapter.

The distribution among living and extinct vertebrates of dentine, enamel and enameloid in their various forms is shown in Fig. 6.1. Enamel and enameloid are at the mercy of the environment; losses by attrition, abrasion and erosion cannot be made good after the tooth comes into function, although in mammals the saliva confers some protective effect against chemical influences.

## COMPARATIVE DEVELOPMENT OF DENTAL TISSUES

In all vertebrates the tooth germ consists of a cap of epithelium which encloses a mass of mesenchymal cells called the dental papilla (Fig. 6.2a). The epithelial cap comprises two layers, the inner and outer dental epithelia, between which may be found variable numbers of less regularly organized cells. The layer of cells at the outer surface of the papilla, next to the inner dental epithelium, differentiates into secretory cells, the odontoblasts, and it is between these cells and the inner dental epithelium that the hard tissues are laid down. In vertebrates possessing enamel the first tissue to appear is the matrix of dentine (Fig. 6.2b). This is made up largely of collagen and is secreted by the odontoblasts. Soon after, the inner dental epithelial cells (the ameloblasts) secrete a layer of enamel matrix on to this first increment of dentine (Fig. 6.2c) and subsequently the two tissues increase in thickness; the enamel towards the inner dental epithelium (centrifugally) and the dentine towards the papilla (centripetally). Enamel when first laid down is a protein matrix already containing some mineral. When this matrix reaches its full thickness the ameloblasts stop secreting the matrix proteins and secrete only mineral ions. The mineral content increases to the point where almost all of the matrix protein is displaced; this protein is resorbed by the ameloblasts. Dentine mineralizes less completely, the matrix is not resorbed and the odontoblasts do not have a biphasic cycle of activity like the ameloblasts.

In fishes and larval urodeles, however, the first extracellular tissue to appear is the matrix of enameloid (Fig. 6.2b′) which, unlike enamel, grows centripetally to reach its full thickness before any dentine is laid down (Fig. 6.2c′). Enameloid matrix contains collagen, which is laid down on its inner surface by the odontoblasts. In teleosts it has been shown that the inner dental epithelial cells simultaneously secrete protein into the matrix. The epithelial protein diffuses into the matrix and has some similarities with the proteins which make up the matrix of mammalian enamel. There is some evidence that the inner dental epithelial cells also contribute to the matrix of enameloid in elasmobranches and larval urodeles although this has yet to be shown conclusively. Until it reaches its full thickness enameloid matrix is completely unmineralized. Mineralization begins at the inner surface as the first increment of dentine is laid down and spreads centrifugally. During this process matrix protein, including the collagen, is displaced; this allows enameloid to become very highly mineralized, like enamel. The

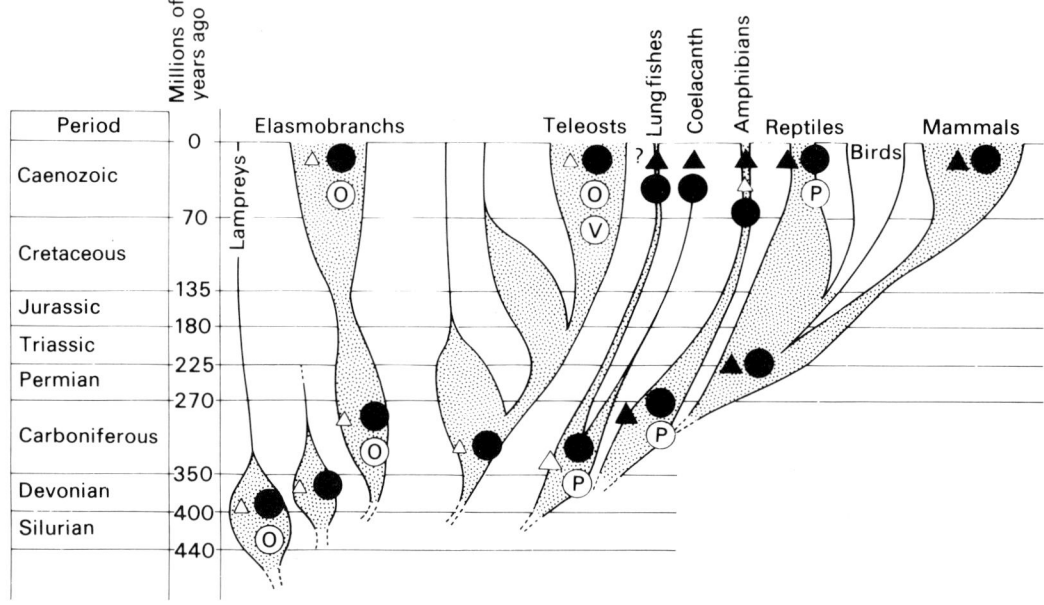

**Fig. 6.1.** Distribution of varieties of dental tissues amongst vertebrates. △, Enameloid; ▲, enamel; ●, orthodentine; Ⓞ, osteodentine; Ⓟ, plicidentine; Ⓥ, vasodentine.

protein is resorbed by the inner dental epithelial cells, which also appear to secrete the necessary mineral.

The orientation of the crystals in enameloid follows that of the matrix collagen fibres. Like dentine enameloid usually contains odontoblast processes. The two tissues thus show a number of similarities and many workers have regarded enameloid as a form of dentine, calling it vitrodentine or durodentine. However, enameloid is distinguished from dentine by the dual origin of the matrix, the high degree of mineralization and the virtually complete absence of protein in the mature tissue.

Clearly, the inner dental epithelial cells have essentially the same cycle of matrix secretion followed by matrix resorption together with mineral secretion during tooth formation in all vertebrates. Whether enamel or enameloid is formed depends on the timing of the activity of the epithelium relative to that of the odontoblasts. Enamel seems to have evolved by delaying the onset of protein secretion by the inner dental epithelium, thereby allowing a layer of dentine to form and start to mineralize first; the epithelial protein is then secreted as a layer of enamel matrix on top of this tissue instead of diffusing into it to form enameloid matrix. In the newts and salamanders this timing changes at metamorphosis from the larval to the adult form: teeth in the young are covered by enameloid while those in the adult are covered by enamel.

In many teleosts the early tooth germ consists simply of an invagination into the oral epithelium, in which the dental papilla is enclosed (Fig. 6.3a). Only during later development does a two-layered sheath of epithelium extend into the connective tissue (Fig. 6.3b). In other teleosts tooth germs form by a similar mechanism in the epithelial sheath surrounding a functional tooth (Fig. 6.3c). In most fishes of this group, however, the epithelial cap develops at the tip of a strand of cells which grow downwards from the oral epithelium into the connective tissue (Fig. 6.3d). In elasmobranchs, amphibians and most reptiles a sheet of epithelium, the dental lamina, grows into the connective tissue and tooth germs form at its inner edge, moving towards the mouth cavity as they develop (e.g. Fig. 6.3e). A dental lamina is present in the crocodiles and mammals for the formation of the first generation of teeth but thereafter tooth germs of replacement teeth originate from subsidiary laminae arising from the epithelium surrounding their predecessors.

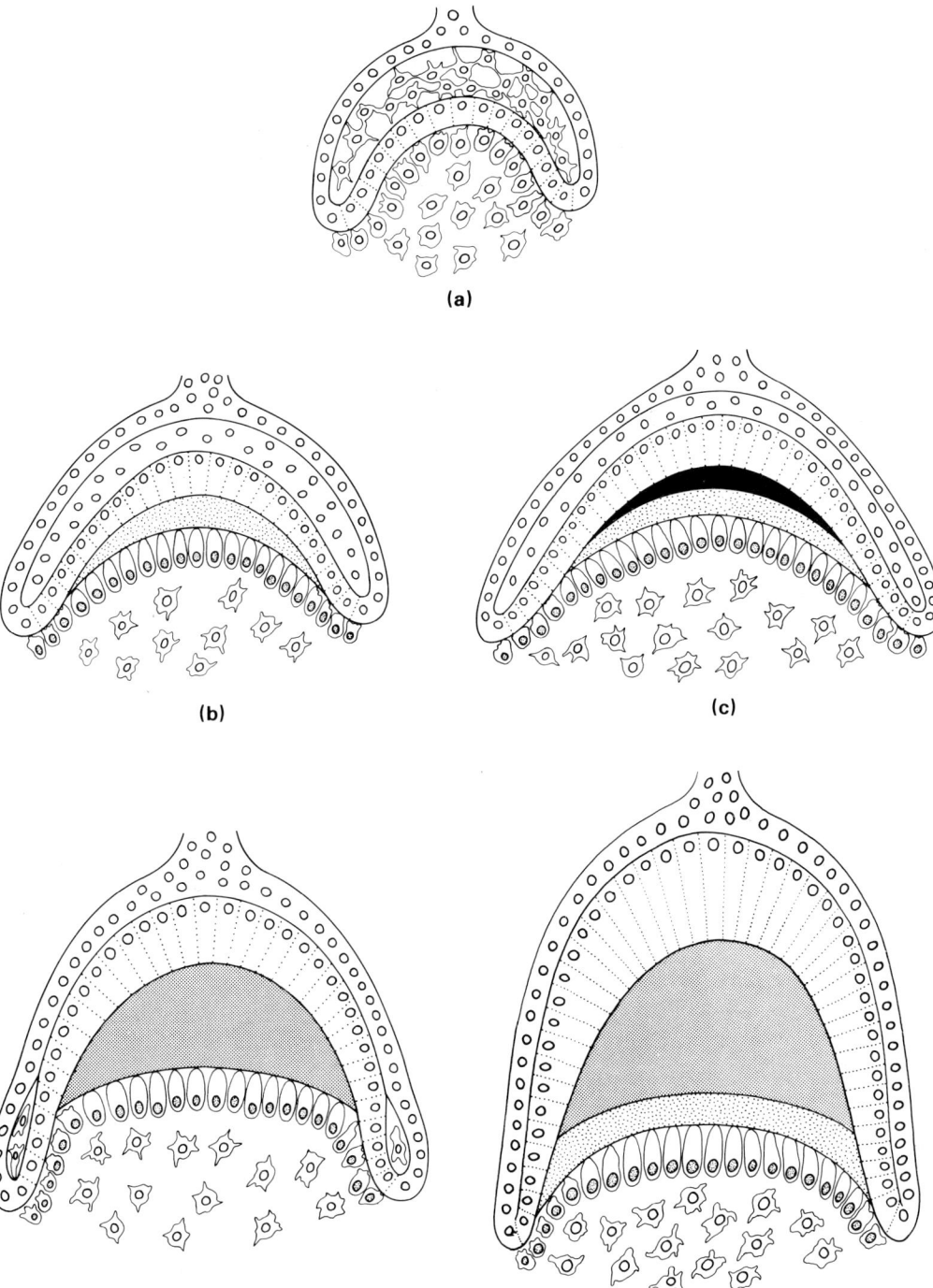

**Fig. 6.2.** The development of enamel (a, b, c) and enameloid (a, b′, c′). ■, Enamel; ▨, enameloid; ▨, dentine.

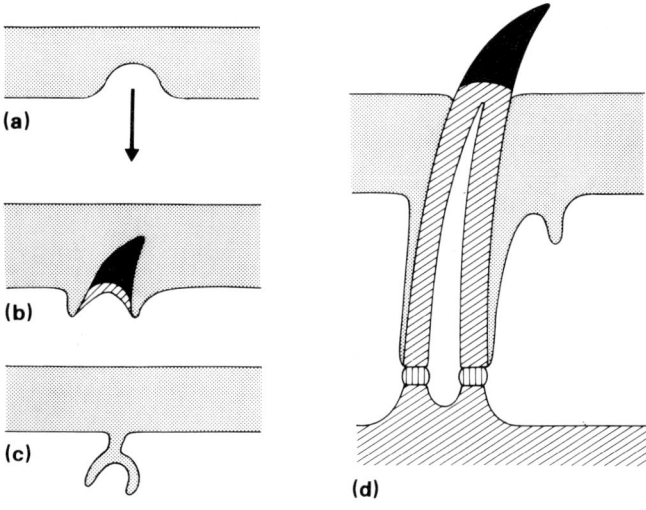
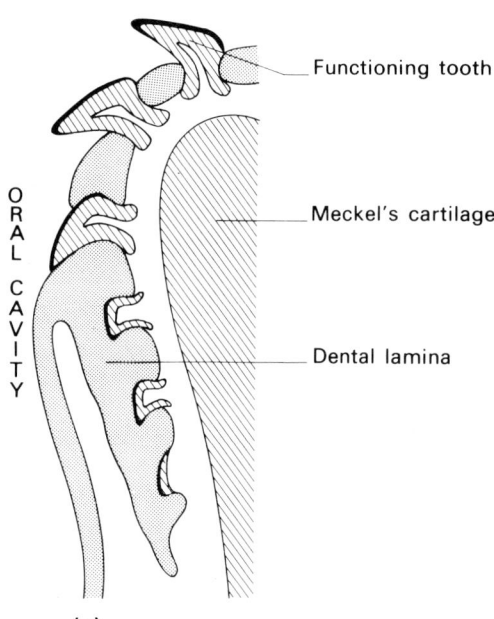

**Fig. 6.3.** (a, b) The dental epithelium is invaginated in the development of some teleost teeth. (c) In others and most tetrapods, the epithelium first grows down. (d) The fully developed teleost tooth, with a tooth germ forming in Hertwig's sheath (left). (e) Tooth development in elasmobranchs.

## COMPARATIVE HISTOLOGY OF DENTAL TISSUES

### Dentine

Dentine is distinguished from other hard tissues with a collagenous matrix, such as bone and cement, by the presence of tubules which, initially at least, contain processes of the odontoblasts. Rudimentary forms of dentine were present in the dermal armour of the primitive agnathan fishes (see Fig. 4.2). In these tissues, known as semidentine and mesodentine, the odontoblasts themselves, as well as their processes, became trapped in the hard tissue. Cells are included in the tooth dentine of some living vertebrates, sometimes by chance, sometimes as a consistent feature.

Dentine takes a number of forms, which can be classified into four types: orthodentine, osteodentine, plicidentine and vasodentine. The first three differ in the arrangement of hard tissue in relation to the pulp cavity, while the fourth type is distinguished by the presence of intradentinal blood capillaries.

ORTHODENTINE

Orthodentine is by far the commonest type of dentine. It is the only type of dentine found in most teeth, where it forms a compact layer surrounding an undivided pulp cavity of fairly simple shape. In some teeth, it forms a shell surrounding an inner layer or mass of one of the other forms of dentine. There exists considerable variation in the morphology and arrangement of the tubules. The tubules in the orthodentine of many elasmobranchs, for instance, are coarse, irregular and highly branched, whereas those of most teleosts and amphibians are very thin and straight, with little branching. The variation in tubule morphology does not seem to be systematic, however. It appears from the available evidence that a hypermineralized peritubular layer (p. 170) may be a consistent feature of orthodentine in all vertebrate classes.

In the orthodentine of most vertebrates the collagen fibres in the matrix are arranged in a network, with the fibres lying mostly in a plane parallel with the formative surface. In the fishes, the dentine also contains a system of coarse bundles of mineralized fibres which run longitudinally down the tooth. Sometimes these longitudinal bundles run throughout the length of the tooth but sometimes they are confined to the basal region. The bundles are very important in tooth attachment, since they emerge from the base of the tooth and link the tooth with the bone (Fig. 7.1).

In vertebrates, mainly mammals, where the teeth are used for a long time without being replaced, dentine not only acts as a supporting tissue for the enamel, but may come to form part of the functioning surface of the tooth as a result of the enamel being worn away in places. Indeed, enamel is never formed in sloths and armadillos, so that dentine is the primary functional tissue. Among reptiles, the agamid lizards have only one generation of teeth. After the loss of the enamel, dentine is exposed but eventually even this is worn away and sharp ridges of bone ultimately replace the teeth as the organs for dealing with food.

There are a number of mammals, for instance, elephants, walruses and hippopotamuses, in which canines or incisors continue growing throughout life and form long tusks. The enamel cap is quickly lost by wear, so that in mature animals the tusks consist entirely of dentine (ivory).

In many herbivores, the dentine is exposed fairly soon after eruption and becomes part of the functioning surface in conjunction with enamel and sometimes cement as well (Fig. 6.4). Since dentine is less hard than enamel, it is worn away

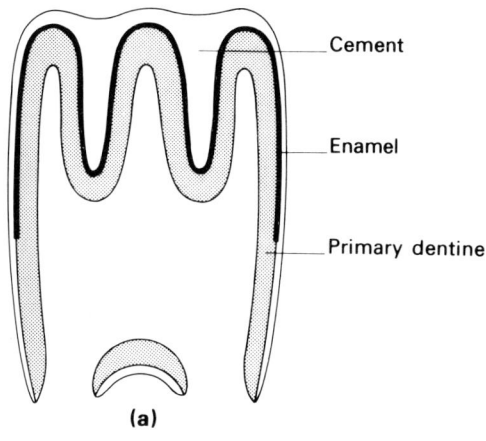

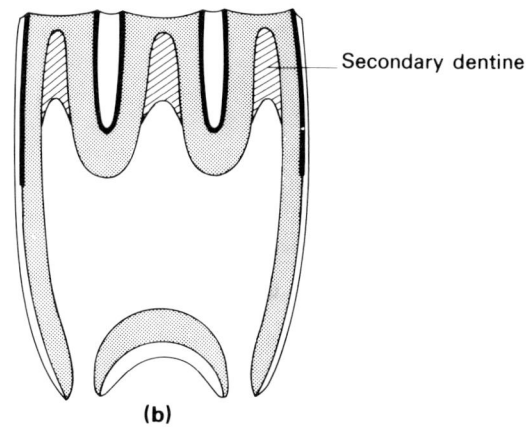

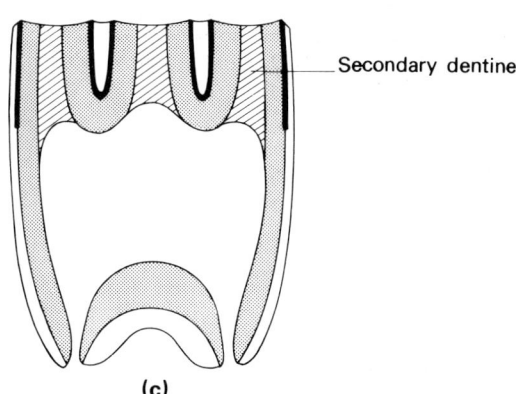

**Fig. 6.4.** Cross-section of a tooth of a herbivore at different stages of wear.

more quickly and this results in a system of elevated enamel ridges supported by dentine at the occlusal surface (Fig. 6.4). In cheek teeth the pattern of ridges may be complex and forms a very efficient grinding surface. A similar process of differential wear is responsible for the production and maintenance of a sharp chisel edge on the incisors of the rodents, lagomorphs and the primate *Daubentonia* (the aye-aye), since these possess enamel only on their labial surface.

In mammals, dentine continues to form after the teeth have erupted when the primary dentine has been completed. This secondary dentine (Fig. 6.4) becomes so thick as to fill the pulp chamber completely in some mammals, notably the toothed whales. Secondary dentine is of great importance in herbivores, omnivores and insectivores since its presence prevents the pulp becoming exposed as a result of the primary dentine being worn away (Fig. 6.4). Secondary dentine is discernible on the occlusal surfaces of teeth from these animals as a dark tissue surrounded by the paler, yellowish primary dentine.

Secondary dentine is not confined to the mammals but is also found in some rays. In these fishes, it is an atubular tissue and does not become exposed at the functional surface.

OSTEODENTINE

Osteodentine is the second most common form of dentine but is almost exclusive to the fishes. Its name derives from a superficial resemblance to spongy bone; the tissue is penetrated by anastomosing tunnels containing pulp tissue. The walls of the canals are, however, not lined by bone but by dentine containing tubules which originate from odontoblasts in the pulp tissue and which radiate from the canals (Fig. 6.5b). Each canal, together with its wall of dentine, is referred to as a denteon, by analogy with the osteons of bone. Where denteons come together, the space between them is filled with coarsely fibrous mineralized tissue which sometimes contains cell lacunae.

Unlike orthodentine, osteodentine is not deposited at the outer surface of the pulp but is laid down within the pulp tissue. In the first stage a meshwork of bundles and sheets of coarse fibres is formed by pulp cells (Fig. 6.5a). These fibres ultimately mineralize to become the interdenteonal tissue. The network of fibres divides the pulp into a system of canals and forms a substrate for the deposition of dentine by odontoblasts which differentiate from the cells previously engaged in laying down the fibre network. The formation of dentine consolidates the walls of the canals, which thus become narrower (Fig. 6.5b).

In rudimentary form, osteodentine was present in the extinct agnathans. It is found in the elasmobranchs, in the holostean fish *Lepidosteus* (the garpike) and in some teleost fishes, such as the pike and the barracuda. In most instances, osteodentine occupies the pulp cavity inside a layer of orthodentine, although in the eagle ray, *Myliobatis*, (see Fig. 4.12) the latter is very thin. In sharks, the basal plate, by which the tooth is attached, is often composed of osteodentine (Fig. 6.5d). Commonly the canals of osteodentine are randomly oriented, an arrangement which enables the tissue to resist forces from any direction. In the eagle-ray the canals and trabeculae all lie vertically, at right angles to the functional surface of the brick-shaped crushing teeth (Fig. 6.5c). This arrangement provides maximum resistance to the compressive stresses set up by tooth function and at the same time is economical of hard tissue. The osteodentine trabeculae are oriented longitudinally in the pike and barracuda.

PLICIDENTINE

Plicidentine appeared among the extinct lobe-finned fishes and labyrinthodont amphibians but among living animals is confined to a few reptiles, such as the monitor lizard *Varanus*. As in osteodentine, the pulp is subdivided but this is due to the folding of the pulp surface, on which the dentine is formed. This results in the formation of lamellae of dentine, running longitudinally down the tooth, which protrude into the pulp cavity (Fig. 6.6a). These lamellae probably act as internal buttresses, strengthening the outer shell of the tooth. Plicidentine has been reported in the teeth of the mammal *Orycteropus* (the aardvark) but this tissue seems to be a form of osteodentine, with numerous subsidiary pulp canals running longitudinally through the tooth.

VASODENTINE

This is found only in some members of certain families of teleost fishes, namely the Gadidae (e.g. the hake) and the Pleuronectidae (e.g. the flounder). It contains blood capillaries and is situated between the pulp and an outer layer of orthodentine. The latter tissue is formed first, in the normal way. The layer of odontoblasts is then penetrated by large capillaries which come to lie next to the forming surface of the dentine.

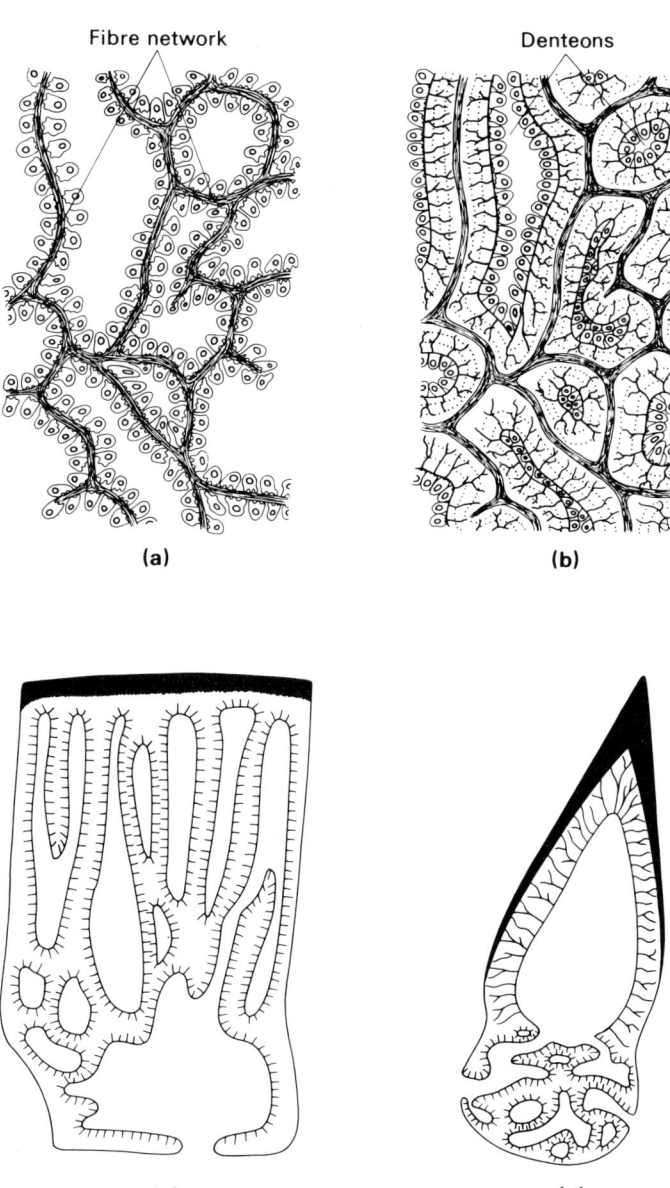

**Fig. 6.5.** (a, b) The development of osteodentine. Osteodentine in (c) *Myliobatis* and (d) a shark.

Continued apposition of dentine traps capillaries in the hard tissue (Fig. 6.6b). The odontoblasts concerned with vasodentine formation have the same cytological features as ordinary odontoblasts but possess a number of microvilli instead of the usual single large process. Vasodentine does not therefore contain tubules but otherwise it has the usual features of fish dentine, with coarse fibre bundles running longitudinally. The capillaries within the vasodentine do not atrophy; they retain their endothelial walls and circulating erythrocytes can be observed in living specimens.

### Enameloid

Enameloid varies a great deal in structure because of differences in the orientation of the apatite crystals.

Crushing teeth, like those of the rays and the primitive Port Jackson shark, *Heterodontus*, are covered with an enameloid layer fairly uniform in thickness on the occlusal surface, thinning off near the edges. The enameloid thus forms a shell resisting compressive forces, being thickest where these forces are concentrated. Frequently

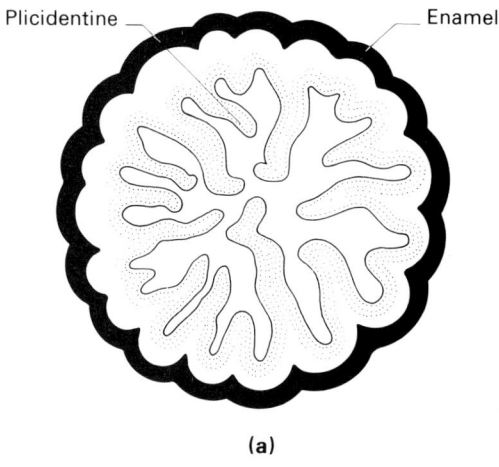

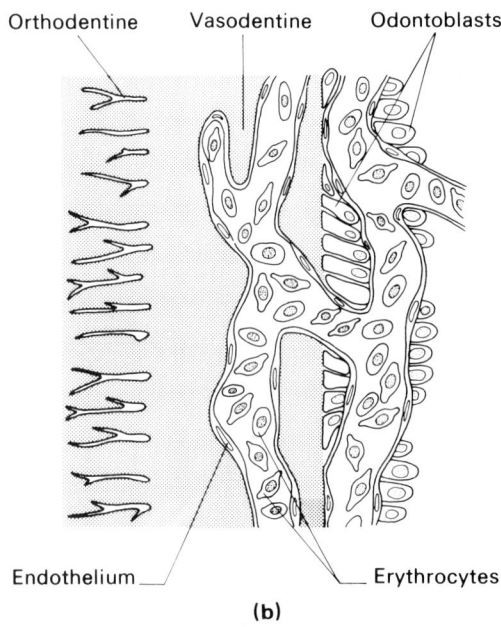

**Fig. 6.6.** (a) Plicidentine; (b) vasodentine.

microscopy reveal the structure shown in Fig. 6.7b. The inner enameloid consists of bundles of crystals running in all directions and interweaving to form a feltwork. The woven structure of this layer resists compressive stresses transmitted from the outer enameloid. This is covered by an outer layer which is largely made up of crystals lying parallel with the surface and organized into sheets which stand perpendicular to the surface, running from the basal region of the tooth towards the tips and cutting edges. When the distribution of the longitudinal sheets over the tooth surface is examined by scanning electron microscopy, patterns like those shown in Fig. 6.7c,d are observed. These patterns follow the predicted lines of stress quite closely. Between these longitudinal sheets penetrate thin bundles of crystals which run out from the dentine at right angles to the surface. Over the whole surface of the enameloid lies a very thin, skin-like layer composed of large single crystals oriented at random within a plane parallel with the surface. This thin layer on the outer surface is responsible for the shiny appearance of shark teeth and is believed to have an important function in preventing the formation of cracks in the underlying enameloid.

Some bony fishes, such as the piranha (see Fig. 4.14), have blade-like teeth for slicing but this is exceptional. Most bony fishes have conical or rounded teeth and the enameloid tends to be concentrated at the tip of the tooth as cap enameloid (Fig. 6.8). The shaft of dentine supporting the cap is covered by a layer which is usefully distinguished as collar enameloid because it has a different structure from the cap enameloid. In most conical teeth the collar enameloid is very thin, often only 1–2 $\mu$m thick, but in the round teeth of fishes with crushing dentitions it is much more substantial, being 50 $\mu$m or more in thickness (Fig. 6.8a).

There are two main forms of cap enameloid. In rounded crushing teeth, like those of the seabreams, the crystals of apatite are gathered in curving bundles which interweave to form a complex woven structure (Fig. 6.8a). This type of enameloid is adapted to resisting the compressive stresses set up by the action of the teeth on food which is often very hard. The thick layer of collar enameloid on these teeth evidently reinforces and gives additional support to the cap enameloid.

In piercing and cutting teeth the cap enameloid has basically the same structure as shark enameloid, with an outer layer made up of longitudinal sheets of crystals, surrounding a central region where the bundles of crystals are interwoven (Fig. 6.8b).

the strength of the shell is increased by the formation of low ridges on the surface (Fig. 6.7a). The crystals within the enameloid, which are often very large (up to $0.2 \times 2\,\mu$m), stand perpendicular to the surface of the dentine (Fig. 6.7a). Forces acting at right angles to the tooth surface are taken up by compression of the crystals.

More complex stresses are set up during function in the fang-like or cutting teeth of sharks and the structure of the enameloid is correspondingly modified. Polarized light and scanning electron

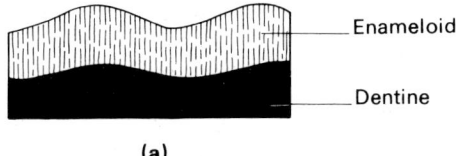

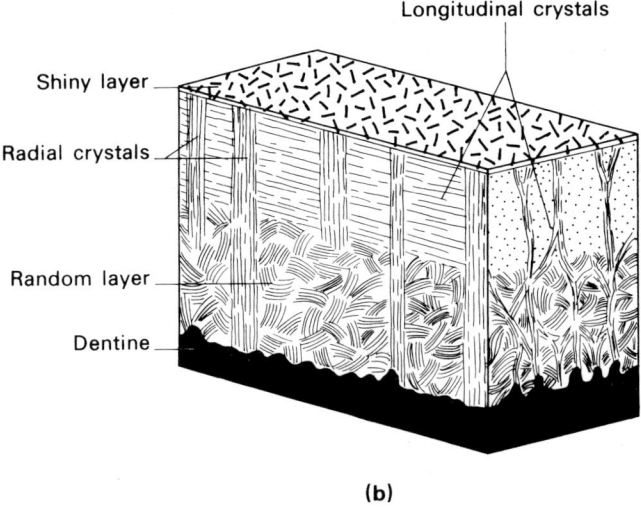

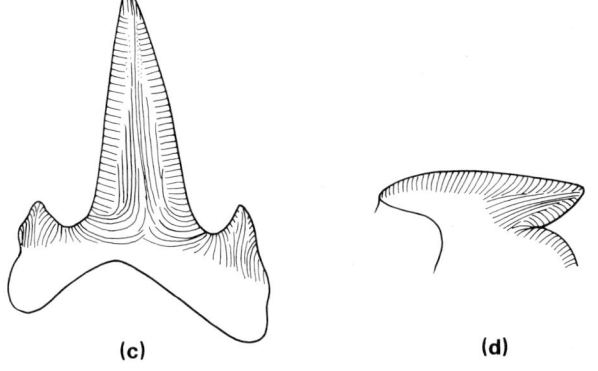

**Fig. 6.7.** (a) Crystals are perpendicular to the tooth surface in enameloid of crushing teeth. (b) Arrangement of crystals in shark enameloid. (c, d) Arrangement of sheets of crystals in shark teeth.

The teeth of teleosts are covered with a thin cuticle which is less highly mineralized than the enameloid underneath. The cuticle frequently contains iron oxide and there may be enough of this substance to colour the tooth surface yellow or orange.

The inner enameloid of fishes generally contains tubules arising from odontoblast processes (Fig. 6.8a,b). These are sometimes very numerous. Other tubules, entering from the outer surface, are also present in some species. These tubules are coarser than dentinal tubules and taper off towards the inside, often branching as they do so (Fig. 6.8a). Enameloid with such tubules is found in a number of sharks and in teleosts with crushing dentitions. Their function is not known.

The larvae of the urodele amphibians have teeth tipped with a cone of cap enameloid, with a very thin layer of collar enameloid down the sides of the teeth. A cuticle pigmented with iron covers the cap. Tooth structure in these animals is thus very similar to that of teleost fishes.

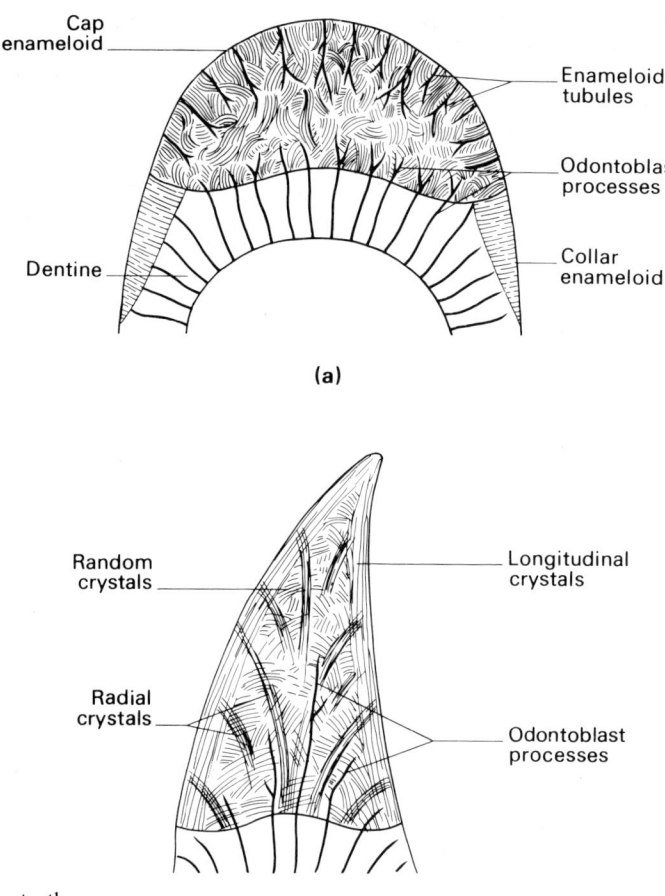

**Fig. 6.8.** Arrangement of enameloid in the teeth of bony fish.

### Enamel

Enamel forms a thin, veneer-like layer on the teeth of the coelacanth and of adult amphibians, but is usually thicker on reptilian teeth. Except in one or two reptilian species the enamel of these groups of vertebrates is non-prismatic and has a simple structure, in which all the apatite crystals stand more or less uniformly perpendicular to the surface. Because of this uniformity, the enamel appears homogeneous in ground sections except for the presence of incremental lines running at a slight angle to the outer surface. The enamel often has a striped appearance in polarized light; this is due simply to slight deviations from the prevailing crystal orientation.

Mammalian enamel is much thicker than in the other tetrapods and is not homogeneous but is built up of rod-like bundles of crystals, the enamel prisms. These may be packed together throughout the enamel or may be separated by interprismatic regions. It must be emphasized that there is no difference in composition between prism bodies and the interprismatic regions; both consist of closely packed apatite crystals together with minute quantities of organic material. The boundaries between neighbouring prisms or between prisms and interprismatic enamel are regions where a more or less abrupt change in crystal orientation corresponds with the optical effect of an edge in sections.

Prismatic enamel seems to have appeared first in primitive mammals from the middle of the Mesozoic era about 150 million years ago. However, in many mammal-like reptiles the enamel crystals were organized into bundles but these were not sufficiently demarcated from the surrounding enamel to form genuine prisms. Prismatic enamel is not strictly confined to recent mammals and their direct ancestors. Among fossil species it was present in the distantly related multituberculates and in the placodonts, large aquatic reptiles with crushing teeth. Recently the enamel of a living reptile, the lizard *Uromastix*, has been shown to be prismatic.

In broad terms, mammalian enamels can be classified into four types, according to the cross-sectional shape and arrangement of the prisms, as shown in Fig. 6.9. This classification is not rigid

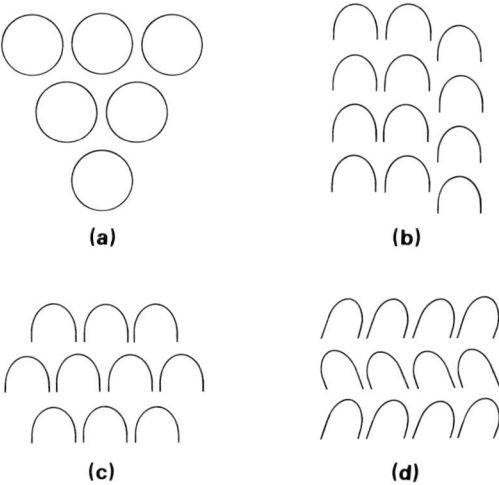

**Fig. 6.9.** Basic arrangements of enamel prisms.
(a) Insectivores, bats, toothed whales, some primates; (b) ungulates, marsupials, rabbits, some rodents; (c) monkeys, apes, man, carnivora; (d) many rodents, e.g. rat.

and more than one prism type can usually be found within any tooth. In places, especially near the inner and outer enamel surfaces, prisms may be absent, the crystals in the outer enamel standing perpendicular to the surface as in reptilian enamel. Enamel prisms rarely follow a straight course but bend and curve to some degree. Sometimes this produces an apparently irregular structure, as in gnarled enamel, but the arrangement of the prisms is usually more orderly. In the incisors of rodents the alternation of prism direction between adjacent rows is particularly highly ordered.

It is not known whether the different shapes and arrangements of prisms impart different properties to the enamel but it seems likely that prismatic enamel is adapted to a wider range of stresses than the simpler reptilian type. Reptilian enamel, because its crystals are uniformly perpendicular to the tooth surface, is probably stronger in compression than in tension. Mammalian enamel, by virtue of the varied crystal orientation, appears to be resistant to both tensional and compressive forces from all directions. Such properties would be particularly valuable during grinding in which complex stress patterns are set up.

In most mammals, as in man, the enamel is penetrated by short tubular enamel spindles arising at the junction with the dentine. However, much longer tubules, extending from the dentine almost to the outer surface, are found in a number of species. Such enamel tubules are present in most marsupials, although they are lacking in the wombat. Among placental mammals they are particularly common in insectivores. They are a constant feature of the enamel of many prosimian primates, but, interestingly, are not found in that of the tree shrews, which are regarded as being close to the ancestral primate stock. They are also found in many mammal-like reptiles.

Enamel tubules are continuous at the enamel–dentine junction with dentinal tubules. One electron microscope study has indicated that, in the very early stages of tooth development in a marsupial (the opossum), odontoblast processes may contact and even fuse with the Tomes processes of ameloblasts and it was suggested that the enamel tubules arise as cytoplasmic processes left behind by the ameloblasts as they deposited enamel. This does not seem to be the case, however, since the tubules undulate and have no consistent relationship with the prisms. Further, a single tubule, if followed for part of its length, may cross from one prism to another, often several times. A more likely explanation seems to be that the tubules arise from the outgrowth of odontoblast processes through the forming enamel at the stage when it is only partly mineralized and gel-like. The function of the tubules, if any, is unknown. It has been suggested that they might have a role in tooth sensitivity, possibly in the detection of pressure, but this hypothesis has not been tested experimentally.

An intriguing feature of the teeth of some mammals is a brown pigmentation of the superficial enamel. The pigment is found in all the teeth of some shrews and in the incisors of many rodents and is due to the presence of ferric iron in large amounts. The iron is not present in a cuticle, as in fishes and amphibians, but forms part of the enamel. It is secreted by the ameloblasts, which accumulate quantities of the iron-bearing proteins ferritin and haemosiderin during the later stages of their life cycle. Iron can be detected chemically in some teeth, such as guinea pig incisors, which are not pigmented. The functional significance of the iron is unknown.

## HUMAN TISSUES

## DENTINE

Dentine makes up the bulk of a tooth. It supports the enamel covering the crown, and is covered in the root regions by cement. At the centre of the tooth lies the pulp tissue, which forms and maintains the dentine. Both the dentine and the pulp are derived from the dental papilla of the tooth germ and, because of their close embryological and functional relationships, the two are often considered together as the pulpodentinal complex.

Dentine is about as hard as bone but considerably softer than enamel. Its pale yellow colour contributes to the colour of the clinical crown because of the translucency of the enamel layer. Like bone, dentine consists of a mainly collagenous matrix mineralized to a moderate degree with apatite, a calcium phosphate. By weight, dentine comprises about 72% mineral, 18% organic matter and 10% water. Histologically, orthodentine, the type of dentine in human teeth, is clearly distinguished from bone by its lack of cell spaces. Instead, it is permeated by numerous tubules which radiate out from the pulp. At least to begin with, each tubule encloses a cytoplasmic process which stems from an odontoblast, a dentine-forming cell.

### Regional differentiation of dentine

In a mature tooth, a number of structurally different regions of dentine can be recognized (Fig. 6.10). The greater part of the dentine in both crown and root is made up of circumpulpal dentine. This is covered by a superficial layer, 10–15 $\mu$m thick. In the crown this layer is known as the mantle dentine and lies immediately next to the amelodentinal junction. The corresponding layer in the root, referred to as the hyaline layer (of Hopewell–Smith) because of its glassy appearance, abuts on to the primary cement and is about 10 $\mu$m thick. At the transition between the hyaline layer and the circumpulpal dentine there is found a diffuse zone, having a dark, speckled appearance in ground section, known as the granular layer of Tomes. The above regions are all formed either before eruption or within 2–3 years thereafter and are collectively known as the primary dentine, to distinguish them from the secondary dentine which forms much more slowly during the later functional life of the tooth. There are regular (or 'physiological') and irregular (or 'pathological') forms of secondary dentine. The structural features of the various regions are described later (the reader is also referred to pp. 260–266).

### Composition of dentine

The major constituents of dentine are shown in

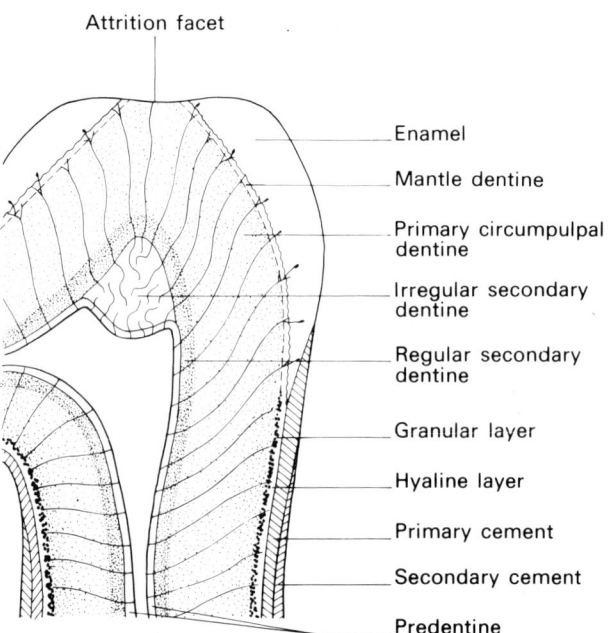

Fig. 6.10. Part of a longitudinal section through a molar, to show the disposition and relative extent of the various regions of dentine.

Table 6.1 (N.B. these are weights for dried dentine).

**Table 6.1.** Composition of dentine (values expressed as weight % of dentine dried at 100°C).

| | | |
|---|---|---|
| *Inorganic matter* | (75) | |
| $CO_2$ | (3) | |
| Ash including: | (72) | |
|   Calcium | (27) | |
|   Phosphorus | (13) | |
|   Magnesium | (1) | |
|   Sodium | (0.5) | |
|   Chloride | (0.1) | |
| *Organic matter* | (20) | |
| Collagen | | (18) |
| Non-collagenous protein | | (0.2) |
| Citrate | | (0.9) |
| Lactate | | (0.15) |
| Chondroitin sulphate | | (0.4) |
| Lipid comprising: | | (0.2) |
|   Fatty acids | (0.18) | |
|   Other lipids | (0.18) | |
| *Residue*—bound water, etc. | | (5) |

ORGANIC MATRIX

Collagen, which accounts for 18% by weight of dried dentine and 90% of the matrix, is the most important constituent. It exists in the form of fibrils, about 50 nm in diameter, arranged in a complex pattern (see below).

Eight to nine percent of dried dentine matrix is non-collagenous and is the residue left after demineralization with EDTA and digestion with collagenase. Only about half of this material is released after treatment with EDTA alone, so that the remainder is probably intimately associated with the collagen. The non-collagenous fraction, consists of a number of proteins, glycosaminoglycans, lipids and organic acids.

MINERAL PHASE

The principal inorganic constituents of dentine are calcium and phosphorus, with smaller amounts of magnesium and carbonate. Sodium and chloride make up a small proportion and trace quantities of a wide range of other elements have also been detected. The molar Ca : P ratio is about 1.55. This departs from the theoretical value of 1.67 for the mineral hydroxyapatite, $Ca_{10}(PO_4)_6(OH)_2$. Studies of dentine by X-ray diffraction and electron diffraction suggest that this is the only crystalline phase in dentine. However, these techniques do not detect amorphous substances and have a poor resolution when the material is poorly crystallized, so that other mineral types, such as carbonates and non-apatitic phosphates, may be present. It appears likely that some of the carbonate may form part of the apatite lattice, by substituting for hydroxyl ions.

**Structure of dentine**

ORGANIZATION OF MATRIX AND MINERAL

To a large extent, the mechanical properties of dentine are influenced by the arrangement of the matrix collagen fibres and by the relationship between the fibres and mineral. Further, the main feature distinguishing between the various regions in the dentine is a difference in fibre orientation. This can be detected by polarizing microscopy.

In circumpulpal dentine, the great majority of the matrix fibres are laid down parallel with the surface of the odontoblast layer, and thus lie at right angles to the dentinal tubules. The fibres lie in planes, indicated in Fig. 6.11, which are not parallel with either the amelodentinal junction or the surface of the pulp chamber, but which have the same orientation as the incremental markings

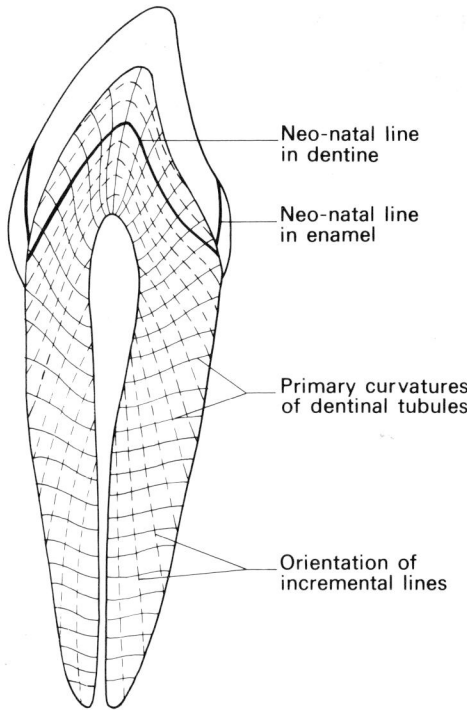

**Fig. 6.11.** Longitudinal section through a tooth to show the primary curvatures of the dentinal tubules and the approximate orientation of the incremental lines, including the neonatal line.

(see below). Dentine may be thought of as being built up of layers: within each layer the fibres form a crisscrossing feltwork. In the crown the preferred orientation of the fibres tends to change between successive layers (cf. adult bone); this gives rise to the von Ebner lines (see below). In the region immediately around each tubule, the fibres tend to deviate and curve around the tubule. In this region, also, there are a few fibres running parallel with the tubules.

In the mantle dentine, a larger proportion of the fibres are orientated parallel with the tubules. These radially arranged von Korff fibres (Fig. 8.22) are embedded in a network of fibres orientated tangentially, as in circumpulpal dentine. The hyaline layer, like the mantle dentine, contains a high proportion of fibres orientated towards the outer surface, although more obliquely than in the mantle dentine. The granular layer lies at the transition between circumpulpal dentine and the hyaline layer where the fibre orientation changes.

The apatite crystals of dentine are much smaller than those of enamel. Their dimensions, estimated by X-ray diffraction and by transmission electron microscopy of ultrathin sections, are: length 20–100 nm; thickness 2–3.5 nm. In ultrathin sections, both needle-like and plate-like forms can be observed but many of the needle-shaped crystals seem to be plates viewed edge-on. The crystals are preferentially aligned parallel with the matrix collagen fibres; this is consistent with observations on developing dentine which suggest that the crystals are initiated within the fibres themselves (p. 264). Calculations from estimates of the internal compartments of dentine indicate that at least 56% of the mineral phase must be situated within the collagen fibres.

Recent work, in which ion-beam etching was used to produce sections for electron microscopical study, have somewhat modified these concepts of the morphology of dentine mineral. The technique of ion-beam etching avoids the mechanical stresses associated with sectioning hard tissues with a diamond knife. The work confirms the thinness of the crystals but suggests that they are much longer than previously supposed, some possibly extending along the full length of collagen fibres. Furthermore, the frequent observation of circular profiles suggests that some mineral may be deposited as tubular structures around microfibrils, subunits of the collagen fibres.

Many of the crystals in dentine are aligned parallel with the matrix fibres. However, throughout the dentine there are present bodies or, more accurately, regions, known as calcospherites, in which the arrangement of crystals is in part independent of the matrix fibres. In a calcospherite, a proportion of the crystals run out radially from a focal point (Fig. 6.12), thus cutting across the direction of the fibres and forming an interpenetrating system with the crystals aligned with the fibres. Calcospherites are not easily visible in ground sections viewed in ordinary light except in localized areas where the dentine filling the space between calcospherites fails to mineralize properly. Such areas of defective mineralization are known as interglobular dentine; the profiles of the calcospherites are visible because of the difference in refractive index between themselves and the interglobular dentine. Interglobular dentine is not seen in all teeth and is most common in the coronal dentine. Although not usually visible in ordinary light, calcospherites are clearly distinguishable in polarized light.

Most calcospherites are spherical but many have an arcade shape, with the round apex of the arcade directed towards the outer surface of the dentine, the opening towards the pulp (Fig. 6.12). The size varies considerably, the arcade forms tending to be larger than the spherical. The size and shape seem to be governed by the rate of dentine formation and by the rate at which new calcospherites are initiated. There is a fairly consistent pattern of distribution within the tooth (Fig. 6.12). In the mantle dentine, the hyaline layer and the superficial circumpulpal dentine, the calcospherites are small, spherical and closely packed. In the middle region of the circumpulpal dentine, they are larger, more widely spaced and arcade in form, but this region tends to be free of calcospherites towards the tooth apex. The inner half to two-thirds of the circumpulpal dentine contains spherical calcospherites.

The mechanism underlying the formation of calcospherites has not been investigated but the presence of these structures is a feature distinguishing dentine from bone and cement; hard tissues in which the crystals are uniformly orientated parallel with the collagen fibres.

Because dentine formation is continuous, there is always present at the pulpal surface a layer of unmineralized dentine matrix, or predentine (Fig. 6.10). In mature teeth dentine is formed very slowly so that the predentine layer is much thinner than in immature teeth where dentine is being formed rapidly.

DENTINE TUBULES

The tubules are an outstanding histological feature of dentine. They radiate out from the pulp

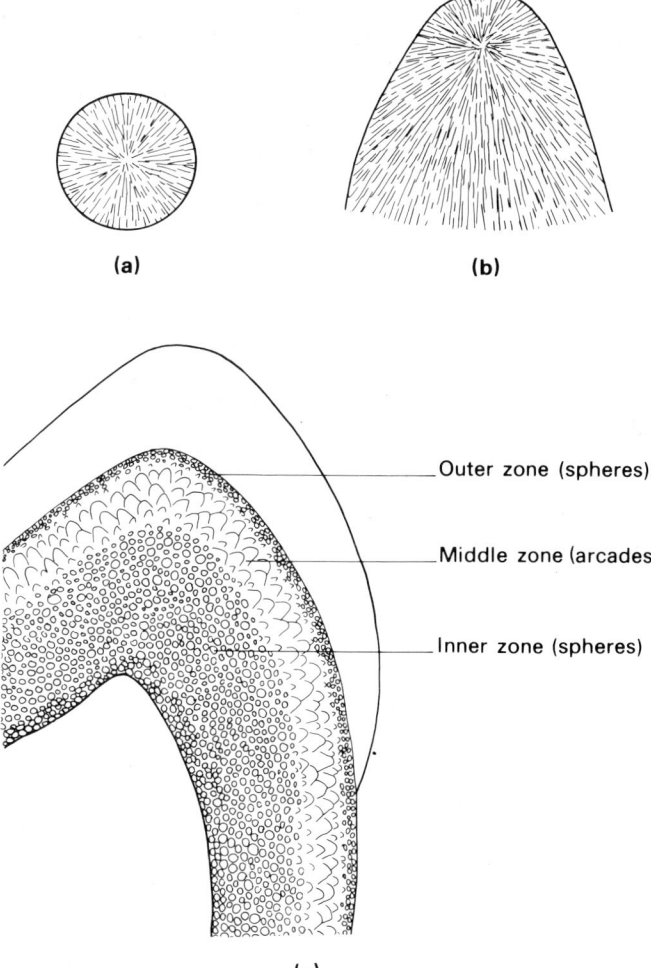

Fig. 6.12. (a, b) The form and crystal orientation of a spherical and an arcade-shaped calcospherite, respectively. (c) Part of a longitudinal section through a tooth, showing the distribution of calcospherites within the dentine.

to the outer surface, tapering somewhat along their length; they are about 4 μm in diameter near the odontoblasts and about 1 μm near their terminal ends, although the diameter is finally determined by the thickness of the peritubular dentine (see below). As the surface area of the dentine is less at the pulpal surface than at the outer surface, the tubules are more widely separated at their outer extremities. Thus, in the outer dentine, there are on average 20 000 tubules/mm$^2$, while in the inner dentine, the density rises to an average of 45 000 tubules/mm$^2$. The tubules occupy about 10% of the total volume of coronal dentine but the relative volume varies between about 4% near the enamel and 28% near the pulp.

The tubules follow a shallow S-shaped course known as the primary curvature (Fig. 6.11), except under the cusps where they are straight. The primary curvature is also much less well marked in the roots than in the crown. Superimposed on the primary curvatures are minor undulations known as the secondary curvatures.

Within the mantle dentine many tubules bifurcate (Fig. 6.13) and some of these branches cross the amelodentinal junction and enter the enamel as enamel spindles. Similar bifurcations appear to be particularly abundant in the outer region of the root dentine, near the granular layer, and it seems probable that the granular appearance of the layer is due to light scattering by air trapped inside dilated or twisted terminal branches of the dentinal tubules, although it has also been suggested that the appearance may be due to defective mineralization.

The tubules give off fine lateral branches. In the circumpulpal dentine these are distinctly less

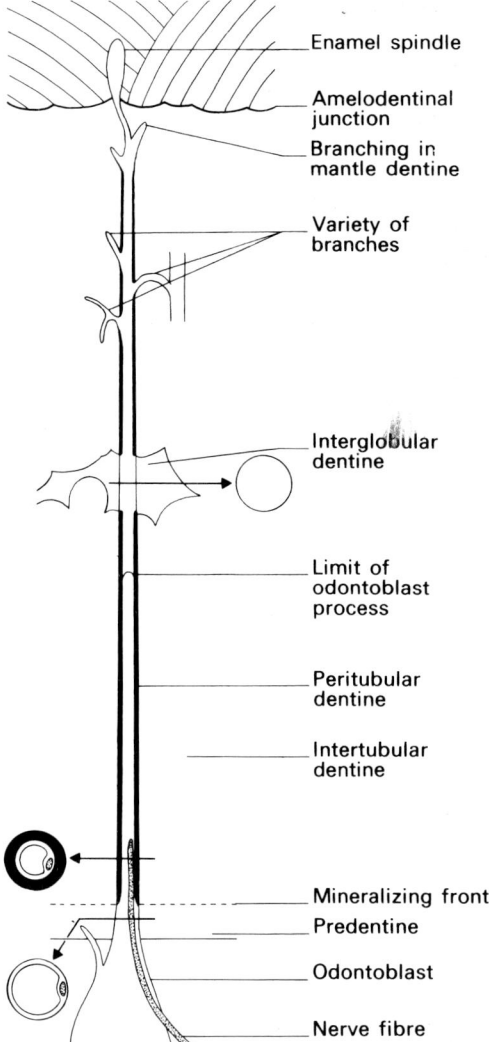

**Fig. 6.13.** Idealized diagram of a dentinal tubule, from pulp to enamel, including features associated with the tubules (not to scale).

common in the coronal region than in the roots; they are usually directed obliquely outwards, but may lie at right angles or even curve back towards the pulp (Fig. 6.13). Sometimes, adjacent tubules are linked by lateral branches.

THE CONTENTS OF DENTINAL TUBULES

During development the dentinal tubules contain cytoplasmic processes from the odontoblasts which line the walls of the pulp cavity. In the mature tooth, however, the true nature of the tubule contents is more obscure, mainly because it is uncertain how well the intratubular structures are preserved by fixation procedures used for preparing specimens for electron microscopy. The question of what the tubules contain is of more than just academic interest because it bears directly on the problem of how sensation in dentine is mediated (p. 193). The data from electron microscopy indicate that an intact process extends only about one third of the way towards the outer surface in mature dentine (Fig. 6.13). The contents of the outer portion vary. Cytoplasmic or membranous fragments are often present just beyond the tip of the process but in the terminal region the tubule contains only fluid or amorphous debris. There have been reports that enzymes and small organic molecules may be found in this fluid.

The odontoblast processes themselves, which are extremely long compared to the cell body, contain microfilaments and microtubules along their length. Other organelles (vesicles, dense bodies and the occasional mitochondrion) are largely confined to the region near the pulp.

In a mature tooth, a very small proportion of the tubules contain fine, unmyelinated nerve fibres, lying alongside the process (Fig. 6.13). Such nerve fibres extend only a short distance into the tubules. In places, junctions have been described between the cell membranes of the process and of the nerve fibre. Intratubular nerve fibres are much more common in the coronal dentine than in the cervical region and are extremely rare in the root dentine. The function of the nerve fibres is not known.

PERITUBULAR DENTINE

During the life of the tooth, a mineralized tissue is laid down on the inner surface of the walls of dentinal tubules (Fig. 6.13). This tissue is known as peritubular dentine although it is, strictly speaking, intratubular. Peritubular dentine is more highly mineralized than the dentine between the tubules (intertubular dentine) and is structurally different. The matrix of peritubular dentine appears amorphous in demineralized specimens viewed in the electron microscope. Collagen fibres are sometimes present between the odontoblast process and the peritubular dentine but these fibres seem to be random inclusions. The mineral phase of peritubular dentine does not have the crystalline morphology of the apatite found in the intertubular dentine but rather seems to be made up of closely packed spherical or polygonal particles, about 25 nm in diameter, which perhaps consist of amorphous calcium phosphate.

Peritubular dentine starts to form as or just after the adjacent intertubular region is mineralized (Fig. 6.13). There is a correlation between the subsequent formation of the tissue and the rate of attrition; in general, the peritubular dentine is thicker in more heavily worn teeth. The tubules commonly become completely occluded with mineral spreading from the walls. At the same time, however, the rate of peritubular dentine formation is not uniform among all the tubules of the same tooth and a proportion of tubules lack a peritubular layer even when attrition is fairly severe. It appears that peritubular dentine is not formed in regions of interglobular dentine.

## STRUCTURAL MARKINGS IN DENTINE

Within the dentine there are found a variety of lines, more or less at right angles to the tubules, as in Fig. 6.11, which reflect the incremental pattern of deposition of the tissue. Some of the lines are related to rhythmic variations in matrix formation and others to differences in mineralization. The markings most consistently present are the von Ebner lines, which are due to diurnal variation in matrix fibre arrangement. They are best seen in ground sections viewed in polarized light, when they appear as alternating dark and light stripes, usually about 5 $\mu$m thick. This appearance indicates that within each stripe or layer the fibres are uniformly oriented, the fibres of one layer lying at an angle to those in adjoining layers. Von Ebner lines tend to be more prominent in the inner two-thirds of the coronal dentine than elsewhere.

Lines due to variations in mineralization are visible in microradiographs of ground sections. The interval between these lines is not constant and consecutive lines can diverge. They often have a more uneven appearance than the smooth von Ebner lines. Because the mineralizing front in forming dentine is not always parallel with the inner surface of the predentine, the incremental lines due to differences in mineralization can lie at an angle to the von Ebner lines. Attempts to correlate the intervals between these incremental lines with the rate of dentine apposition have been unsuccessful.

In teeth which begin to mineralize *in utero*, there is often a very pronounced line in the dentine (and in enamel), which appears brown in ordinary light. This neonatal line (Fig. 6.11) reflects the physiological disturbances associated with birth. Similar prominent lines can be produced experimentally by administering a range of substances (e.g. high doses of tetracycline) during tooth formation. Such lines are referred to as calciotraumatic lines because they result from gross disturbances of dentine mineralization.

Areas are occasionally seen where the secondary curves of the dentinal tubules lie in register; this produces an optical appearance of lines, known as the contour lines of Owen, orientated at an angle to the tubule direction. The lines of Owen are more widely spaced than other lines (up to about 50 $\mu$m apart) and the spacing is variable.

## SECONDARY DENTINE AND STRUCTURAL CHANGES IN PRIMARY DENTINE

As mentioned previously, there are two varieties of secondary dentine. They differ both in structure and in the circumstances of their formation. Regular secondary dentine forms continuously but slowly throughout life, causing a progressive reduction in the size of the pulp cavity. In structure, it is almost indistinguishable from primary circumpulpal dentine of which it is, essentially, a continuation. However, the junction between the two tissues is frequently marked by a change in direction of the dentinal tubules which can be regarded as a form of Owen line.

Irregular secondary dentine tends to form in association with areas exposed to some form of injury, such as caries or abrasion (Fig. 6.14), and is

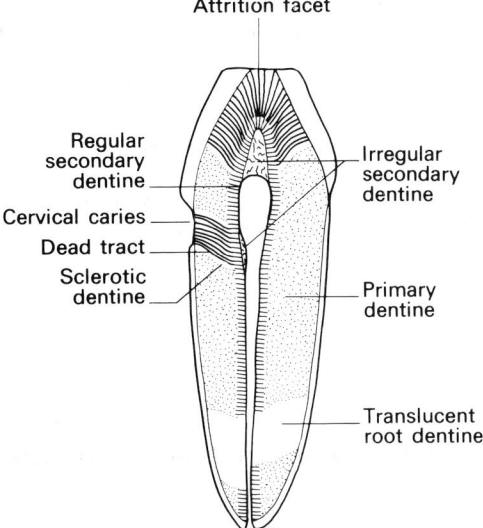

Fig. 6.14. Longitudinal section through a tooth, indicating the arrangement of dead tracts, sclerotic dentine and irregular secondary dentine in relation to external stimuli (attrition and caries), and the location of translucent dentine in the roots.

often linked with structural changes in the primary dentine (see below). Because of this association with injury, irregular secondary dentine is sometimes referred to as 'pathological' secondary dentine but this appears to be a misnomer, since the tissue can form in teeth which appear sound, or in areas of a tooth away from the site of injury. Irregular secondary dentine derives its name from the often distorted pattern of matrix fibres, clearly seen in polarized light, from the reduction or loss of tubules, and from the disturbed arrangement of those tubules which remain (Fig. 6.10). The presence of these features is associated with the fact that irregular secondary dentine is laid down very quickly.

Dentine, because of its association with the pulp, can be modified to some extent in response to various stimuli. The formation of secondary dentine is one manifestation of this and the increase in peritubular dentine in response to attrition is another. Other changes occur in response to ageing and to injury.

The principal change in dentine associated with ageing is the formation of translucent dentine in the roots (Fig. 6.14). In areas affected by this process the tubules become completely occluded by mineral, probably by a process closely resembling peritubular dentine formation, their contents acquiring the same refractive index as the intertubular dentine. Thus, when a ground section is prepared and placed in a medium such as water, with a refractive index different to that of dentine, affected regions of dentine appear translucent, in contrast to the opaque appearance of dentine containing patent tubules (Fig. 6.15). The extent of translucent areas in root dentine has been used

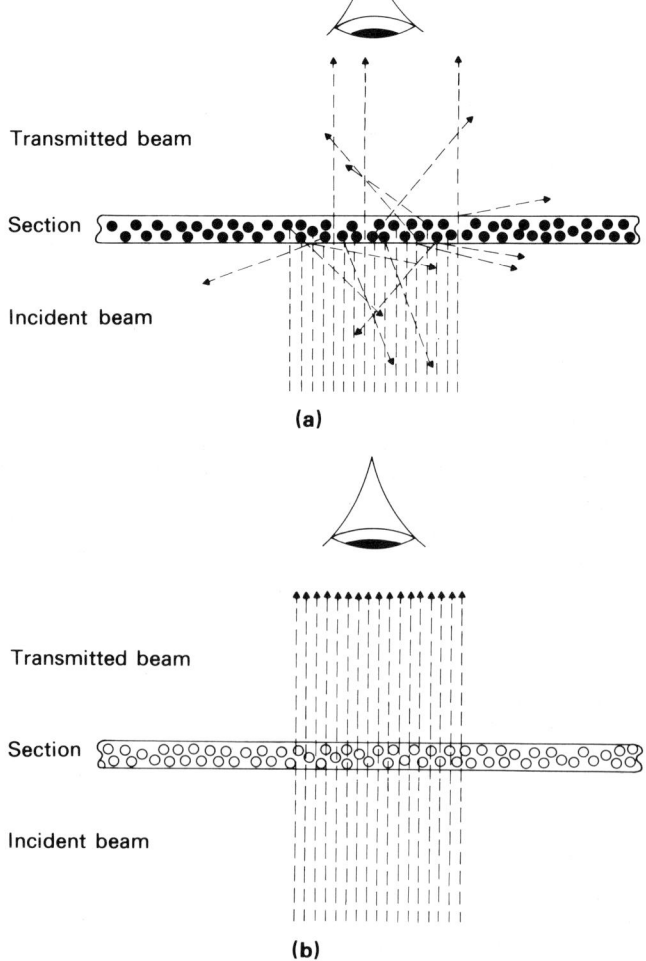

Fig. 6.15. The optical basis for the appearance of translucent or sclerotic dentine when examined in water. (a) In unaffected dentine the tubules imbibe water (shown as black circles). Most of the light passing through the section is scattered by refraction or reflection at the boundary between the tubule and the intertubular dentine, because of the sudden change in refractive index. The tissue thus appears opaque. (b) In translucent or sclerotic dentine, the tubules are occluded by mineral of a similar refractive index to the intertubular dentine and thus do not become filled with water. Consequently, the incident light is not scattered and passes through the section so that the tissue appears transparent.

as a criterion for estimating age from dental material (p. 356).

Loss of tooth substance, e.g. by attrition or caries, can provoke two responses in the primary dentine, the response being apparently governed by the severity of the stimulus. Relatively mild stimuli tend to induce sclerosis of the dentinal tubules in the affected region. Sclerosis, like the formation of translucent dentine, involves the infilling of tubules by mineral. The mineral which occludes the tubules has a fine texture like that of peritubular dentine. In primary dentine affected by caries, the intratubular mineral usually appears to be apatite but within some tubules platelike crystals which have been identified as octocalcium phosphate, $Ca_8H_2(PO_4)_6 \cdot 5H_2O$, are deposited. The occlusion of tubules by mineral in dentine sclerosis is considered to be brought about by the odontoblasts but the details are not known. Sclerosis is a defensive reaction, inhibiting the penetration of bacteria and their products along the tubules and thus protecting the pulp.

Under the influence of more severe stimuli, the formation of a dead tract in the primary dentine is a common response (Fig. 6.14). In a dead tract, the odontoblast processes atrophy and the tubules are sealed at their pulpal ends by the deposition of irregular secondary dentine. When a ground section is mounted in balsam, unaffected dentine becomes translucent because the medium can penetrate the tubules but in a dead tract the sealed tubules remain filled with air (or xylene vapour from the mounting medium) so that the area remains opaque. A dead tract is usually bordered by a zone of sclerotic dentine (Fig. 6.14). The formation of the plug of secondary dentine represents a defensive reaction to the injurious stimulus which is severe enough to prevent the infilling of tubules by mineral which would occur under less drastic conditions. The sclerosis adjacent to the dead tract is a response to the same stimulus but attenuated by distance.

The existence of a dead tract is not necessarily evidence of injury however. A dead tract can develop even in an unerupted tooth. In such circumstances, it is believed that death of odontoblasts is brought about by some internal factor. For instance, the odontoblasts at a pulp horn could degenerate because of crowding and this would lead to the formation of a dead tract.

MINERALIZATION IN THE PULP

The pulp is frequently a site for the formation of mineralized bodies of two types, known as denticles and pulp stones. The former are smooth-surfaced and tend to be spherical. They have a laminar structure and grow by mineralization of collagen fibres laid down tangential to the surface, and so resemble spheres of dentine. However, tubules are not necessarily present. Denticles may be free in the pulp or attached to the inner surface of the dentine, in which they may become embedded by continued dentine formation. Pulp stones are more irregular in form and enlarge by deposition of mineral on the predominantly longitudinal connective tissue fibres of the pulp. Although both denticles and pulp stones appear to grow by mineralization of collagen, there is some evidence that they are initiated by mineralization of amorphous material, which has not so far been identified. The presence of mineralized bodies in the pulp tends to be associated with some form of irritation but apparently healthy pulps can also mineralize.

**Properties of dentine in relation to function**

MECHANICAL PROPERTIES

Enamel is well adapted to grinding and cutting food because it is hard and highly incompressible. At the same time, it is a brittle substance, so that a tooth made entirely of enamel would probably fracture quite readily under the stresses of mastication. However, the enamel is relieved of a large proportion of these stresses by the presence of the underlying dentine, which is not only more compressible but also has greater tensile and compressive strength than enamel, due to the presence of, respectively, collagen and ground substance proteoglycans. A tooth may thus be visualized, in mechanical terms, as a cap of a rigid material cushioned by a core of a more elastic substance.

Dentine has not only a supporting function but a masticatory function. Attrition of the enamel exposes dentine on the occlusal surface and the two tissues act in concert in the reduction of the food. This function is more readily appreciated in herbivorous mammals (p. 345) or in primitive man (p. 385) than in modern civilized populations. Under the influence of a coarse diet, the dentine wears faster than the enamel, leading to the formation of concave grinding surfaces surrounded by sharp cutting edges.

Dentine probably owes its strength to its heterogeneous structure. It seems likely that the tubules and interfaces between the various structural elements of dentine act as 'crack stoppers'. A crack stopper is an interface, weaker than the bulk of the material, which is opened up by the action of

**Table 6.2.** Comparison of the physical properties of dentine and enamel.

| Property | Dentine | Enamel |
|---|---|---|
| Specific gravity | 2.14 | 2.9–3.0 |
| Hardness, Knoop number | 63.9 | 296.1 |
| Young's modulus | 12 GN m$^{-2}$ | 131 GN m$^{-2}$ |
| Compressive strength | 262 MN m$^{-2}$ | 76 MN m$^{-2}$ |
| Tensile strength | 29–65 MN m$^{-2}$ | 30–35 MN m$^{-2}$ |
| Rigidity modulus (cf. Young's modulus) | 0.62 GN m$^{-2}$ | — |

MN = N × $10^6$
GN = N × $10^9$

the stresses concentrated at the tip of a moving crack. The opening up of the interface dissipates the stress and this slows down or stops the propagation of the crack. The crack-stopper mechanism is the factor usually responsible for the toughness of strong non-metallic materials of which fibreglass is a well known example.

The existence of this mechanism in the tissue is supported by observations on experimentally fractured dentine. For moist dentine fractured at room temperature, failure seems to be due primarily to the mineralized fibres pulling out of the tissue, indicating that the fibres themselves are stronger than the forces binding them together.

Dentine was previously thought to be uniformly strong in all directions. However, more recent work shows that specimens fracture more easily at an angle to the tubules than parallel with the tubules. This is probably due to the greater ease of crack propagation between the fibres, which are parallel with the incremental lines, than through the fibres. Dentine seems to be well adapted to withstanding compressive forces on the crown, as the incremental layers run almost parallel with the dentine surface (Fig. 6.11). The orientation of the dentine fibres possibly has a further useful mechanical effect. Enamel tends to fracture between the prisms rather than across them, so that cracks would run inwards. Such cracks would be stopped by the dentine because of the change in direction of the plane of greater weakness.

Experimental evidence suggests that dentine is much more susceptible to shearing forces than to compression or tension. This indicates that dentine may be more liable to fracture when subjected to such forces as those set up as molar surfaces sweep past each other in contact, or those resulting from excessive torsion applied to the roots during tooth extraction.

For reference purposes, some of the physical properties of dentine, compared with those of enamel, are listed in Table 6.2.

BIOLOGICAL PROPERTIES

In contrast to enamel, dentine remains vital throughout life by virtue of its contact with the dental pulp. One consequence of this is that dentine is capable of mediating sensation. Furthermore, the effects of attrition or injury can be countered to some extent by changes in the dentine. These changes include: the slow progressive deposition of regular secondary dentine which tends to maintain the tissue thickness; the formation of dead tracts, sclerotic dentine and irregular secondary dentine under areas affected by abrasion, attrition or caries; finally, the formation of peritubular dentine in response to attrition and age.

# ENAMEL

## Physical characters

Many of the physical properties of enamel have been measured. Most importantly, and predictably, it has been shown to be the hardest of vertebrate tissues but it is also rather brittle. Its hardness gives it considerable resistance to the abrasive effects of mastication. Damage to the enamel, because of its brittleness, is to a large extent prevented by the elasticity of the underlying dentine which absorbs any crushing forces. Because dentine is very elastic, the crushing force is probably dissipated by a slight distortion of the dentine which then returns to its original shape.

Enamel is about 95% by weight hydroxyapatite, 4% water, and less than 1% organic material. It is thickest over the working surface of the tooth and thinnest where it is least exposed to wear: over the tips of cusps it can be about 2.5 mm thick tapering to knife-edge at the cervical margin. It is also hardest at the tips of cusps and incisal edges and least hard at the cervical margin.

The colour of enamel varies from the dense white of deciduous teeth to steadily deepening glassy shades of yellow and grey-blue in the ageing dentition. The colour is probably related to the translucency of enamel and to the colour of the underlying dentine. The more heavily mineralized and the thinner the enamel, the more transparent it is and the more the colour of the underlying dentine can be seen. The less heavily mineralized the enamel, the more whitely opaque it becomes with the result that the underlying colour of the dentine is obscured and the enamel appears white. Thus, because deciduous teeth are less well mineralized than permanent teeth they are whiter. In very old permanent teeth the enamel is thinner due to abrasion thereby making more visible the underlying dentine: old teeth are therefore yellower than young permanent teeth but perhaps the darker colour is due to a darker dentine in the aged.

Enamel contains so little apart from hydroxyapatite that when it is demineralized the tenuous unsupported matrix becomes dispersed through the acid. Therefore demineralized, wax-embedded sections of teeth or of teeth and jaws rarely contain even fragments of enamel matrix; instead there remains a space which was once occupied by the enamel. Enamel structure can only usefully be studied in ground sections under the light microscope, in undemineralized sections under the electron microscope, and in fractured, etched, or naturally exposed surfaces under the scanning electron microscope.

### Enamel prisms

#### TERMINOLOGY

At an ultrastructural level enamel consists of long crystals, perhaps 1 $\mu$m or more long, of hydroxyapatite with a somewhat flattened hexagonal cross-section of about 40 nm diameter. These crystals are roughly parallel to each other and so closely packed that they occupy about 88% of the volume (Fig. 6.16), the remaining 12% containing water, proteins, glycoproteins, glycosamino-

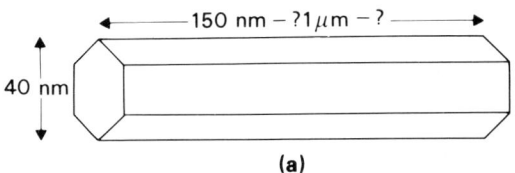

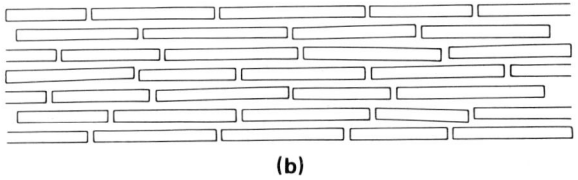

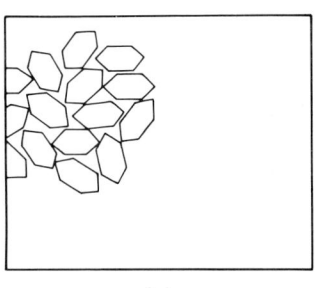

Fig. 6.16. Enamel crystals. (a) Single crystal. (b) Crystals packed together, cut in longitudinal plane (nearly parallel to each other and closer than shown). (c) Crystals sectioned in transverse plane.

glycans, citrate and lipid. Because hydroxyapatite is so much denser than the remaining constituents, enamel is about 96% (by weight) mineral.

The hydroxyapatite crystals are far too narrow to be resolved by the light microscope. With this instrument enamel seems to consist of closely packed rods (prisms), about 5 $\mu$m wide which are roughly perpendicular to the enamel surface and extend uninterrupted from close to the enamel–dentine junction to close to the enamel surface (Fig. 6.17a).

When viewed in a plane tangential to the surface of the tooth the appearance is less easy to analyse. Apart from a region near the enamel–dentine junction where the prisms (rods) may sometimes be circular, their borders are c-shaped, the open end of the 'c' invariably facing cervically (Fig. 6.17b). This appearance is interpreted in two ways. The c-shaped border is always called a prism sheath but the region enclosed by the sheath is called either the prism body or, more briefly, the prism. The reason for this difference is as follows. One way of describing enamel is to join (in the imagination) the free ends of a prism sheath to the adjacent prism sheaths. This 'creates' close-packed keyhole-shaped prisms having bodies and tails (Fig. 6.17c). The other way is to close the prism sheaths to form roughly circular prisms. This 'creates' prisms separated by an interprismatic region (Fig. 6.17d). It can be seen that the prism tails of the first system are equivalent to the interprismatic region of the other system. Both descriptions are imperfect because one incorrectly separates the tail of a prism from the bodies of adjacent prisms and the other incorrectly separates prisms from their interprismatic region. The following account uses the system based on prisms and interprismatic regions but it must be remembered that the prism is continuous with the interprismatic region (Fig. 6.17b) and, what is even more important, that the composition of the prism is, as far as is known, identical to that of the interprismatic region.

### CRYSTAL ORIENTATION

The hydroxyapatite crystals are arranged in a regular pattern which matches the appearance of prisms. Imagine looking into a roughly cylindrical prism from the surface of a tooth (Fig. 6.17a). As a first approximation, the crystals all 'funnel' away from the sides of the prism down to a region situated in the midline on the cuspal edge of the prism (Fig. 6.17e). This describes the appearance of intraprismatic crystals in the longitudinal (Fig. 6.17g,h) and transverse planes of the tooth (Fig. 6.17f). In the interprismatic region beneath each prism the same deviations are continued (Fig. 6.17f,g,h).

### PRISM SHEATHS

It will be noted that a prism sheath is always found, and is only found, at boundaries where there is an abrupt change in crystal orientation. A sheath is a region of microporosity where the ends of one closely packed cluster of crystals (in the interprismatic region) unevenly abut against the sides of another closely packed cluster (the prism itself). This irregular crystal-free boundary is about 0.1 $\mu$m wide, a dimension which is so narrow that prism sheaths are beyond the resolution of the light microscope yet they can easily be seen. The most satisfactory explanation for this paradox points out that the sheath is protein, which has a refractive index of about 1.3, while the prism and interprismatic region, being largely hydroxyapatite, have a refractive index of about 1.6. Incident light is reflected away from the viewer if it grazes this boundary at angles less than about 35° (the critical angle), accounting for the widened 'image' of a prism sheath (Fig. 6.18).

### THE SIZE AND SHAPES OF PRISMS

There is a structureless region, which is up to about 5 $\mu$m wide, adjacent to the dentine and another structureless region, ranging from 0 $\mu$m to 12 $\mu$m wide in permanent teeth and up to 40 $\mu$m in deciduous teeth, at the tooth surface (Fig. 6.17). The absence of structure near the dentine seems to be related to an irregular arrangement of crystals. In contrast, all the crystals are parallel to each other in the structureless surface regions. The absence of abrupt changes in crystal orientation accounts for the absence of prism sheaths and possibly for the fact that the surface of the enamel is the most heavily mineralized.

Near the enamel–dentine junction prisms are about 3 $\mu$m wide, have irregular shapes, and are widely separated by the interprismatic region (Fig. 6.19a). At about 50 $\mu$m further out the prisms have enlarged at the expense of the interprismatic region and are arranged in roughly horizontal and vertical rows (Fig. 6.19b). This pattern rapidly changes into one in which the horizontal rows are staggered (Fig. 6.19c). The prisms steadily increase in size as they extend towards the tooth surface where they are about 6 $\mu$m wide. Close to the tooth surface the prism borders are either irregular (Fig. 6.19d), or the surface layer is structureless (Fig. 6.17). The average width of a prism is 4–5 $\mu$m.

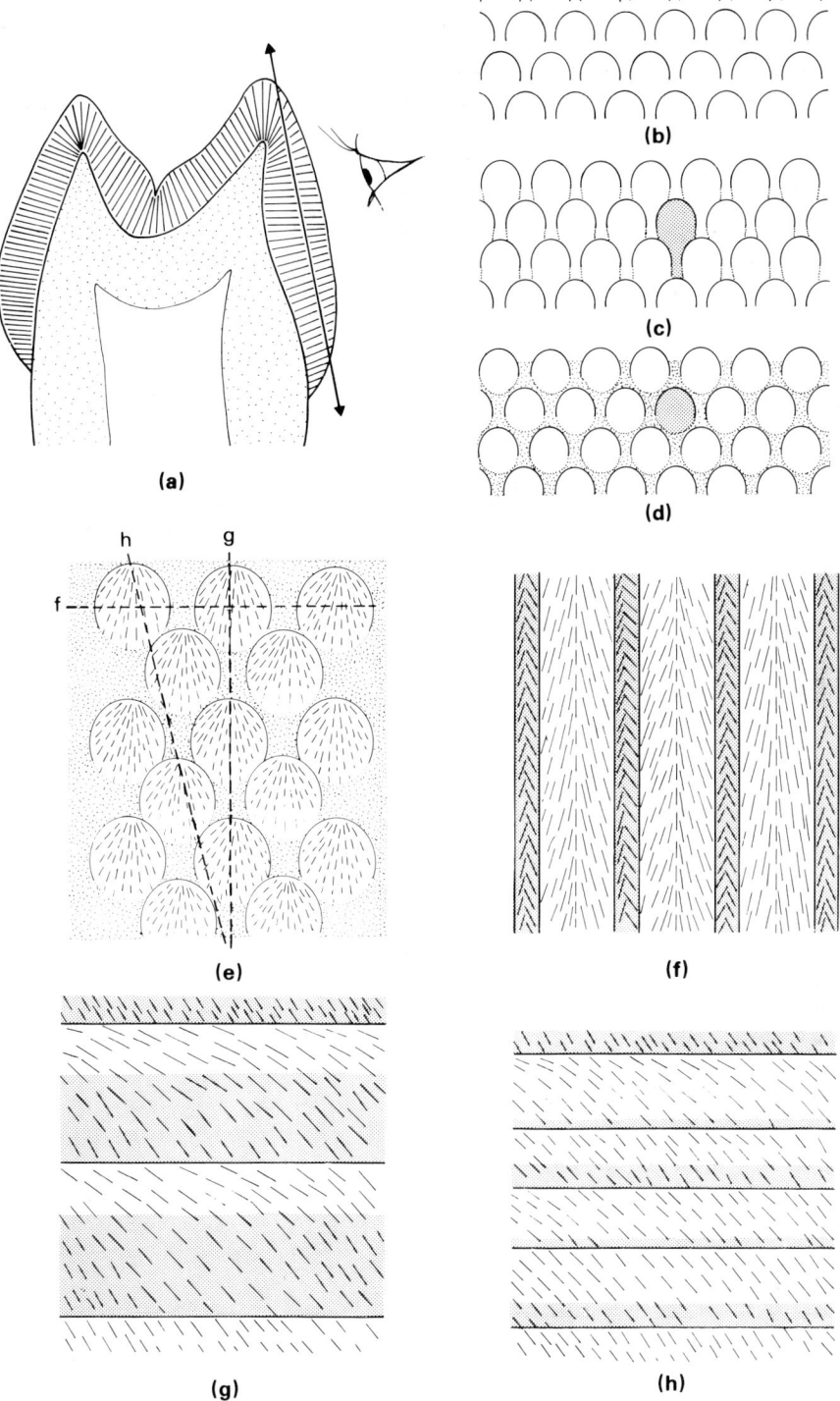

**Fig. 6.17.** (a) Enamel prisms seen in longitudinal section of a tooth. (b) The appearance of prisms viewed from the surface of a tooth (a) when sectioned roughly perpendicular to their long axes. (c) In one interpretation of (b) the cervical borders of the curved lines are continued (dotted lines) to meet the subjacent lines. This creates interlocking keyhole-shaped prisms (shaded). (d) In the interpretation used in this text the cervical borders in (b) are joined (dotted lines) to create roughly circular prisms (shaded) surrounded by an interprismatic region (stippled). (e) If sufficiently magnified under an electron microscope crystals can be seen in prisms sectioned as in (b). When viewed from the direction indicated in (a) the crystals inside a prism are directed away from the viewer towards a point (deep in the paper) at the cuspal edge of the prism. (f, g, h) The appearances of cut surfaces sectioned in the planes indicated in (e).

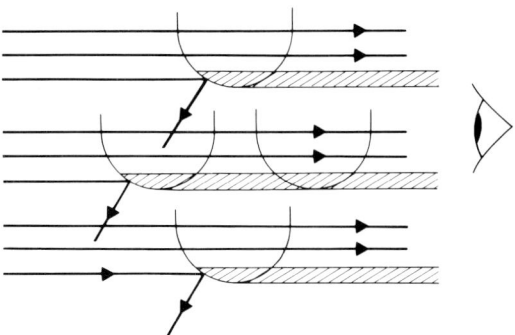

**Fig. 6.18.** The prism sheath. Light is reflected from the sides of the prisms so that the eye sees widened dark lines.

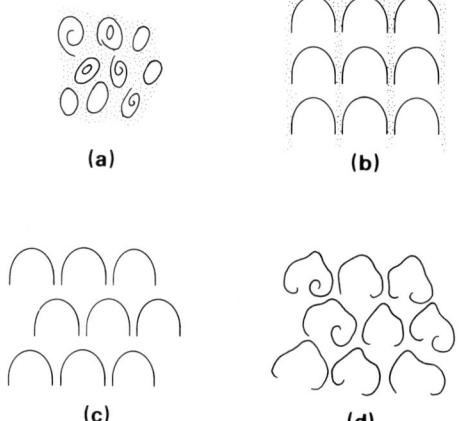

**Fig. 6.19.** The appearance of human enamel prisms in cross-section: (a) close to the enamel–dentine junction; (b) at about 50 μm from the enamel–dentine junction; (c) within most of the enamel; (d) in some regions at the surface of the enamel. [Generally agreed interprismatic regions are stippled in (a) and (b).]

CROSS STRIATIONS

At intervals of about 4–5 μm along its length each prism is marked by a cross-striation (Fig. 6.20a). These are thought to be incremental lines, possibly corresponding to a diurnal variation in the rate at which the enamel is secreted. It has been observed that prisms frequently undulate along their courses, the undulations having a periodicity of about 4–5 μm (Fig. 6.20b). A similar appearance has also been interpreted as alternating varicosities and constrictions (Fig. 6.20c). Although these changes in outline probably correspond with the cross-striations neither necessarily accounts for the appearance of the dark lines:

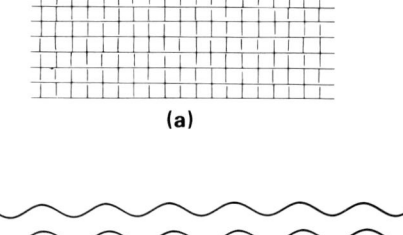

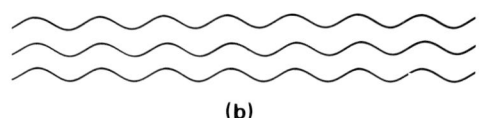

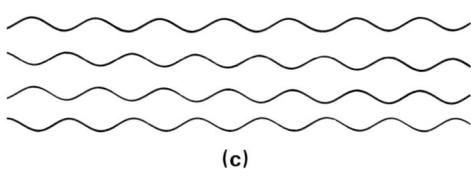

**Fig. 6.20.** (a) Enamel prisms passing from left to right are marked by cross-striations. The marking probably corresponds with the undulations (b) but some workers consider that prisms are alternately varicose and constricted (c). It may be noted that if the lines correspond with variscosities (for example) the latter interpretation would lead to staggered cross-striations.

perhaps there is some change in crystal size or orientation, or in the degree of mineralization of a prism at each cross-striation.

PRISM ARRANGEMENT

Although human prisms are arranged in a simple pattern, it is one which is difficult to visualize in three dimensions. Imagine looking down the length of a prism from the surface of a tooth (Fig. 6.21a). In such a view each prism would be seen to bend from side to side but not to bend up and down: some start out towards the left, others to the right (Fig. 6.21b). Now consider a vertical row of prisms setting out from the enamel–dentine junction in their course towards the surface of the tooth. Passing from above downwards there is a gradual change in the directions at which prisms start out from the enamel–dentine junction, changing from right to left to right and so on (Fig. 6.21c). Now superimpose on Fig. 6.21c the side to side bending of each prism (Fig. 6.21b) to produce Fig. 6.21d. The prisms within a horizontal row are roughly parallel (Fig. 6.21e). Finally, if we polish the left side of the block in Fig. 6.21e, the flat surface would have the appearance shown in Fig. 6.21f. This is the typical appearance of an enamel

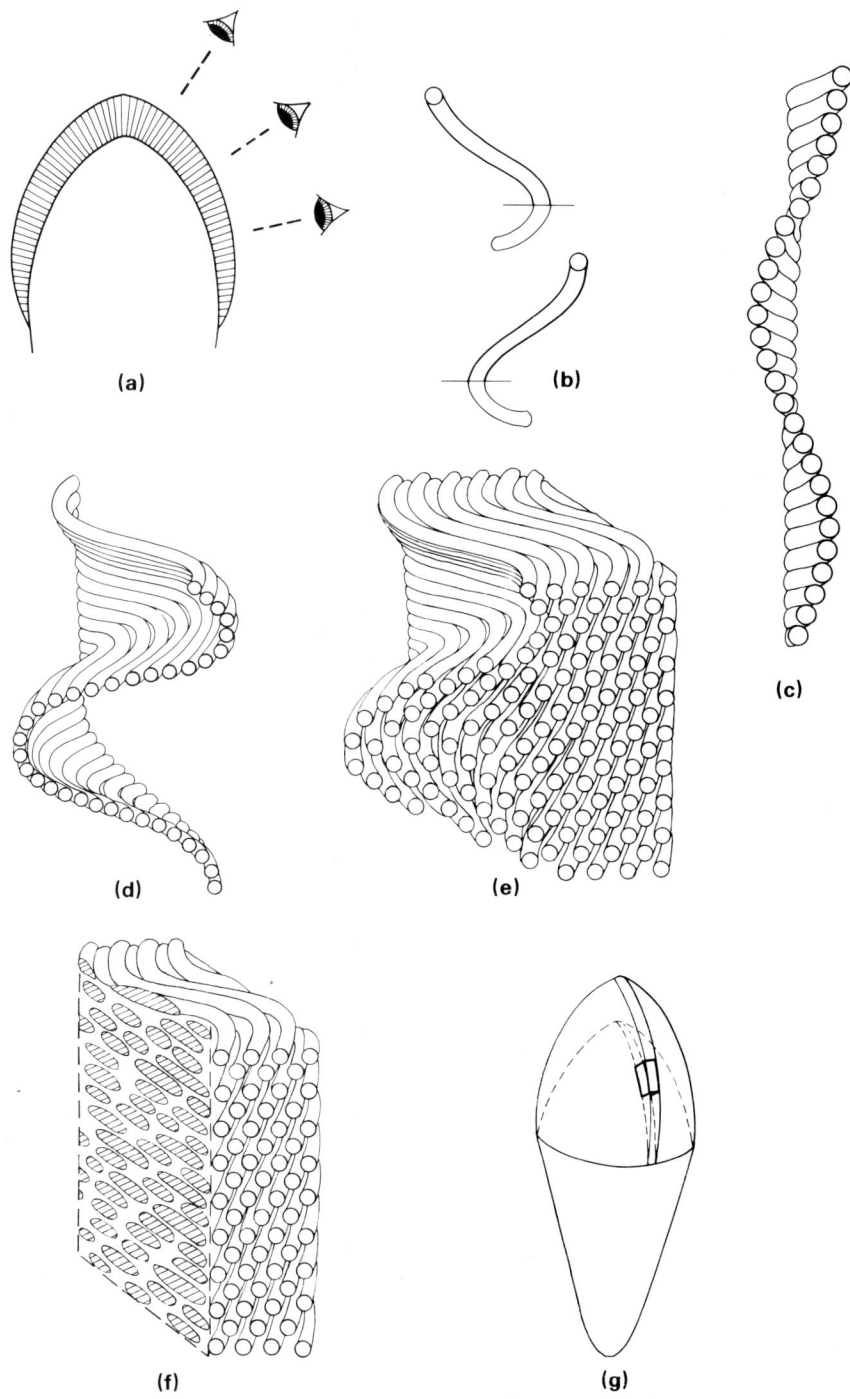

**Fig. 6.21.** The arrangement of enamel prisms. When viewed end on (a) prisms bend to the right and left (b). Starting from the enamel–dentine junction each prism has a direction which differs slightly from adjacent prisms (c). If each prism takes about $1\frac{1}{2}$ turns (b), the appearance (d) is seen for a single vertical row. (e) A rectangular block of prisms [sectioned in (f)] in which all the fragments of prisms on the left have been removed (the orientation of the block is shown in (g)).

surface in a ground longitudinal section of a tooth when the surface has been etched and stained. However, without this treatment the sides of prisms, as opposed to their cuspal borders, are usually invisible in longitudinally sectioned teeth because light does not graze the sides of prisms at angles less than 35°.

*Hunter–Schreger bands*

At the end of the 17th century Hunter and Schreger independently observed that light is reflected from the surface of a polished longitudinal section of enamel to produce the light and dark bands which are now called the Hunter–Schreger bands (Fig. 6.22a). The bands, which cover about two-thirds the thickness of enamel are due to the regular changes in prism direction described above. Much of the light directed onto an enamel section passes through it (if this were not so a ground section of enamel would appear black when viewed by transmitted light). However, some light is reflected by the enamel and obeys the normal laws of reflection. Although it may be the submicroscopic crystals which reflect the light it is easier to understand the origin of the bands by imagining that it is the sides of prisms which reflect it.

The bending of prisms is represented in Fig. 6.21. When incident light is directed from the left side of the page the left sides of each 'wave' appear bright and the right sides dark (Fig. 6.22b). If light is directed from the right side, the dark and bright bands exchange places. In the outer one third all the prisms are roughly parallel to each other with

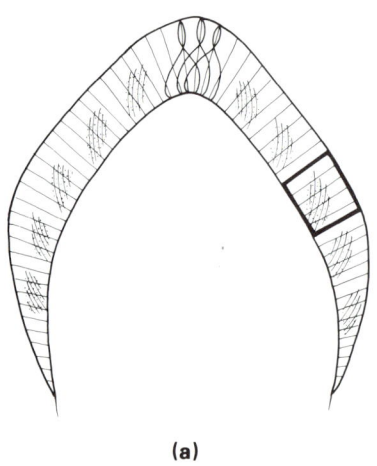

(a)

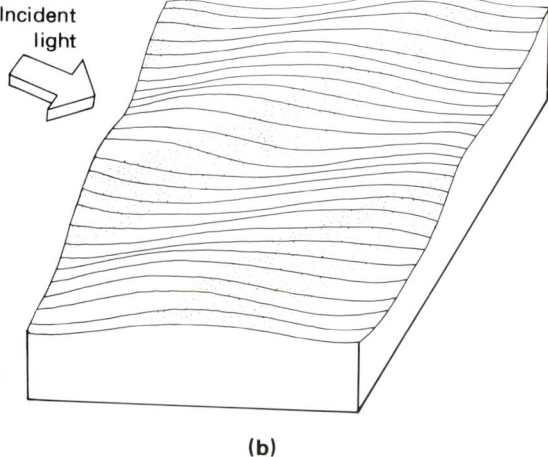

(b)

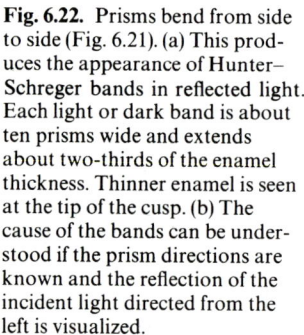

**Fig. 6.22.** Prisms bend from side to side (Fig. 6.21). (a) This produces the appearance of Hunter–Schreger bands in reflected light. Each light or dark band is about ten prisms wide and extends about two-thirds of the enamel thickness. Thinner enamel is seen at the tip of the cusp. (b) The cause of the bands can be understood if the prism directions are known and the reflection of the incident light directed from the left is visualized.

the result that this region does not produce Hunter–Schreger bands. Each light (or dark) band is about ten prisms wide (~ 50 μm).

PRISM DECUSSATION

It can be visualized that as horizontal rows of prisms bend from side to side, each row crosses and is itself crossed by vertically adjacent rows. This crossing of prisms is known as prism decussation. An end-on view of several prisms is shown in Fig. 6.23a. As they pass out towards the surface the horizontal rows of prisms slide over each other until each row has slipped one prism width over an adjacent row (Fig. 6.23a,b,c,d).

In terms of the prism/interprismatic region terminology this behaviour is easy enough to visualize (prisms 1, 11 and 21). But in terms of the keyhole prism terminology the behaviour is less simple. As the middle row slides over the top row, the tail of prism 4 is distorted to the left (Fig. 6.23b). But the slight change between Figs. (6.23b,c) requires the tail to be withdrawn from between prisms 13 and 14 and then to be extended down between prisms 14 and 15. In the intermediate position (Fig. 6.23e), when the tail has been withdrawn, it is necessary to describe an interprismatic region (stippled in Fig. 6.23e).

*Cuspal enamel*
Prisms in cuspal enamel are arranged in a similar way to those at the sides of teeth. Viewed from the tip of the cusp, the prisms, arranged in circular bands, alternately spiral in clockwise and anti-clockwise directions around an axis passing longitudinally through the centre of the tooth (rather than bending to left and right). When a tooth is sectioned longitudinally the sectioned 'spirals' produce a twisted arrangement of prisms which is called gnarled enamel (Fig. 6.22a), a name which inaccurately implies that the structure is irregular. It has been speculated that this arrangement of prisms strengthens the cusps.

*Cervical enamel*
In the cervical region of both deciduous and permanent teeth the prisms are roughly horizontal although they may deviate about 10° either upwards or downwards, and outwards (Fig. 6.22a).

**Incremental lines**

In common with all other mineralized tissues enamel is thought to be laid down in increments, thin lines known as incremental lines separating each increment.

CROSS-STRIATIONS

The cross-striations of enamel prisms have been described above. The cross-striations of one prism are almost always in line with the cross-striations

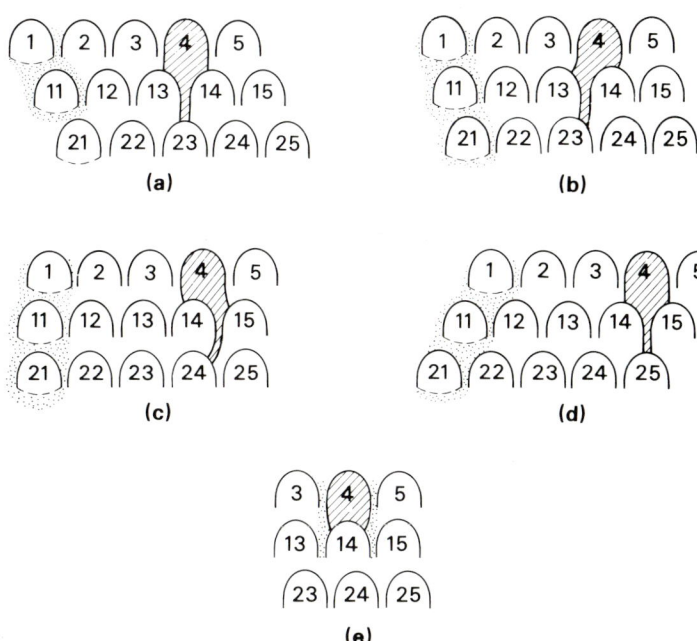

Fig. 6.23. (a) A cross-section of three rows of prisms about 150 μm from the enamel–dentine junction. At intervals of 100 μm further towards the tooth surface (b, c, d) it can be seen that the rows are sliding over each other. In one terminology the prisms are considered to be circular and surrounded by an interprismatic region (prisms 1, 11 and 21). A problem arises with the keyhole terminology (prism 4). (c) As the rows slide over each other the tail of the keyhole must be withdrawn from between prisms 13 and 14, and replaced between prisms 14 and 15. (e) At the intermediate position it is necessary to describe interprismatic sheets.

of adjacent prisms. Each increment of prism is about 4–5 μm long (Fig. 6.20).

BROWN STRIAE OF RETZIUS

The brown striae of Retzius (Retzius lines) are incremental lines, usually brown, seen in ground sections of enamel. In transverse sections they look like the growth rings in a tree trunk (Fig. 6.24a). In longitudinal sections the first stria to be formed outlines a cap of enamel over the tip of the dentine cusp (Fig. 6.24b). All subsequent striae are roughly parallel to this stria. Thus, at the sides of teeth the striae are slightly curved as they pass obliquely outwards and cuspally towards the enamel surface.

Retzius lines vary in thickness from a few microns to 100 μm or more, and they may be separated from each other by about 16 μm up to 100 μm or more. The unworn surface of a tooth is furrowed where each Retzius line meets the enamel surface (perikymata: see below).

The Retzius lines become increasingly difficult to see as light microscope magnifications are increased until with a × 100 objective they 'disappear'. This has made it very difficult to discover what changes in prism structure are responsible for the appearance of the striae. Based on three-dimensional reconstructions it has been shown that in association with some striae prisms bend to the left or right in the transverse plane of the tooth. Based on their appearance in longitudinally sectioned teeth it has been argued that prisms bend down towards the cervix of the tooth when they enter a striae. The prism sheaths within striae appear much darker than those in the adjacent enamel.

Microradiographs and polarization microscopy both suggest that Retzius lines may be either more or less mineralized than adjacent enamel.

The striae appear brown when viewed by transmitted light but blue when viewed by reflected light. This indicates that they preferentially scatter short, as opposed to long, wavelengths of light (Fig. 6.25). In order to scatter blue light the striae should contain structures or spaces whose sizes are comparable to the wavelength of light. This suggests that the brown striae correspond with some change in the size or orientation of crystals.

Very narrow 'splits' near the enamel surface seen in recent electron and scanning electron micrographs have been interpreted as Retzius lines. These studies lead to the conclusion that, at least near the tooth surface, striae may be gaps between rows of crystals.

It seems that the pattern of Retzius lines is the same in all teeth remembering, for example, that the last lines developing towards the cervical margin of a first permanent molar (crown completed at about 3 years) are equivalent to the first Retzius lines developing in the cusp of a second permanent molar (crown starts to mineralize at about 3 years). This suggests that Retzius lines develop in response to systemic influences such as illness, the intensity of the line being proportional to the severity of the influence.

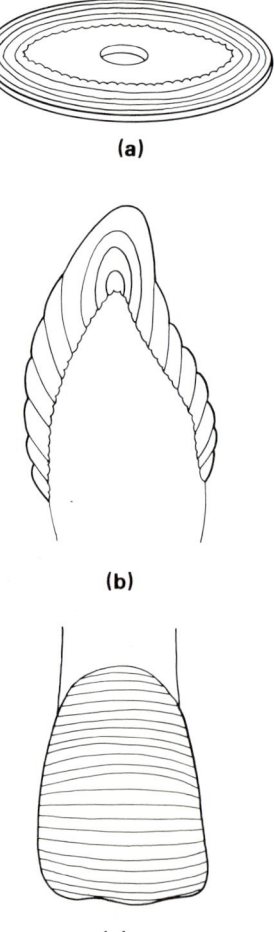

**Fig. 6.24.** Retzius lines in (a) transverse section and (b) longitudinal section. (c) Perikymata.

PERIKYMATA

A newly erupted tooth is surrounded by furrows parallel to the enamel/cement junction, each furrow marking the line at which a brown stria

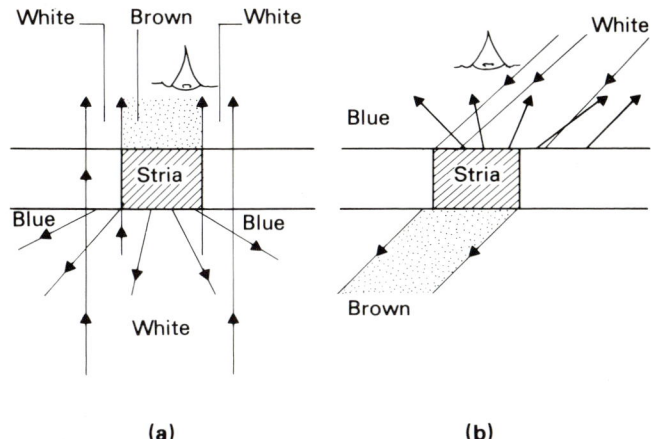

Fig. 6.25. 'Blue' light is scattered by the striae and 'brown' light transmitted. Therefore, by transmitted light striae appear brown (a), and by reflected light appear blue (b).

meets the surface (Fig. 6.24c). These perikymata troughs are separated by perikymata crests. The surface of a tooth is later worn flat.

NEONATAL LINE

The well developed, homogeneous enamel formed in the carefully controlled environment of the embryo differs from later formed enamel, the two being separated by a well marked stria of Retzius known as the neonatal line. Neonatal lines consist of poorly mineralized enamel developed while the newborn infant is losing weight as it adjusts to its new environment. They are seen in all deciduous teeth and in the first permanent molars; that is, those teeth which begin to mineralize before birth.

**Tufts, lamellae and spindles**

These three structures share a major heading because (a) they are entirely organic, at least when they develop, (b) they are not part of the prisms, and (c) they are easily seen in ground sections.

TUFTS

In transverse ground sections of enamel structures which resemble tufts of grass weave outwards from the enamel–dentine junction through up to one third of the thickness of the enamel (Fig. 6.26a). Each 'leaf' of a tuft seems to correspond with a thickened prism sheath.

The real shape of the tufts is best seen in longitudinal ground sections which are cut tangential to the surface of the dentine (Fig. 6.26b). Such sections reveal that each tuft consists of several long splayed-out 'ribbons' (viewed from their edges): the 'leaves' of a tuft seen in transverse sections are 'cuts' through the splay of ribbons. Each ribbon consists of vertically connected thickened (organic) prism sheaths (Fig. 6.26c).

Microradiographs and hardness tests show that for two or three prism widths to each side of a tuft the enamel is less mineralized than adjacent enamel which does not contain tufts.

LAMELLAE

Lamellae are thin sheets of organic tissue which pass from the surface of the enamel (tufts do not reach the surface) usually as far as the enamel–dentine junction (Fig. 6.26d) and occasionally into the dentine. From their orientation, roughly parallel to the long axis of the tooth, it can be visualized that lamellae are best studied in transverse sections of teeth.

There are three possible types of lamellae. First, a lamella may be the result of a developmental fault in which, for some reason, a sheet of enamel matrix fails to mineralize. Second, following the development of its full thickness but before it is fully mineralized, the enamel may be compressed and then split. Cells from the reduced enamel epithelium could be sucked into the crack and subsequently die thereby producing a sheet-like organic flaw. Third, in elderly people the enamel sometimes cracks: debris from the saliva penetrates the crack producing the last type of lamella.

The frequency of each type of lamella, and even the existence of all three types, is open to argument. In ground sections lamellae can easily be confused with cracks caused by grinding the section. The only convincing way of distinguishing between cracks and lamellae is to demineralize the section: in such a preparation, cracks disappear but lamellae remain.

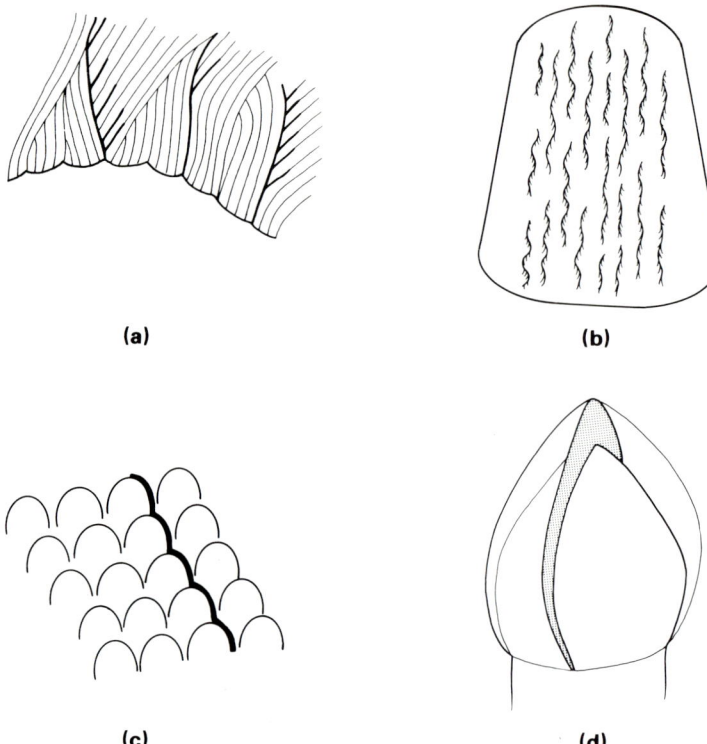

**Fig. 6.26.** (a) Tufts seen in a transversely sectioned tooth. (b) Tufts as they would appear if they could be seen through the buccal enamel of an incisor tooth. (c) A high power view of a small part of a tuft seen in (b). (d) A lamella.

SPINDLES

Enamel spindles (Fig. 6.27) almost certainly develop around processes of odontoblasts which have grown between the cells of the internal enamel epithelium before the start of amelogenesis (they are not often parallel to the prisms). These tubular extensions become 'fossilized' during amelogenesis. They are most commonly seen at the tips of cusps either in longitudinally sectioned teeth or in sections which cut transversely through the tip of the cusp. They are usually about 30–40 $\mu$m long.

FISSURES AND PITS

Fissures are the crevices which separate the cusps of cheek teeth. They extend for a variable depth through the enamel. It can be visualized that as the ameloblasts move outwards from the concave surface between two dentine cusps they become progressively more crowded. Sometimes this crowding leads to an early end of amelogenesis with the result that the enamel at the depth of a fissure is thin (Fig. 6.27c): such a fissure may be very narrow and it is possible that it could retain protein from dead ameloblasts. The same is true for pits, in upper lateral incisors for example. Other fissures may be narrower (Fig. 6.27d).

**Enamel–dentine junction**

The enamel–dentine junction appears scalloped in all planes of section, the concavities facing towards the enamel. It can be visualized that the dentine surface is covered by minute depressions into which fit domes of enamel. Spindles and tufts arise from the enamel–dentine junction, lamellae often reach it and may pass across it.

Unlike the light microscope, under the electron microscope the enamel–dentine junction is very poorly defined, appearing to be a no-man's land in which the collagen fibres and small crystals of dentine are mixed with the large crystals of enamel. For a few microns the enamel is less well mineralized than in the bulk of the tooth.

It has been argued that the shape of the

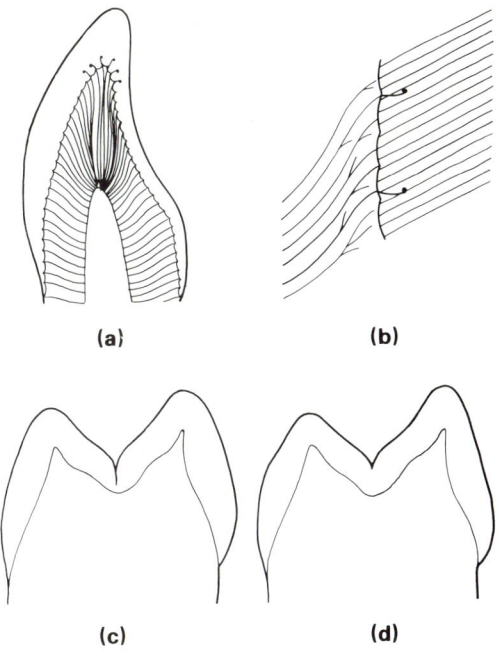

Fig. 6.27. (a) Enamel spindles near tip of cusp. (b) The spindles are parallel to the long axes of ameloblasts at the beginning of amelogenesis. (c) A deep fissure and (d) a shallow fissure.

enamel–dentine junction has the advantage that it minimizes the possibility of enamel being sheared off the underlying dentine. However, the strength of the junction is more likely to depend on the blending of enamel and dentine tissues.

### Enamel surface

The enamel surface is extremely important because, being exposed to the oral cavity, it is the site of the initial carious attack and, for at least part of our lives, it must form an effective attachment to the oral epithelium which protects the underlying mesoderm (Fig. 7.25).

Apart from just after the teeth have been brushed with abrasives, all the enamel is covered by acquired organic integuments—cuticles, pellicles and plaque (p. 280).

Under the light microscope the surface of young enamel is furrowed by the perikymata (Fig. 6.24). Generally speaking prisms reach the surface in the perikymata troughs but fail to reach the surface of the perikymata crests. However, this arrangement and the thickness of the non-prismatic layer are variable. Microradiographs reveal that the surface enamel is more heavily mineralized than the rest of the enamel. Fluoride can be taken up at the surface (Table 6.4).

At an ultrastructural level, the regions where prisms reach the surface are covered by shallow pits, each pit corresponding to the end of a prism.

Less commonly, the surface is marked by larger depressions or dome-shaped protuberances which can be up to $\mu m$ wide.

### Vital or dead

It can be argued that because of its rock-like structure and, more importantly, the absence of cellular processes, let alone cells, enamel is a dead tissue comparable to keratin squames or to the outer bark of trees: indeed, like these tissues, enamel provides a protective covering. However this may be too narrow a view of enamel tissue. By far the majority of bone and cement tissue does not consist of cells or cell processes; it is extracellular. And the majority of the dentine is 'outside' the processes of odontoblasts. Yet, with the exception of the deepest layers of cement, these extracellular tissues are considered to be 'living'. For each of these examples the argument hinges on the fact that although the extracellular regions, by definition, lack cells, the tissue as a whole possesses cells which appear to be specialized for its maintenance. In each case it is the formative cells which later maintain the tissue, presumably by controlling the contents of the fluid which percolates into and out of the extracellular regions. However, enamel loses its formative cells, the ameloblasts and related cells of the enamel organ, to the reduced enamel epithelium (Fig. 8.42) which, apart from those contributing to the junctional epithelium (Fig. 7.25), are shed into the oral cavity. Therefore, if enamel is considered to be vital it is unusual because it does not retain its formative cells in the role of maintenance cells. This role must be undertaken by other cells.

Bone provides an excellent example of the reaction of the body to 'dead' extracellular tissue. In the very unpleasant condition of osteomyelitis, infection sweeps through the bone killing the osteocytes. Following recovery from the acute infection it appears that the body recognizes the absence of osteocytes and the 'dead' nature of the bone. Osteoclasts are differentiated and, by resorption, separate the living bone from the dead bone which is now pushed out through the skin.

Clearly the above is not the fate of enamel, although it was once argued that teeth erupt because enamel, being a dead tissue, is extruded from the body! However, it could be that the enamel is 'protected' from rejection by the underlying vital dentine. In the following situation dentine and cement can be used to prevent rejection of a foreign substance. In order to replace a lens in the eye, a thick transverse section is cut from the root of a patient's canine, the pulp is removed from the disc of tooth and a plastic lens cemented in its place. The disc consisting of lens and tooth is now transferred into the eye where the cement becomes attached to the surrounding tissues thereby maintaining the foreign lens. In this case the dead lens is attached to the body via an intermediate 'live' tissue, the cement. But no intermediary is required in the case of enamel; junctional epithelium forms a direct attachment. However, this argument in favour of enamel vitality may not be valid because epithelia can attach to glass, for example, in tissue culture conditions.

Returning to the argument that an extracellular tissue can only be considered vital if its structure is, in some way, maintained by cells, clearly dentine with its odontoblasts and subjacent pulp would be important for the maintenance of enamel. However, in order to be maintained, it must be shown that fluid can pass into the enamel.

In a striking experiment the enamel surface of extracted teeth was covered with oil. Within a few hours droplets of fluid appeared beneath the oil on the surface of the enamel. It can be concluded that water, and therefore probably any small molecules, can penetrate enamel (however, it is possible that the water was absorbed from the atmosphere). The permeability of enamel can also be demonstrated by sealing dyes or radioactive tracers into the pulps of extracted teeth. After a few days the dye, for example, penetrates the dentinal tubules and for a variable distance into the enamel. Dyes reach the surface of young dog teeth but penetrate far less into human teeth. In particular they pass into the spindles, lamellae and tufts of young human teeth. The enamel of older teeth rapidly becomes increasingly impermeable. However, this suggests the possibility that the organic matrix of, at least, young enamel could be maintained by the body (or even protected in some way against caries). In order to test this it might be possible to show that the enamel matrix of root-filled teeth (teeth whose pulp has been removed and replaced by an inert filling material) is different from that in normal teeth. Certainly, root-filled teeth appear to be more brittle than normal teeth but this change may be attributed more to 'death' of the dentine rather than the overlying enamel.

To a very limited extent enamel is also permeable from its surface. Thus, enamel can 'absorb' stains from the oral cavity although it is possible that these stains merely attach to or lie in the small pits at the ends of prisms which reach the surface.

Although the surface of the enamel is, to all intents, impermeable to large dye molecules, it is permeable to ions. For example, radioactive iodine placed on the surface of a cat's canine was subsequently detected in its thyroid gland. This suggests the possibility that calcium or phosphate ions might enter or leave enamel under appropriate conditions. However, although theoretically possible there is little doubt that the amounts are negligible. For example, calcium tablets are not prescribed for a pregnant mother in order to prevent the removal of calcium from her teeth to nourish the foetus. Alarming amounts of calcium can indeed be removed from the mother's skeleton, but not from her teeth.

Although enamel does not seem to lose mineral ions to the body, ions are certainly exchanged with the saliva. Such ion exchange may be isoionic (e.g. calcium for calcium) or heteroionic (e.g. strontium for calcium). This is the rationale for topical applications of fluoride and for the use of fluoride toothpaste: under these conditions it seems probable that fluoride ions are exchanged for hydroxyl ions in the crystal lattice of apatite. However, they may also enter the enamel matrix. Once again young enamel is more reactive than old enamel.

Finally, it is sometimes possible for enamel which has become partially demineralized by caries to become remineralized. Presumably the demineralized enamel is more permeable than is normal enamel to mineral ions in the saliva.

In each of the above cases the reactivity of enamel is probably best viewed as physicochemical rather than biological. In other words, by most criteria enamel can be considered a dead tissue which is not rejected by the body.

**Clinical considerations**

Enamel is lost in the face of caries, and by attrition, abrasion and injury. Caries starts as a process in which enamel crystals are dissolved by the acidic by-products of bacterial metabolism. Enamel crystals are more soluble at their ends than their sides from which it can be visualized that caries advances more rapidly down the cores of prisms than the interprismatic region. Clearly the structure of the surface enamel must, in part, determine how prone a tooth is to carious attack.

The protein sheets in enamel, the lamellae and tufts, are probably unimportant in the original caries attack but may be important when the cavity has enlarged and contains secondary, perhaps proteolytic, bacteria.

Much of a practising dental surgeon's life is spent preparing cavities for fillings. The cavities are designed for maximum strength. Enamel is brittle, tending to shear along planes between prisms. This suggests that the crossing of prisms, which produces the Hunter–Schreger band appearance, reduces the tendency of enamel to split (in that masterpiece of biological design, the rodent incisor, adjacent rows of prisms cross each other at right angles reducing to its absolute minimum the tendency for enamel to shear). When cutting cavities the operator must ensure that all the enamel prisms at the edges of the cavity have their inner ends lying on dentine: unsupported prisms tend to chip off the surface leaving cracks which are prone to a new carious attack. It is often difficult to ensure that all prisms are supported at the edges of cavities which depend on undercuts for retaining the filling material; e.g. amalgam (Fig. 6.28).

It is now possible to bond some types of filling material to the enamel surface, a technique which is particularly valuable for cavities near the cervical margin. For this purpose the enamel is etched with acid. Just as with caries, the acid penetrates more rapidly down the prisms than the interprismatic region (although, surprisingly, the reverse is true for some acids) leaving a pitted surface to which some filling materials can be effectively bonded.

Narrow and deep fissures probably retain food and bacteria despite the most determined oral hygiene. They are therefore very prone to caries. It is a common prophylactic treatment to seal these fissures with an inert material before they can become carious.

Enamel which has been lost due to attrition can only be replaced by crowns or inlays. It requires very considerable practice and judgement to match the colour of a crown to the colour of the patient's teeth. Surprising though it may be, different teeth have an enormous range of fugitive but obviously different colours.

The importance of heteroionic exchange in the effectiveness of fluoride treatment has been described above.

## PULP

The pulp cavity consists of a pulp chamber and one or more pulp (root) canals terminating at apical foramina. Pulp horns (cornua) extend towards the incisive edge or cusp regions. The cavity is enclosed by dentine except at the apical foramen where it is continuous with the periapical part of the periodontal ligament. Part of the root

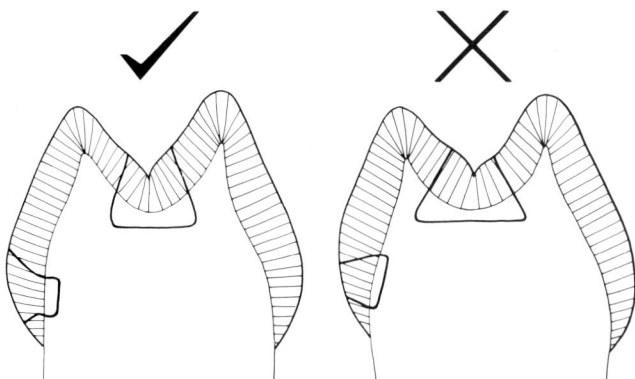

Fig. 6.28. In order to retain a filling material the walls of cavities are undercut. Care is taken to ensure that prisms are supported (right) rather than unsupported (left).

canal immediately adjacent to the apical foramen may eventually be lined with cement. The pulp chamber contains a soft connective tissue, the dental pulp. The apical foramina and root canals allow vessels and nerves to enter and leave the pulp chamber.

The shape of the pulp cavity varies from tooth to tooth and changes with age as primary and subsequently secondary dentine are produced (Fig. 6.10). In permanent teeth the size and number of the pulp horns is correlated with the degree to which the cusps are developed so that in general premolars have two pulp horns and molars have four. The pulp horns diminish rapidly in size with age due to the formation of secondary dentine which may be deposited in this region before the apical foramina are fully formed. In deciduous teeth, the pulp cavities are relatively larger and the pulp horns are higher than in permanent teeth.

The root canal leads from the pulp chamber to the apical foramen. A single root may have two root canals and accessory canals may form a delta-like system towards the apex of the tooth. The apical foramen is the last part of the pulp cavity to develop; it is formed 1–1.5 years after eruption in deciduous teeth and 2–3 years after eruption in permanent teeth. The size of the foramen is progressively reduced with age by the deposition of secondary dentine and cement on its pulpal aspect.

**Structure of pulp**

Like all connective tissues the pulp contains cells, fibres, ground substance, vessels and nerves.

CELLS

*Odontoblasts*
Odontoblasts function primarily as secretory cells. They synthesize and secrete collagen and the ground substance of primary and secondary dentine. The structure of odontoblasts changes during the life of the tooth. When dentinogenesis is at its height, the cells are large with a bulky cytoplasm containing copious amounts of granular endoplasmic reticulum so that they stain pale blue with haematoxylin. As dentinogenesis slows down the odontoblasts take on a stratified appearance (Fig. 6.29) and become less active. The bulk of cytoplasm is decreased, and it contains fewer ribosomes and less RNA. It is important to realize that odontoblasts remain capable of synthesizing the organic component of dentine throughout the life of the cell. It is likely in practice that some odontoblasts die as the result of damage to the tooth by carious attack, fracture of dentine, conservative dentistry or as part of the ageing process. In a healthy pulp odontoblasts continue their reduced activities to an advanced age of the tooth.

Odontoblasts are incapable of mitosis and do not differentiate or dedifferentiate into any other type of cell. In the subodontoblastic layer, there is a pool of precursor cells which can divide and differentiate into odontoblasts should the need arise, as for example after the death of existing odontoblasts. If new odontoblasts are produced in this way they are formed without the organizing influence of the internal enamel epithelium. Probably as a result of this, such odontoblasts lack the precise orientation of the first formed cells and they produce irregular secondary dentine.

*Subodontoblast cells*
On the pulpal side of the odontoblast layer in a very young tooth there is a cell-rich layer of subodontoblastic cells. These are mainly fibroblasts but included in this layer are the supposedly undifferentiated cells.

A few years after the tooth erupts, a zone in which cells are scarce appears between the odontoblasts and the subodontoblastic cells. The space is sometimes called the cell-free layer (of Weil) and is most prominent in the crowns of the teeth. Beneath is a cell-rich layer.

*Fibroblasts*
The most numerous cells of the pulp are fibroblasts or fibrocytes. They do not differ in structure from those found in connective tissues elsewhere. Pulp is a comparatively cellular connective tissue but the number of fibroblasts decreases with age (Fig. 6.29d) and the activity of those remaining also declines.

Pulp fibroblasts synthesize and secrete collagen, reticulin and the proteoglycans (protein-glycosaminoglycan complexes) and proteins of pulp ground substance.

*Mesenchyme cells*
These cells are supposedly present in all connective tissues and have been mentioned in relation to the origin of some odontoblasts.

*Defence cells*
Pulp contains lymphocytes and other white cells derived from the blood together with tissue histiocytes. No mast cells are present.

# Dental Tissues

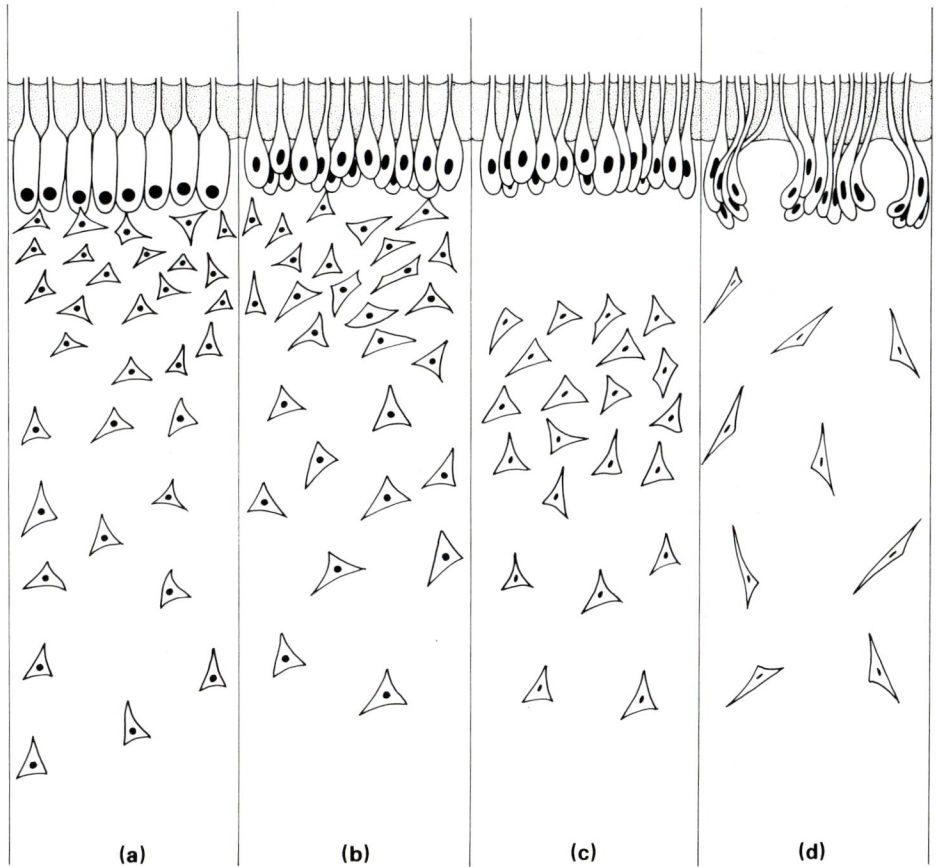

**Fig. 6.29.** (a) Appearances of pulp and odontoblasts at the beginning of dentinogenesis; (b) later in dentinogenesis; (c) 2 or 3 years after the tooth has erupted; (d) in an old tooth.

*Perivascular cells*

Cells found near capillary blood vessels in pulp are called pericytes. No special significance is now attached to them and they resemble perivascular cells in general.

Pulp contains no fat cells.

FIBRES

In pulp, elastic fibres and oxytalan fibres are absent. Young pulp especially contains few fibres: those present are collagen and reticulin. Usual staining methods (e.g. van Gieson's picro-fuchsin) show that the amount of collagen increases with age. Silver stains show reticulin, especially in relation to blood vessels, but they also reveal immature collagen and von Korff fibres.

GROUND SUBSTANCE

Several glycosaminoglycans (as components of proteoglycans) are present in the dental pulp. Hyaluronic acid appears to predominate in human teeth but chondroitin sulphates are important especially during dentinogenesis.

BLOOD SUPPLY

The arteries enter the pulp at the apical foramen and through any accessory foramina. On entering the pulp the vessels are so small and thin-walled that they can be regarded as arterioles. Their walls contain a little smooth muscle. Soon after entering the pulp canal the arterioles branch out and run longitudinally through the periphery of the pulp.

They give rise to capillaries which loop towards the odontoblasts. Blood vessels may usually be seen within the odontoblast layer but patent vessels do not enter the dentine. The capillaries drain into venules which run more centrally in the pulp chamber and drain through the apical foramen.

In general the veins draining the teeth run with the corresponding arteries but with a greater degree of anastomosis. The blood from the maxillary teeth may drain forward through the infra-orbital foramen to join the facial vein or back into the pterygoid plexus. Blood from the mandibular teeth may also drain forward through the mental foramen to join the facial vein or back via the mandibular foramen into the pterygoid plexus.

Some doubt has been expressed about the existence of lymphatics in the dental pulp but it seems reasonable to accept that they drain this connective tissue in the same way that they drain others. They drain to the submandibular and deep cervical lymph nodes.

### NERVE SUPPLY

The pulpal nerves enter or leave the apical foramina. There are two types of nerves present: sensory nerves in which all impulses appear to be related to pain (in man) and sympathetic nerves which control the smooth muscle of the blood vessels.

The sensory nerves of the pulp canal consist of several separate trunks of both myelinated and unmyelinated fibres which run into the coronal pulp in the company of the arterioles. The fibres disperse towards the odontoblast layer and near the 'cell-free zone', beneath the odontoblasts, they branch and intermingle to form the plexus of Raschkow. Small branches, mainly unmyelinated, arise from this plexus and pass between the odontoblasts to form a plexus over and in the predentine. From this plexus a few terminal branches pass a short distance into dentinal tubules, where they run beside or in a recess in the odontoblast process. Intratubular nerve fibres appear to be quite rare in the root dentine. When the fibres end they come into close contact with the odontoblast process with a localized interdigitation of the nerve and cell plasma membranes (see also under development and ageing of pulp).

Postganglionic (unmyelinated) sympathetic nerves, whose cell bodies are in the superior cervical ganglion, enter the pulp as a perivascular net and remain closely related to the arterioles.

They supply the smooth muscle of the blood vessels.

## SENSORY MECHANISMS OF DENTINE AND PULP

### Sensations produced by stimulating teeth

It is generally believed that the only sensation produced by stimulating nerves within teeth is pain. This is the case for all forms of stimulus which have been tested with the possible exception of electrical, which, at or just above threshold, produces a pricking or throbbing sensation which most people do not describe as painful. Only if a stimulus spreads beyond dentine and pulp to affect receptors in gingival or periodontal tissues, as may happen with thermal or mechanical stimuli, can the subject identify accurately the type of stimulus being applied. The sensations of touch and pressure which result from mechanical stimulation of teeth do not involve receptors in dentine or pulp. The touch thresholds of teeth from which the pulps have been removed are not different from those of intact teeth.

#### OTHER RESPONSES TO STIMULATION OF INTRADENTAL NERVES

Stimulation of nerves in teeth produces reflex responses in the muscles of mastication. These consist of a reduction in elevator activity and in cats, but not apparently in man, contraction of depressor muscles. In man, the threshold of the reflex response in the masseter is about the same as the sensory threshold and it appears that both responses depend on activating the same group of nerves.

#### STIMULI WHICH PRODUCE PAIN FROM INTACT TEETH

Mechanical, thermal and electrical stimuli are capable of producing pain when applied to intact enamel. The enamel is non-vital and the pain is due to excitation of nerves in the underlying dentine or pulp. Large compressive or shearing forces, as are produced when forceps are applied to extract a tooth, excite nerve endings in the teeth as well as the periodontal tissues and produce pain. With thermal stimuli applied to intact enamel, the thresholds for pain are about 45°C for hot and 27°C for cold.

## THE SENSITIVITY OF EXPOSED DENTINE

When a cavity is cut through the enamel with a bur, the moment at which the amelodentinal junction is reached is usually associated with the sudden onset of pain. If the cavity is deepened further, it seems that the sensitivity of the dentine is at first less than that at the amelodentinal junction and then increases again as the pulp is approached. Not only does the sensitivity of an exposed dentine surface appear to depend upon the depth of the cavity, but also on the condition of the underlying pulp. A freshly prepared cavity in a healthy, intact tooth, or a tooth with just minimal caries of the enamel, seems to be much less sensitive than one prepared in a tooth in which caries has penetrated to the dentine and produced some inflammatory reaction in the pulp. Also, a freshly prepared cavity in a tooth with a normal pulp is much less sensitive than the same cavity 1 week later if it has been filled with the temporary filling material gutta percha for the intervening period. Gutta percha does not make a good seal with the cavity walls and pulpal inflammation develops due to penetration of material from the mouth.

Clinical experience also indicates that the sensitivity of dentine tends to decrease with age, although it appears to vary considerably between individuals of the same age. The coronal dentine of permanent teeth is sensitive to stimulation even when the tooth is only partially erupted and root formation is incomplete. The dentine of deciduous teeth tends to be less sensitive than that of permanent teeth. Dentine is, of course, insensitive in a tooth from which the pulp has been removed.

Pain may be produced by stimulating exposed dentine with a sharp probe, by heating or cooling it, by drying it with a stream of air, absorbent paper or cotton wool, or by applying to it certain solutions such as strong sugar solutions. The pain producing properties of a large number of substances has been tested in human volunteers by applying them in solution to occlusal cavities cut just into dentine in minimally carious premolars. The solutions which caused pain did so with a frequency which was related to their osmotic pressures (Fig. 6.30) and was independent of their chemical composition. Some solutions which cause pain when applied to the exposed nerve endings in skin, such as acetylcholine, histamine and bradykinin, produce no pain in dentine. Neither local anaesthetics nor protein precipitants when applied topically to dentine affect its sensitivity.

Dentine which is exposed between the enamel and the gingival attachment in the cervical region of a tooth may be very sensitive to thermal, mechanical or osmotic stimuli. The sensitivity of dentine under these conditions appears to be similar to that of dentine overlying inflamed pulp in an occlusal cavity, although there is no evidence that the sensory mechanisms are the same in both situations.

## THE SENSITIVITY OF PULP

Pulp which is exposed either as a result of a tooth being fractured in an accident or during cavity preparation is extremely sensitive and even gentle mechanical stimulation produces severe pain. For this reason, very few experiments have been carried out on the sensitivity of the pulp in man. It has been shown however that solutions of acetylcholine and histamine, which do not cause pain

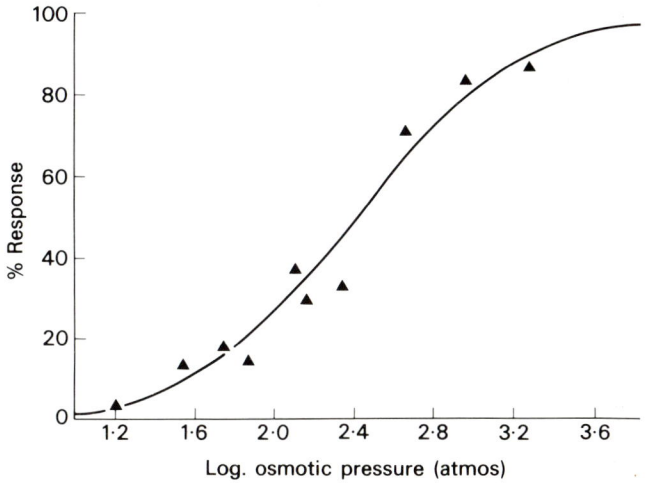

Fig. 6.30. The relationship between osmotic pressure of a wide range of different solutions and the % of applications to dentine which produced pain. The solutions were applied to freshly cut dentine. (Data from Anderson D. J. & Matthews B. (1967) *Archives of Oral Biology* **12**, 417).

from the outer dentine cause pain when applied to inner dentine.

**The innervation of dentine and pulp**

The afferent nerves in pulp include both non-myelinated and small myelinated fibres with diameters up to about 6 μm and conduction velocities from less than 1 m/s$^1$ to about 40 m/s$^1$ (Fig. 6.31). They have their cell bodies in the ipsilateral trigeminal ganglion and project to both the spinal and main sensory nuclei of the trigeminal nerve in the brain stem. From these nuclei connections have been demonstrated to the thalamus and cerebral cortex.

The pulpal vasculature is supplied by sympathetic vasoconstrictor fibres with cell bodies in the superior cervical ganglion. It appears that the fibres travel at first with the branches of the external carotid and then join the appropriate dental nerves. The vasoconstrictor endings are of the α-adrenergic type.

There may also be other efferent fibres supplying the pulp. Possible functions include active vasodilatation, regulation of the rate of dentine formation, modulation of the excitability of afferent nerve endings, as well as trophic influences; but the evidence for these is as yet incomplete.

There is an extensive network of branched nerve terminals close to the surface of the pulp, deep to the odontoblast cell bodies. This is the plexus of Raschkow. From this plexus, some nerve terminals cross the cell-free layer of Weil, pass between the odontoblasts and form a second branched network on the predentine surface. This is the subodontoblastic plexus. A few of the terminals can be traced for up to 0.5 mm or so into the dentinal tubules of permanent teeth, although not before the time at which root formation is complete. There are many such intratubular fibres above the pulp cornu but otherwise only 1–10% of tubules in the coronal dentine contain nerve terminals. In fully formed teeth, the odontoblast processes extend only one third to half of the distance from the cell body to the amelodentinal junction and there is no evidence of any vital

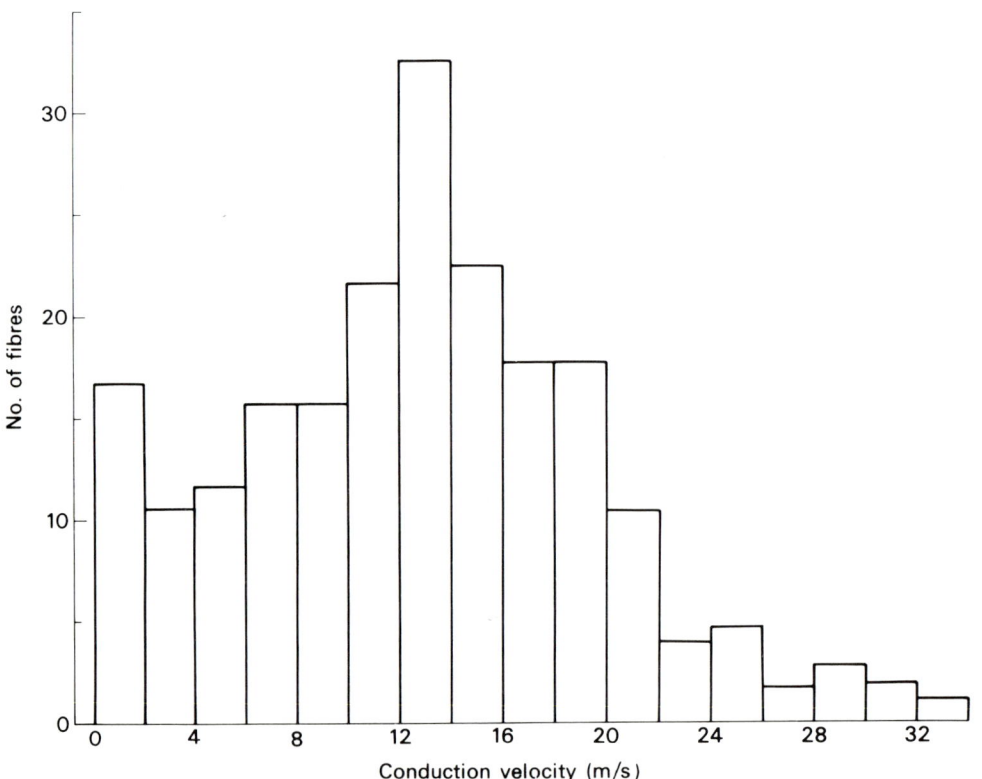

**Fig. 6.31.** The distribution of conduction velocities of 214 pulpal nerve fibres which were isolated for recording in experiments on dogs. Those with conduction velocities less than 2 m/s were presumed to be non-myelinated. (Data from Matthews, B. (1977) *Journal of Physiology* **264**, 641–664).

cellular material in the outer dentine. In some places, what appear to be nerve terminals form specialized junctions with odontoblasts. These may merely provide mechanical or metabolic support or they could constitute electrical synapses.

POSSIBLE RECEPTOR MECHANISMS

It is not known how the stimuli which produce pain from dentine excite nerve endings. There are three principal hypotheses:
1  Nerve endings in the inner dentine are excited directly by the applied stimuli.
2  Mechanosensitive nerve endings in the region of the pulp/dentine junction are excited indirectly by displacement in each direction of dentinal tubule contents (the hydrodynamic hypothesis).
3  The odontoblasts, being electrically coupled to nerves, function as receptors.

From the histological evidence it must be concluded that the sensitivity of the outer dentine is due to nerve endings being excited at some distance from the point of application of the stimulus. This same conclusion is consistent with the physiological studies in which it was shown that solutions which cause pain when applied to exposed nerve endings in skin, do not cause pain when applied to dentine and that neither local anaesthetics nor protein precipitants such as silver nitrate caused any detectable desensitization when applied to outer dentine.

It must be assumed that the sensitivity of the outer dentine to mechanical and osmotic stimuli is due to the movement of tubule contents which in turn causes excitation of nerve endings or receptors in the inner dentine or superficial layers of the pulp. The apparent hypersensitivity of the amelodentinal junction during cavity preparation might be due to a rapid initial movement of the contents when the tubules are first opened, or to branching of tubules in this region resulting in a larger number being affected by a stimulus than when the same stimulus is applied at a deeper level.

Thermal stimuli applied to either intact teeth or to exposed dentine in man excite nerves before there is a significant temperature change at the pulp surface, suggesting that receptors in the dentine are involved. However, because a temperature change produces different degrees of expansion or contraction in the dentine matrix and in the tubule contents, a movement of tubule contents rather than the temperature change itself might be responsible for exciting the receptors. In this case, the receptors involved might not be in the dentine.

It has been shown that many of the stimuli which cause pain from dentine also cause displacement of tubule contents in extracted human teeth. Unfortunately, it is not yet possible to make these measurements *in vivo* and correlate them directly with pain.

In experimental animals it is possible to record action potentials from pulpal nerves. Recordings have been made from single pulpal nerves during the application of thermal and chemical stimuli. These studies indicate that all the nerve endings in teeth do not have the same properties; for example, those which respond to cooling do not respond to heating or to chemical stimuli (Fig. 6.32). Also, those which respond to the application of solutions to dentine appear to respond to the changes in ionic composition of the extracellular fluid around them rather than any osmotic effects (Fig. 6.33). Topically applied local anaesthetics readily abolish the response of intradental nerves to chemical stimuli in cats. Thus, there are several discrepancies between the properties of the nerve endings which have been studied in experimental animals and the properties which have been assumed for the receptors associated with pain in man. Some of the differences may be due to substances diffusing more readily into cat than human dentine but it may also be that some of the nerves studied in animals are involved in functions other than evoking pain.

CONCLUSIONS

The available evidence indicates that there are receptors in the outer pulp and possibly also the inner dentine which can be excited by changes in temperature, by changes in chemical composition of the extracellular fluid or by deformation resulting from displacement of dentinal tubule contents. The sensitivity of the outer dentine depends on stimuli causing changes which are transmitted passively through to those more deeply situated receptors.

# CEMENT

Cement (or cementum in the Latin form) is a bony tissue that covers the roots, and sometimes the crowns, of teeth and provides an anchorage for the fibres of the periodontal ligament. It is, therefore, a component of two functional units: the tooth and the periodontium (Fig. 6.34).

Cement contributes to the size and strength of the tooth and protects the encased dentine of the root. Coronal wear is compensated by continued formation of cement at the root apex, thus

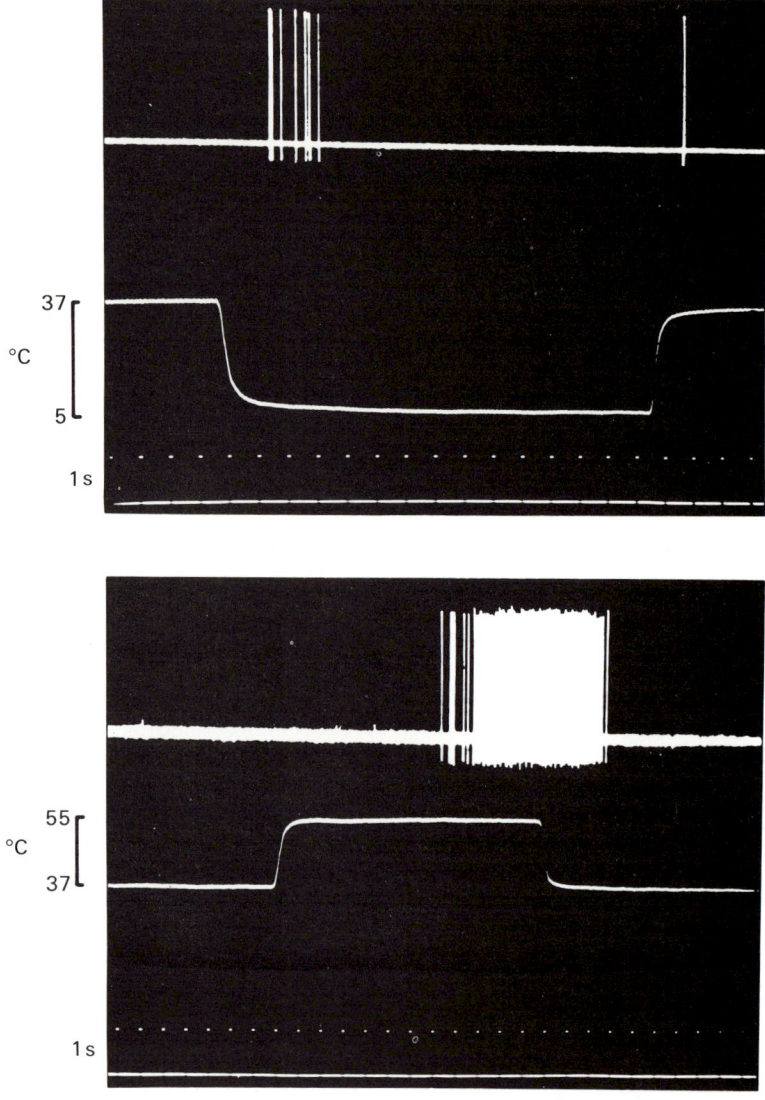

**Fig. 6.32.** Records obtained from two single pulpal fibres isolated from the inferior dental nerve in dogs. Thermal stimuli were applied to coronal dentine of a lower canine. (upper) Response of a fibre to cooling. This fibre did not respond to heating of the exposed dentine surface to 55°C. (lower) Response of another fibre to heating. This fibre did not respond to cooling of the exposed dentine surface to 5°C. Receptors with these characteristics do not respond to 6 mol/kg $CaCl_2$, which causes pain in man (point at log OP = 3.2 in Fig. 6.30) and which causes fluid movement from dentine, in the same direction as a cold stimulus. (Data from Matthews B. (1977) *Journal of Physiology* **264**, 641–664).

lengthening the root, and the tooth is able to respond to changing functional demands by the selective apposition, resorption and repair of cement. Due to this continuous activity, the size and shape of a tooth is never finalized during its functional life.

As a component of the periodontium, cement is essential for normal eruption, and for the support and maintenance of a tooth in function. It links the tooth, through the periodontal ligament, with the surrounding teeth, gingiva and alveolar bone. Changes in function, distribution or health of any of the other tissues in the periodontium of the tooth provoke a response from the cells

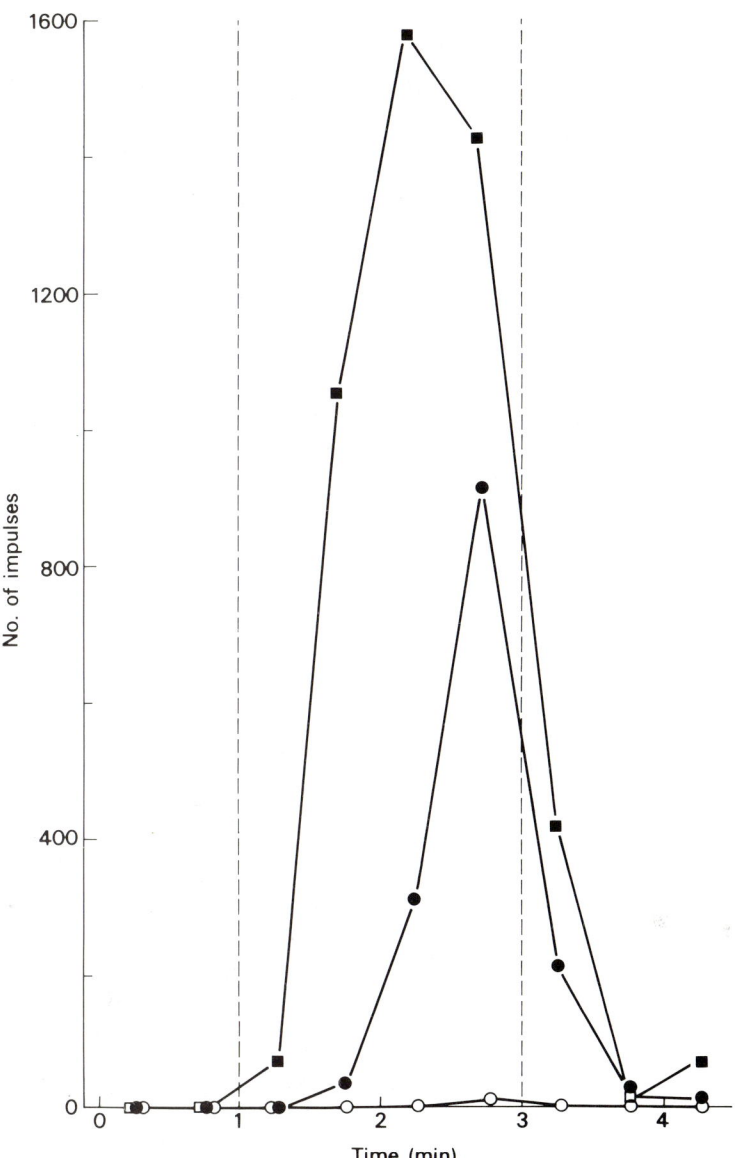

**Fig. 6.33.** Total impulse counts recorded from a group of intradental nerves during successive 30 s intervals for 1 min prior to stimulation, during 2 min application of a solution to exposed dentine, and for 1.5 min after the solution was washed away. The data were obtained from a cat's tooth with a layer of approximately 0.15 mm of dentine remaining over the pulp. ■, 2.5 mol/dm$^3$ NH$_4$Cl; ●, 2.5 mol/dm$^3$ NaCl; ○, 4.0 mol/dm$^3$ dextrose. The dextrose solution has an osmotic pressure of approximately 240 atm, while that of the other two is approximately 130 atm (for details of osmotic pressures see Horiuchi H. & Matthews B. (1973) *Archives oral Biology.* **18**, 175). Data from Horiuchi H. & Matthews B. (1976) *Pain* **2**, 49.

responsible for making or removing cement. The continued viability, recruitment and activity of its surface cells makes cement the most accommodating tooth tissue. Adaptability is a necessary requirement for a member of the periodontium.

### Physical characteristics and distribution

Cement is light cream in colour, readily distinguishable from the much whiter, shinier enamel. In bulk, for example on a sperm whale's tooth, it is also easy to distinguish cement from dentine,

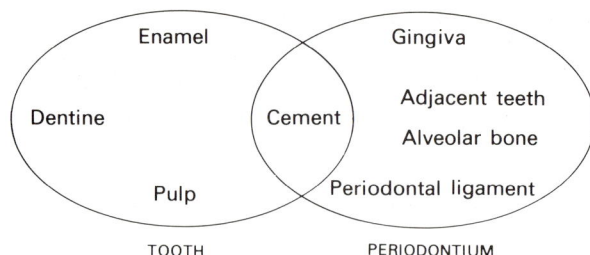

**Fig. 6.34.** Cement is a component of two functional units: the tooth and the periodontium.

which is yellower, but on a human tooth cement is rarely present in sufficient quantity and is not so dissimilar in colour and texture. Cement is less hard than either enamel or dentine, and is thought to be similar in most of its mechanical characteristics to bone. However, because the layer of human cement is so thin, values for its tensile strength, compressive strength and elasticity are not readily obtainable and have not been correlated with the varying texture of the tissue.

Cement coats the roots of human teeth as a thin layer of uneven thickness. The enamel–cement junction is usually irregularly scalloped and as a rule extends further occlusally between longitudinal ridges of enamel (Fig. 6.35). Cement may just overlap the enamel of the crown at the cervical margin or meet the enamel edge to edge. Less frequently a gap separates enamel and cement, and dentine forms part of the surface of the tooth. The ratios for the occurrence of these three relationships are generally given respectively as 6 : 3 : 1. However, very few studies have been made of the frequencies of the three possible junctions, and none comparing tooth types, variations around single teeth or comparing the whole dentitions of individuals or races. Available information is therefore scanty and may not be generally applicable.

Cement has an extensive smooth junction with dentine, being deposited initially on the dentine template. The exact position of this junction becomes obscured when both tissues are mineralized. If enamel pearls (Fig. 6.35) form next to the dentine on a root they may be overlaid with cement at a later time. The root surface of an extracted tooth is generally smooth to the touch but not featureless. A series of shallow horizontal undulations is often present on the surface of the coronal two-thirds of the root. These may reflect a lack of synchrony between the rates of root growth and eruption in the prefunctional stage of eruption. The apical surface of the root and the interradicular area of the multirooted teeth are usually rougher and more irregular than the rest (Fig. 6.36). The cement may thicken abruptly and unevenly in these regions of the root. The irregularity of the root surface tends to increase with age, and is generally greater in multirooted teeth.

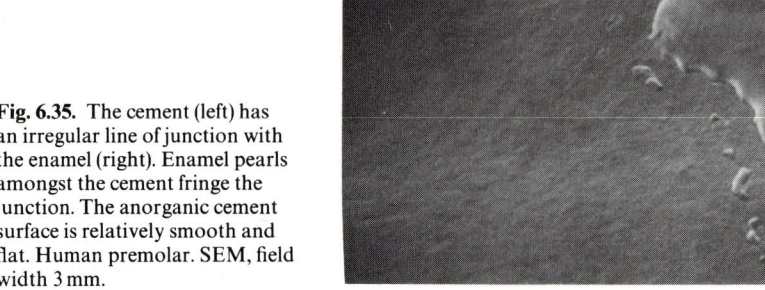

**Fig. 6.35.** The cement (left) has an irregular line of junction with the enamel (right). Enamel pearls amongst the cement fringe the junction. The anorganic cement surface is relatively smooth and flat. Human premolar. SEM, field width 3 mm.

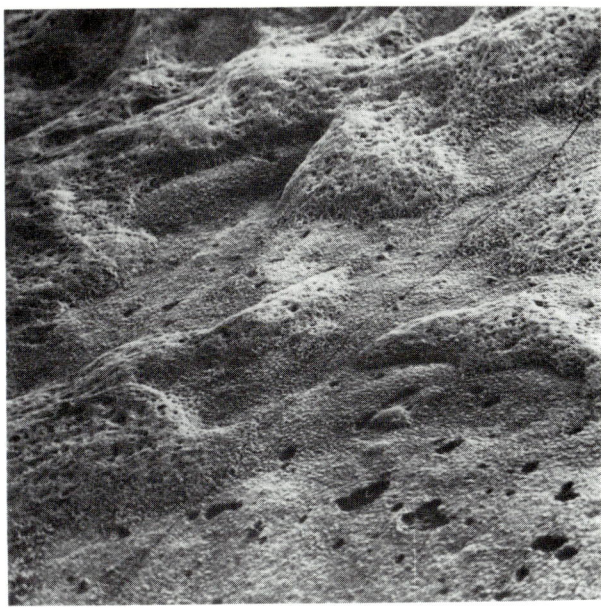

**Fig. 6.36.** Large numbers of small resorption bays are present in the flat acellular cement surface which was 'resting'. Extensive irregular deposits of forming cellular cement were extending over the former surface. Repair cement has partly filled one resorption bay and extended on to the surrounding unresorbed surface. Anorganic third molar root tip from 21-year-old. SEM, field width 1 mm.

Some human teeth, particularly multirooted ones, have an irregular deposition of cement along the line of junction of parts of the epithelial root sheath in the interradicular area and running down the length of the root, giving the appearance of raised cobbled seams. The development of the ridge lags slightly behind that of the rest of the developing rim of the root so that it is associated with a notch. Capillary loops and even occasional epithelial cells may be incorporated in interradicular areas in such lines of junction and imperfect junctions may give rise to accessory root canals.

Cement is thinnest in the cervical part of the root, and forms a fairly thin, even layer in the coronal half to two-thirds (Fig. 6.35). This layer is only about 10–20 $\mu$m thick in the cervical and midroot regions of a newly erupted human premolar. It may thicken very gradually and evenly from the cervical margin in an apical direction. The thickness of cement on the apical part of the root depends upon the type, age and functional history of the tooth, but may reach several hundred micrometres. The apical cement on young anterior teeth with closed apices may be very thin and regular, but that on older cheek teeth is relatively thick and uneven. In older teeth the extra apical cement increases the length of the root and forms the wall of the extended pulp canal. Thicker cement is also found in the furcation areas of multirooted teeth.

Large knobs of cement are sometimes deposited on roots, and may join the roots of multirooted teeth. This condition, referred to as hypercementosis, may also affect unerupted, impacted teeth. A more localized overproduction of cement, often extending along the line of the oblique fibre groups of the periodontal ligament, results in cemental spurs on the roof surface. Rarely, small bony nodules develop in the periodontal ligament close to the root surface. These may be overrun by deposits of cement and become incorporated in the tooth as cementicles.

**Chemical characteristics of cement**

Cement is a calcified connective tissue. It contains about 65% mineral (wet weight); less than either enamel or dentine. The mineral is an impure form of hydroxyapatite. The crystals in cement are considered to be similar in size and shape to those of bone. In transmission electron micrographs of ultramicrotomed sections they appear as needles or plates about 60 nm long. It is probable, however, that in life the mineral particles are much more extensive than this, forming long tubular coats to the microfibrils of collagen.

The organic phase of cement contains collagen fibres and ground substance. Collagen is the major protein found in human cement and may constitute 20% or more of the tissue. The type of collagen is similar to that found in bone. The ground substance of cement contains proteoglycans but little is known of their character or how closely they resemble those of bone or dentine.

Both the physical and chemical characteristics of cement vary within any one tooth. The very thin acellular cement in the cervical and midroot regions of human teeth may be as highly mineralized as peripheral root dentine, and often has a quite different structure from that of the bulkier, often less well mineralized, apical cement. However, the latter tissue is easier to collect and separate from dentine for analysis. Data for the levels of mineralization in different types and zones of cement are still required.

**Structure of cement**

It has been traditional to describe two types of cement, acellular and cellular. This classification is simple, easy to make and useful but it ignores the most important variation in the structure of cement which is the composition of its matrix.

Cement may contain any of the normal components of connective tissues; that is, cells and an intercellular matrix containing fibres and a ground substance. The amount of each component may range from almost nil to abundance, and a spectrum of tissues often exists within the same tooth. With such a continuous variation it can readily be seen that the way in which one chooses to classify any particular cement is arbitrary. The following classification is based on the fibrillar component of cement as that is its main functional asset.

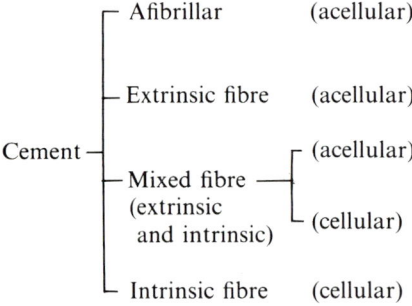

All the above combinations of organic components are found in human cement. Extrinsic fibres and intrinsic fibres differ in their origin, orientation and function.

Extrinsic fibres are formed outside the cement by fibroblasts of the periodontal ligament and are incorporated within the cement as it increases in thickness. They are also known as the perforating fibres of Sharpey. These fibres are continuous with the fibres of the ligament and form its anchorage to the tooth. The extrinsic fibres lie approximately perpendicular to the cement surface.

Intrinsic fibres are laid down in the plane of the developing surface of cement by cementoblasts. They have never been a part of the periodontal ligament and are not continuous with the fibres of the ligament. They form part of the matrix in which the extrinsic fibres are housed.

AFIBRILLAR CEMENT

Afibrillar cement consists only of a mineralized ground substance and is usually so sparse that it cannot be detected by light microscopy. In human teeth it may be found overlying the cervical enamel for a distance of a few micrometres (Fig. 8.43) and as a very thin layer between the dentine and fibrillar cement, particularly below extrinsic fibre cement. The layer may be continuous or discontinuous and uneven in thickness, or the tissue may be present as isolated islands on either enamel or dentine. As its name suggests, the matrix contains no collagen fibres and it is always acellular.

Afibrillar cement is usually well mineralized and can be likened in structure to peritubular dentine or perilacunar bone. The mineral is distributed more or less evenly throughout the tissue although there may be minor variations in constitution marked by incremental lines. Afibrillar cement may contribute to the radiodense line seen at the dentine–cement junction.

FIBRILLAR CEMENT

Fibrillar cement may contain only extrinsic fibres derived from the periodontal ligament; both extrinsic fibres and intrinsic fibres produced by the cementoblasts; or only intrinsic fibres.

*Extrinsic fibre cement*
Extrinsic fibre cement has sometimes been called primary cement, for it is characteristic of much of the first-formed cement laid down during early root formation and prior to functional occlusion. It forms very slowly and evenly and produces a smooth root surface (Fig. 6.35). The extrinsic fibres are cemented by a ground substance which is thought to be produced by cementoblasts. There are no cells and no intrinsic fibres lying between the extrinsic fibres which are so closely packed in the cement that they form a continuum of parallel elements.

The extrinsic fibres in this type of cement are always well mineralized: unmineralized cores or regions do not remain within the fibres. Incremental lines are present and are usually parallel to the dentine-cement junction and the root surface, and approximately at right angles to the fibres. They outline some past position of the surface and probably indicate compositional or structural variations related to an altered rate of apposition of cement or eruption of the tooth. Microradiographic studies demonstrate variations in the mineral density of layers of differing widths within such cement. The level of mineralization may sometimes equal, and even exceed, that of the adjacent dentine. It has been suggested, and is widely accepted on the basis of a single study of the thickness of cement in teeth of differently aged people, that the thickness of the cement increases at a constant slow rate throughout life. A survey of the longitudinal data imprisoned in the cement of each tooth in the form of incremental lines suggests that this is not so. It would be intriguing to find out whether cement formation in northern man ever showed seasonal annuli such as are present, for example, in sperm whales, English foxes and some Canadian caribou.

*Mixed (extrinsic and intrinsic) fibre cements*

Mixed fibre cements contain fibres of two different origins. The extrinsic fibres are derived from the periodontal ligament but the intrinsic fibres are, together with the ground substance, contributed by the cementoblasts. The proportion of the fibrous matrix from this source varies greatly. Indeed, acellular mixed fibre cement is often confused with extrinsic fibre cement when examined by light microscopy because the small intrinsic-fibre component goes unrecognized (Fig. 6.37). However, it is always readily discernible by electron microscopy because the orientation of the sets of fibres is distinctive. The extrinsic fibres penetrate through the depth of the tissue; the intrinsic fibres are oriented within planes approximately parallel to the developing surface.

*Extrinsic fibres.* The inclusion of intrinsic fibres into the substance of the cement delineates and separates the extrinsic fibre bundles. The latter vary in cross-sectional diameter but, in human molar cement, with a 40% extrinsic fibre component, they are 6 or 7 $\mu$m across. They may be ovoid or round in cross-section and be incorporated singly, in groups, in horizontal rows around the root (Fig. 6.38) or in vertical rows at the apex. They tend to be rounder in cross-section where widely separated, and more irregular in shape when closely packed. The extrinsic fibres lie in the cement and leave its surface at the same angle as the fibres of periodontal ligament with which they are continuous. Changes of the directions of extrinsic fibres in different layers of cement indicate variations related to eruptional or functional changes in the direction in which fibres have been pulled at that site on the root surface at different times. Much of the past life history of the tooth is recorded in this way as, unlike bone, cement is infrequently absorbed.

*Intrinsic fibres.* The intrinsic fibres are smaller and resemble the collagen fibres of lamellar bone in size, reaching 1–2 $\mu$m in diameter. In cement

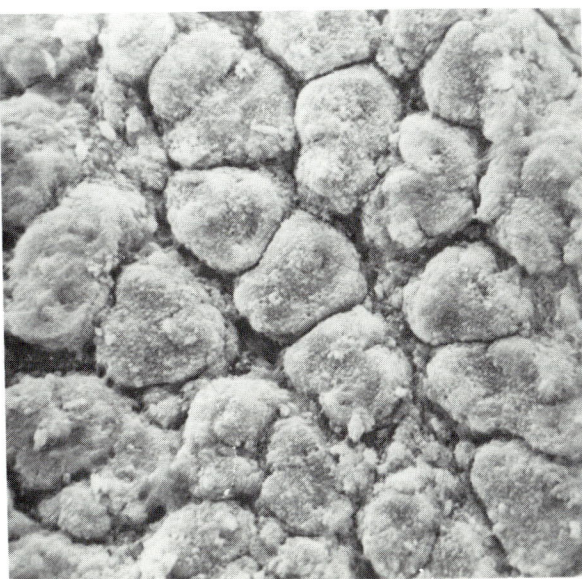

**Fig. 6.37.** In this anorganic preparation of the midroot surface of a human premolar, the mineral ends of the extrinsic fibres are seen as projections. Close packing of the extrinsic fibres has led to a flattening of their adjacent sides. The intrinsic fibre component of the mixed fibre cement is low and no cells were being incorporated. SEM, field width 30 $\mu$m.

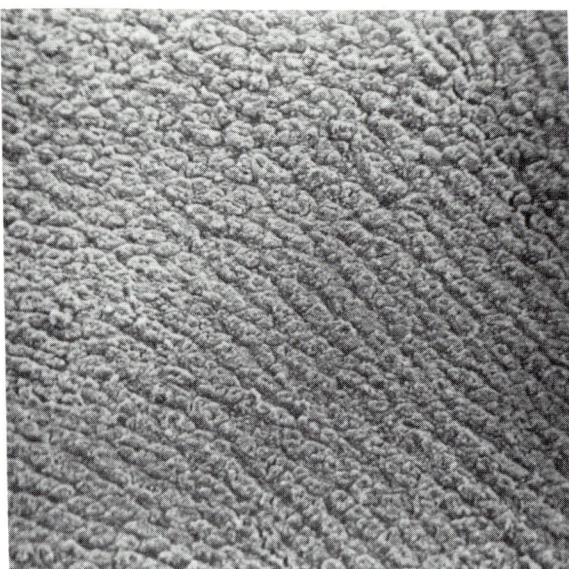

**Fig. 6.38.** Long horizontal rows of extrinsic fibres pattern the anorganic cement surface. The mineral level in the central regions of the extrinsic fibres lags behind the peripheral area. Mixed fibre cement of premolar from 19-year-old man. SEM, field width 200 μm.

containing a high proportion of extrinsic fibres, the intrinsic fibres pack in between and around the perforating extrinsic fibres and show little order themselves. As the distance between the extrinsic fibres increases, the intrinsic fibres are larger and tend to run parallel for greater distances and over larger areas (Fig. 6.39), although those immediately adjoining the extrinsic fibres may still encircle them (Fig. 6.40). It is probable that the freedom of groups of cementoblasts to move with respect to the surface they are forming controls the degree of organization of the intrinsic fibres in the cement. With a high proportion of intrinsic fibres extensive patches of cells may function and move synchronously. The orientation of domains of fibres can change in successive layers of cement producing a lamellar arrangement of the intrinsic fibres.

*Mineral content.* The extent of mineralization in mixed fibre cement varies, particularly with respect to the extrinsic fibres. Depending upon the appositional rate at the time of their inclusion into

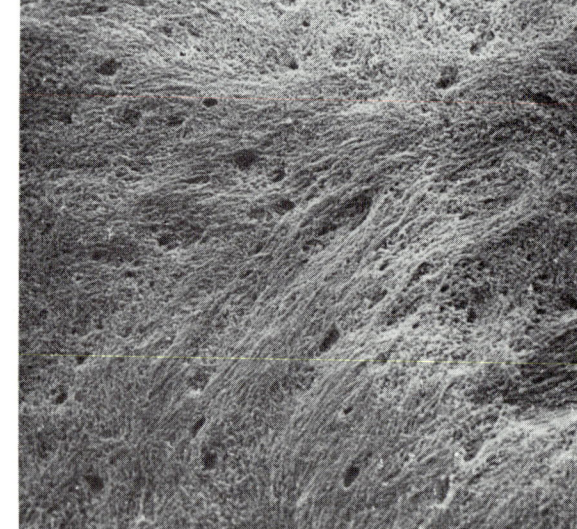

**Fig. 6.39.** Extrinsic fibres are sparse and marked by patches of small depressions in this apical, cellular cement. The intrinsic fibres run in groups of parallel fibres in the plane of the surface. Arrows point to some of the cementocyte lacunae in mineral surface of forming cement. Anorganic root tip of upper third molar from 55-year-old man. SEM, field width 475 μm.

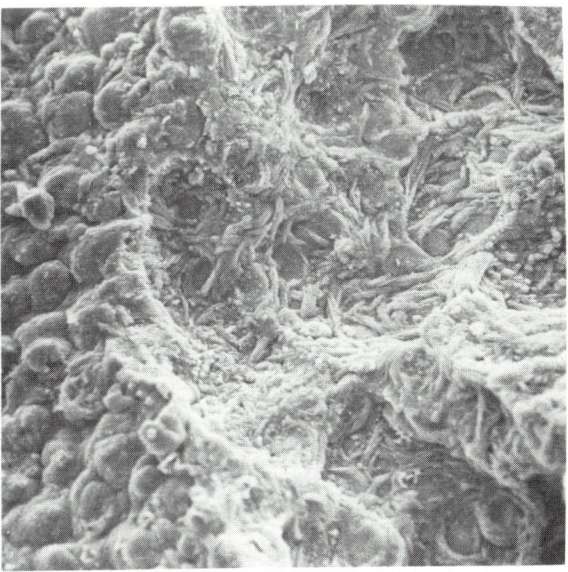

**Fig. 6.40.** Extrinsic fibres that had been fully mineralized are seen end on at the bottom of a large deep resorption bay in the midroot region of an upper third molar of a 60-year-old man. Intrinsic fibres wrap around the extrinsic ones. The intact cement surface (left) had been undermined by the resorption and was resting. Anorganic preparation of mixed fibre cement. SEM, field width 85 μm.

the tissue, the extrinsic fibres may be fully mineralized, retain unmineralized segments or cores, or be incompletely mineralized throughout the fibres for part or all of their lengths (Fig. 6.41). The slower the deposition of cement the more highly mineralized the tissue becomes, and the greater the likelihood that the extrinsic fibres will be completely mineralized.

*Incremental layers.* The rate at which cement is formed depends upon the activity of the cementoblasts. When the rate is slow and the intrinsic fibre component is small the incremental layers are even and thin and no cells are incorporated (Fig. 6.42). As the proportion of intrinsic fibres rises the thickness of the cement layer increases more rapidly and the incremental layers, and hence the cement surface, are less regular (Fig. 6.43). A rapid production of intrinsic matrix and consequent embedding of extrinsic fibres also leads to the incorporation of cells within the cement. The increments in cellular cement are generally patchy and uneven and the incremental lines are more widely spaced: the plane of the root surface is rarely parallel with the plane of the dentine–cement junction.

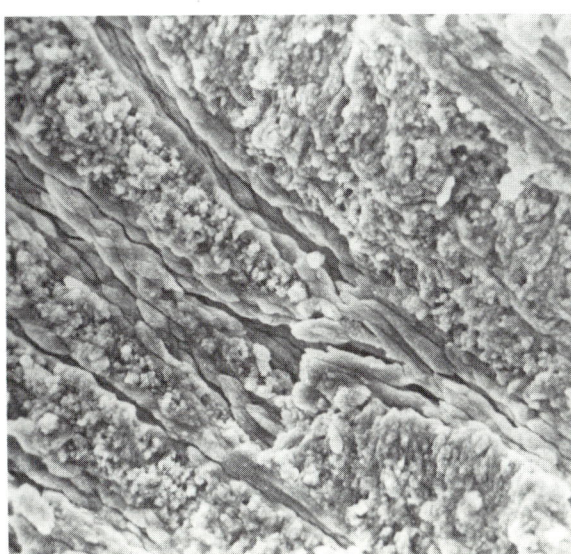

**Fig. 6.41.** Fractured, anorganic, mixed fibre cement showing diagonally running extrinsic fibres that have unmineralized cores and partly mineralized peripheries. The spindle-shaped mineral segments are mostly fused end to end, but some remain separate. The intrinsic fibres lie in layers approximately perpendicular to the extrinsic fibres. SEM, field width 50 μm.

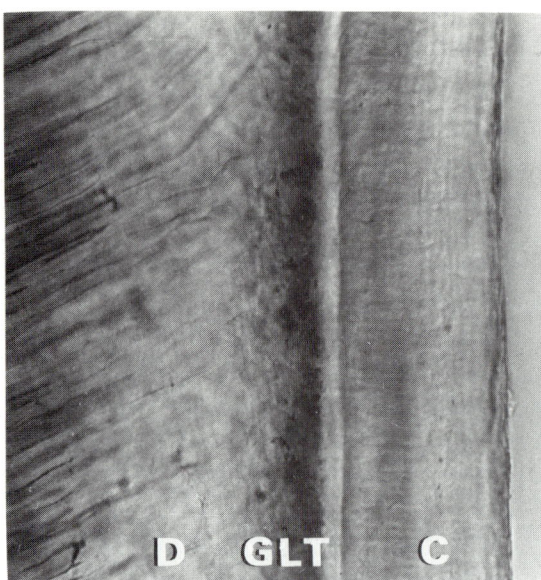

**Fig. 6.42.** Thin layer of evenly deposited acellular cement on midroot region of a human permanent canine. Faint striations parallel to the cement–dentine junction and the tooth surface are incremental lines. D, Dentine; GLT, granular layer of Tomes, C, cement. L/M, field width 450 μm.

As the rate of production slows, the number of cementoblasts trapped by the tissue is reduced and the cement may become acellular. Layers of acellular and cellular cement may alternate on a root surface, indicating variations in the appositional rate (Fig. 6.43). The thickness of unmineralized matrix, the precement (or cementoid) at the surface also varies with the appositional rate and is greatest during cellular cement formation. Cellular cement is characteristically found at the root apices and interradicular areas of human teeth where the cement is thickest. It is associated with an increase of tooth movement; either rapid eruption and lengthening of the root, or increased functional movements. In the lower part of the root even the cement immediately overlying the dentine may contain cells, indicating a rapid deposition of tissue during the formation and growth of that part of the root. These cells may be of epithelial or cementoblastic origin.

*Intermediate cement*. Epithelial cells from the root sheath may be incorporated in human cement close to the dentinal surface. The cells fail to move from the developing root surface and become embedded in the rapidly forming cement. Tissue containing epithelial cells, either singly or in clusters, is termed intermediate cement. It is generally only found in the apical one-third of the roots of human cheek teeth. Otherwise the cells of cement are cementocytes and originate from embedded cementoblasts. It is often difficult to distinguish between the two types of cells using light microscopy, but their ultrastructural appearances are quite dissimilar. Degenerative changes have been observed in epithelial cells soon after their incorporation into cement. The cytoplasmic volume is reduced, bundles of tonofilaments become thicker and more prominent and the granular endoplasmic reticulum is reduced.

*Cementocytes*. Cementocytes within precement closely resemble cementoblasts. They have a rich rough endoplasmic reticulum, a well developed Golgi apparatus, many mitochondria and several cell processes. Microfilaments and microtubules are plentiful. Their structure suggests that they might be more properly called precement cementoblasts rather than cementocytes. Cementocytes embedded in calcified matrix have fewer organelles and are considered to be much less active. The cytoplasmic organelles and the cytoplasmic volume both decrease in relation to the depth of a cementocyte within the cement. Cells far from the cemental surface, and hence their nutritional supply, may be dead.

The embedded cells are housed in spaces in the cement, called lacunae, whose shapes are determined by the restraints of the surrounding fibres at the time that they develop (Fig. 6.44). If the extrinsic fibres are sparse the lacunae are oval with a long axis in the same direction as the intrinsic fibre orientation. A rounder outline results from more random intrinsic fibres. If the extrinsic fibres border the site of incorporation of a cell then the cell outline will often accommodate itself to the

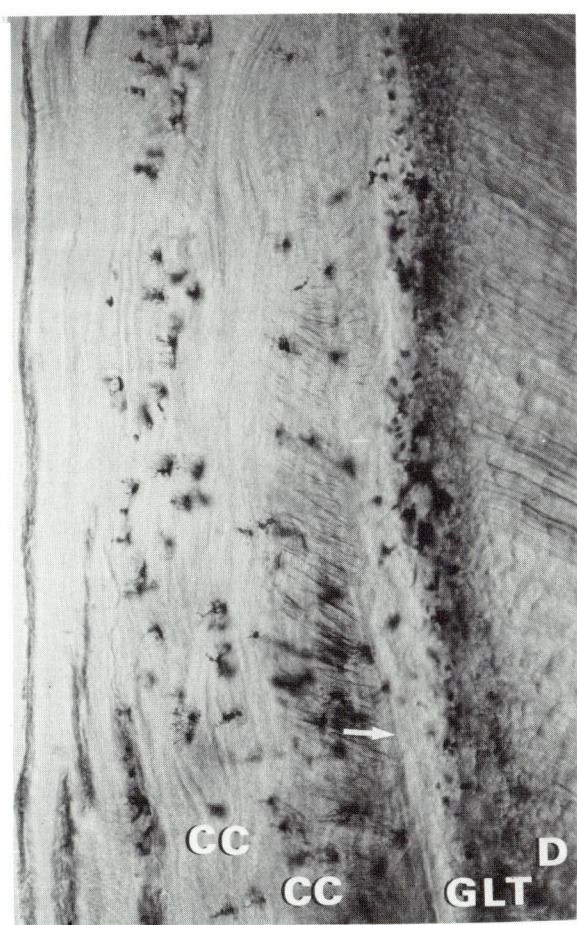

**Fig. 6.43.** Thicker, more irregularly deposited cement from apical region. Layers of cellular cement are interspersed with acellular cement. The site of a previous, extensive, resorbed surface is marked by a reversal line (arrowed). Longitudinal ground section of a human permanent canine. CC, Cementocyte lacunae; GLT, granular layer of Tomes; D, dentine. L/M, field width 450 μm.

side of one or several fibres and its lacuna has a stellate shape. The collagen fibrils in the lacunar wall are usually fine with a random pattern (Fig. 6.45) and mineralize just ahead of the matrix level housing the lacuna.

The cementocytes have cell processes that radiate out from the lacunae through canaliculi in the matrix. These are longer and more numerous towards the surface of cement (Fig. 6.46). It is probable that this is due to a greater maintenance of contact of the newly incorporated cementocytes with the overlying cementoblasts rather than other cementocytes, and because the nutritive source is one-sided. The inclusion of cells into cement is a much more erratic process than the incorporation of cells into lamellar bone, and the pathways of the canaliculi are more irregular. The extensive interconnecting canalicular system essential to the maintenance of adult bone cells is absent. Gap and tight junctions are developed where processes from cementocytes contact each other or cementoblast processes.

A space exists between the cell membrane of the cementocyte and the calcified lacunar wall. This pericementocytic space contains an amorphous ground substance in which there may be occasional collagen fibrils. The amorphous ground substance may also extend inside the cementocyte canaliculi. The collagen fibre pattern of the inner calcified wall of a lacuna is occasionally obliterated in older cement by a thin deposit of mineralized ground substance, equivalent to perilacunar bone.

*Intrinsic fibre cement*
Large patches of cement that are devoid of extrinsic fibres sometimes develop in the apical regions of older human teeth (Fig. 6.44). This cement is cellular and contributes to the substance

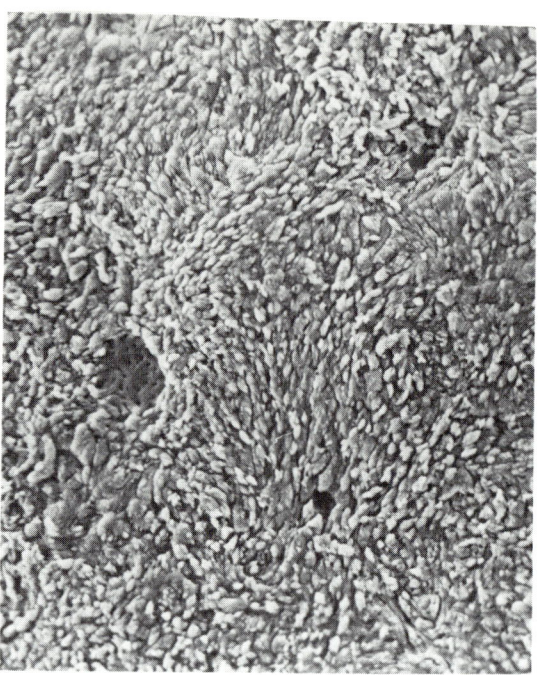

Fig. 6.44. Cementocyte lacunae in the mineral surface of the cement of a human permanent lower first molar. Openings and paths of canaliculi can be seen in the wall of lacuna (middle left). One lacuna (lower right) is almost entirely embedded in calcified cement. The field comprises only intrinsic fibres, so that the lacunar shape relates only to these. The fibres are incompletely mineralized at this level of forming cement but their directions can be deduced from the long axes of the mineral particles within them. Anorganic preparation. SEM, field width 100 μm.

of the tooth but does not serve as part of its supporting system. The lack of extrinsic fibres may be only transitory, during the early stage of repair of a resorbed area, or it may represent a permanent reduction in the attachment area. Apical regions of the roots of old teeth commonly have only a patchy inclusion of groups of extrinsic fibres, much like regions of the alveolar bone. Lamellar formation then occurs in the intrinsic fibre matrix.

### The cement–epithelial junction: exposed cement

The junctional epithelium (Fig. 7.25) of the tooth may overlie cement. This is not uncommon, in the absence of any inflammatory change, with the afibrillar cement that overlaps enamel. Rootward migration of the epithelium over cement that contains extrinsic fibres is secondary to a loss of attachment of the ligament in the cervical regions.

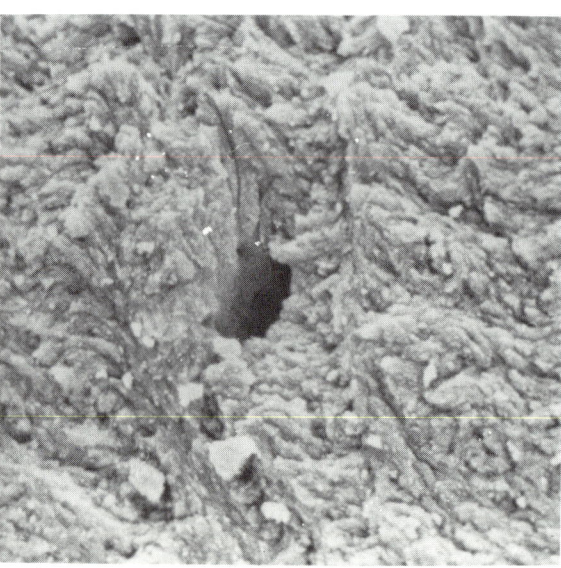

Fig. 6.45. Human cement fractured through a lacuna. The collagen fibrils in the wall of the lacuna are fine and random. Canaliculi can be seen radiating from the lacuna through the mixed fibre matrix towards the surface (upper left). SEM, field width 40 μm.

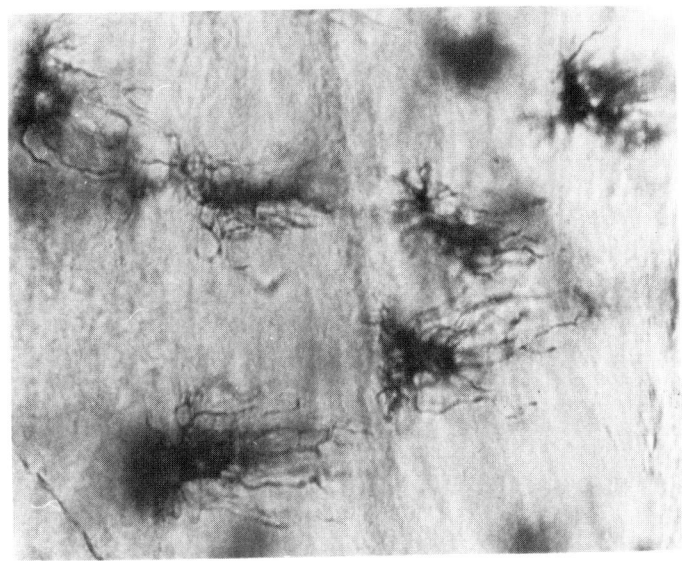

Fig. 6.46. Most of the canaliculi radiate from the lacunae towards the surface of the cement (to the right). Longitudinal thick ground section of human canine. L/M, field width 90 μm.

Cement may become exposed to the oral environment if the loss of attachment of fibres and the apical migration of the epithelium continue. Exposed cement resists wear very poorly compared with the much harder enamel. The cement surface usually becomes more highly mineralized and richer in some ions, such as $F^-$, acquired from the oral cavity. Plaque and calculus may accumulate on its surface, lodged initially in crevices marking the boundaries of the extrinsic fibres. The exposed cement may also become carious. Caries proceeds preferentially perpendicular to the surface: demineralization and destruction of matrix follow the line of the extrinsic fibres of the exposed cervical cement.

The junctional epithelium also migrates over the cement in exfoliating deciduous teeth. Some hold that this is a physiological process designed to assist in the exfoliation, but it is much more likely to be due to inflammation of the soft tissues at that time.

## BIOCHEMISTRY OF THE DENTAL TISSUES

Of the three dental calcified tissues, the dentine and cementum both have a very similar chemistry to bone tissue. Enamel differs from these mainly in the components and amount of the organic structures: in enamel considerably less than 1% of the whole is organic, with 95% mineral and 4% $H_2O$. In contrast, dentine and cementum, like compact bone, have organic contents of 20% and 30%. The main mineral component, calcium hydroxyapatite (Book 1), is about three times heavier than the organic structures and the actual volume occupied by the organic matrix is considerably larger than the weight analyses suggest at first. In dentine, cementum and bone 40–60% or more of the tissue volume is actually occupied by the organic components. In enamel the organic structures fill about 1.4% of the space, and water 11.5%.

Hydroxyapatite is the mineral component common to all the human calcified tissues, though the crystal sizes in enamel are considerably larger, by a factor of ten, than in the other mineralized tissues.

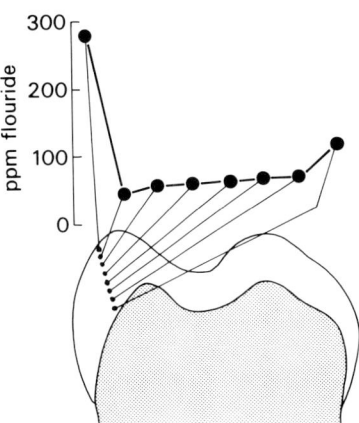

Fig. 6.47. Fluoride distribution across section of human molar enamel.

## Separation of dental tissues for analysis

For the purposes of analysis and further investigations, it is necessary first to separate the dental tissues from one another. There are various approaches to this problem depending on the particular tissue sought and the ultimate purpose of its isolation.

One approach to obtaining enamel and/or dentine separately is first to grind the cementum from the roots of cleaned extracted teeth, and then to dry them in an oven at 100–120° C. Large portions of the enamel cusp may then be easily cracked off or ground from the underlying dentine. The inner aspects of the enamel shells obtained are then drilled out to remove attached dentine organic matter. The dentine cusps and roots, now denuded of enamel, may then be split open, the dry pulps removed and, if required, the walls of the pulp chambers drilled out. If fresh tissue is required for any purpose, the same technique may be applied using low temperatures and eliminating the drying stage. This allows fresh pulp and root dentine to be collected but does not separate crown enamel from the underlying cusp dentine, to which it remains firmly attached.

This hand dissection method is necessarily tedious and laborious and an alternative approach is to reduce the whole extracted (sound) teeth to a fine powder using a ball mill, or a similar unit, maintaining low temperatures throughout grinding. Use is then made of the differing densities between the calcified tissue components to separate them using a differential flotation technique. Enamel has a density of 2.95–3; dentine 2.14; and cement 2.07. Suitable mixtures of bromoform and acetone, or tetrabromethane and acetone, are prepared with a density midway between that of dentine and enamel (e.g. 2.5). Suspension of the powdered tooth preparation in this medium, sometimes aided by low speed centrifugation, causes the heavier enamel particles to sink, and the dentine and cementum to float together. Collection of the latter and reflotation in a fluid of density 2.10 would theoretically separate the cementum from the dentine particles. In practice, the latter separation is only partially successful, although the first stage can yield enamel of claimed 99% purity. Nevertheless, some of the enamel particles are attached to fragments of dentine. With dentine containing 20% organic matter quite small levels of it as a contaminant can seriously obscure studies on the organic components of enamel powders prepared by this flotation technique.

With recent advances in microanalytical technology, accurate analyses can be made on very small amounts of tissue. This has enabled microtechniques (e.g. discs of tissue punched out of longitudinally sectioned teeth) to obtain directly for analysis small samples from each dental tissue (microgram to milligram range), which are quite free from contamination by the others.

## The organic components of enamel

### ADULT TISSUE

After eruption the tooth enamel surface acquires by adsorption organic matter from the oral salivary environment. Thus the enamel surface of adult teeth possess a higher organic content, deriving largely from acquired cuticle or pellicle components, which are not true tissue constituents. The organic enamel matrix proper contains both a water soluble (12–25%) and a water insoluble (70–80%) fraction. Amino acid analyses of the protein components in these three enamel fractions are shown in Table 6.3; the water insoluble fraction is mainly composed of tuft protein.

The presence of eight residues per 1000 of hydroxyproline in the water soluble fraction may reflect collagen contamination. Apart from the technical difficulties in obtaining pure enamel described above, there may well be small 'pockets' of collagen encapsulated within enamel tissue during its formation. The high glycine content may also be due to such collagen contamination. The insoluble protein is unevenly distributed in the tissue with greater amounts nearer the dentine–enamel junction in the enamel tuft and spindle regions. It is a very inert highly insoluble protein, resembling in physical properties the keratins. On this basis, coupled with some early inaccurate amino acid analyses, enamel protein was originally classified as a eukeratin. This view is now obsolete, though on the basis of inertness and certain tenuous affinities with the keratins of oral epithelium it is, for want of a better terminology, described as *pseudokeratin*.

The nature of the carbohydrate components in adult enamel tissue is obscure, apart from the acquired glycoprotein and polysaccharide components involved in cuticle–pellicle formation.

### FETAL TISSUE

In the early stages of enamel formation, the organic content is as high as 20% and the constituents of this fetal enamel, largely protein,

**Table 6.3.** Amino acid composition of human enamel proteins (results expressed in residues/1000).

|  | Adult | | | Foetal (Amelogenins) |
|---|---|---|---|---|
|  | Water soluble | Water insoluble | Acquired pellicle |  |
| Cystine (half) | 4 | 20 | 13 | 0 |
| Hydroxyproline | 8 | 2 | 0 | 0 |
| Aspartic acid | 54 | 79 | 71 | 30 |
| Threonine | 42 | 52 | 43 | 38 |
| Serine | 119 | 82 | 46 | 63 |
| Glutamic acid | 106 | 136 | 133 | 142 |
| Proline | 137 | 81 | 44 | 251 |
| Glycine | 193 | 62 | 81 | 65 |
| Alanine | 53 | 69 | 146 | 20 |
| Valine | 32 | 52 | 53 | 40 |
| Methionine | 34 | 22 | 12 | 42 |
| Isoleucine | 19 | 23 | 30 | 33 |
| Leucine | 66 | 111 | 64 | 91 |
| Tyrosine | 23 | 51 | 14 | 53 |
| Phenylalanine | 33 | 49 | 29 | 23 |
| Hydroxylysine | 4 | 6 | 0 | 0 |
| Lysine | 26 | 40 | 51 | 18 |
| Histidine | 19 | 27 | 19 | 65 |
| Arginine | 28 | 36 | 42 | 23 |
| Ornithine |  |  | 26 |  |
| Muramic acid |  |  | 21 |  |
| Diaminopimeic acid |  |  | 4 |  |
| Hexosamines |  |  | 53 |  |

fraction are very different from those found in the mature calcified adult tissue. Disc electrophoresis and gel chromatographic studies have shown the fetal enamel proteins to be a heterogeneous complex, consisting of at least three major protein components with twelve or more minor constituents. Their behaviour suggests that they collectively comprise a complex aggregation-disaggregation system of protein units.

As a group these fetal enamel proteins are termed the *amelogenins*, and their right to such a separate identity is supported by the amino acid analyses given in Table 6.3. These analyses are of the total amelogenin complexes, though analysis of a few of the individual components have also been reported.

From Table 6.3 it will be seen that the amelogenin complex is characterized by the following compositional features:
1  Large levels of proline (Pro)—25% of the total residues.
2  High acidic amino acid levels (20%).
3  Histidine (His) present as the predominant basic amino acid.
4  Absence of hydroxylysine (Hyl), hydroxyproline (Hyp) and cystine (Cys).
5  Low glycine content.

The absence of Hyl, Hyp and the low Gly content in amelogenins show them to be lacking in any collagen type components, and the absence of cystine indicates the absence of keratins. The very high Pro content of 25% is amongst protein structures. The only other known proteins with this characteristic are some of the parotid secretion glycoproteins with 30% or more Pro, which are also similar in possessing high acidic amino acid levels. In contrast to the amelogenins these parotid proteins have quite high Gly levels and low His values. Nevertheless, the similarities are sufficiently strong to suggest the possibility that such high Pro proteins may play some key role in enamel mineralization processes in both the pre- and post-eruption stages.

Comparison of amelogenin analyses with those from the adult tissues show clear differences. Most marked is the inverse ratio between Gly and Pro respectively, and the higher His and Ser levels in the amelogenins.

An unsolved problem is the nature of the mechanisms involved in the change from fetal to adult protein structures. How does the 20% content in the young enamel reduce to less than the 1% found in the adult tissue? Why is there a completely dissimilar amino acid composition?

One explanation offered is that the amelogenin complex contains one (or at most a few) specific protein which forms a calcification template that remains in the tissue after mineralization and maturation is complete. As crystal growth proceeds, the other amelogenin proteins behave like an amorphous thixotropic gel and are squeezed out and removed. An example of a thixotropic gel is in 'non-drip' paints which, when under pressure from the paint brush, change from a semi-solid state to a liquid one that flows evenly over surfaces, returning to semi-rigid form when the brush pressure is removed. In a similar way it is envisaged that pressure is exerted on the thixotropic amelogenin complex proteins by the progression of mineralization which therefore causes them to flow as a liquid and be extruded in to the tissue surroundings.

THE ORGANIC COMPONENTS OF DENTINE

As already noted, the composition of the dentine closely resembles that of bone. The collagen structure and composition is essentially the same, though there is evidence that dentine collagen may be even more highly cross-linked. The presence of a greater number of Hyl residues and of a higher organic phosphate content is consistent with the possible formation of larger numbers of cross-links. This would account for the fact that dentine is even more difficult to solubilize and extract than bone.

Studies on the non-collagenous matrix components in human dentine show them to be very similar, though not quite identical, to bone. There is the same range of small molecular weight components and also glycoprotein fractions resembling those found in bone tissue.

**Fluoride**

Fluoride is unevenly distributed in enamel. The concentrations are highest at the surface and fall precipitously over the outer 100 or 200 $\mu$m (Fig. 6.47): within the main body of the enamel the levels are relatively low. Near the enamel–dentine junction there is a slight rise in concentration. This pattern is found shortly before eruption. It can be altered after eruption by either a loss of surface enamel due to wear or a small gain by ion exchange throughout life from food, water and tea, especially on surfaces commonly covered by dental plaque. This means that over the tooth surface the fluoride concentration in surface enamel varies from high levels in the cervical region to lower levels at the biting surface. There may also be differences between fluoride concentrations on the labial and lingual surfaces. In young adults the fluoride levels in the whole thickness of enamel and in surface enamel are related to the fluoride intake during the period of tooth development (Table 6.4). In regions where the water supply

**Table 6.4.** Mean fluoride concentrations (parts/$10^6$) in enamel of young adults from different communities.

| F in water supply (parts/$10^6$) | Enamel | |
|---|---|---|
| | Surface | Interior |
| 0.1 | 499 | 42 |
| 1.0 | 889 | 129 |
| 3.0 | 1930 | 152 |
| 5.0 | 3370 | 570 |

From Isaac S., Brudevold F., Smith F.A. & Gardner D.E. (1958) The relation of fluoride in the drinking water to the distribution of fluoride in the enamel. *Journal of Dental Research* **37**, 318.

contains fluoride at levels of 1–2 parts/$10^6$, there is clear evidence of its beneficial effect in reducing dental caries by about 50%.

One explanation offered for the mode of action of fluoride stems from observations that fluorapatite is more resistant to acid dissolution than hydroxyapatite. Within limits the greater the substitution of F for OH in the apatite lattice the greater this effect. An outcome of this is the use of concentrated fluoride solutions (1% F and above) to boost surface fluoride. These prophylactic agents may be applied topically to teeth about twice a year in the dental surgery. The main reaction at the surface is a double decomposition with formation of calcium fluoride. Some fluorapatite is also formed.

$$Ca_{10}(PO_4)_6(OH)_2 + 20 F^- \rightarrow$$
$$10CaF_2 + 6PO_4^{3-} + 2 OH^-$$

$$Ca_{10}(PO_4)_6(OH)_2 + 2F^- \rightarrow$$
$$Ca_{10}(PO_4)_6F_2 + 2 OH^-$$

The effectiveness of these procedures in reducing dental caries is beyond question, but there is considerable variation in the degree of reduction claimed for them.

## MOTTLING

With 2 parts fluoride/$10^6$ and above in the water supply the permanent teeth have a mottled appearance—sometimes called dental fluorosis. With 2 parts F/$10^6$ in the water the condition is mild and as the concentration increases the mottling becomes more unsightly. There is discolouration ranging from opaque flecks in mild cases to dark brown areas with hypoplasia of the enamel when the mottling is severe. These defects are permanent and are seen in people who have ingested fluoride when the enamel was forming; adults moving into high fluoride areas do not show mottling. The development of dental fluorosis involves some as yet undetermined effect on the ameloblasts. More of the enamel matrix is retained during maturation and this leads to an increase in the porosity of the enamel and possibly to subsequent penetration of it by oral fluids and pigment. There is evidence to show that when mottling is severe, caries incidence increases.

## FURTHER READING

ANDERSON D.J., HANNAM A.G. & MATTHEWS B. (1950) *Physiology Review* **50**, 171.

APPLETON J. & WILLIAMS M.J.R. (1973) Ultrastructural observations on the calcification of human dental pulp. *Calcified Tissue Research* **11**, 222.

BERRY D.C. & POOLE D.F.G. (1974) Masticatory function and oral rehabilitation. *Journal of oral Rehabilitation* **1**, 191.

BOYDE A. (1974) Transmission electron microscopy of ion beam thinned dentine. *Cell and Tissue Research* **152**, 543.

BOYDE A. (1975) Scanning electron microscopy of enamel surfaces. *British medical Bulletin* **31**, 120.

CHRISTNER P. ROBINSON P. & CLARK C.C. (1977) A preliminary characterization of human cementum collagen. *Calcified Tissue Research* **23**, 147.

DARLING A.I. & MENDIS B.R.R.N. (1975) Response of human dentine to attrition. *Journal of Dental Research 54* Special issue A, Abstract no. L439.

FEARNHEAD R.W. (1967) *Structure and Chemical Organisation of Teeth*. ed. Miles, A.E.W., Vol. 1: p. 247. New York: Academic Press.

FRANK R.M. & STEUR P. (1977) Étude ultrastructurale du cément cellulaire chez le rat. *Journal de Biologie Buccale* **5**, 121.

FURSETH R. (1967) A microradiographic and electron microscopic study of the cementum of human deciduous teeth. *Acta Odontologica Scandinavica* **25**, 613.

FURSETH R. (1969) The fine structure of the cellular cementum of young human teeth. *Archives of Oral Biology* **14**, 1147.

FURSETH R. (1974) The fine structure of a cellular cementum in young human premolars. *Scandinavian Journal of Dental Research* **82**, 437.

GARBEROGLIO R. & BRANNSTROM M. (1976) Scanning electron microscopic investigations of human dentinal tubules. *Archives of Oral Biology* **21**, 355.

HALSTEAD L.B. (1974) *Vertebrate Hard Tissues*. London: Wykeham Publications.

HEROLD R.C. (1970) The fine structure of vasodentine in the teeth of the white hake *Urophycis tenuis* (Pisces, Gadidae). *Archives of Oral Biology* **15**, 311.

HEROLD R.C. (1971) Osteodentinogenesis. An ultrastructural study of tooth formation in the pike, *Esox lucius. Z.Zellforsch. mikr.Anat.* **112**, 1.

MATTHEWS B. (1976) *British Dental Journal* **140**, 57.

MEREDITH SMITH M. & MILES A.E.W. (1971) The ultrastructure of odontogenesis in larval and adult urodeles: differentiation of the dental epithelial cells. *Z.Zellforsch. mikr. Anat.* **121**, 470.

MILES A.E.W. (1967) *Structural and Chemical Organization of Teeth*. 2 vols. London: Academic Press.

OSBORN, J.W. (1973) Variations in structure and development of enamel. In *Dental Enamel*, Oral Science Reviews, Volume 3, p. 3. Copenhagen: Munksgaard.

PEYER B. (1968) *Comparative Odontology*. Chicago: University Press.

RASMUSSEN R.T., PATCHIN R.E., SCOTT D.B. & HEUER A.H. (1976) Fracture properties of human enamel and dentine. *Journal of Dental Research* **55**, 154.

RENSON C.E. & BRADEN M. (1975) Experimental determination of the rigidity modulus, Poisson's ratio and elastic limit in shear of human dentine. *Archives of Oral Biology* **20**, 43.

RYGH P. (1977) Orthodontic root resorption studied by electron microscopy. *Angle Orthodontist* **47**, 1.

SCHMIDT W.J. & KEIL A. (1971) *Polarizing Microscopy of Dental Tissues*. (Trans. Poole D.F.G. & Darling A.I.). London: Academic Press.

SELVIG K.A. (1965) The fine structure of human cementum. *Acta Odontologica Scandinavia* **23**, 423.

SHELLIS R.P. (1976) The role of the inner dental epithelium in tooth formation in fishes. In *Proceedings of the 4th Symposium on Dental Morphology*. London: Academic Press.

SHELLIS R.P. & BERKOVITZ B.K.B. (1976) The dental anatomy of piranhas (Characidae), with special reference to tooth structure. *Journal of Zoology (London)*

SYMONS N.B.B. ed. (1968) *Dentine and Pulp*. Edinburgh: Livingstone.

TEN CATE A.R. (1972) An analysis of Tomes' granular layer. *Anatomical Record* **172**, 137.

TYLDESLEY W.R. (1959) The mechanical properties of human enamel and dentine. *British Dental Journal* **106**, 269.

YILMAZ S., NEWMAN H.N. & POOLE D.F.G. (1977) Diurnal periodicity of von Ebner growth lines in pig dentine. *Archives of Oral Biology* **22**, 511.

# CHAPTER 7

# Tooth Support

## EVOLUTION

The supporting tissues of teeth play as important a part in the efficiency of the dentition as the structure and morphology of the teeth themselves. Although a great variety of tooth supporting mechanisms exists among the vertebrates, each adapted to a different function, all types of tooth attachment are mediated primarily by collagen which is mineralized to a greater or lesser extent. The degree of mineralization, together with the shape and arrangement of the hard and soft parts of the attachment tissues are the factors influencing the properties of the supporting mechanism. In addition to sharing a common structural basis, most forms of tooth attachment develop in a similar way; the cells responsible for laying down the attachment tissues are derived, at least in part, from the cells of the dental papilla. This is clearly seen in the fishes, amphibians and most reptiles, where the teeth are attached at only their basal ends to the skeleton, the cells forming the attachment tissues being differentiated after the tooth has been formed. The emergence of socketed teeth in some reptiles and in the mammals was a phylogenetic novelty and involved changes in the pattern and timing of the formation of the supporting tissues relative to that of the tooth itself.

## TYPES OF TOOTH SUPPORT AND THEIR PROPERTIES

In functional terms, two broad classes of tooth support can be distinguished: rigid and deformable. The former is found only in non-mammalian vertebrates and shows less variation of form.

In a rigidly attached tooth the region of union with the bone is completely mineralized. This condition is referred to as ankylosis (Fig. 7.1a; 7.4b,c). Where teeth are ankylosed, the stresses of biting must be taken up by rigid hard tissues and the shape of the tooth may be modified in such a way as to absorb stress more efficiently. In animals which crush their food with squat, blunt teeth the ankylosis prevents sideways displacement of the tooth. In some carnivorous animals, where the teeth tend to be long and pointed, they often increase rapidly in cross-sectional area towards the base, which gives maximum strength against lateral forces exerted by a struggling prey.

In deformable attachments, the teeth are joined to bone by unmineralized collagen fibres, either directly or by way of an intermediate mineralized tissue (Figs. 7.1b–d, 7.2, 7.3). The degree of tooth mobility is governed by the length of the fibres and by the area of tooth surface over which they are inserted. The fibres may be short, permitting only slight tooth movement, or may be long enough or so arranged as to permit considerable movement.

It is useful to distinguish two types of fibrous attachment, although the distinction is largely a formal one. In some animals there is a direct fibrous attachment between tooth and a bone of attachment which merges, sometimes indistinguishably, with the bone of the jaw (Fig. 7.1b). Here the unmineralized fibres are embedded at one end into the dentine of the tooth and at the other into the bone of attachment. A special modification of the direct fibrous attachment is found in the elasmobranch fishes, which lack bone. In this group the fibres anchor the teeth to a sheet of other fibres which run over the surface of the jaw cartilage underneath the tooth rows (Fig. 7.2). Other types of tooth support may be referred to as indirect fibrous attachments. In this type the fibres are embedded into a special mineralized tissue. This mineralized tissue attachment may be (a) united with the bone but be of different structure, when it is known as a pedicel (Figs. 7.1c, 7.4a), or (b) be united with the dentine of the tooth, when it is known as cement (Fig. 7.1d).

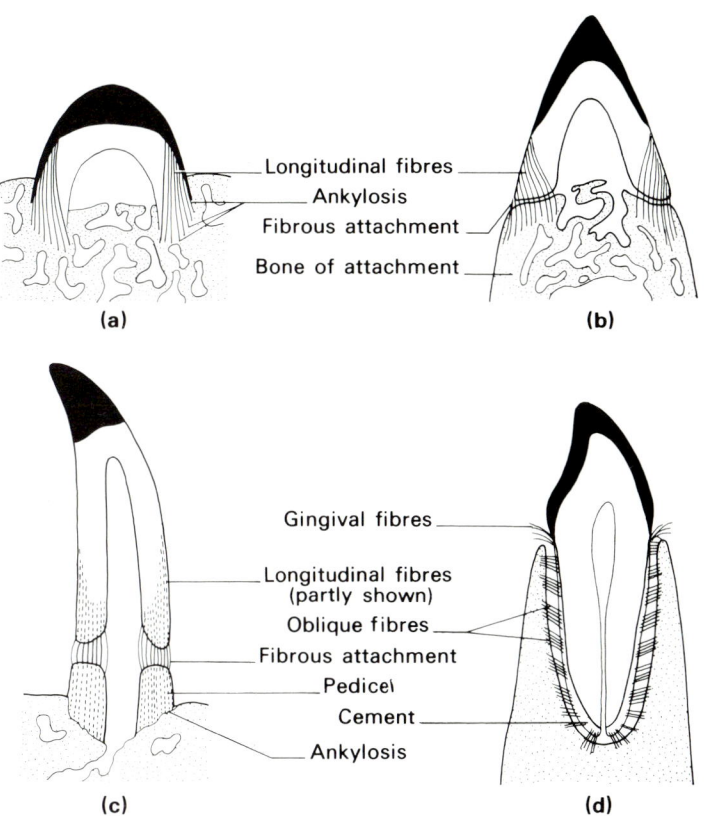

**Fig. 7.1.** Forms of attachment: (a) ankylosis in a teleost; (b) direct fibrous attachment in piranha; (c) indirect fibrous attachment (pedicel) in a teleost; (d) indirect fibrous attachment (gomphosis) in a mammal.

## THE FORMATION OF ATTACHMENT TISSUES

The development of the gomphosis is described in detail elsewhere (p. 283), so that the concern here will be with the other forms of attachment. Collagen fibres continuous with the dentine of the tooth are a prominent feature in these attachment tissues. This continuity is achieved by a two-stage process: first, the fibres are laid down and second, calcification of this collagen 'blends' it with the tooth substance. In ankylosis and in the direct fibrous attachment, a large proportion of the fibres are laid down by fibroblasts of the pulp and the connective tissue around the base of the tooth germ. Later, dentine formation extends into the basal region and incorporates part of these fibres. Their free ends extend out of the dentine and bone (bone of attachment) is laid down around them or, in the case of the elasmobranchs, the fibres become embedded in the sheet of fibres below the teeth. In ankylosis the 'bony mineralized' ends meet the 'dentine mineralized' ends to form a mineralized union. Bone is sometimes laid down around the sides of the lower portion of ankylosed teeth thereby reinforcing the attachment. In the direct fibrous attachment, on the other hand, bone formation stops short of the base of the tooth, leaving a zone of unmineralized fibres. It is obvious that there is a close similarity between the development of these two forms of attachment.

The development of the indirect, pedicellate attachment differs slightly from this pattern. In the formation of a pedicel, Hertwig's sheath (Fig. 8.46) continues to grow down beyond the lower limit of the dentine and odontoblasts continue to differentiate on its inner surface. The odontoblasts lay down against the inside of the sheath longitudinally oriented fibres continuous with the fibres of the dentine matrix. Later, the portion of this fibrous tissue further from the tooth mineralizes and becomes the pedicel, while the fibres between the tooth and the pedicel fail to mineralize. By the time that the pedicel has almost been completed, its base is close to the bone of the jaw and the deposition of hard tissue in this region cements the pedicel to the bone.

It is appropriate at this point to discuss the term bone of attachment, which is sometimes used simply to mean the bone on which the teeth rest but is sometimes used to mean the pedicel as well. From the developmental point of view, the pedicel is closely related to dentine, not to bone. In its mature state, it sometimes has a dentine-like structure but more often its structure is indeterminate, containing only a few tubules and occasionally a small number of included cells in lacunae. Both developmental and structural considerations thus lead to the view that the term 'bone of attachment' is not applicable to the pedicel. The use of the term for the bone underlying the teeth is, however, useful, for this bone has distinctive characteristics. In terms of structure, it is usually spongy and is often quite distinct from the bone forming the body of the jaw, which tends to be dense and compact. In terms of development, each newly erupting tooth seems to stimulate the development of its own bone of attachment which is resorbed when the tooth is shed.

## ADAPTIVE RADIATION OF TOOTH SUPPORTING STRUCTURES

### Elasmobranchs

In these fishes, the dentine of the tooth merges at the base with a structure known as the basal plate (Fig. 7.2). This may be composed either of orthodentine or osteodentine. The fibres anchoring the teeth to the sheet of fibres overlying the jaw cartilage are inserted into a basal plate whose shape varies considerably. The plate is always perforated by one or more channels allowing access of blood vessels to the pulp.

The attachment is in principle flexible but the mobility of the teeth varies widely in different types of elasmobranchs. In the flat crushing teeth of rays (Fig. 4.12) the functional dentition consists of several rows of teeth arranged in a pavement and the teeth tend to be quite firmly fixed. Other elasmobranchs, the dogfishes and sharks, have more mobile teeth, especially the carnivorous species. These animals usually have only a single tooth row in function at any one time (Fig. 4.11). The basal plate has an ovoid shape so that tooth mobility is governed only by the restraints of the attachment fibres. The mobility of the teeth seems

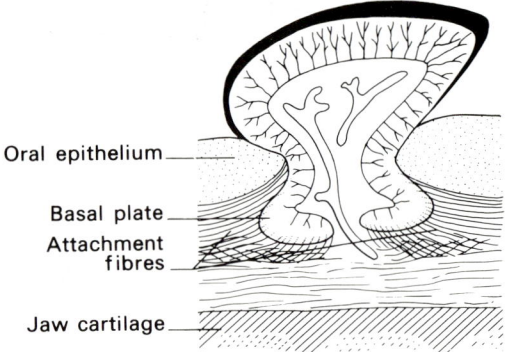

**Fig. 7.2.** Fibrous attachment in a shark.

to be correlated with the great stresses set up by the exceptionally violent sawing action of the dentition.

### Teleosts

Many of these fishes have rigidly attached teeth. The attachment may be by ankylosis or by a direct fibrous attachment in which the attachment fibres are very short. Rigidly attached teeth are more common among fishes with crushing dentitions adapted to dealing with a hard diet such as crustaceans, molluscs or corals. Examples of these fishes are the wrasses (Fig. 7.1a), the sea-breams which include the well-known sheep's-head fish, *Sargus ovis* (Fig. 4.14), the parrot fishes and some flat fishes, such as the plaice. Among the wrasses, the ankylosis of the teeth is frequently reinforced by bone deposited around the sides of the teeth and even within the pulp chamber.

Mobile teeth are found among a large number of teleosts. Familiar examples are the eels (Fig. 7.1c), many members of the cod family and the sea basses. The teeth are sometimes capable of a certain amount of movement in all directions but usually movement is more or less restricted to the labiolingual plane.

Considerably more mobile teeth are found in the hake, the pike, the angler fish and others: these are called hinged teeth. Inward tilting of the tooth around its hinge aids the ingestion of prey by allowing easier access into the oral cavity whereas outward movement erects the teeth thereby trapping the prey. The hinge mechanism is probably best known in the hake and serves as a very good example of the adaptability of tooth attachment. In the hake, the teeth can be depressed lingually through almost 90° by gentle pressure. The hinge is a highly modified direct fibrous attachment (Fig.

# Tooth Support

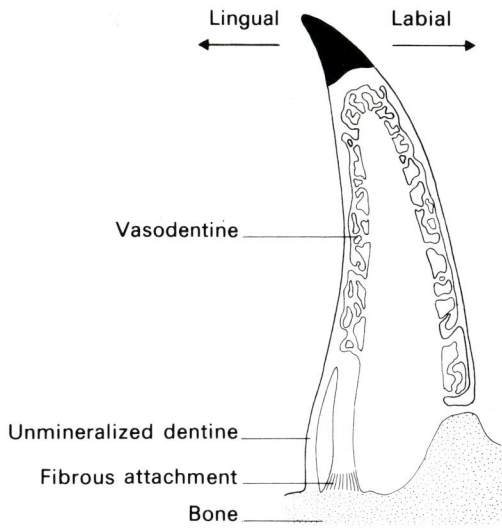

Fig. 7.3. Hinged attachment in hake.

7.3). However, the fibres arise only from the inner layers of the wall of the tooth and are absent over part of the circumference on the labial surface. Outside the lingual half of the ring of attachment fibres there is a sheet of an additional fibrous tissue—apparently unmineralized dentine—which runs from the outer layer of the mineralized dentine of the tooth into the bone of attachment. The fibres of which it is composed are strongly bonded together and the tissue is stiff and elastic. When the tooth is depressed, it rotates about the fibrous attachment and the semicircular sheet of unmineralized dentine is buckled. When the load is removed the elastic recovery of this tissue provides a force restoring the tooth to its upright position. The tooth is prevented from moving in a labial direction by the presence of a raised shelf of bone under the labial half of the tooth and by the inextensibility of the sheet of unmineralized dentine on the lingual surface.

## Amphibians

In the living members of this class, a pedicellate tooth attachment (Fig. 7.4a) is almost universal. Generally, the attachment fibres appear to be rather short, so that the teeth are not very mobile. Whereas in teleosts, the tooth tends to be much longer than the pedicel, the reverse is the case in the amphibians. The pedicel is attached to the bone in a pleurodont fashion (see next section). A few species appear to lack the division between tooth and pedicel but this condition seems to be secondary rather than primitive.

## Reptiles

Among living reptiles ankylosis is the prevalent mode of tooth attachment. Between the tooth and the bone is a layer of coarse textured tissue which contains lacunae and tubules. This does not seem to be cement, as is often suggested, but a tissue formed by both odontoblasts and osteoblasts which have come together after completing the dentine of the tooth and the bone of attachment. The ankylosis thus has much the same structure as in teleost fishes.

Two forms of ankylosis are distinguished in reptiles, according to whether the tooth is attached to the crest of the jaw (acrodont attachment; Fig. 7.4b) or to the lingual surface of the bone (pleurodont attachment; Fig. 7.4c). Pleurodont attachment is found in the majority of lizards, while acrodont attachment is found in snakes and a few lizards, most notably the members of the family Agamidae.

Socketed teeth were present in many reptiles which are now extinct. These included the dinosaurs and primitive birds, the pterosaurs and the groups ancestral to the crocodiles and mammals. The only living reptiles with this type of attachment are the Crocodilia (crocodiles, alligators and caimans). In structure, the gomphosis of these animals (Fig. 7.4d) is very similar to that of mammals.

## Mammals

The particular value of a gomphosis is that the teeth can be moved through the jaws to compensate for changes due to growth or tooth wear without their efficiency being affected.

Each mammalian tooth has, at most, a single replacement meaning that each tooth has to function for much longer than one in a polyphyodont dentition. In non-mammalian vertebrates the teeth last for months in some species but in others are replaced at intervals measured in weeks or even days; in mammals the life span of the tooth usually extends into years. This creates a problem at the potentially weak point where the tooth protrudes through the body surface. In non-mammalian vertebrates, the mucosa surrounding the teeth shows no structural differentiation from that in the rest of the mouth and does not adhere firmly to the teeth. Bacteria and toxins may thus be able to enter the body at the junction between tooth and epithelium fairly freely, being hindered only by the mucus secreted by the epithelium. When the teeth are replaced fairly frequently, this may be of little long-term significance. In the

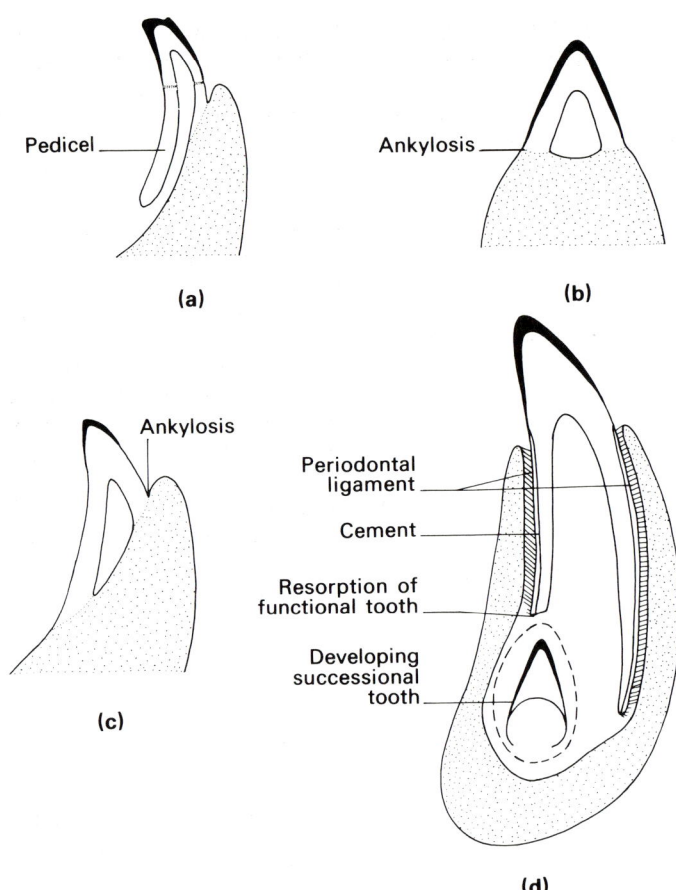

**Fig. 7.4.** (a) Pedicellate attachment in amphibians. Acrodont (b) and pleurodont (c) ankylosis in reptiles. (d) Socketed attachment of crocodilian tooth.

crocodiles, however, which replace their teeth relatively slowly, there is evidence that the circumdental (gingival) epithelium becomes progressively infiltrated with white cells as the tooth ages and that bleeding may occur through the damaged epithelium around a tooth near the end of its functional life. In the mammals, specializations of the gingival mucosa and of the epithelial attachment to the tooth have evolved. These seem to provide a much more efficient barrier to microorganisms and their products.

Cement covers the surface of the hypsodont crowns of the cheek teeth in rodents, lagomorphs, elephants, and ungulates. (Fig. 7.5). The enamel of hypsodont teeth extends far into the bone of the jaw. Were the enamel not covered by cement the tooth could not be efficiently attached to the jaws.

In order to compensate for wear the teeth of all mammals erupt, to a greater or lesser extent, throughout life. In some animals the wear is so extensive that it needs to be compensated by the continuous formation of new tooth substance: for example, the incisors and sometimes the molars of rodents and lagomorphs. Since there is no generally accepted theory of tooth eruption it is not

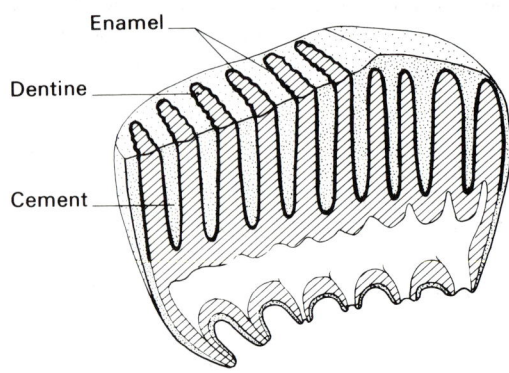

**Fig. 7.5.** Longitudinally sliced molar of elephant, showing cement covering.

possible to say what the role of the attachment tissues in the continuous eruption of these teeth is but it is certain that teeth of this type could only have evolved in a group having teeth supported in sockets. No other form of tooth attachment allows the teeth to grow once they have become attached to the bone.

## ALVEOLAR BONE

The body of the mandible is divided into basal bone and an alveolar process by an imaginary line which passes horizontally just below the bony tissue lining the sockets of the teeth (Fig. 7.6). The

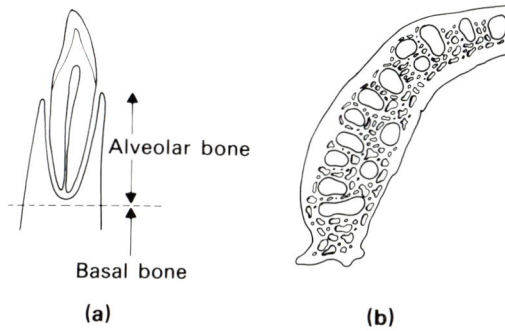

**Fig. 7.6.** (a) The cortical plate of alveolar bone (black) lines the tooth socket (lamina dura) and extends onto the buccal and lingual surfaces of the bone. (b) Horizontal section through alveolar bone in the upper jaw.

alveolar process contains alveoli (little holes) in which the teeth lie. The concept of separate alveolar bone is justified because it focuses attention on that bone which is intimately related to, and immediately supports, the teeth. The unique physiological demands to which alveolar bone is subjected by the sudden pressures involved in grinding and tooth–tooth contacts leads to reactions which are rather different from other bony tissue. Nevertheless, with the exception of a narrow strip of bone containing the embedded parts of periodontal fibres, its histological structure is the same as basal bone and all other lamellated bone in the body. Obviously the maxilla also has an alveolar process.

### Development (Chapter 3)

A rigid application of the definition of alveolar bone would lead to the conclusion that alveolar bone cannot exist without tooth sockets: and indeed alveolar bone does seem to depend on teeth for its existence. In a developmental anomaly, (total) anodontia, not only are no teeth formed, nor is the bone which would normally surround them. In a normal individual the alveolar bone develops around the tooth germs and only deepens (grows) in association with active eruption: after the teeth are lost the alveolar bone is gradually lost. These data suggest that in some unknown way the teeth influence the development and maintenance of the bone which surrounds them. In an experimental situation tooth germs have been enucleated from the jaws and cultured in different sites of the body, such as muscle, skin or the anterior chamber of the eye. Even under these conditions 'alveolar' bone developed around the teeth. It has been suggested that the osteoblasts differentiate from cells adhering to the enucleated tooth germ.

In summary, alveolar bone is stimulated to develop by the presence of teeth and by their eruption. In the absence of teeth it is resorbed.

### Structure

#### GENERAL

Like all bones the alveolar process consists of an outer layer of compact bone surrounding an inner region of trabeculated bone (Fig. 7.6). The compact bone on the labial and lingual surfaces is indistinguishable from the adjacent compact layers of the basal bone. From the alveolar crest, the most coronal edge of the alveolar process, the compact layer turns inwards to line each alveolus (tooth socket). This lining layer has been called the lamina dura because of its dense appearance, common to all compact bone, on radiographs; alveolar bone proper because it provides the most direct bony support of the tooth; and a cribriform plate because it is perforated by numerous vascular canals. Trabeculated bone between the lamina dura and the buccal (and lingual) cortical plates of the alveolar process blends indistinguishably with trabeculae of the basal bone. Adjacent teeth are separated by interdental septa of bone, and the roots of multirooted teeth by inter-radicular septa. Where adjacent teeth are close, the interdental septa terminate as interdental crests of bone and where teeth are more widely separated there are interdental tables of bone (Fig. 7.7).

Just as in all bones, the cortical plate of alveolar bone is covered by a periosteum but this is modified to become the periodontal ligament where it covers the lamina dura.

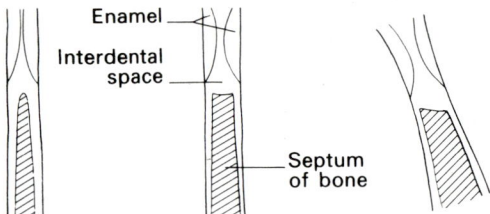

**Fig. 7.7.** Variations in the shape of interdental septa of bone.

REGIONAL VARIATIONS AND RELATIONS

*Maxilla*
The relations between the teeth and maxillary bone vary along the jaw (Fig. 7.8). Over anterior teeth the buccal cortical plate of alveolar bone is generally fused with the adjacent lamina dura so that the apices of the teeth are close to the bony surface: in many dried skulls it can be seen that part of the buccal surface of the canine root is not even covered by bone. Inflammatory exudate associated with apical abscesses of anterior teeth usually perforates the thin buccal plate and swells into the lip region. Occasionally the apex of the lateral incisor is more deeply placed.

Passing back from the premolars the buccal alveolar bone thickens and begins to contain some trabeculae, particularly over the roots of molars where the zygomatic arch begins. Abscesses of cheek teeth generally swell into the soft tissues either above or below the attachment of buccinator.

Palatally the bone is thicker and trabeculae generally separate the lamina dura from all regions of cortical bone covering the oral surface of the hard palate. Here the incisive papilla, canal and nerves are close to the central incisor, and the greater palatine nerves and vessels are near the cheek teeth.

The apex of the central incisor is sometimes very close to the floor of the nose; that of the shorter lateral incisor is further from, although still beneath, the nasal cavity. The maxillary antrum lies above the cheek teeth. Its wall usually curves upwards before it reaches the first premolar although a large antrum can extend this far forwards. Posteriorly the antrum may hollow out the tuberosity of the maxilla to such an extent that this region is fractured when the third molar is extracted. The distance between the antrum and the roots of the cheek teeth varies. In some people the antrum is so far away as to be unimportant in any dental surgery; in others the antrum may be so large that the roots of the second premolar to the second molar actually lie inside it and are covered

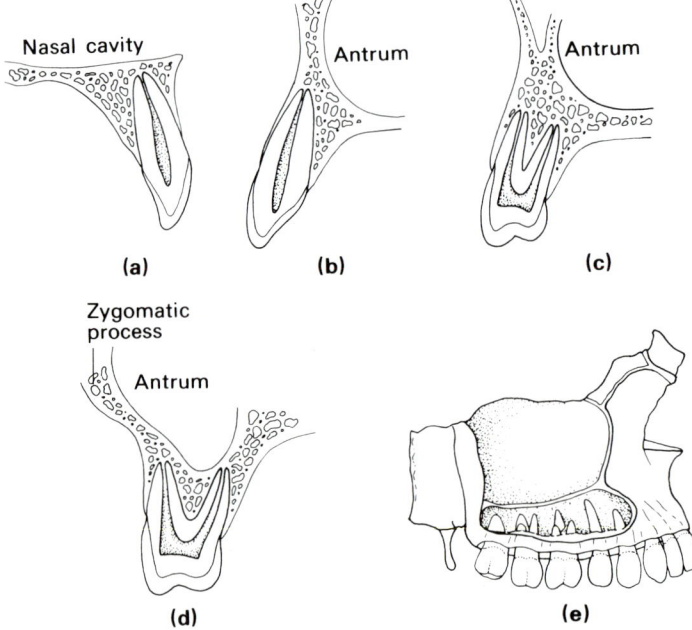

**Fig. 7.8.** Sections through upper (a) incisor, (b) canine, (c) first premolar and (d) first molar. In (b) and (d) the antrum is exceptionally large. Bone has been dissected away in (e) to show the relation of the roots of the teeth to a large antrum.

by antral mucosa. An infection of the antrum (sinusitis) can now stimulate the nerves entering the roots of these teeth producing a sensation of toothache.

The canine is implanted in a buttress of bone separating the nasal cavity from the maxillary sinus.

*Mandible*

The buccal plate of alveolar bone in the lower jaw is similar to that in the upper jaw with the difference that in the lower jaw the external oblique ridge is responsible for thickening the plate posteriorly. The lingual plate of bone is thin all round the jaw (Fig. 7.9).

The mental nerve emerges from between the roots of the lower premolars. Before undertaking any bone surgery in this region, such as may be required for removing the roots of teeth, it is essential that the mental nerve and vessels be located and isolated so that they are not damaged during the operation. If the nerve is cut, the adjacent lower lip will probably be 'anaesthetized' for life.

The thick buccal plate of bone makes a buccal approach less attractive for the surgical removal of lower third molars since a considerable amount of bone may need to be removed before the tooth can be exposed. However, despite the thinness of the lingual bone, the lingual approach is potentially more hazardous. Not only is it less accessible because of the tongue but, of far greater importance, the lingual nerve runs forwards just beneath the oral mucosa adjacent to the roots, and sometimes the crown, of an impacted molar. Prior to removing bone lingually, the lingual nerve must be identified and suitably protected.

The inferior dental nerve is a further hazard. Although the roots of the molar teeth shorten posteriorly, the nerve rises and the associated neurovascular bundle may be in contact with the roots of the third molar and even be totally surrounded by them (the developing roots grow to surround the bundle). Under these conditions, unless extreme care is taken, the nerve and artery are cut in two when the roots are extracted. As an immediate problem the haemorrhage may be difficult to control, and in the long term it is very doubtful whether any sensation will ever return to the lower lip.

Abscess cavities associated with the roots of lower teeth may discharge through the bone either lingually or buccally. In both cases the infection may break through a sinus (a canal eroded in the bone) in the cortical bone above or below muscle attachments: if it is buccal and above, the resultant swelling lies in the buccal sulcus and if it is below, it lies in the neck. The mylohyoid muscle is the 'watershed' lingually. If the sinus opens above the mylohyoid, the swelling lies in the mouth under the tongue: if below the mylohyoid, the swelling spreads down the neck.

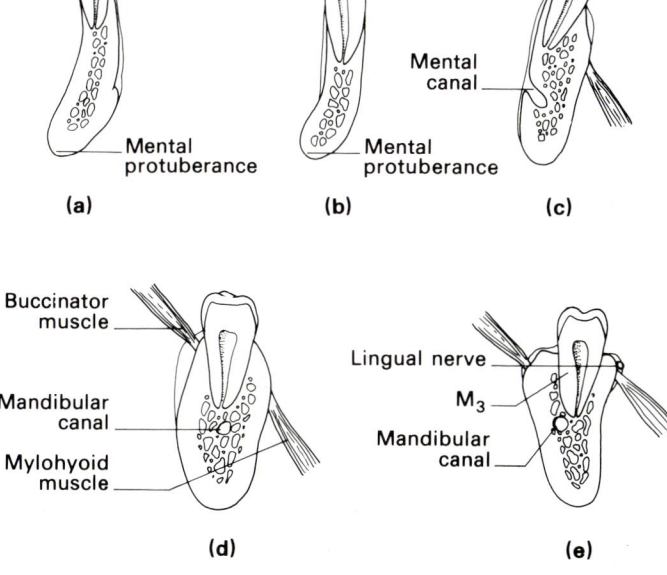

Fig. 7.9. Sections through lower (a) incisor, (b) canine, (c) second premolar, (d) second molar and (e) third molar.

## Mechanics

Stresses applied to the teeth are passed to the alveolar bone via the periodontal ligament and from here to the jaw bones and thence to the skull. For example, it has been shown that if the jaws are clenched, the sutures joining the skull bones may either be widened or narrowed (stretched or compressed) depending on their positions.

A study of the construction of the upper jaw suggests that forces can be transmitted along three buttresses, the frontal process of the maxilla, the zygomatic arch and the pterygoid plates (Fig. 7.10).

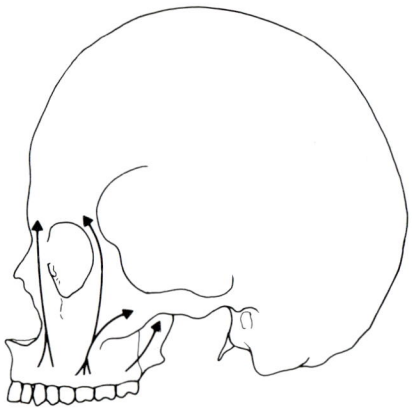

**Fig. 7.10** Forces applied to the maxillary teeth are transmitted to the cranium in the direction of the arrows.

It is probable that very little force is applied to the articular fossa on the temporal bone via the mandibular condyle (Fig. 10.3) so that masticatory forces would be transmitted (a) via bone to the muscles of mastication and thence to the cranium and (b) via the upper teeth to the maxillary bone and thence to the cranium.

## Histology

Alveolar bone initially develops as a lattice of woven bone without cortical plates. It is subsequently replaced by lamellated bone. The buccal and lingual cortical plates, consisting of circumferential and concentric (Haversian system) lamellae, and the intervening trabeculated bone appear to have the same histology as any lamellated bone.

The degree of development of the trabeculae in alveolar bone is related to the stress applied to the teeth. They are much diminished around a tooth which lacks an opponent, and are heavily developed around teeth which are heavily stressed. The trabeculae are constantly being remodelled. The marrow spaces contain haemopoietic tissue (red marrow) in the young but during childhood this is replaced by fatty tissue (yellow marrow).

The buccal and lingual cortical plates are covered by periosteum which blends with the lamina propria of the gingiva to become a mucoperiosteum. The remaining (alveolar) mucosa is separated from the periosteum by the loose connective tissue of a submucosa.

The interdental bone is often perforated by transalveolar fibres (Fig. 7.15).

## Lamina dura

The lamina dura, which is considerably thinner than the buccal and lingual cortical plates, also consists of circumferential lamellae, adjacent to the periodontal ligament, and concentric lamellae (Fig. 7.11). It is perforated by numerous canals containing arteries and veins connecting the periodontal ligament to the interdental arteries and veins, and by the apical vessels and nerves of the tooth.

The principal fibres of the periodontal ligament pierce the lamina dura and occupy tunnels within it. The penetrating fibres are Sharpey fibres. The matrix of the bone containing Sharpey fibres often differs from that of the remaining bone; it consists of coarser and fewer fibres with the result that it stains less heavily with collagen stains. This is known as bundle bone. The bundle bone (reduced collagen matrix) is not found lining the whole of the lamina dura. It is particularly developed on the walls of sockets away from which teeth are moving. Thus if a tooth is drifting mesially, bundle bone tends to be deposited on the distal wall of the socket. The reduced, coarser, matrix may be associated with more rapid movements of teeth.

In a radiograph of a healthy tooth the lamina dura can be seen as a continuous thin white line surrounding the whole root and separated from it by a thin black line, the periodontal ligament. An infected pulp can often be diagnosed due to the presence of a disruption of the lamina dura around the apex of the tooth. This is related to osteoclastic removal of bone in response to infection spreading into the adjacent periodontal ligament. A widening of the thin black line associated with the periodontal ligament on radiographs is commonly associated with advanced periodontal disease.

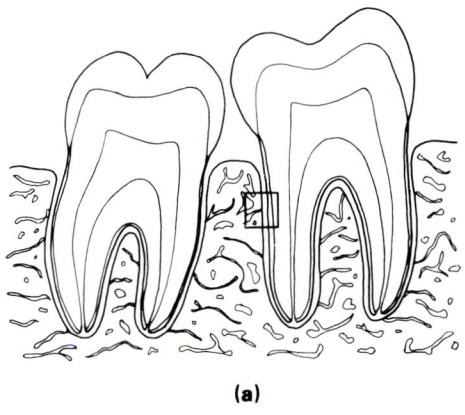

**(a)**

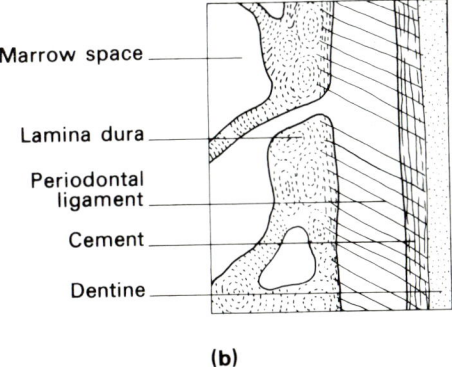

**(b)**

**Fig. 7.11.** (a) Section through two lower molar teeth showing the lamina dura and trabeculated bone. (b) The lamina dura consists of concentric and circumferential lamellae.

## PERIODONTAL LIGAMENT

The periodontal ligament is the connective tissue which lies between the roots of teeth and their alveolar walls and is derived from the dental follicle. It is said to be primarily concerned with tooth support, maintaining the relationships of teeth to the surrounding hard and soft tissues during mastication. Above the level of the alveolar crest the ligament is continuous with the lamina propria of the gingiva and at the apical foramen it is continuous with the dental pulp. 'Periodontium' is a collective term referring to the periodontal ligament, gingiva, alveolar bone and cement.

Radiographically, the periodontal ligament appears as a thin, radiolucent line between the root surface and the lamina dura of the alveolar bone. The average width of the periodontal ligament is about 0.2 mm (0.15–0.3 mm) but this is likely to vary in different individuals, in different teeth of the same individual and at different levels in the same tooth. The width is liable to be greater in teeth subjected to considerable occlusal stress than in teeth subjected to minimum stress and in unerupted teeth. The periodontal spaces of deciduous teeth are wider than those of permanent teeth. The periodontal ligament is thinner near the fulcrum of physiological tooth movements, which is located about one third along the length of the root from the apex.

Like other soft connective tissues, the periodontal ligament consists of cells and an extracellular matrix composed of fibres and a gel. The ligament has a rich vascular and nerve supply and a high turnover rate for some of its elements.

### Fibres

A number of fibre types have been described in the periodontal ligament, namely collagen, oxytalan, reticulin and elastin.

#### COLLAGEN

Collagen fibres form the most conspicuous element within the ligament. Many of them are gathered together in bundles whose diameter may be of the order of 5 $\mu$m. In longitudinal section these fibres are differently orientated in different parts of the root. Such groupings have been termed the principal fibres of the periodontium to distinguish them from smaller, non-aligned 'indifferent' collagen fibres lying between the principal fibres. The larger blood vessels lie in regions between the principal fibres.

The following principal dento-alveolar (meaning 'tooth to bone') fibre groupings have been described in longitudinal sections of the periodontal ligament (Fig. 7.12).

*Apical group.* These fibres radiate out perpendicular to the apex of the root; coronally they merge with the oblique group.

*Oblique group.* These fibres occupy the middle third of the ligament passing from the root obliquely upwards and outwards to the alveolus; coronally they merge with the horizontal group. The oblique fibres do not usually run in a strictly radial fashion in the transverse plane. Their irregular arrangement in this plane is thought to limit the amount of rotary movement of the tooth (Fig. 7.13).

*Horizontal group.* These fibres, lying just below

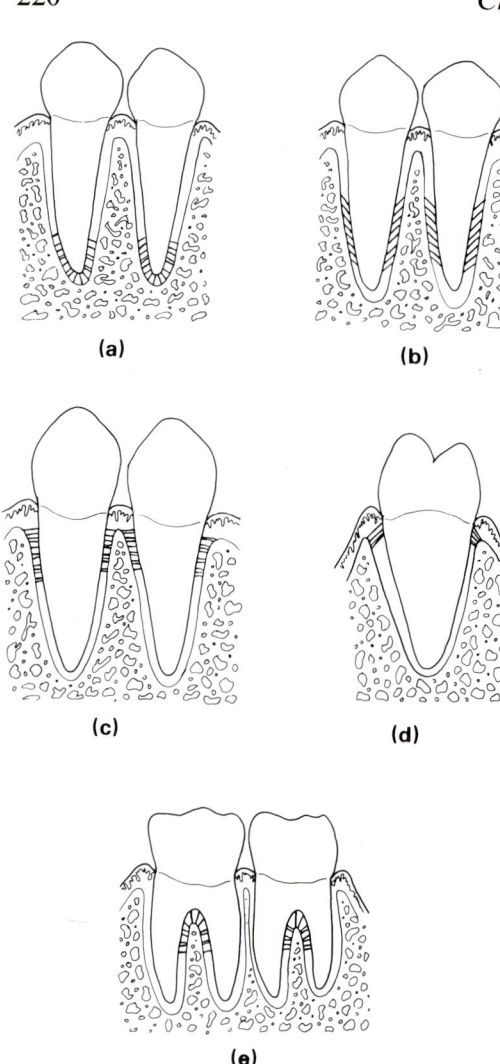

**Fig. 7.12.** Diagram showing the orientation of the principal periodontal ligament collagen fibre bundles: (a) apical; (b) oblique; (c) horizontal; (d) alveolar crest; (e) interradicular.

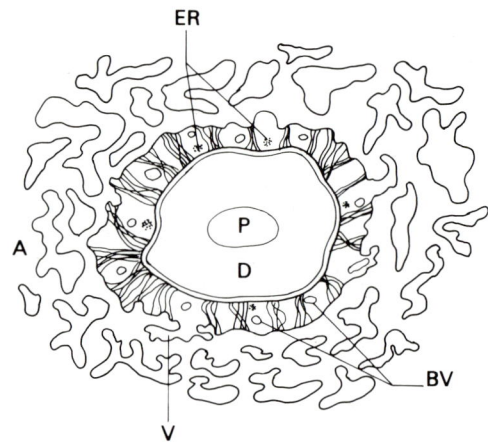

**Fig. 7.13.** Cross-section of a root showing the radial arrangement of the principal collagen fibre bundles between which are seen blood vessels (BV). Many of these vessels enter the periodontal ligament through openings in the alveolar wall known as Volkmann's canals (V). D, dentine; P, pulp; A, alveolar bone; ER, epithelial rests.

the level of the alveolar crest, pass horizontally across the ligament from the lower portion of the coronal third of the root to the alveolus.

*Alveolar crest group.* Lying primarily in the buccolingual plane these fibres are attached to the root above the level of the alveolar crest. Fibres with a somewhat similar orientation have also been illustrated in the mesiodistal plane (see Fig. 7.15).

*Interradicular group.* In teeth with more than one root, these fibres fan out from the crest of the interradicular bony septum to the adjacent part of the root surface.

The course of the collagen fibres from cement to bone is described as being wavy and it has been suggested that during functional stress the fibres are stretched, thus allowing for slight movements of the teeth despite the inelastic nature of collagen fibres. As yet there is no positive evidence (*in vivo*) to support the truth of these statements. A greater number of bundles containing fewer fibrils are attached to the cement in contrast to a lesser number of bundles containing more fibrils passing into the alveolar bone (Fig. 7.14).

There has been considerable debate concerning the distance that individual principal fibres extend across the periodontal ligament. There are two main views concerning this question. The first suggests that the periodontal ligament fibres span the ligament in three portions, one part attached to the alveolar bone, another part attached to the cement and a central component splicing them together. The central portion, referred to as the 'intermediate plexus', is thought to be a region where the two peripheral components can be separated and respliced to provide the necessary adaptation for tooth movement. The intermediate plexus should be visible throughout the life of continuously erupting teeth due to constant separation of fibres and resplicing as the tooth slides past the bone, but be visible only during the main phase of active eruption in non-continuously

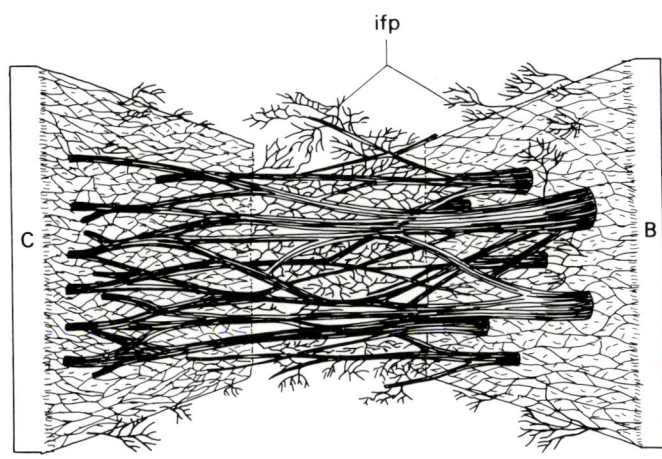

**Fig. 7.14.** Diagrammatic representation of the collagen fibres of the periodontal ligament showing the relationship of the indifferent fibre plexus (ifp) to the principal fibre bundles which are the larger structures passing between bone (B) and cement (C). Note the different size of principal fibre bundles at the bone and cement surfaces. [From Shackleford J. M. (1971). The indifferent fibre plexus and its relationship to principal fibres of the periodontium. *American Journal of Anatomy* **131**, 427.]

erupting teeth. A modification of this view is that the cemental fibres directly interlace with the alveolar fibres without the intervention of a third, specifically different, intermediate group of fibres. The presence of an intermediate plexus has yet to be established beyond doubt. The occasional appearance of such a plexus in longitudinal sections has been interpreted as the result of oblique sectioning of the principal fibre bundles. However, a functional zone of shear may be present to allow for tooth movements without being readily visible histologically.

The alternative to the above view is that, in passing from cement to alveolar bone, the majority of closely packed collagen fibres become more loosely arranged and branch and join neighbouring fibres (Fig. 7.14).

*Indifferent fibre plexus*
In addition to principal fibres, the periodontal ligament is also said to contain collagen fibres with a more random orientation. These have been described as forming an 'indifferent fibre plexus'. The spatial arrangement of this indifferent plexus has been studied by scanning electron microscopy. Characteristically, it is composed of small collagen fibres, approximately 50 nm in diameter, which probably represent individual fibrils. They course in every direction throughout the periodontal ligament and are joined with the larger principal fibres by intermediate size fibres to form a continuous fibrous matrix (Fig. 7.14). However, this plexus may be an artefact related to the method of specimen preparation.

*Attachment of the periodontal ligament fibres*
The ends of the principal collagen fibres of the periodontal ligament which are embedded in cement and alveolar bone are termed 'Sharpey's fibres' (in common with fibres from muscle tendons which are inserted into bone). It was previously thought that Sharpey's fibres were simply inserted into the outermost part of the alveolar bone. However, recent evidence indicates that a more complex arrangement exists in this region. In the cervical portions of the interdental septum, Sharpey's fibres entering bone in the mesiodistal plane may pass straight through to become continuous with fibres from the root of the adjacent tooth (Fig. 7.15); similar fibres are seen in interradicular bone except that here the fibres link roots of the same tooth. In the buccal and lingual planes Sharpey's fibres may again pass through the entire thickness of the alveolar bone and intermingle with the overlying periosteum or with the lamina propria of the gingiva. The term 'transalveolar fibres' has been given to describe these fibres. More apically, however, especially in the cheek teeth where the alveolar bone is cancellous or where there are numerous Haversian systems, transalveolar fibres are not seen. The distribution of these fibres in mouse molars is illustrated in Fig. 7.15. In these teeth the alveolar bone is primarily of the lamellated type and therefore transalveolar fibres are seen to best advantage. As a general rule, transalveolar fibres are coarser and less numerous than the fibres of the periodontal ligament with which they are continuous. Thus, at least in the cervical portions of the roots of man, there may be transalveolar fibres which, together with the transseptal fibres, form a 'ligamentous' band by which every tooth in the arch is interconnected.

The following principal gingival fibre groups have been described (Fig. 7.16).

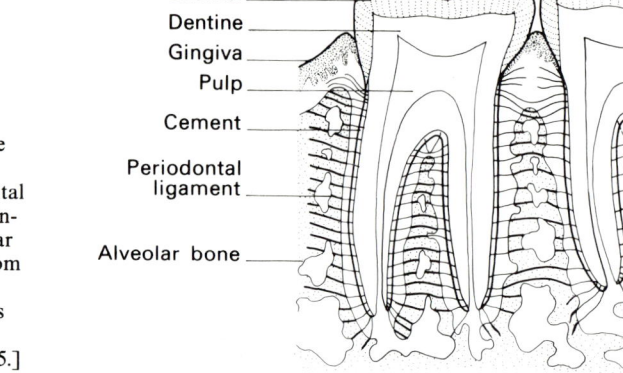

**Fig. 7.15.** Diagram to show the manner in which the various principal fibres of the periodontal ligament of the mouse pass uninterruptedly through the alveolar wall (transalveolar fibres). [From Cohn S. A. (1972). A re-examination of Sharpey's fibres in alveolar bone of the mouse. *Archives of Oral Biology* **17**, 255.]

*Transseptal group.* This group lies in the mesiodistal plane passing horizontally from the root of one tooth above the alveolar crest to be inserted into the root of the adjacent tooth.

*Dentoperiosteal group.* This group arises from the root at the same level as the transseptal group but lies in the buccolingual plane. The fibres pass downwards over the alveolar crest and are inserted into the periosteum of the alveolus beneath the gingiva.

*Dentogingival group.* This group arises from the root surface above the alveolar crest and its fibres radiate out to be inserted into the lamina propria of the gingiva. The uppermost fibres curve upwards to lie beneath the crevicular epithelium, the middle group passes outwards almost horizontally while the lowermost course between the gingiva and alveolar bone and have been reported to extend sufficiently for them to terminate in close association with the facial musculature.

*Alveologingival group.* These fibres pass from the alveolar crest coronally into the overlying lamina propria.

*Circular group.* These fibres lie in the lamina propria of the gingiva coronal to the level of the alveolar crest and, as the name suggests, encircle the tooth. Some fibres are attached to cement, others to the alveolar crest. Circular fibres from one tooth may intermingle with those of the adjacent teeth.

*Interdental group.* These fibres pass longitudinally in the buccolingual plane within the lamina propria of the gingival papilla and may fan out at the buccal and lingual surfaces.

*Longitudinal and vertical gingival groups.* Longitudinal fibres extend in a mesiodistal direction throughout the whole extent of each dental arch and meet distal to the last molar tooth. They lie in the lamina propria of buccal and lingual gingiva a short distance below the gingival margin and may extend to the mucogingival junction. Vertical fibres arise in the alveolar mucosa or attached gingiva and pass coronally, the bundles frequently being traceable to the connective tissue of the marginal gingiva and interdental papilla.

*Semicircular group.* These fibres arise from the cement near the cement enamel junction, traverse the free (marginal) gingiva and insert into a comparable position on the opposite side of the tooth at a level just apical to the circular fibres.

*Transgingival group.* These fibres arise from the cement of one tooth and traverse the free marginal gingiva of an adjacent tooth. Some of the relationships between these fibre groups are indicated in Fig. 7.17.

In summary it can be seen that collagen fibres run in almost every possible direction between teeth and the tissues which contain them.

The relative inaccessibility of the periodontal ligament means that, as yet, there is little information concerning its chemical composition. Evidence suggests that in cattle, the total protein content of the periodontal ligament expressed for dry weight is about 80% with collagen accounting for about 48%, a slightly smaller figure being quoted for erupting teeth. Approximately 90% of periodontal ligament collagen is insoluble indicating that the rapid rate of collagen synthesis must be associated with a rapid rate of maturation into insoluble fibres.

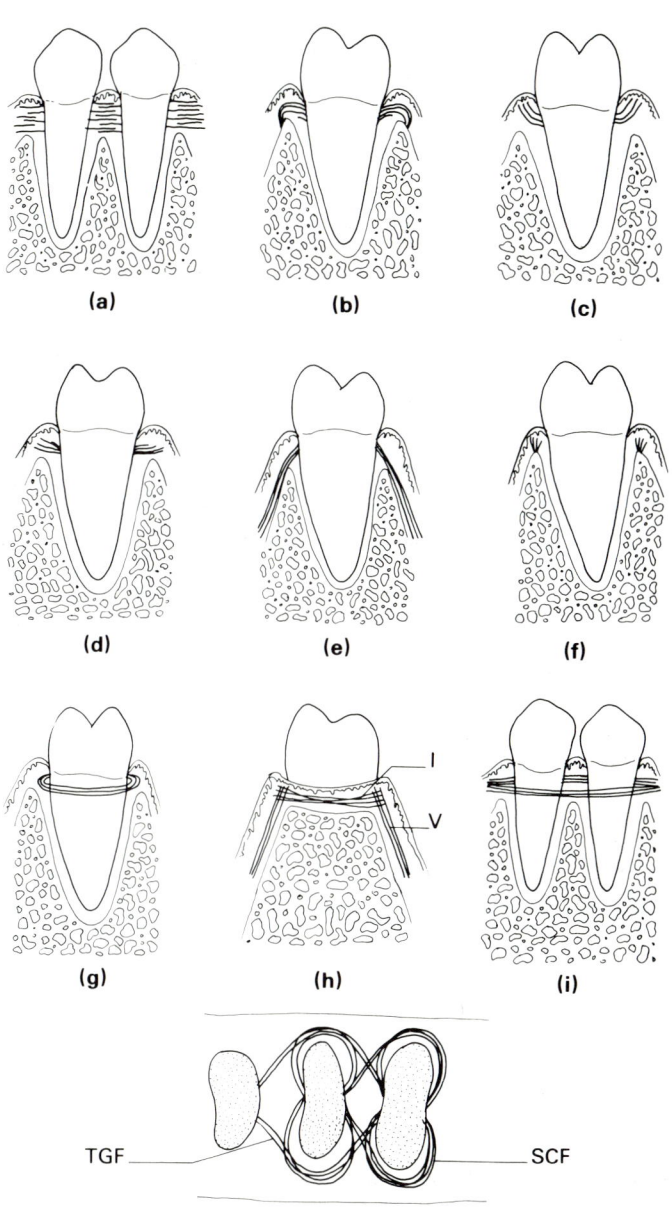

Fig. 7.16. Diagram to show the arrangement of the principal collagen fibre groups of the gingiva: (a) transseptal; (b) dentoperiosteal; (c, d, e) dentogingival; (f) alveologingival; (g) circular; (h) interdental (I) and vertical (V); (i) longitudinal; (j) semicircular (SCF) and transgingival (TGF).

## OXYTALAN FIBRES

Though collagen is the predominant fibre type in the periodontal ligament, the presence of an additional fibre type, oxytalan, which is more resistant to acid solution than is collagen, has recently been described. Oxytalan fibres at the light microscopic level can be distinguished from collagen by special staining techniques. An important stage in demonstrating oxytalan fibres involves an initial oxidation process.

Oxytalan fibres form a delicate network throughout the ligament, the diameter of the fibres varying but sometimes reaching values of the order of 5 μm. Characteristically, they are more numerous near the tooth than the alveolar bone and are said to reach densities of tens of thousands per square millimetre. They tend to be aligned parallel to the long axis of the tooth. The ends of some, but by no means all, of the oxytalan fibres are embedded in cement. However, only very rarely are they embedded in alveolar bone.

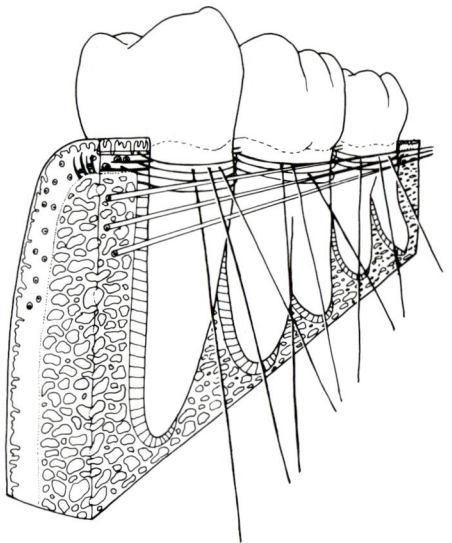

**Fig. 7.17.** Diagram showing the relationship between periodontal ligament and gingival fibres.

Collections of oxytalan fibres are present around blood and lymph vessels.

At the ultrastructural level the oxytalan fibre is readily distinguishable from collagen: oxytalan fibres are not banded and they consist of fibrils arranged parallel to the long axis of the fibre. Each fibril is approximately 15 nm in diameter and an interfibrillar, amorphous material is present in variable amounts.

Though easily distinguishable from collagen, oxytalan fibres are less readily distinguished from elastin fibres and even less so from pre-elastin fibres. Very little is known about the composition and function of oxytalan fibres. The observation that more and larger oxytalan fibres are observed around the necks of teeth in firm occlusion and around teeth used as bridge abutments (supporting false teeth) suggests that they may develop in response to stresses placed upon the teeth. Because they are often aligned close to blood vessels it has been hypothesized that the oxytalan system may be part of a mechanism that regulates blood flow. At present, however, the role of oxytalan fibres remains controversial.

ELASTIN AND RETICULIN FIBRES

These constitute the remaining fibres found in the periodontium. Elastin fibres in the human periodontal ligament are generally restricted to the walls of the blood vessels, though the ligament of some other mammals contains more elastin fibres. In these latter cases the distribution of elastin fibres is similar to that of oxytalan fibres in the human periodontal ligament. Reticulin fibres are related to basement membranes.

### Gel

The gel, which is presumed to be secreted by periodontal fibroblasts, consists mainly of glycosaminoglycan–protein complexes (proteoglycans) and water but also includes carbohydrates, lipids, proteins and glycoproteins. It is associated with many important functions which are, as yet, poorly understood: these include ion binding and ion exchange, water binding, control of collagen fibrogenesis and fibre orientation. Variation in the quality and quantity of the various constituents of the gel imparts different physical and chemical properties to different types of connective tissue.

Hyaluronic acid, chondroitin-4-sulphate, chondroitin-6-sulphate, dermatan sulphate and heparan sulphate have all been identified in the periodontal ligament. The ratio of sulphated glycosaminoglycans to hyaluronate is higher in young than adult humans; chondroitin sulphates decrease and dermatan sulphate increases with age. In cattle hyaluronic acid decreases relative to chondroitin sulphate following tooth eruption.

### Cells of the periodontal ligament

Cells covering the surface of both alveolar bone and cement are considered as an integral part of the periodontal ligament. The type of cell lining the surface of alveolar bone varies according to the activity prevalent at that particular time. Thus, if bone is being deposited, osteoblasts may form a conspicuous layer of cuboidal cells. In 'resting' bone the surface cells are more fusiform in shape. If bone is being resorbed then osteoclasts, which are generally large, multinucleated cells, can be seen lying in recesses termed Howship's lacunae. Cementoblasts overlie the cement of the root. Their shapes resemble those of osteoblasts and similarly vary in accordance with the rate of cementogenesis. When cement is resorbed, giant cells, apparently similar to osteoclasts and lying in resorption lacunae, are seen. Such cells are sometimes called cementoclasts.

FIBROBLASTS

The predominant connective tissue cell in the periodontal ligament, the fibroblast, secretes the collagen and gel. In tissues with a low turnover of collagen, such as tendons, the fibroblasts have reduced amounts of intracytoplasmic organelles. In this form they probably only maintain a minimal extracellular secretion and they are called fibrocytes. In the periodontal ligament, however, because of the rapid turnover of collagen, there is no such morphological separation into fibroblasts and fibrocytes. There is evidence that a single cell type, the fibroblast, is associated not only with the formation and maintenance of the connective tissue fibres and, presumably, the gel, but also with its resorption.

The morphology of periodontal fibroblasts can vary from being round in outline to fusiform (Fig. 7.18). Research in to the three-dimensional shape

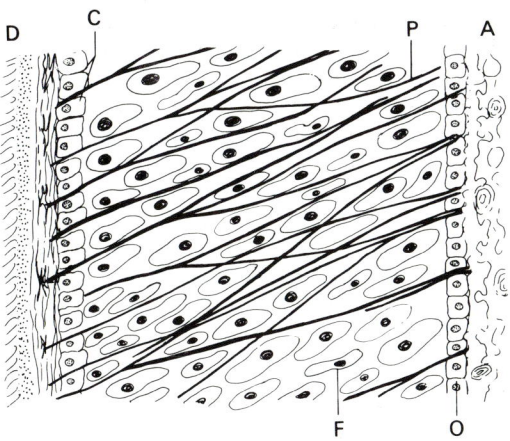

**Fig. 7.18.** Diagram showing the general disposition of some of the cells of the periodontal ligament. A, alveolar bone; C, cementoblasts; D, dentine; F, fibroblasts; O, osteoblasts; P, principal collagen fibres.

of periodontal fibroblasts suggests that they are disc-shaped with an irregular outline. Apart from the usual organelles, fibroblasts may also possess elongated, membrane-bound profiles containing collagen fibrils apparently undergoing dissolution: this is the evidence which indicates that the cell, in addition to secreting collagen, is also involved in resorbing it. It seems that a fibroblast phagocytoses a collagen fibril to form a phagosome: the phagosome fuses with a primary lysosome to become a phagolysosome within which the fibril is ultimately broken down. Acid and alkaline phosphatase activity have been observed within these collagen-containing phagolysosomes. It thus seems probable that a cell may be secreting collagen at one surface and resorbing it at another. The quality and quantity of intracytoplasmic organelles varies according to the metabolic activity within the ligament. These organelles are likely to be most conspicuous in young erupting teeth (and especially in teeth of continuous growth) and least conspicuous in old teeth which are not in occlusion. Cell contacts have been described between periodontal fibroblasts, namely desmosomes and gap junctions, though their functions are not understood.

EPITHELIAL CELLS (RESTS OF MALASSEZ)

Aggregations of epithelial cells surrounded by a basement membrane are regarded as a normal feature of the periodontal ligament: they are remnants of the epithelial root sheath (of Hertwig). In routine sections they may appear pseudotubular, cluster-like or in the form of strands, but tangential or serial sections show that much of this system is in the form of an epithelial network which parallels the long axis of the root (Fig. 7.19). The majority of epithelial cells lie close to the cement. A possible continuity has been described between epithelial cell rests and the reduced enamel epithelium before eruption and the junctional epithelium after eruption. The cells decrease in number with age.

Classifications of the epithelial cells have relied upon morphology and cellular activity. Accordingly, a small resting type, a profilerating type, a differentiating type and a degenerating type have been described. Differences have been observed in the distribution of epithelial cells according to site and age. During the 1st and 2nd decades they are more prevalent in the apical zone whereas between the 3rd and 7th decades the majority are located cervically in the gingiva above the alveolar crest. However, in the latter region they may be derived from epithelium associated with the gingival crevice. It seems that some epithelial cells proliferate (as evidenced by their uptake of the marker tritiated thymidine) while others degenerate, accounting for their reduced numbers with age. Histochemical and electron microscope studies reveal little activity in the epithelial cells in which case the term 'resting' may be appropriate. They may sometimes form a nidus for calcification, giving rise to small, localized calcifications termed cementicles.

The cell rests are clinically important because stimuli such as inflammation may trigger them to proliferate, ultimately to contribute to a cyst or granuloma. Those in the cervical region of the tooth may be important in certain phases of

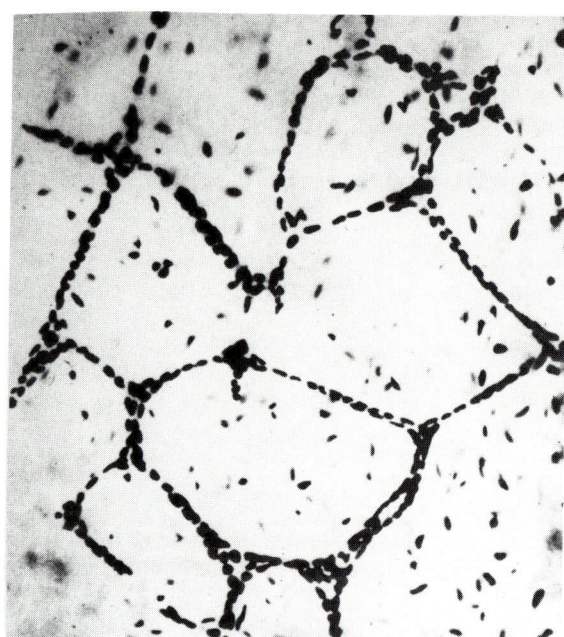

**Fig. 7.19.** Tangential section through the epithelial rests showing them to be in the form of an epithelial network.

periodontal disease. In tissue culture explants of the periodontal ligament, the cell rests have been induced to proliferate. The results show that epithelial cells proliferate in an atmosphere of high $CO_2$, low $O_2$ tension because of their ability to undertake anaerobic glycolysis.

OTHER CELL TYPES

In order to give rise to the various types of formative cells found in the periodontal ligament, progenitor (undifferentiated) mesenchyme cells are presumed to be present throughout the periodontal ligament. It is not known whether there is a separate progenitor type for each cell population.

Mast cells are present in varying concentrations within the periodontal ligament and can be identified by their characteristic cytoplasmic granules. Mast cells contain amongst other things heparin, histamine and serotonin. Their precise function is poorly understood.

Macrophages (defence cells) in the periodontal ligament are best demonstrated after the injection of foreign material such as carbon particles which are ingested by these cells. Inflammatory cells such as lymphocytes are almost always evident towards the cervical margin.

## Vascular supply

ARTERIES

The rich blood supply to the periodontal ligament is derived primarily from the appropriate superior and inferior dental arteries; cervically they anastomose with branches from other arteries (e.g. palatine and lingual arteries) which supply the gingiva. The periodontal arteries enter the ligament primarily as a series of perforating arteries through Volkmann's canals in the alveolar bone; branches entering at the apex have also been described (Fig. 7.20). The major vessels lie between the principal fibre bundles close to the wall of the alveolus and are said to have an average diameter of 20 $\mu$m. The vessels branch and anastomose to form a capillary plexus around the teeth. Glomeruli-like structures, said to be arteriovenous shunts, have been described within the ligament. Due to the diffuse origins of the arterial supply the periodontal ligament can survive following removal of the root apex.

In the region of the alveolar crest the vascular system is specialized. Here the vessels of the periodontal ligament anastomose with those of the encircling gingiva. From this vascular circle capillaries resembling renal glomeruli and arteriovenous shunts, are given off into the attached gingiva at regular intervals. The function of these gingival glomeruli is not clear; they may be required to maintain the integrity of the junctional epithelium. The onset of periodontal disease is accompanied by changes in this vascular bed. Such an arrangement of gingival rete is not present in continuously growing teeth.

The following information is based on the assumption that perforations in the alveolar walls

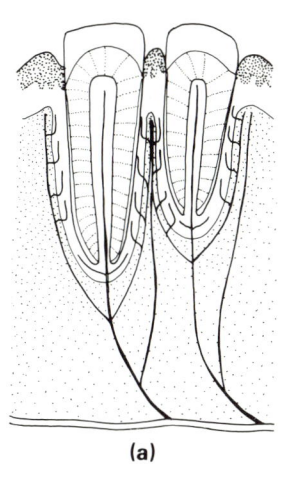
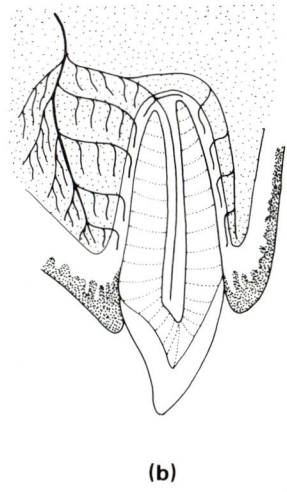
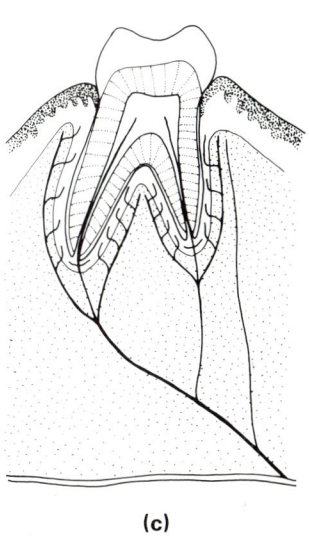

**Fig. 7.20.** Diagram of the distribution pattern of the arteries to the periodontal ligament in (a) single rooted teeth of the lower jaw, (b) single rooted teeth of the upper jaw and (c) molar teeth. [From Hayashi S. (1932) Untersuchungen über die arterielle Blutversorgung des Periodontiums. *Deutsche Monatsschrift für Zahnheilkunde* **50**, 145.]

of human teeth indicate the distribution of arteries supplying the periodontal ligament:

1  The blood supply increases gradually along the jaw towards the molar teeth (there is a close similarity in supply between equivalent teeth in upper and lower jaws).
2  In single-rooted teeth the blood supply is greatest in the cervical third, less in the apical third and least in the middle third; in multirooted teeth the supply is equal in the middle and apical thirds.
3  The mesial and distal surfaces have a slightly better supply than the buccal and lingual surfaces, but the difference is small.

4  For lower molars the blood supply is less for the distal than for the mesial root.

Variations in the distribution of blood vessels presumably indicate differences in the requirements of different regions.

### VEINS, LYMPHATICS AND TISSUE FLUID

Less is known about the distribution of veins and lymphatics within the periodontal ligament. The veins generally accompany the arteries. Networks of veins are especially prominent beneath the attached epithelium, at the root apex and in the bifurcation area of multi-rooted teeth. Veins also pass through the alveolar walls into intra-alveolar venous networks. Lymph capillaries originate as blind endings within the ligament and connect with the lymph vessels which may continue in three directions; over the alveolar crest into the submucosa, through the alveolar bone or through the root apex.

Human incisor teeth at rest undergo small pulsatile displacements from the neutral position towards the labial side synchronous with the arterial pulse; the displacement is of the order of 0.4 $\mu$m with a much smaller axial component. Tissue fluid pressure within the periodontal ligament appears to be about 10 mm Hg above atmospheric, a figure higher than that recorded for most body situations. Whether this relatively high tissue fluid pressure is associated with the mechanism of tooth support and/or eruption is not known.

One study described short-term tissue fluid pressure changes within the periodontal ligament when abnormal (and apparently increased) loads were placed on a tooth. After 2 days, tissue fluid pressures were almost double the control values of 10 mm Hg; in light microscopic sections, however, the ligament presented a normal or near normal histological appearance.

**Nerves**

The nerves supplying the periodontal ligament come from the appropriate superior and inferior dental nerves, while the gingiva receives additional nerves (palatine, lingual and buccal nerves).

Nerves enter the periodontal ligament from two directions. Some enter at the apex of the root and pass up through the periodontal ligament. Others enter the middle and cervical portions of the ligament through openings in the alveolar walls. Both large and small diameter nerve fibres are present, the larger fibres being myelinated and the smaller ones being myelinated or non-myelinated. The apex is especially richly supplied with nerves.

The periodontal ligament is thought to possess nociceptors and mechanoreceptors. For example, pain is produced by piercing the periodontal ligament or when teeth contact an unexpected hard object in the food during chewing. The discharge of afferent impulses from mechanoreceptors has been recorded from nerve fibres dissected free from the dental nerves: the discharge varies according to the direction and amplitude of the displacing force. Some mechanoreceptors adapt rapidly to a maintained stimulus (Fig. 7.21a) whereas others continue to discharge for long periods (Fig. 7.21b). The sites of the nerve endings involved have not been precisely determined. Although specialized nerve endings have been demonstrated histologically by some authors, and electrophysiological experiments on animals have shown that endings of the mechanoreceptor type can be excited by mechanical stimulation of the teeth, there is no irrefutable evidence that the histological and electrophysiological studies are dealing with the same endings. For example, some of the mechanoreceptors could be situated in the alveolar bone and periosteum.

Several differently shaped nerve endings have been described. There is general agreement that the ligament contains a rich supply of branching and coiled 'free nerve endings'. However, there is less agreement about more specialized endings. Thus, some authors report no specialized endings while others simply note 'knob-like' swellings at the ends of nerves. An electron microscope study appears to show two main types of specialized nerve endings: (a) simple mechanoreceptors of approximately $10 \times 10$ $\mu$m, consisting of single, myelinated nerve fibres surrounded by cell bodies (not of nerves) and terminating as encapsulated unmyelinated nerve fibres; (b) compound mechanoreceptors, approximately $35 \times 45$ $\mu$m, consisting of encapsulated, myelinated nerve fibres which lose their myelin sheaths and encircle the adjacent myelinated nerve fibres; a cluster of compound mechanoreceptors may form a complex about 100–150 $\mu$m wide. An arterial system seems to supply nutrition for the compound receptors whilst an arcade of veins surrounds the neural complex (Fig. 7.22). However, further work is necessary before such structures can be identified with certainty as mechanoreceptor nerve endings.

Many problems face the investigator studying the mechanisms which control blood flow in the periodontal ligament and for this reason little is known about the subject. There is some evidence to support the view that sympathetic vasoconstrictor fibres may be involved. If this is so it remains to be discovered whether such nerves enter the periodontal ligament as a plexus around the vessels or are incorporated with the dental nerves.

**Turnover of connective tissue components**

Two aspects of turnover can be considered: passive turnover which involves breakdown of the

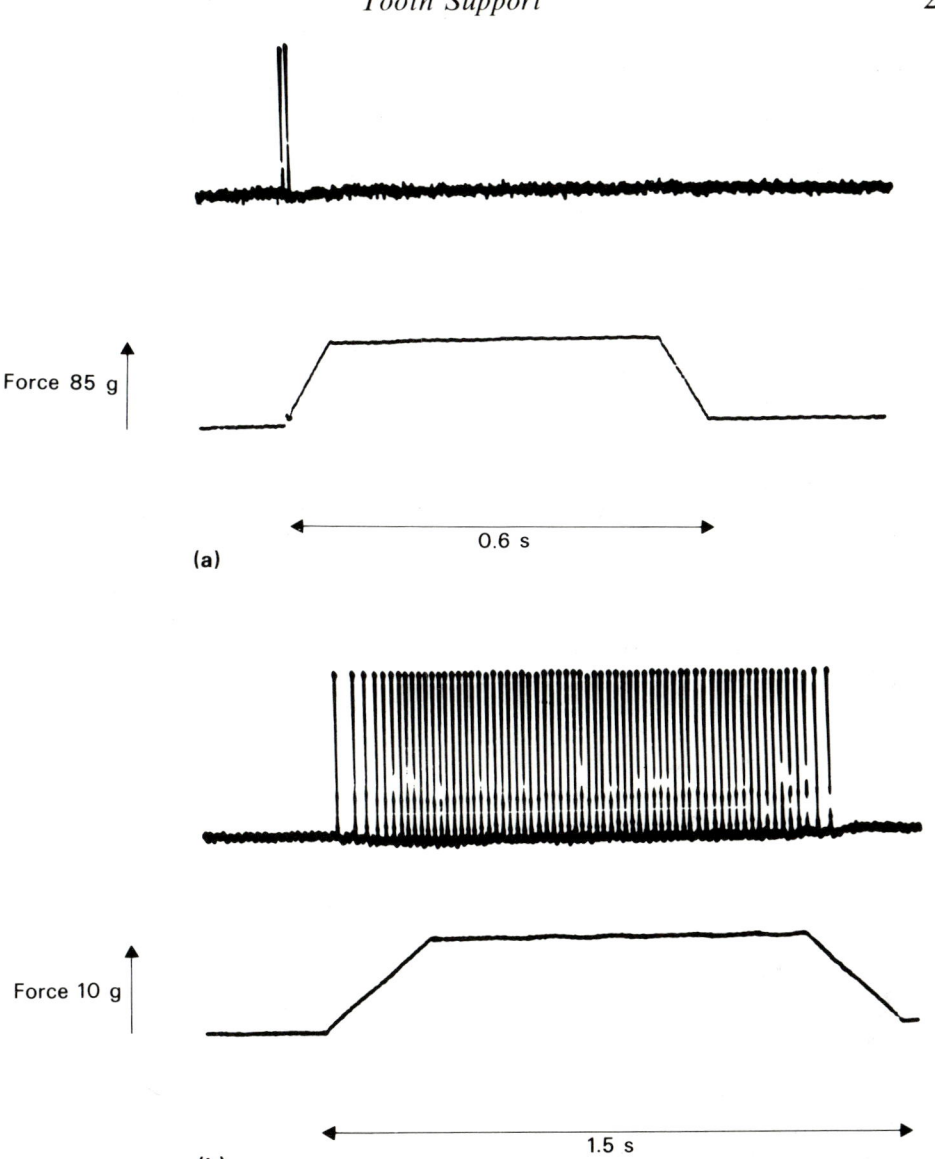

**Fig. 7.21.** Examples of the responses of single periodontal mechanoreceptors. The upper trace in each case represents the response and the lower trace represents the force applied to the teeth: (a) rapidly adapting unit; (b) slowly adapting unit.

older molecules and their replacement by identical but newly synthesized ones without any corresponding alteration in tissue structure, and remodelling in which shape and structure are modified probably in response to function. In the periodontal ligament both processes occur but cannot readily be separated.

COLLAGEN

Turnover of collagen is appropriately studied by assessing the quantities of labelled hydroxyproline which can be recovered from a tissue. However, this is difficult for periodontal ligament, where usually only small amounts of tissue can be obtained. Hence an alternative approach has involved quantitative autoradiography of tissue sections following injection of tritiated proline or glycine on the assumption that these substances will be incorporated into newly-synthesized collagen. However, proline and glycine are also incorporated into non-collagenous elements of

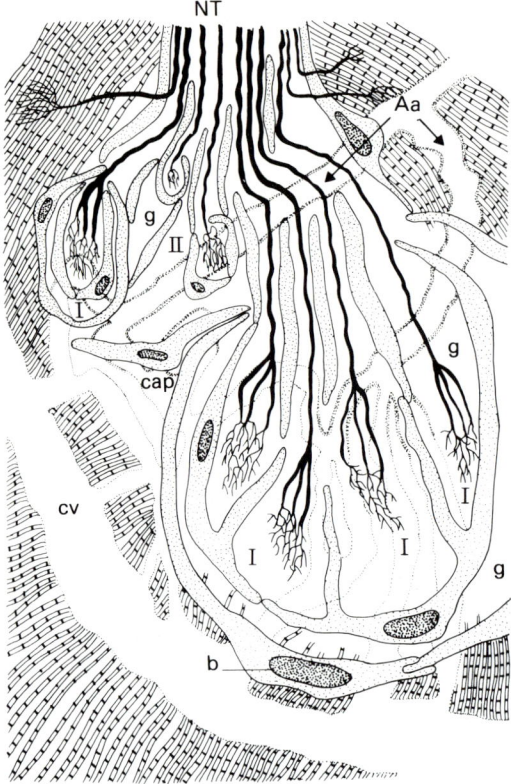

**Fig. 7.22.** Diagram showing periodontal neural tissue. I, Compound mechanoreceptors occurring singly or forming a cluster (complex); II, Simple mechanoreceptor. NT, distal part of periodontal nerve trunk; Aa, afferent arteriole; cv, collecting vein; cap, capillary system; b, cell bodies and processes of capsular cells forming a reticulum; g, ground substance; f, dense fibrous tissue. [From Griffin C. J. & Harris R. (1974) Innervation of human periodontium. I. Classification of periodontal receptors. *Australian Dental Journal* **19**, 51.]

the periodontal ligament such as the gel. In an attempt to distinguish labelled collagen from labelled non-collagenous components, control sections have been treated with collagenase. The evidence suggests that a considerable amount of the label is incorporated into collagen and the following data have been obtained.

Collagen turnover within the periodontal ligament is faster than in most other connective tissues; it appears faster in the young than in adults and can vary in different parts of the ligament. In the fully-erupted molars of growing rats, collagen half-lives have been reported of $6\frac{1}{2}$, $4\frac{1}{2}$ and $2\frac{1}{4}$ days in the alveolar crest, mid-root and apical areas respectively. Other studies report a collagen half-life of 3 days (continuously erupting guinea pig molars), 5 days (continuously erupting rabbit molars), 20 days (marmoset molars) and 23 days (mouse molars). By quantifying labelled hydroxyproline, it has been proposed that, for the rat, the half-life for periodontal collagen in the molar is about 1 day compared with 3 days for the continuously growing incisor. This indicates that such turnover rates are not directly related to rates of axial tooth eruption.

Fibroblasts of the periodontal ligament take up $S^{35}$-sulphate, a precursor of glycosaminoglycans, which is rapidly transferred to the extracellular compartment. This label disappears from the tissues within a month, indicating a rapid turnover of at least some components of the gel.

The mechanism whereby the periodontal ligament supports the tooth and yet also allows it to move has still to be elucidated: the problem is especially difficult to understand during the rapid phase of tooth eruption. Though some authors suggest that the alveolar portion of the ligament may have a higher turnover rate than the cemental portion, quantitative (autoradiographic) studies indicate that the rate of collagen turnover is about equal throughout the whole width of the periodontal ligament in any particular zone, a finding which tends to invalidate the concept of an intermediate plexus. Rather, it suggests that tooth movement is associated with reorganization of the full width of the ligament. Even with full-width remodelling, with the exception of cementoblasts, it is not known what portion of the periodontal ligament moves with the tooth during eruption. However, in the case of the continuously growing rodent incisor, the view has been forwarded that the cemental part of the ligament moves with the tooth and the alveolar part remaining stationary. This implies a zone of tissue shear between the two parts of the ligament (the modified view of an intermediate plexus described above).

In addition to the extracellular components, the cells of the periodontal ligament are also replaced. This is indicated by studies which show that some cells, presumably undifferentiated mesenchyme cells, take up tritiated thymidine. Later they may give rise to new protein synthesizing cells of the ligament. With increasing age there is a decrease in the number of cells synthesizing DNA (i.e. the cells taking up tritiated thymidine).

Turnover of the connective tissue elements of the periodontal ligament may be necessary to allow teeth to move: the following is an account of

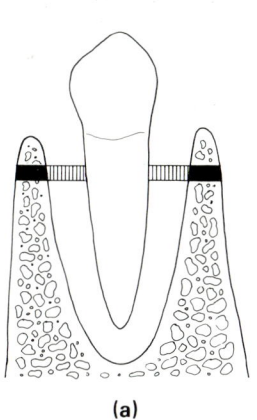

**Fig. 7.23.** Schematic diagram illustrating the possible histological changes associated with drift. (a) Before drift: periodontal ligament fibres indicated by vertical lines and adjacent collagen fibres in bone by solid black line. (b) After drift: original outline is dotted in. On the side towards which the teeth are moving (traditionally termed the pressure side) bone matrix fibres are continually exposed from the resorbing surface and become incorporated within the periodontal ligament some of whose original fibres are lost during remodelling to maintain normal thickness; continued bone deposition at a deeper level incorporates new collagen (clear zone). On the side away from which the teeth are moving (traditionally termed the tension side) bone deposition progressively incorporates the outer fibres of the periodontal ligament, requiring remodelling to add fibres (horizontal lines) to maintain a normal width of ligament. [Modified from Kraw A. G. & Enlow D.H. (1967) Continuous attachment of the periodontal membrane. *American Journal of Anatomy* **120**, 133.]

the possible histological changes associated with drift (or movement in the horizontal plane) of teeth (Fig. 7.23). On the side towards which the teeth are moving the alveolar bone is resorbed, its surface being pitted with scalloped concavities containing osteoclasts. In areas close to vascular bundles entering the bone, the principal fibres of the periodontal ligament are destroyed. In other areas, however, resorption of the alveolar wall leaves behind a trail of undisturbed collagen fibres that were once a component part of the bone matrix, but which become progressively uncovered as the inorganic bone crystals are removed. These uncovered fibres are, by definition, now contained in the periodontal ligament. The bone underlying resorbing surfaces is often extensively (internally) remodelled. On the opposite alveolar bone surface, away from which the tooth is moving, the reverse is happening. Thus, the successive layers of new bone deposited by osteoblasts incorporates the peripheral fibres of the periodontal ligament which become new Sharpey's fibres of attachment.

Apart from physiological drift, teeth can be made to move by the controlled application of forces generated, for example, by metal springs. Such treatment is the basis of orthodontics. Ideally, the tissue changes should be kept within the limits of those developed during physiological drift. When sufficient force is applied to a tooth to cause it to move, one surface of the alveolar bone is resorbed, traditionally referred to as the 'pressure' side, while on the opposite or 'tension' side bone is deposited. The terms 'pressure' and 'tension' should not be used in a functional sense since no studies have been carried out to determine whether, or for how long, the components of the periodontal ligament are under pressure or tension during force application. Orthodontically-produced tooth movement can be distinguished histologically from physiological drift by the appearance of a hyalinized (clear, structureless) zone within the periodontal ligament on the 'pressure' side, the degree and duration of hyalinization probably being related directly to the amount of force. The hyalinized zone is a localized, sterile, necrotic area. The cells in this area gradually break down and the normal fibrocellular structure becomes replaced by a homogenous, acellular mass. The hyalinized tissue is later invaded and replaced by cells and vessels proliferating from the adjacent periodontal ligament. The necrotic tissue of the hyalinized zone is removed by cells which include macrophages and foreign body, giant cells. Eventually a normal appearance is re-established within the periodontal ligament. The precise stimulus for the bone activity observed during tooth movement is not known though it probably involves changes in the microenvironment. One possibility is piezoelectric effects. Another is changes in the pH of the tissue fluid following constriction of vessels on the 'pressure' side and dilation on the 'tension' side.

**Functions of the periodontal ligament**

These are primarily related to tooth support.
1  Its cells are responsible for the formation and maintenance of cement and the tooth attachment surface of alveolar bone.
2  By the turnover of its components, especially collagen fibres, it probably allows for tooth movement and adjustments to changing functions.
3  Its sensory nerves probably transmit information which is especially important for the control of mastication.
4  It appears to be responsible for generating the eruptive force though the precise mechanism has not been elucidated (p. 310).

In its supportive role the periodontal ligament maintains the relation of the teeth to the surrounding hard and soft tissues. By limiting the movements of teeth during mastication it protects the tissues at sites of pressure. Studies on tooth mobility in both the axial and horizontal directions indicate that similar mechanisms support the tooth in both cases. It is found that there is no simple linear relationship between tooth displacement and the applied force. When force is suddenly applied to a tooth there is an initial rapid displacement followed by a slow creep phase. Similarly, when the load is removed, there is an initial rapid recovery followed by a slower creep back to the first position. This non-linear response to loading implies that more than one mechanism is involved in tooth support and the view that tensioning of the principal collagen fibres of the ligament provides the sole support is no longer tenable. If tension alone were responsible, axial loading would be expected to pull inwards the alveolar margins as the tooth was pushed into the socket; in fact the margins are pushed out, presumably by tissue fluid expelled from the ligament by the intruding tooth. Since the periodontal ligament under load is neither perfectly elastic nor perfectly viscous but acts as a complex of the two, it is said to be visco-elastic. It seems likely that during mastication tooth movement is resisted by compression of the periodontal ligament. In the case of the rat incisor, for example, it has been postulated that there are three phases in tooth support: (a) by the interstitial fluid acting as a squeeze film; (b) by the creation of cirsoid aneurysms resulting from the strangulation of vessels by displaced collagen fibres (in the walls of which are heteroporosities through which fluid passes under high pressure); (c) by diffusion of fluid through the walls of the vessels as they are subjected to increased pressure by the displaced root.

From studies on tooth mobility in monkeys, which involved cutting collagen fibres with a blade, there is evidence that areas of the periodontal ligament under 'tension' and areas under 'compression' are of approximately equal importance in supporting a tooth. The function of collagen in the support mechanism is still unclear: however, following administration of drugs which prevent cross-linking of collagen (e.g. lathyrogens), teeth become loosened in their sockets and developing roots may become distorted due to their impaction into the bone by occlusal forces which the weakened periodontal ligament cannot support.

When a vasoconstrictor (noradrenaline) is injected locally around the incisor teeth of monkeys the mobility of teeth is decreased. This suggests that the vascular-tissue fluid system is involved in the tooth support mechanism: it may also aid in the subsequent recovery of the tooth. However, these and other views must remain theoretical until more information is available concerning the reactions of the components of the periodontal ligament under load.

**Clinical features**

Certain conditions, such as gingival inflammation, can lead to destructive changes within the periodontal ligament and adjacent alveolar bone, resulting in an increased tooth mobility which, unless suitably treated, eventually leads to tooth loss. In such situations, the collagen appears to be destroyed by bacterial collagenases.

The effects on the supporting tissues which result from lack of function (i.e. due to extraction of opposing teeth) are not yet clear. One view suggests that the principal fibres of the periodontal ligament become considerably disorganized with accompany loss of alveolar bone. An alternative view is that the changes are far less obvious and important.

Though the periodontal ligament lies sandwiched between two calcified tissues, it is only rarely calcified. This might be due to the nature of the collagen or gel or to the presence of inhibitors of calcification. The rare condition in which alveolar bone is in 'bony' continuity with cement is termed ankylosis. Tooth ankylosis has been reported following traumatic injury to the teeth and their supporting structures. Experimentally, ankylosis may be produced following reimplantation of teeth, thermal injury to the periodontium, root canal treatment and high crown placement. Occasionally teeth remain, or become, 'submerged' in alveolar bone. Sometimes these teeth are ankylosed but whether the ankylosis is a cause or an effect of the condition is not known.

In the case of reimplantated and transplanted teeth, considerable importance is attached to retaining portions of the periodontal ligament on the tooth. In the absence of periodontal ligament, the tooth becomes attached by ankylosis. Apparently a gomphosis can only develop if some original periodontal tissue is present. Thus, in one human study, teeth which were to be reimplanted were first cultured for at least 1 week so as to permit the attached periodontal ligament cells to proliferate. Following their reimplantation, these teeth became surrounded by a normal supporting apparatus rather than an ankylosis (judged by radiographs).

## GINGIVA

Changes in knowledge and understanding of the structure and physiology of tissues at the dentogingival junction, during the last 50 years, have led to some problems in terminology. Current knowledge relating to the dentogingival junction has been reviewed critically (Schröeder & Listgarten 1971) and the terminology proposed is used here.

The oral mucosa can be divided into three zones: the gingiva and covering of the hard palate, often called the masticatory mucosa; the dorsum of the tongue covered by specialized mucosa; and the remaining zones covered by lining mucous membrane.

The gingiva is the part of the oral mucosa which surrounds the necks of the teeth and alveolar processes of the jaws (Fig. 7.24). It is limited coronally by the gingival margin and apically by the mucogingival junction. Internally it is limited by the dentoperiosteal fibre bundles (Fig. 7.16c). Studies of adolescent human gingiva have shown that it comprises about 31% epithelium and 69% connective tissue. Approximately 75% (by weight) of gingiva is water. The gingival epithelium can be divided into three zones (Fig. 7.25):
1 Oral epithelium extending from the mucogingival junction to the gingival margin (i.e. the imaginary line passing through the most coronal aspect of the gingiva);
2 Oral sulcular epithelium lining the gingival sulcus. The gingival sulcus is the shallow groove surrounding each tooth, which is limited coronally by the sulcular orifice and apically by the free surface of the junctional epithelium. The oral sulcular epithelium morphologically resembles the oral epithelium.
3 Junctional epithelium attaching the gingiva to the tooth. The actual junction of this epithelium to the tooth surface is termed the epithelial attachment. The most coronal extension of the junctional epithelium, which lines the bottom of the gingival sulcus, is its free surface and is the surface from which cells desquamate.

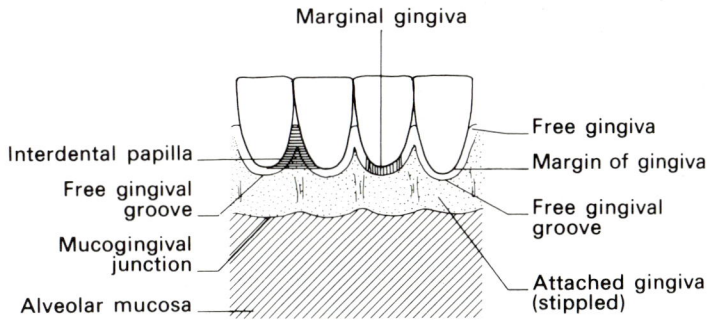

**Fig. 7.24.** Terminology of gingival tissues.

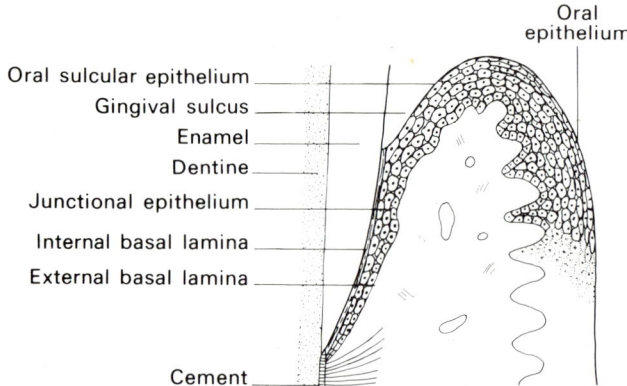

**Fig. 7.25.** Diagrammatic representation of the dentogingival junction.

## Normal clinical features

In health the gingiva is pink, firm, stippled to a variable degree and scalloped to conform to the contour of the underlying alveolar process and teeth (Fig. 7.24). The colour depends on the vascular supply, the level of keratinization and thickness of the epithelium, and the presence of pigment-containing cells. In dark-skinned individuals physiological melanin pigmentation may be present as patches, or more diffuse areas, of brown to purplish colouration.

The gingiva can be divided into free and attached regions.

### FREE GINGIVA

The free gingiva extends from the gingival margin, to the base of the gingival sulcus. In man, the gingival margin is generally slightly rounded. Clinically, a shallow furrow can usually be found between the gingival margin and the enamel surface. This is the orifice of the sulcus. The clinical gingival sulcus (1–3 mm) is usually deeper than the histological gingival sulcus (0–2 mm) depending on the type of periodontal probe used and the pressure exerted during probing.

The margin of the gingiva, like the enamel–cement junction, follows an undulating course around the tooth, the interdental part being the most occlusally located. In the anterior part of the mouth, where the contact area between teeth is small, the interdental gingiva may form a pyramid. Between posterior teeth, and on occasion between anterior teeth, particularly in children where the teeth have not fully erupted, the interdental gingiva may consist of two papillae, one facial and one oral to the contact area. In such circumstances the interdental gingival margin is saddle-shaped in the facial oral direction, and is termed the interdental 'col' (Fig. 7.26). The free gingiva is generally smooth as opposed to stippled (Fig. 7.27).

### ATTACHED GINGIVA

The attached gingiva extends from the coronal border of the free gingiva to the mucogingival junction. In approximately 50% of cases the free gingiva is demarcated from the attached gingiva by the gingival groove, which is a shallow V-shaped depression running parallel to the gingival margin and at a variable distance from it (0.5–2.0 mm: i.e. the depth of the gingival sulcus). The gingival groove is an inconstant feature, whose presence is thought to be dependent on the arrangement of the principal collagen fibre bundles running from cervical cement to the free and attached gingiva. The attached gingiva is firmly bound down to alveolus and cervical cement by collagen fibres, and to enamel by the junctional epithelium. Unlike the free gingiva, the

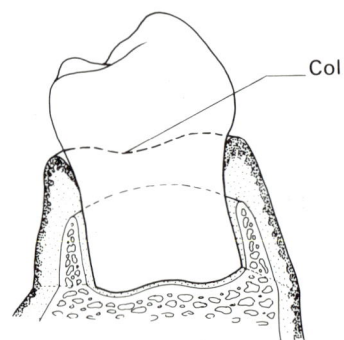

**Fig. 7.26.** Mesial view of a lower first molar showing the col.

attached gingiva is stippled, having a surface resembling orange peel. The stippling is produced by elevations and depressions of the surface, which relate to the configuration of the underlying epithelial–connective tissue junction. Stippling may vary between and within individuals, and also with age. The attached gingiva varies in width, both within and between individuals. In some areas it may be 1 mm or less whilst in others it may be 6–8 mm wide, it is usually widest in the maxillary anterior region.

## Structural features of gingiva

The gingiva consists essentially of a central lamina propria of collagenous connective tissue covered by stratified squamous epithelium, which shows differing levels of keratinization.

### LAMINA PROPRIA

The lamina propria of the gingiva comprises about 54% collagen fibres and 46% intercellular substance, cells, vessels and nerves. On the basis of total extractable hydroxyproline, normal human gingiva has been reported to contain 2.2% salt-soluble collagen and 4.5% acid-soluble collagen. Using $^{14}$C-proline it has been shown by autoradiography that collagen turnover in the marmoset is extremely rapid when compared with other connective tissues, i.e. skin, palate and tendon of the same animal. Reticulin fibres are found in a network around vessels, in the subepithelial connective tissue, with a few branching fibres running throughout the lamina propria. Although there are numerous elastic fibres in the connective tissue of alveolar mucosa, there are few in gingiva. Those present are usually in the connective tissue underlying oral rather than junctional epithelium. The oxytalan fibre (so named because it resists acid digestion) may be a young elastic fibre and it can also be demonstrated in gingiva following special staining; its specific function is unknown.

Anchoring fibrils have recently been described in gingival connective tissue and are found closely related to the basal lamina separating the lamina propria from the epithelium. They are short, curved fibrils 20–40 nm thick which fan out into filaments as they near the lamina densa. They seem to traverse the lamina densa and lamina lucida in the vicinity of the hemidesmosomes of the basal keratocytes. The fibrils may thus aid anchorage of the epithelium to the underlying connective tissue.

*Gingival fibre bundles*
The lamina propria of the gingiva contains a system of collagen fibre-bundle groups which, by stabilizing the gingiva against the tooth and alveolar bone, are thought to provide the rigidity necessary to withstand the forces of mastication. These fibre bundles have been observed by conventional light microscopy (Fig. 7.16). Future studies using the scanning electron microscope should increase knowledge and understanding of these fibre-bundle groups because with this instrument they can be viewed in three dimensions.

During the early stages of gingival inflammation, marked pathological changes can be noted in these fibre bundles and there is a substantial reduction in the quantity of collagen present. Changes are also apparent in neighbouring fibroblasts.

*Mast cells and leucocytes*
Mast cells are distributed throughout the body and are quite numerous in the gingiva. They contain a variety of biologically active substances such as histamine, heparin, proteolytic and other enzymes, which probably play a role in tissue maintenance and repair. Macrophages and occasional lymphocytes and plasma cells are also present in gingival connective tissue and are part of the defence mechanism of the host. They are most commonly seen in the connective tissue adjacent to the base of the gingival sulcus, often as perivascular foci.

### GINGIVAL EPITHELIUM

The gingiva is covered with stratified squamous epithelium. In man the oral epithelium of the attached and free gingiva is of the keratinizing type (Fig. 7.27). The junctional epithelium does not keratinize, neither does the adjacent oral sulcular epithelium. The aspect of the sulcular epithelium adjacent to the oral epithelium of the free gingiva, shows a limited tendency to keratinize.

*Oral epithelium*
The oral epithelium of the gingiva is thicker than the junctional or sulcular epithelium, and is fairly uniform in thickness. The underside of oral epithelium is characterized by a series of ridges of varying depth and thickness, which surround the interdigitating connective tissue papillae. The two tissues are separated by a basal lamina and the general arrangement gives a greatly increased surface area to facilitate diffusion of oxygen and nutrients into the epithelium as well as stability to

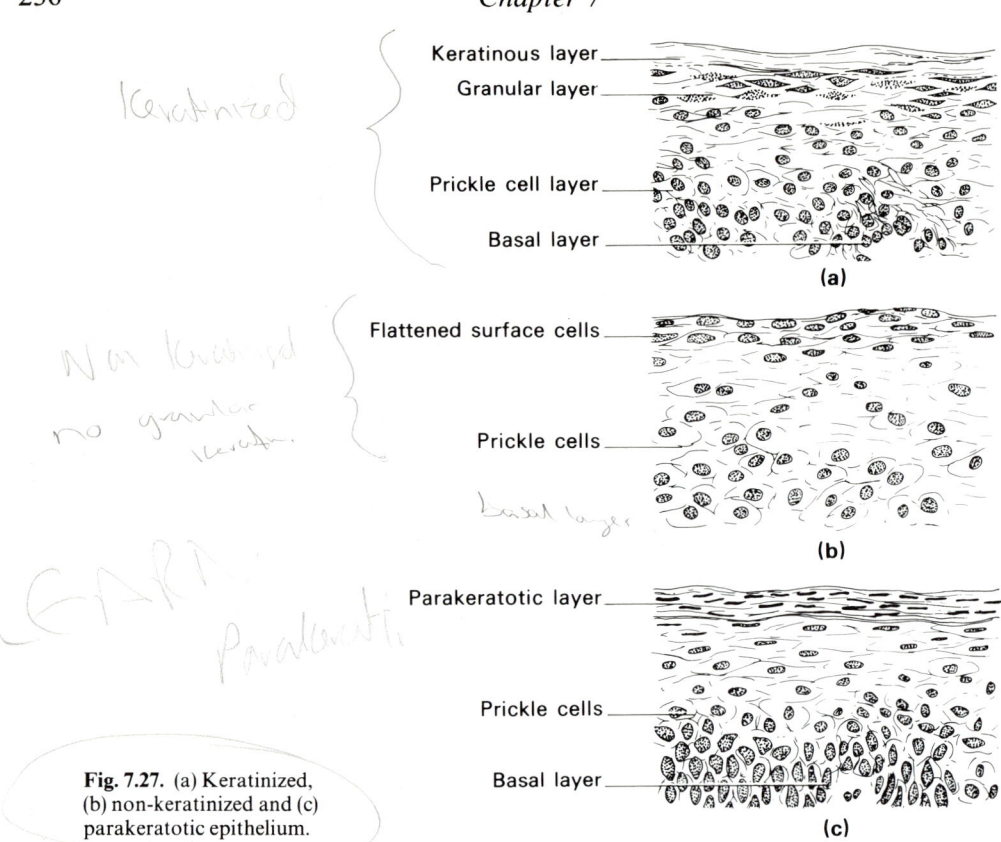

**Fig. 7.27.** (a) Keratinized, (b) non-keratinized and (c) parakeratotic epithelium.

resist separation, particularly from shearing forces.

The general arrangement and ultrastructural features of the oral epithelium of gingiva, the special junctions between neighbouring cells, and their attachment to the basal lamina are basically the same as those described for oral mucosa (Book 1). The stratum spinosum makes up the major part of the tissue. Superficial to this are several layers of flattened cells with keratohyalin granules in their cytoplasm (stratum granulosum). The cornified surface layer is composed of greatly flattened and densely packed cells containing keratin. In some specimens neither nucleus nor cell organelles can be seen and such complete maturation is termed orthokeratinization (Fig. 7.27a). In human gingival epithelium quite frequently this process does not go to completion. The nucleus remains visible in the cornified layer, which is less well defined, as is the granular layer. This is termed parakeratinization (Fig. 7.27c). The most superficial cells are lost by desquamation although the precise mechanism by which the desmosomes rupture is not known.

A regular feature of oral epithelium is the presence of melanocytes. As gingiva is variably exposed to sunlight it may be possible that melanosomes serve a function in addition to protection from ultraviolet radiation.

*Oral sulcular epithelium*

The characteristics of the sulcular epithelium vary according to the part of the sulcus being studied (Fig. 7.25). The epithelium lining the coronal aspect of the sulcus is similar to the oral epithelium of the gingiva, but usually a less complete level of keratinization is achieved. The epithelium lining the deeper aspect of the gingival sulcus has many features similar to those of the junctional epithelium (see below). The sulcular epithelium is probably less permeable than junctional epithelium, but more permeable than the orthokeratinized oral epithelium, which is also thicker.

*Junctional epithelium*

Junctional epithelium in man is a stratified squamous epithelium from 10–20 cells thick which does not keratinize. It has some features in common with oral epithelium but cytologically the two epithelia are quite distinct. Junctional epithelium consists of a basal layer of cuboidal or slightly flattened keratocytes with no melanocytes. The basal cells are attached to the underlying connective tissue by hemidesmosomes (Fig. 8.42) and a basal lamina but, in contrast to oral epithelium, the border between epithelium and lamina propria does not have a series of interdigitating epithelial ridges and connective tissue papillae, being relatively flat. Anchoring fibrils are, however, present in the underlying connective tissue. A stratum granulosum and stratum corneum are absent; thus the bulk of junctional epithelium consists of prickle cells which are elongated with their long axis parallel to the tooth surface. In contrast to oral epithelium, the prickle cells and basal cells of junctional epithelium have a more prominent and better developed endoplasmic reticulum and golgi apparatus. Fewer and less dense aggregations of tonofilaments are seen and the number of desmosomes is reduced. The intercellular space is wider and neutrophil polymorphonuclear leucocytes are occasionally dispersed throughout the width of the junctional epithelium. Lysosome-like bodies may also be identified in the intercellular zone. Occasionally a lymphocyte or monocyte may be seen. Such leucocytes can be found in the epithelium lining other parts of the alimentary canal and represent an important part of the host defence system.

The junctional epithelial cells facing the tooth surface are characterized by hemidesmosomes at intervals along their plasma membranes and attach the epithelium to the enamel crystallites via a basal lamina. The basal lamina at the dentogingival junction, in contrast to that between oral epithelium and gingival connective tissue, does not have an obvious lamina lucida. It is relatively electron dense and its overall thickness is similar to the combined widths of the lamina lucida and lamina densa beneath oral epithelium and other basal laminae.

Junctional epithelium may be attached to enamel, afibrillar or fibrillar cement, dental cuticle or dentine. The structure of the attachment is similar in all instances. It thus seems clear that the basal lamina is a product of the epithelial cells and that if keratinization took place, the concomitant loss of intracellular organelles would remove the machinery for production of the basal lamina.

The biological seal provided by the epithelial attachment is essential for maintaining the health of the host tissue. The health deteriorates following the multiplication and extension in an apical direction of microorganisms in dental plaque; the effect is to damage the epithelial attachment thereby extending the gingival sulcus into a pathological pocket. The teeth are eventually lost because of irreversible damage to the periodontium unless appropriate treatment is instituted to halt deepening of the pocket.

Following complete surgical removal of junctional epithelium a new non-keratinized junctional epithelium and epithelial attachment re-forms. Regeneration presumably takes place from the oral epithelium. Junctional epithelium grown in a chamber embedded in a subcutaneous site, away from its normal environment, regains its capacity to keratinize. Thus it seems that the morphological characteristics which are so essential for epithelial attachment to enamel and which distinguish junctional from oral epithelium are determined by environmental factors (phenotype) rather than being genetically determined (genotype). In the case of non-keratinized alveolar mucosa, current evidence suggests that the connective tissue determines the properties of the ectoderm and that it is this mesoderm which is genetically determined.

**Dentogingival junction**

The previous description of oral sulcular and junctional epithelium derives from recent work in which plastic-embedded specimens of human teeth and gingiva have been studied using the electron microscope. It greatly clarifies and replaces the differing and controversial views put forward in the past 150 years, and illustrates the beneficial impact of new technology on old and important problems. Dentists regularly probe the dentogingival junction to assess the state of periodontal health or disease, and restorations are frequently placed in this area. A sound knowledge of its structure and physiology is thus essential.

Up to 1921, although literature relating to the dentogingival junction was limited, there seemed to be general agreement that a definite space separated gingival epithelium and enamel. Only the connective tissue fibres of the gingiva were thought to be attached to adjacent structures; cement and bone.

In 1921, Gottlieb proposed that an 'epithelial attachment' was also present. He argued that during tooth formation there is an organic union between ameloblasts and the enamel. Although there was disagreement on points of detail, Gottlieb's view was accepted by the majority, and it was not until 1952 that any real challenge was mounted. In that year Waerhaug completed a series of experiments on humans and animals. He postulated that there is no firm attachment of epithelium to enamel. He believed that a physiological pocket or crevice is formed when the tooth erupts and that the epithelium forms a 'cuff' around the tooth. Orban (1956) suggested that an 'attached epithelial cuff' was present.

More recently, the electron microscope has given much improved resolution, and plastic embedding techniques have allowed sections of the dentogingival junction to be prepared with both enamel and gingiva *in situ*. In addition, much has been learned about the physiology of epithelium using radioactive tracers to study the dynamics of cell turnover. Growth of epithelial cells in culture has provided additional information relating to the mechanisms and physiology of cell adhesion.

Schröeder and Listgarten (1971) presented detailed evidence to support the concept of a basal lamina and hemidesmosome attachment at the dentogingival junction and described the development of the structure in human tissues.

**Aspects of gingival physiology and biochemistry**

All portions of gingival epithelium and connective tissue are replaced by continuous cellular activity and cell turnover. The relative rates of turnover between various tissues and between various portions of the gingival epithelium have been clarified in the last 10 years using radiolabelled substances and autoradiography to detect the location of the isotope.

Using $^3$H-thymidine as a nuclear marker of dividing cells, it has been clearly demonstrated that oral epithelium, like epithelium elsewhere, is a renewing cell population. This implies that under normal circumstances the rate at which cells are lost from the surface is balanced by cell division in the germinative layer. Values are not yet available for human tissue but a turnover time of 4–6 days for the junctional epithelium of marmosets has been reported. The turnover in the interdental region is similar to the rate reported for junctional epithelium elsewhere. As the junctional epithelium can only desquamate from the area forming the base of the gingival sulcus, which is narrow when compared to the length of the basal layer, desquamation from this area is high when compared to oral epithelium. This probably acts as a mechanism for clearing bacteria attached to superficial cells.

In recent years much interest has been focused on the passage of substances from gingival connective tissue into the mouth and also the inward penetration of substances. Leucocytes pass from gingival vessels, through connective tissue into the healthy gingival sulcus, and it seems probable they migrate towards chemotactic substances which are produced by plaque bacteria and which penetrate gingival tissue. They are present in small numbers in clinically healthy tissue but greatly increase during gingival inflammation.

Flourescein (a dye which fluoresces under ultraviolet light), administered intravenously, can be collected on filter paper strips inserted at the dentogingival junction. This evidence for an outward passage of fluid from gingiva was initially suggested as being a physiological activity. However biochemical studies of sodium, potassium and calcium levels, and plasma protein investigations, have suggested that such fluid is an inflammatory exudate and thus a feature of damaged tissue.

There is probably greater interest in the passage of molecules in the opposite direction. $^3$H-labelled albumin (mw 68 000) has been shown to penetrate junctional but not oral epithelium, in animals. It was found to follow an intercellular route, small amounts reaching the gingival connective tissues.

Horseradish peroxidase does not penetrate keratinized, rodent oral epithelium, but histochemical and ultrastructural studies have clearly shown that it can easily penetrate junctional epithelium.

The various gingival epithelia probably exert a selective control on the passage of substances into and out of gingival tissue. Products from bacterial plaque growing at the dentogingival junction are thought to be important in the pathogenesis of periodontal disease. Techniques are now available to label chemically characterized bacterial products, and to determine their capacity to penetrate gingival tissues. In this regard it should be remembered that antigenic bacterial products have to penetrate against the outward flow of gingival exudate. Cellular and humoral defence mechanisms tend to counter penetration, disease resulting only when homeostasis fails.

Current knowledge relating specifically to gingival chemistry is patchy. Few controlled biochemical studies have been reported and there are extensive gaps in our knowledge of structural proteins, lipids, amino acids, steroids, purines and pyrimidines. Limited information is available concerning energy metabolism. Chemical studies of gingiva have been mainly histochemical and have dealt, largely qualitatively, with the identification and localization of enzyme activity, particularly with regard to carbohydrate metabolism and acid hydrolytic enzymes.

# INNERVATION, BLOOD SUPPLY AND LYMPHATICS

## Innervation

The trigeminal nerve (fifth cranial nerve) provides the main sensory innervation of the oral cavity; its mandibular division supplies the dental tissues in the lower jaw and its maxillary division those in the upper jaw. In the lower jaw a single nerve branch, the inferior dental nerve, supplies all the teeth in its own quadrant whereas the upper teeth are supplied in each quadrant by two or three main branches from the maxillary nerve.

### MANDIBULAR TEETH AND PERIODONTIUM

The inferior dental nerve is the terminal branch of the posterior part of the mandibular division of the trigeminal. This nerve arises in the infratemporal fossa deep to the lower head of the lateral pterygoid muscle. On emerging from behind this muscle, it lies within the pterygomandibular space near the sphenomandibular ligament (Fig. 7.28). Here it gives off a mylohyoid branch which is predominantly a motor nerve to the mylohyoid muscle and anterior belly of the digastric, but may have a sensory twig entering the mandible in the mental region which is said to participate in the nerve supply to the lower incisors. The inferior dental nerve enters the ramus of the mandible through the mandibular foramen which is centrally positioned in the ramus, lying 2 cm below the mandibular notch. Since this nerve lies very close to the ramus for approximately 5 mm before entering the mandibular foramen, there is little leeway in cutting horizontally through the ramus without damaging the nerve: for example, when surgically correcting abnormal mandibular protrusion or retrusion.

The course of the inferior dental nerve on entering the mandibular foramen is illustrated in Fig. 7.29. The distribution of nerves to the premolars and molars is variable, the branches either coming directly from the nerve or indirectly through alveolar branches. In rare instances the nerve to the mandibular third molar may arise from the inferior dental nerve before it enters the mandibular canal. In any individual the mandibular canal remains in a relatively fixed position with respect to the lower border of the mandible throughout life. The canal is often closely related to the roots of the mandibular molars. Indeed, the roots of lower third molars may even be perforated by the contents of the

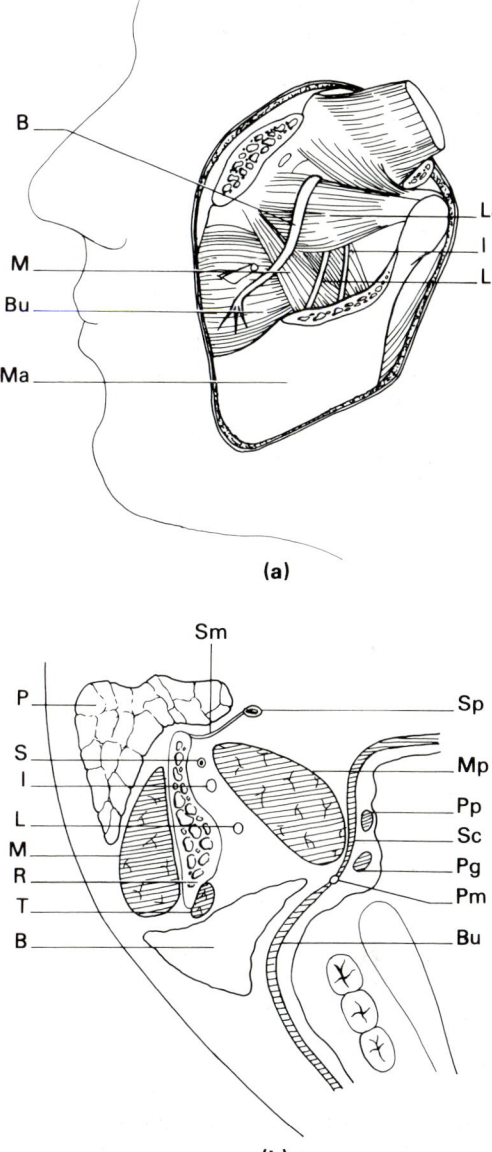

**Fig. 7.28.** (a) Lateral view of the infratemporal fossa showing the course of the inferior dental, lingual and buccal nerves. Ma, mandible; La, lateral pterygoid muscle; M, medial pterygoid muscle; Bu, buccinator muscle; I, inferior dental nerve; L, lingual nerve; B, buccal nerve. (b) Transverse section through pterygomandibular region. R, ramus of mandible; M, masseter muscle; Mp, medial pterygoid muscle; P, parotid gland; Sc, superior constrictor muscle; Bu, buccinator muscle; B, buccal pad of fat; Pm, pterygomandibular raphe; L, lingual nerve; I, inferior dental nerve; Sp, styloid process; Sm, stylomandibular ligament; S, sphenomandibular ligament; T, temporalis muscle; Pp, palatopharyngeus muscle; Pg, palatoglossus muscle.

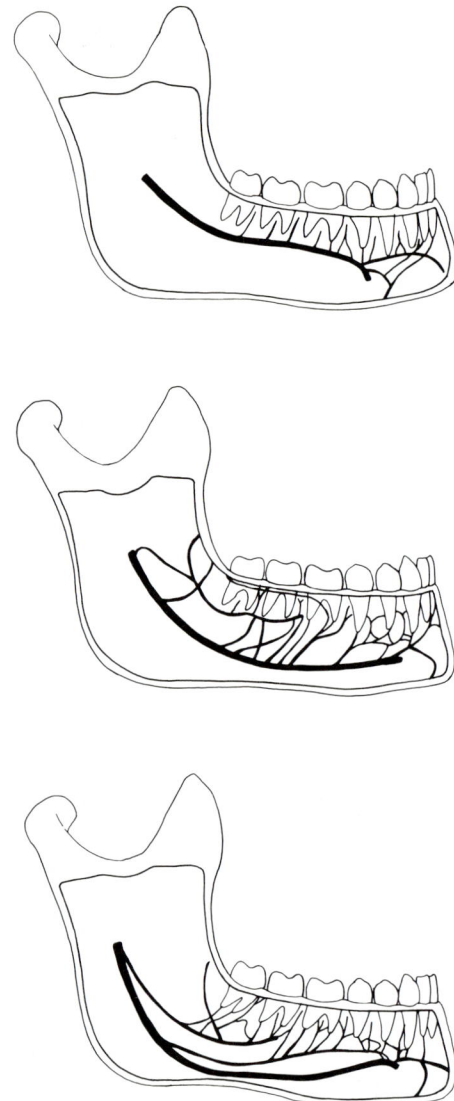

**Fig. 7.29.** Variations in the course of the inferior dental nerve. [Modified from Carter R. B. & Keen E. N. (1971) The intramandibular course of the inferior alveolar nerve. *Journal of Anatomy*, **103**, 433.]

mandibular canal. Therefore, when extracting these teeth care must be taken to prevent damaging the inferior dental nerve. Following tooth extraction and subsequent resorption of alveolar bone, the inferior dental nerve may lie very close to the oral mucosa and this could explain the altered sensitivity of the mucosa during mastication sometimes complained of by endentulous patients.

Communications between the inferior dental nerve and/or its molar branches and nerves from the temporalis and lateral pterygoid muscles have been described, the nerves penetrating the mandible through foramina in the region of muscle attachments. It has been suggested that such nervous connections might explain the 'escape-pain' phenomenon; that is, in approximately 5% of patients the inability to anaesthetize the teeth after the main trunk of the inferior dental nerve has been blocked at the mandibular foramen by the injection of local anaesthetic solution.

In the premolar region the main trunk of the inferior dental nerve divides into mental and incisive nerves. The mental nerve, which is to supply the skin of the chin and lower lip, the mucosa of the lip and the adjacent gingiva, leaves the body of the mandible at the mental foramen. Before passing through the mental foramen the mental nerve runs for a short distance in an intraosseous mental canal. Fig. 7.30 illustrates the variation in the relationship of the mental foramen to the teeth. In an adult with a full dentition the mental foramen usually lies midway between the upper and lower borders of the mandible.

During the 1st and 2nd years of life, as the prominence of the chin develops, the opening of the mental foramen alters in direction from facing forwards to facing upwards and backwards. In the adult it faces directly backwards.

The incisor and canine teeth are supplied by the incisive nerve which runs forwards in an intraosseous incisive canal. This nerve may also supply the first premolar tooth. Further variations are common, however, and the canine may be supplied directly by the inferior dental nerve.

An intricate plexus of nerves, the incisor plexus, whose fibres are derived directly from the mental

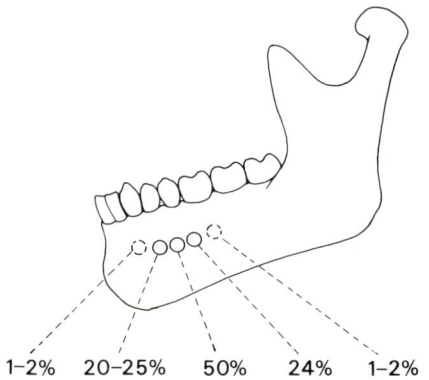

**Fig. 7.30.** Diagram showing the variable position of the mental foramen in Caucasians. (From Hollingshead W. H. (1968) *Anatomy for Surgeons* Vol. 1. Head and Neck. 2nd Edition. Maryland: Harper and Row.)

nerves, may be seen lying near the buccal surfaces of the roots of the incisors. Nerves from this plexus are thought to supply the buccal periodontium of the mandibular incisors. Whilst overlap between the right and left incisor plexuses has been observed, no overlap in distribution across the midline has been reported for the incisive nerves themselves.

The buccal gingiva is supplied by the mental nerve, the (long) buccal nerve and twigs directly from the inferior dental nerve trunk. As previously indicated, the buccal gingiva in the incisor region is supplied directly by the mental nerve and/or via the incisor plexus. In the majority of cases the buccal nerve supplies buccal gingiva as far forwards as the second premolar and first molar, the intervening region receiving fibres from perforating interdental branches of the inferior dental nerve. However, the area supplied by the buccal nerve may extend forward into the region of the canine and backward into that of the third molar. The buccal nerve is the terminal branch of the anterior part of the mandibular nerve. It arises behind the upper head of the lateral pterygoid and, passing between the two heads of this muscle, crosses the anterior border of the ramus at about the level of the occlusal plane. The nerve crosses the upper part of the retromolar fossa and breaks up into a number of branches within the buccinator muscle, (N.B. this sensory nerve does not provide motor fibres to the buccinator muscle).

The lingual gingiva is supplied by branches of the lingual nerve. The lingual nerve is derived from the posterior part of the mandibular nerve behind the lateral pterygoid muscle. Here it receives the chorda tympani branch of the facial nerve, which is concerned with the perception of taste in the anterior two-thirds of the tongue and with secretomotor activity to the submandibular and sublingual salivary glands. In the plane of the mandibular foramen the lingual nerve lies on the medial pterygoid muscle anterior to the inferior dental nerve (Fig. 7.28). It leaves the pterygomandibular space (the space between the mandible and the pterygoid muscle), passing downwards and anteriorly to lie close to the lingual alveolar plate of the third mandibular molar tooth (Fig. 7.9e). At this point the nerve lies immediately beneath the oral mucosa and thus is easily damaged during surgical procedures in this region. Before curving forwards into the tongue the nerve lies above the origin of the mylohyoid muscle and lateral to the hyoglossus. Apart from conveying fibres of the chorda tympani to their destinations, the lingual nerve is distributed to the

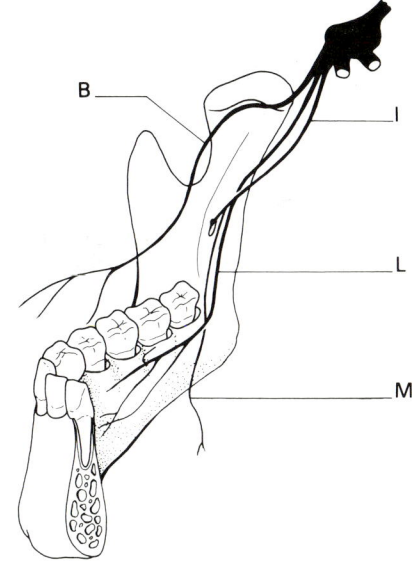

**Fig. 7.31.** Diagram illustrating the relationships of the inferior dental (I), lingual (L), buccal (B), and mylohyoid (M) nerves.

lingual gingiva, the floor of mouth and the anterior two-thirds of the tongue. Fig. 7.31 illustrates the relationships of the inferior dental, buccal and lingual nerves to the mandible and to each other.

MAXILLARY TEETH AND
PERIODONTIUM

The maxillary teeth and periodontium are supplied by the superior dental, infraorbital, nasopalatine and anterior palatine nerves from the maxillary division of the trigeminal plus occasional twigs from the buccal nerve of the mandibular division.

The superior dental nerves which supply the teeth consist of three main groups, posterior, middle and anterior superior dental nerves (Fig. 7.32).

The posterior superior dental nerve arises from the maxillary nerve in the pterygopalatine fossa. At a variable distance from its origin the nerve divides into two or three branches (Fig. 7.33). The dental branches of the nerve enter the posterolateral wall of the maxilla and run in narrow, posterior superior dental canals above the roots of the molar teeth. One branch, the gingival branch, does not enter the bone, however, but runs downward and forward along the outer surface of the maxillary tuberosity.

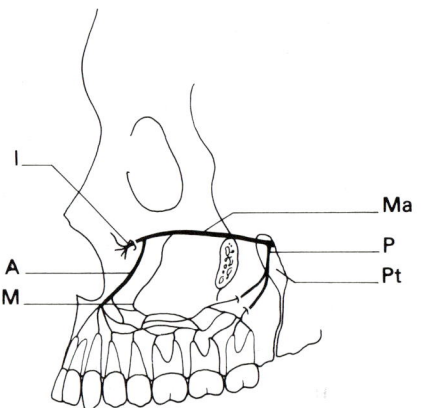

**Fig. 7.32.** Diagram showing the superior dental nerves and the associated dental plexuses. Ma, maxillary nerve; I, infraorbital nerve; Pt, pterygopalatine fossa; P. M. and A, posterior, middle and anterior superior dental nerves, respectively.

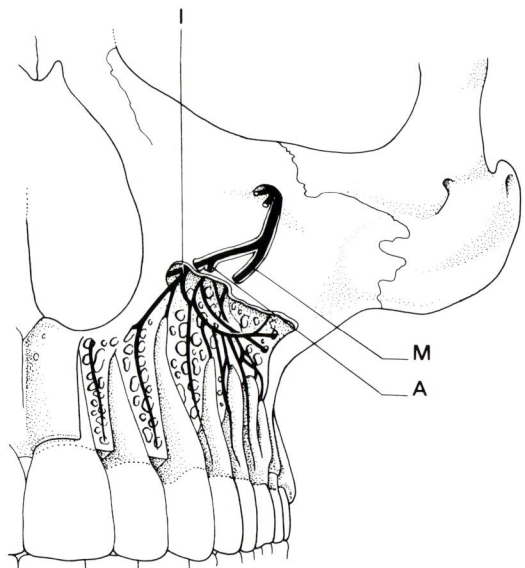

**Fig. 7.34.** Diagram showing course of the anterior and middle superior dental nerves. I, infraorbital nerve exiting infraorbital foramen; A, anterior superior dental nerve in canalis sinuosis; M, middle superior dental nerve.

The middle superior dental nerve is found in about 70% of subjects. In general the nerve arises from the infraorbital nerve in the floor of the orbit but may also arise from the maxillary nerve in the pterygopalatine fossa. The nerve may run in the posterior, lateral or anterior walls of the maxillary antrum and it terminates above the roots of the premolar teeth.

The anterior superior dental nerve arises from the infraorbital nerve, within the infraorbital canal, generally as a single nerve but occasionally as two or three small branches. The nerve leaves the infraorbital canal towards its terminal part and then, diverging laterally from the infraorbital nerve, it runs in the anterior wall of the maxillary sinus in the so-called 'canalis sinuosus' (Fig. 7.34). It terminates near the anterior nasal spine after giving off a small nasal branch.

As the superior dental nerves approach the teeth they become small, variable and difficult to trace. The nerves form a number of plexuses above the roots of the teeth from which it is not possible to trace accurately fibres of a given dental nerve to a particular tooth. As a general rule, the molars are supplied by the posterior dental branches, the premolars and canine by the middle dental branches and the incisors by the anterior branches.

The buccal gingiva is supplied posteriorly by the gingival branches from the posterior superior dental nerves and the buccal branch of the mandibular nerve. The labial mucosa of the more anterior teeth is supplied by labial branches of the infraorbital nerve.

The palatal gingiva is supplied by the anterior palatine and nasopalatine nerves. The anterior palatine nerve supplies the greater part of the palatal gingiva, the nasopalatine nerve supplying a small anteromedial portion behind the central

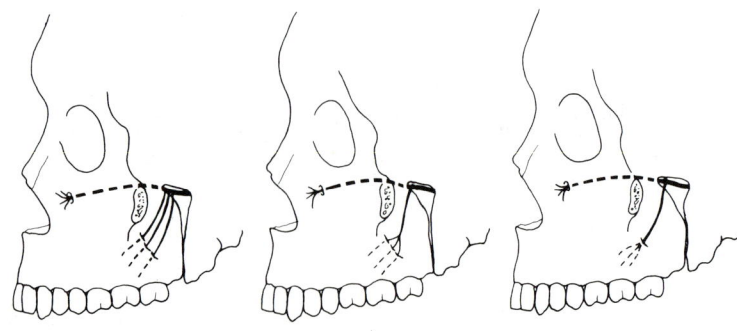

**Fig. 7.33.** Diagram showing variations in extra bony course of posterior superior dental nerve.

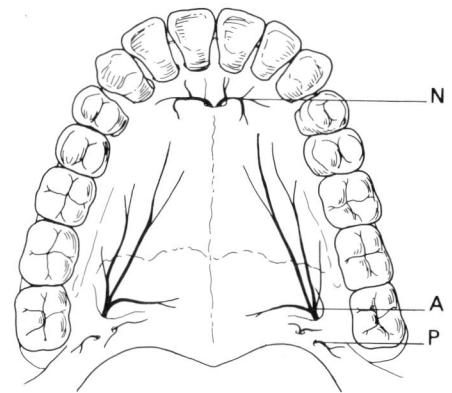

**Fig. 7.35.** Diagram showing nerves supplying the palate. A, anterior palatine nerve; P, posterior palatine nerve; N, nasopalatine nerve.

incisors (Fig. 7.35). Both nerves are dervied from the pterygopalatine ganglion, the anterior palatine nerve entering the palate through the greater palatine canal and the nasopalatine nerve through the incisive foramen.

APPLIED ANATOMY

The teeth and associated structures can be anaesthetized either by infiltrating anaesthetic solution close to the desired site of action, or by depositing the solution around the main nerve trunk at some distance from the operative site (a nerve block). The choice between these two techniques depends upon the density of the alveolar bone surrounding the roots of the teeth, the accessibility of the nerve trunks for blocking techniques and the area required to be anaesthetized. Thus, because of the solidity and thickness of buccal alveolar plates associated with lower molar teeth, nerve-blocking techniques are usually required in these regions. In contrast, the deep course of the anterior and middle superior dental nerves within the maxilla precludes satisfactory nerve-blocking methods; fortunately, the porosity of the bone makes infiltration satisfactory. In periodontal and oral surgery, the large areas needed to be anaesthetized may be best accomplished by a nerve-blocking technique.

The common intra-oral nerve blocks used in dentistry are the inferior dental, lingual, buccal, posterior superior dental, infraorbital, anterior palatine and nasopalatine nerve blocks. The inferior dental and lingual nerves are blocked as they course through the pterygomandibular fossa. The buccal nerve is blocked as it passes across the anterior border of the coronoid process of the mandible. Alternative sites for blocking the lingual and buccal nerves are on the lingual and buccal sides of the mandibular third molar. Very rarely, the inferior dental nerve may be blocked by an extra-oral approach either through the mandibular notch or medial to the lower border of the mandible. The posterior superior dental nerve which lies on the posterior surface of the maxilla in the infratemporal fossa is best approached not by direct injection around the nerve but indirectly by depositing local anaesthetic solution at the upper border of the buccinator just posterior to the anterior root of the zygomatic process and then manipulating the anaesthetic fluid towards the nerve. The infraorbital block can be approached intra-orally or extra-orally (where infection may prohibit an intra-oral approach) by injection around the infraorbital foramen. The anterior palatine nerve may be blocked anywhere along its course behind the operative site. The nasopalatine nerve is blocked around the incisive foramen.

**Blood supply**

ARTERIAL

The chief arteries to the teeth are derived from the maxillary artery and essentially follow the dental nerves.

*Mandibular teeth and periodontium*
The inferior dental artery which supplies the mandibular teeth is derived in the infratemporal fossa from the first part of the maxillary artery. Its subsequent course corresponds closely to that of its accompanying nerve. The mylohyoid branch is given off before the inferior dental artery enters the mandibular foramen. The inferior dental artery passes through the mandibular foramen to enter the mandibular canal and terminates as the mental and incisive arteries.

Posteriorly the buccal gingiva is supplied by the buccal artery, a branch of the second part of the maxillary artery, and perforating branches from the inferior dental artery. Anteriorly the buccal gingiva is supplied by the mental artery and perforating branches of the incisive artery, both derived from the inferior dental artery. The lingual gingiva is supplied by perforating branches from the inferior dental artery and the lingual artery.

*Maxillary teeth and periodontium*
The posterior superior dental artery arises from the third part of the maxillary artery just as the latter enters the pterygopalatine fossa. It accom-

panies the corresponding nerve on the posterior aspect of the maxilla, coursing tortuously over the maxillary tuberosity before entering bony canals to supply molar and premolar teeth. The artery also gives off branches to the adjacent buccal gingiva, maxillary sinus and cheek. Occasionally this artery is derived from the buccal artery. Where present, the middle superior dental artery arises from the infraorbital artery which is itself a branch of the third part of the maxillary artery. The middle superior dental artery runs in the lateral wall of the maxillary sinus terminating near the canine tooth where it anastomoses with the anterior and posterior superior dental arteries. The anterior superior dental artery also arises from the infraorbital artery and runs downwards in the anterior wall of the maxillary sinus, accompany its nerve within the canalis sinuosus, to supply the anterior teeth. As with the superior dental nerves, the dental arteries form plexuses.

The buccal gingiva around the posterior maxillary teeth is supplied by gingival and perforating branches from the posterior superior dental artery and the buccal artery. The labial gingiva of anterior teeth is supplied by labial branches of the infraorbital artery and perforating branches of the anterior superior dental artery.

The palatal gingiva is supplied primarily by branches of the anterior palatine artery which emerges through the greater palatine foramen and is a branch of the third part of the maxillary artery. It accompanies the anterior palatine nerve and enters the incisive foramen where it anastomoses with the nasopalatine artery. Unlike the nasopalatine nerves, the nasopalatine artery does not extend through the incisive canal into the palate.

VENOUS

The venous drainage of dental structures is extremely variable and complex. Small veins from the teeth and alveolar bone pass into larger veins which surround the apex of each tooth or into veins running in the interdental septa. In the mandible the veins are then collected into one or more inferior dental veins which themselves may drain anteriorly through the mental foramen to join the facial vein or posteriorly through the mandibular foramen to join the pterygoid plexus. In the maxilla the veins may drain anteriorly into the facial vein or posteriorly into the pterygoid plexus, both of which connect with the cavernous sinus (Fig. 7.36). The facial vein anastomoses with the angular vein in the medial corner of the eye, which itself drains to the ophthalmic veins and thence to the cavernous sinus. The cavernous sinus is connected inferiorly, through the base of the skull, with the pterygoid plexus of veins. Because the angular vein is without valves, blood can drain from here either into the facial vein or the cavernous sinus. If the facial vein is blocked by, for example, the swelling of an abscess over the canine, venous blood from this region can be carried into the cavernous sinus. The possibility of transporting infection to the cavernous sinus, which may lead to dangerous cavernous sinus thrombosis, makes a dental surgeon very careful when treating abscesses which might be related to the facial vein.

No detailed description is available concerning the venous drainage of the gingiva though it may be assumed that the buccal, lingual, anterior palatine and nasopalatine veins are involved;

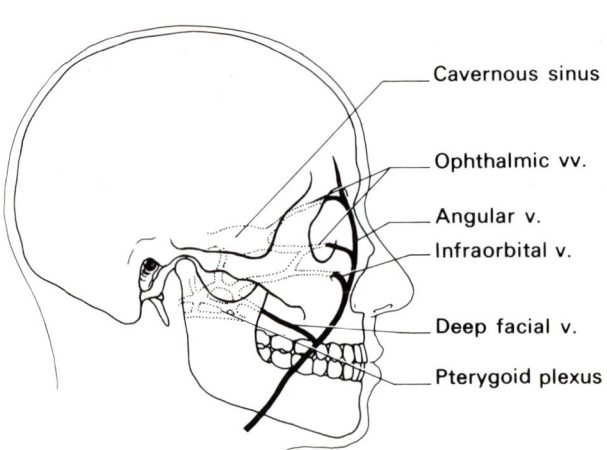

**Fig. 7.36.** Connections of the pterygoid plexus and facial veins to the cavernous sinus.

apart from the lingual which drains directly into the internal jugular vein, these veins run into the pterygoid plexus.

**Lymphatics**

LYMPHATIC DRAINAGE OF THE DENTAL TISSUES (Fig. 7.37)

Despite considerable variation in the anatomy of the lymphatic drainage of orodental structures,

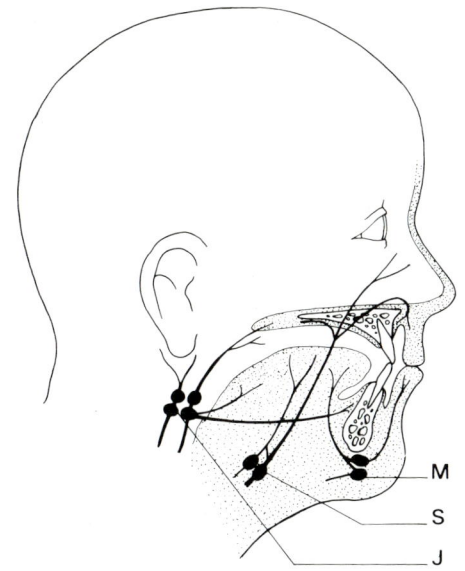

Fig. 7.37. Regional lymphatic drainage of the oral structures. J, jugulodigastric nodes; S, submandibular nodes; M, submental nodes.

particularly the course of the lymph vessels, a knowledge of the generalized pattern of such drainage is essential in the diagnosis, prognosis and treatment of oral infections and tumours.

The lymph vessels draining the pulp and periodontal ligament have a common outlet. As a rule those vessels draining the incisors and canines pass anteriorly, those draining the molars run posteriorly, whilst the vessels from the premolars may pass anteriorly or posteriorly. The lymph vessels of all teeth, except for the lower incisors, pass directly into the submandibular lymph nodes on the appropriate side; lymph from the lower incisors drains into the submental lymph nodes. The great variation of lymphatic drainage is, however, indicated by the fact that lymph from molar teeth may pass directly into the jugulodigastric group of nodes.

The lymph vessels of the labial and buccal gingiva of the upper and lower teeth unite to drain into the submandibular nodes, though in the labial region of the lower incisors they may drain into the submental lymph nodes. The vessels of the lingual gingiva drain into the jugulo-digastric group of nodes either directly or indirectly through the submandibular nodes.

Occasionally, lymph from the cheek teeth drains into a buccal (facial) lymph node which itself drains into the submandibular lymph nodes.

From the regional submandibular and submental lymph nodes, lymph vessels pass directly to deep cervical lymph nodes.

## FURTHER READING

ADATIA A.K. (1976) Regional nerve block for maxillary permanent molars. *British Dental Journal* **140**, 87.

ANDERSON D.J., HANNAM A.G. & MATTHEWS B. (1970) Sensory mechanisms in mammalian teeth and their supporting structures. *Physiology Reviews* **50**, 171.

CARTER R.B. & KEEN E.N. (1971) The intramandibular course of the inferior alveolar nerve. *Journal of Anatomy* **103**, 433.

FITZGERALD M.J.T. (1956) The occurrence of a middle superior alveolar nerve in man. *Journal of Anatomy* **90**, 520.

HOLLINGSHEAD W.H. (1968) *Anatomy for Surgeons. Vol. 1. Head and Neck* 2nd Edition. Maryland: Harper & Row.

JONES F.W. (1939) The anterior superior alveolar nerve and vessels. *Journal of Anatomy* **73**, 583.

SICHER H. & DUBRUL E.L. (1970) *Oral Anatomy*, 5th ed. St. Louis: Mosby.

STARKLE C. & STEWART D. (1931) The intramandibular course of the inferior dental nerve. *Journal of Anatomy*, **65**, 319.

WARWICK R. & WILLIAMS P.L. (eds.) (1980) *Gray's Anatomy*, 36th ed. London: Longman.

# CHAPTER 8

# Development of Dentition

## EARLY STAGES OF TOOTH DEVELOPMENT

Early in development the embryonic oral cavity is lined by an epithelial layer of low columnar cells which become squamous and stratified over the regions which later develop the lips, cheeks and teeth. This epithelial layer is separated from the underlying mesenchymal tissue by a basement membrane. At about the 6th week of intra-uterine life, a condensation of mesenchymal (ectomesenchymal) cells accumulates immediately beneath the oral epithelium and heralds the onset of tooth development. In association with this mesenchymal condensation there is a plexus of blood capillaries, a characteristic of regions undergoing significant morphogenesis. During the 6th week, the oral epithelium proliferates into the mesenchymal condensation to form an ingrowing sheet of epithelium termed the primary epithelial band. During the 7th week, the free margin of the primary epithelial band develops two distinct processes: the vestibular and dental laminae (Fig. 8.1). The vestibular lamina develops on the labial side of the dental lamina and subsequently contributes to the development of the oral vestibule which delineates the cheeks and lips from the tooth-bearing regions (Fig. 1.31). The dental lamina gives rise to the teeth.

The dental lamina now deepens and lengthens: it is not known whether the deepening results from active invagination of the lamina or upward proliferation of the mesenchyme. The dental lamina appears as an arch-shaped band of tissue which follows the line of the developing jaws. From its free edge, a number of epithelial swellings, the enamel organs, develop, each being surrounded by dense mesenchyme (Fig. 8.2). By the 10th week, five developing tooth germs are present in each jaw quadrant, the developing deciduous teeth. Backward growth of the dental lamina produces the tooth germs of the permanent molar teeth. The first permanent molar appears at about the 16th week (the second and third permanent molars appear long after birth).

For descriptive purposes, tooth germs are classified into bud, cap and bell stages according to the degree of morphodifferentiation and histodifferentiation of their enamel organs.

The growth of a tooth germ can be considered in two phases. During the first phase leading up to the late bell stage, the tooth germ changes rapidly both in its size and shape; cells are dividing and morphogenetic processes are taking place. In the second phase, at and following the late bell stage, hard tissues are formed, the shape having already been established. During this phase, growth in size is related mainly to the deposition of enamel, the rate of cell division falling.

**Bud stage** (Figs. 8.3a and 8.4)

Here the enamel organ appears as a simple, spherical to ovoid, epithelial ball of cells which are poorly morphodifferentiated and histodifferentiated. Compared with the overlying oral epithelium, however, the cells of the tooth bud contain more RNA, less glycogen, and have greater oxidative enzyme activity. The surrounding mesenchymal condensation has become more conspicuous.

**Cap stage**

EARLY CAP STAGE (Fig. 8.3b)

By the 11th week, morphogenesis has progressed and the deeper surface of the enamel organ invaginates to form a cap-shaped structure. Though the enamel organ is still rather poorly histodifferentiated, the more rounded central cells are becoming distinguishable from the cuboidal peripheral cells.

LATE CAP STAGE (Figs. 8.3c and 8.5)

By about $12\frac{1}{2}$ weeks, the central cells of the enlarging enamel organ have become separated, though maintaining contact by processes ending

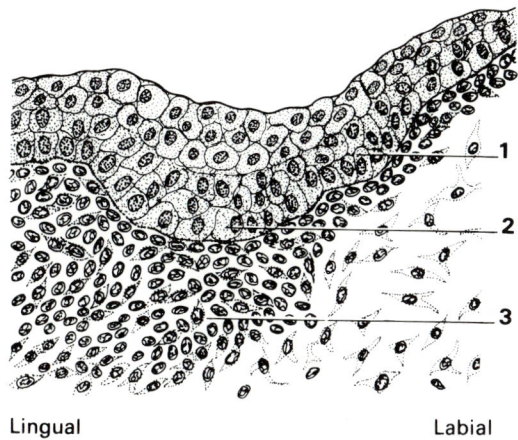

Lingual          Labial

**Fig. 8.1.** Transverse section through the primary epithelial band showing its early division into the labial, vestibular lamina (1) and the lingual, dental lamina (2). Note the associated mesenchymal condensation (3).

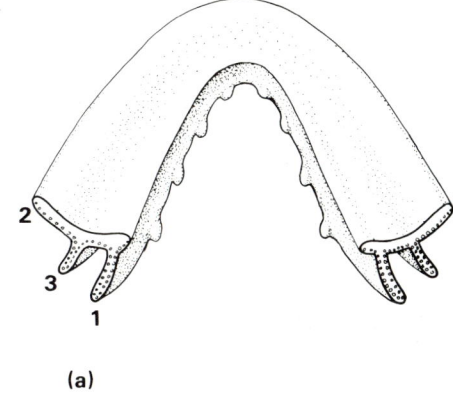

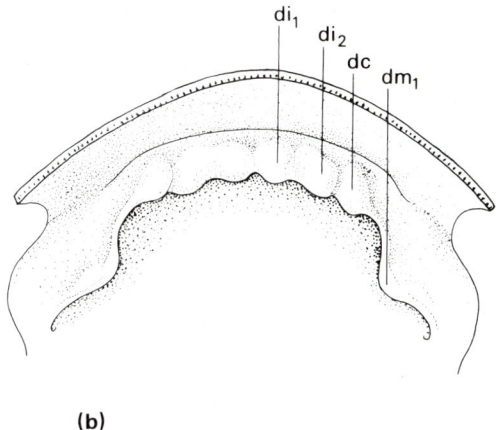

**Fig. 8.2.** (a) The dental lamina (1) is an arch-shaped invagination of oral epithelium (2), lateral to which is the vestibular lamina (3). All mesoderm has been deleted from this diagram. Swellings along the free edge of the dental lamina represent the developing enamel organs. (b) An actual reconstruction (from serial sections) of the developing oral epithelium in the lower jaw of a 2.5 cm CR length human embryo seen from below. The deciduous incisors ($di_1$, $di_2$) canine (dc) and first molar ($dm_1$) are beginning to develop. (After Ooë T. (1956))

in desmosomes. The resulting tissue, consisting of stellate (star-shaped) cells, is termed the stellate reticulum and its intercellular spaces contain considerable quantities of glycosaminoglycans. The full thickness of the stellate reticulum is not developed until the bell stage. The internal enamel epithelial cells lining the inner, concave surface of the 'cap' become more columnar whilst the external enamel epithelial cells remain cuboidal. The cells of the internal enamel epithelium manufacture more RNA and their hydrolytic and oxidative enzyme activity increases as they become taller. The mesenchymal cells continue to proliferate and surround the enamel organ. The part of the mesenchyme lying beneath the internal enamel epithelium is termed the dental papilla whilst that surrounding the tooth germ forms the dental follicle.

## Bell stage

EARLY BELL STAGE
(Figs. 8.3d and 8.6)

Continued growth of the enamel organ converts it into a bell-shaped structure. The central region is now clearly differentiated into the stellate reticulum and an additional layer of flattened cells, the stratum intermedium, is evident between the stellate reticulum and the internal enamel epithelium. The dental papilla and follicle become more clearly demarcated at this stage.

The enamel organ of the early bell has four cell layers:

*The external enamel epithelium*
This layer is one cell thick. Its cells are more rounded or cuboidal than the cells of the internal enamel epithelium. The external enamel epithelial cells are joined to each other and to the cells of the stellate reticulum by desmosomes. Hemidesmosomes lie along the outer surface of the cells attaching them to the basement membrane. The external enamel epithelial cells contain only moderate amounts of rough-surfaced endoplasmic reticulum, mitochondria and Golgi

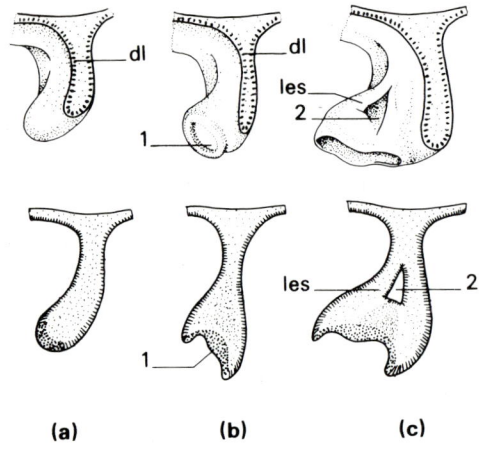

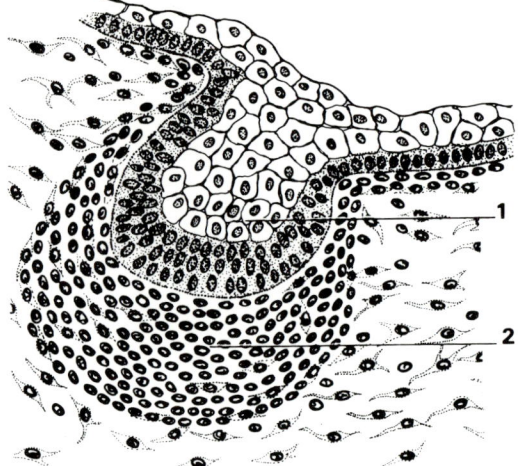

**Fig. 8.4.** Section through a developing tooth germ at the bud stage: 1, enamel organ; 2, mesenchymal condensation.

development, the capillaries lie in depressions in the external enamel epithelium. The external enamel epithelium is thought to be involved in maintaining the shape of the enamel organ and, more obviously, in exchanging substances between the enamel organ and the dental follicle. As a constituent of the epithelial root sheath (p. 261) it can be presumed to play a part in root formation.

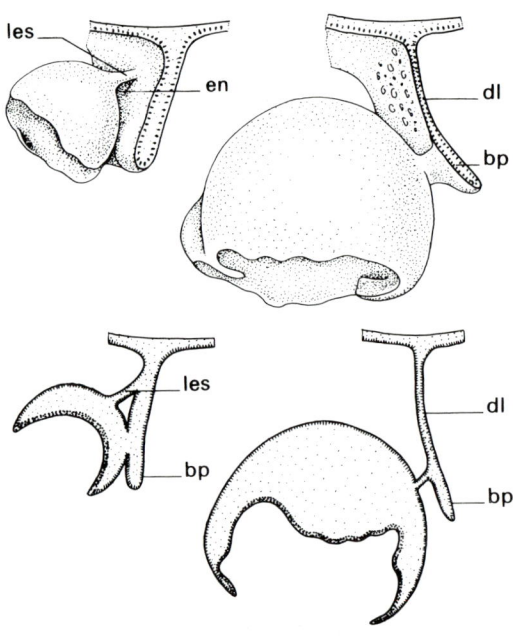

**Fig. 8.3.** Five stages (a–e) in the development of a tooth germ from bud to advanced bell stages: 1, enamel knot; 2, enamel niche; dl, dental lamina; les, lateral enamel strand; en, enamel niche; bp, permanent tooth buds. The upper drawings and three-dimensional representations; the lower drawings represent the appearance of typical sections. (After Sicher & Tandler (1941)).

material, and contain alkaline phosphatase. Within the cytoplasm adjacent to the basement membrane are small vesicles which are thought to be pinocytotic. A rich capillary plexus surrounds the external enamel epithelium. At later stages in

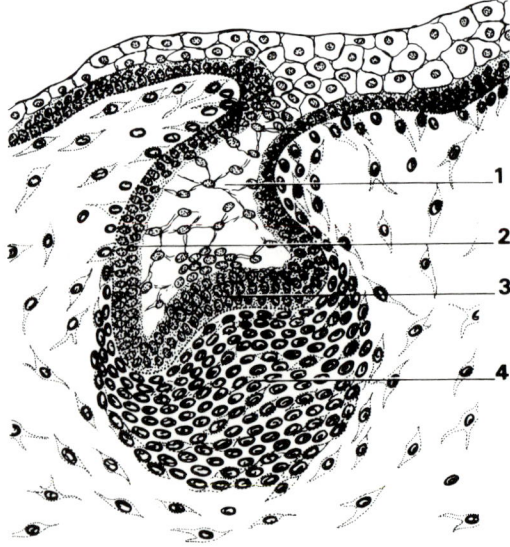

**Fig. 8.5.** Section through a developing tooth germ at the late cap stage. 1, stellate reticulum; 2, external enamel epithelium; 3, internal enamel epithelium; 4, dental papilla.

# Development of Dentition

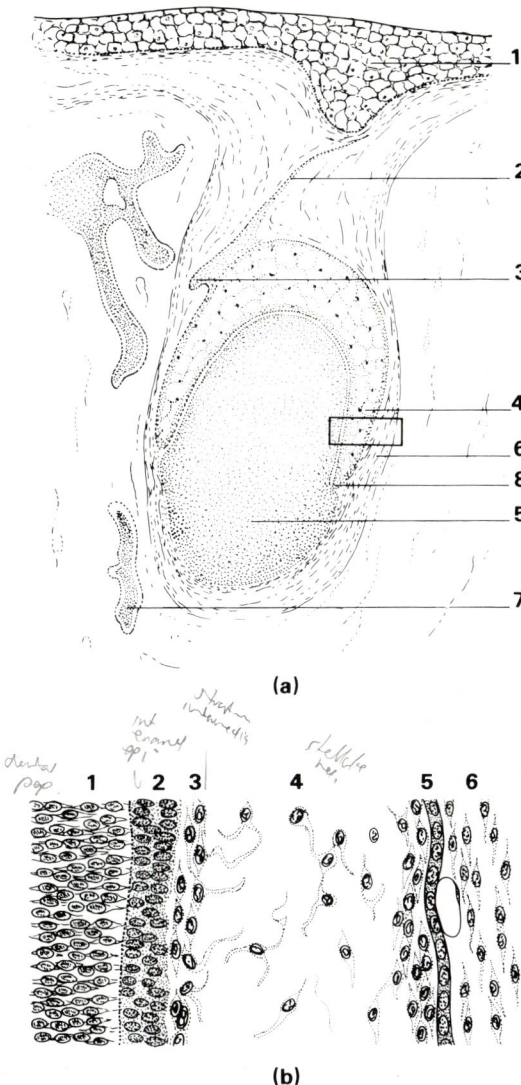

**Fig. 8.6.** (a) Low power view of section through a tooth germ at the early bell stage: 1, oral epithelium; 2, dental lamina, 3, developing permanent tooth; 4, enamel organ; 5, dental papilla; 6, dental follicle; 7, bone of developing alveolus; 8, cervical loop. (b) High power view of region indicated in (a): 1, peripheral cells of dental papilla; 2, internal enamel epithelium; 3, stratum intermedium; 4, stellate reticulum, 5, external enamel epithelium; 6, dental follicle.

## Stellate reticulum
This tissue is most fully developed at the bell stage. The interstitial spaces become fluid-filled, presumably due to osmotic effects arising from the high concentration of (extracellular) glycosaminoglycans. The cells of this layer characteristically have a central body which contains the nucleus and long, branching, cytoplasmic processes. The cells of the stellate reticulum contain little endoplasmic reticulum, but the presence of Golgi material, microvesicles and microvilli on the cell surface has been interpreted as indicating that the cells contribute to the secretion of the extracellular material. Numerous tonofilaments are present. The cells contain alkaline phosphatase but only small amounts of RNA and glycogen. Two main functions have been ascribed to the stellate reticulum, mechanical and nutritive.

*Mechanical.* This relates to the protection of the underlying dental tissues against physical disturbance and to the maintenance of tooth shape. It has been suggested that the hydrostatic pressure generated within the stellate reticulum is balanced by the pressure generated by the growing dental papilla. A change in either of these pressures would lead to a change in the outline of the internal enamel epithelium which could be of importance during morphogenesis of the crown.

*Nutritive.* This relates to the uses of glycosaminoglycans by the enamel forming cells: for example, these glycosaminoglycans could be passed into the developing enamel.

## Stratum intermedium
This consists of two or three layers of flattened cells lying over the internal enamel epithelial cells and later the ameloblasts. The cells of the stratum intermedium resemble those of the stellate reticulum, though their intercellular spaces are smaller and they contain more alkaline phosphatase than those of the stellate reticulum. It has been suggested that the stratum intermedium may be concerned with the synthesis of proteins, with the transport of materials to and from the ameloblast and/or with the concentration of materials.

## Internal enamel epithelium
These cells form a single layer lining the concavity of the bell-shaped enamel organ. They become increasingly columnar. Their large, ovoid nuclei lie initially near the middle part of the cell. A small Golgi complex is situated in the basal part of the cell (adjacent to the stratum intermedium). There are only a few organized membranous structures in the distal cytoplasm (neighbouring the dental papilla) though it contains numerous free ribosomes. Desmosomes connect the cells of this layer together and to the stratum intermedium. The internal enamel epithelium is separated from the peripheral cells of the dental papilla by a basement membrane and a cell-free zone 1–2 μm

wide. The cells of the internal enamel epithelium are loaded with RNA but, unlike the stratum intermedium and stellate reticulum, do not contain alkaline phosphatase.

The most obvious function of the internal enamel epithelial cells is related to their future formation of enamel. Before the formation of enamel, the internal enamel epithelial layer is said to play an important part in the determination of crown form due to its intrinsic growth pattern (see below). The internal enamel epithelial cells induce the adjacent cells of the dental papilla to form odontoblasts. Following amelogenesis, the cells contribute to the formation of the reduced enamel epithelium which is involved in developing the epithelial attachment.

Though early on in development cells divide throughout the enamel organ, at later stages mitosis becomes more restricted and is particularly noticeable at the margins of the enamel organ, the cervical loop. The epithelial cells that comprise this wedge-shaped region where the external and internal enamel epithelia become continuous have a high nuclear:cytoplasmic ratio and, though they vary in shape, they contain remarkably similar organelles, which include numerous free polyribosomes and a sparse rough-surfaced endoplasmic reticulum and Golgi material. Mitotic figures have only been seen in the central zone of the cervical loop, between the external and internal enamel epithelia, rather than at its tip. With the completion of enamel formation the cervical loop continues growing and produces the epithelial root sheath.

*Dental papilla*
The differentiation of the dental papilla is less striking than that of the enamel organ. The cells of the dental papilla have a variety of shapes and profiles. They contain more rough-surfaced endoplasmic reticulum and Golgi material than the internal enamel epithelial cells and numerous free ribosomes are present. No desmosomes are seen between the cells. Only a few delicate extracellular fibrils are present. Small vessels start to invade the dental papilla at this stage preparatory to hard tissue genesis. The dental papilla produces abundant glycosaminoglycans.

*Dental follicle*
Interposed between the growing tooth germ and the wall of the developing bony crypt is the mesenchymal tissue of the dental follicle in which three layers can generally be distinguished. The inner layer is a vascular, fibrocellular condensation, three to four cells thick, immediately surrounding the tooth germ. The outer layer is a vascular mesenchymal layer which lines the developing alveolus. The middle layer is made up of loose connective tissue with no marked concentration of blood vessels. The majority of cells in the dental follicle at the bell stage contain only a few cytoplasmic organelles. The subsequent development of the dental follicle is discussed elsewhere (p. 283).

*Enamel knot, enamel cord and enamel niche*
During the early stages of tooth development, these three transitory structures may be seen in association with the enamel organ.

*The enamel knot* (Figs. 8.3b and 8.7) is a localized mass of cells produced by rapid multiplication of the cells in the centre of the internal enamel epithelium. Characteristically it bulges into the dental papilla at the centre of the tooth germ. It was once thought that the enamel knot played a role in the formation of crown pattern by outlining the central fissure. This has not been substantiated and its role is unknown though the enamel knot appears to contribute cells to the enamel cord.

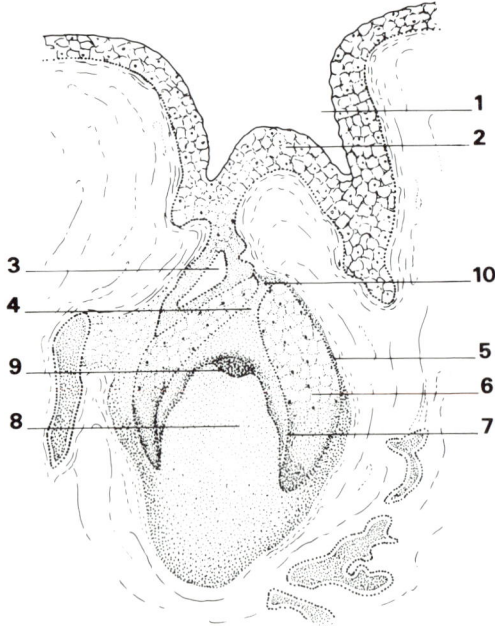

**Fig. 8.7.** Section through a developing tooth showing the transitory enamel knot (9), enamel cord (4) and enamel niche (3). These structures are not necessarily present in all teeth, nor are they necessarily all present at the same time: 1, vestibule; 2, oral epithelium; 5, external enamel epithelium; 6, stellate reticulum; 7, internal enamel epithelium; 8, dental papilla; 10, enamel navel.

*The enamel cord* (Fig. 8.7) is a strand of cells seen at the bell stage of development which extends from the stratum intermedium into the stellate reticulum, generally reaching the external enamel epithelium. Where present, the enamel cord overlies the incisal edge of a tooth or the apex of the first cusp to develop (primary cusp). When it completely divides the stellate reticulum into two, it is termed the enamel septum. Where the enamel cord meets the external enamel epithelium a small invagination termed the enamel navel may be seen. The cells contributing to the enamel cord are conspicuous within the surrounding stellate reticulum cells because of their increased cell density and/or the elongation of their nuclei in the plane of the cord. It has been suggested that the enamel cord may be involved in the process by which the cap stage is transformed into the bell stage, acting as a mechanical tie and/or that it is a focus for the origin of stellate reticulum cells.

*The enamel niche* (Figs. 8.3c, d and 8.7). The tooth germ may appear to have a double attachment to the dental lamina by means of lateral and medial enamel strands. These strands enclose a funnel-shaped depression containing connective tissue which is termed the enamel niche. Its significance is unknown.

LATE BELL STAGE (Figs. 8.8 and 8.9)

This stage, associated with the formation of dental hard tissue, begins at about the 18th week of intrauterine life. The further stages in development which concern the formation of the dental hard tissues are described elsewhere.

During the bell stage of development, an epithelial lamina appears on the lingual side of the enamel organ. In the case of the deciduous teeth, these lingual downgrowths (Figs. 8.3e, 8.6a and 8.9) give rise to enamel organs of permanent teeth which subsequently pass through the same developmental stages as the enamel organs of deciduous teeth. Since the enamel organs of the permanent molars show similar undifferentiated lingual downgrowths, this has been considered evidence in support of the view that the permanent molars are members of an ancestral deciduous dentition. However, even the enamel organs of permanent teeth which have deciduous predecessors develop undifferentiated lingual downgrowths, though these rapidly degenerate. Thus, these downgrowths may either be regarded as a normal feature of development or as evidence of a successive, but reduced, dentition.

In an attempt to elucidate the biochemical actions and reactions within and between the tissues of the developing tooth germ, a number of histochemical studies have been undertaken. The centre of the undifferentiated (ectodermal) bud (Fig. 8.10) is rich in alkaline phosphatase while

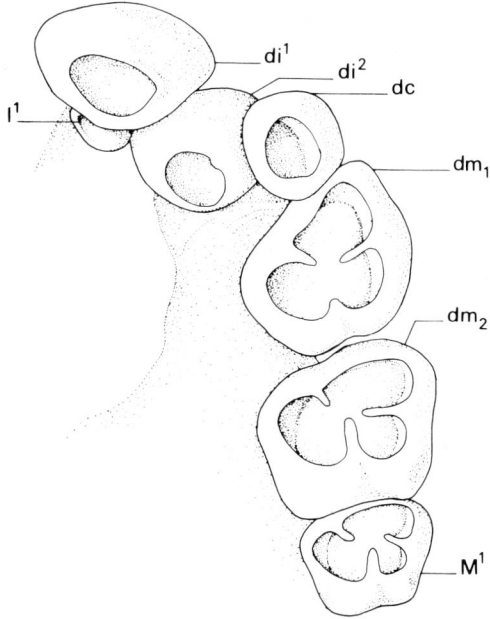

**Fig. 8.8.** A reconstruction (from serial sections) of the developing oral epithelium in the upper jaw of a 26.5 cm CR length human embryo viewed from above. The deciduous teeth are at the bell stage. In addition, the enamel organs of the permanent first incisor ($I^1$) and molar ($M^1$) are present. (After Ooë T. (1956))

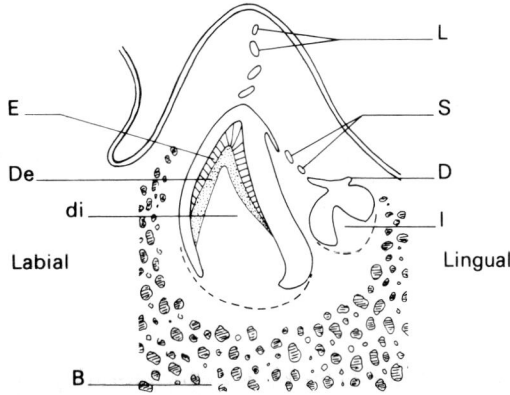

**Fig. 8.9.** A sagittal section through the incisor region showing a deciduous incisor (di) in which both enamel (E) and dentine (De) are forming, the developing permanent incisor (I), the remains of the dental lamina (L) and the successional lamina (S), a lingual downgrowth (D) from the permanent incisor and developing alveolar bone (B).

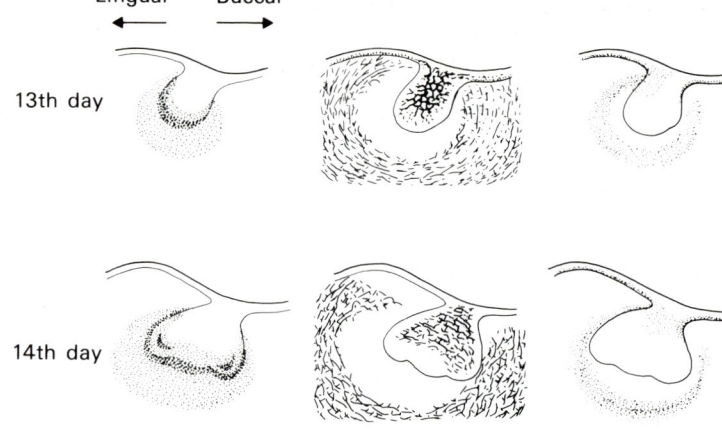

**Fig. 8.10.** Changes in the localization of RNA, alkaline phosphatase and glycogen in the first mandibular tooth germ of the mouse embryo between the 13th and 14th day. (After Pourtois (1961))

RNA is particularly concentrated in the peripheral layer. Small amounts of glycogen are restricted to the neck of the bud. The adjacent mesenchyme shows only a small amount of RNA while alkaline phosphatase and glycogen are absent.

At later stages of development alkaline phosphatase is found in all layers of the enamel organ except for the internal enamel epithelium and is particularly conspicuous in the stratum intermedium. RNA becomes mainly concentrated in the differentiating ameloblasts whilst glycogen persists in the neck of the enamel organ and also accumulates in the differentiating ameloblasts. Alkaline phosphatase appears in the subodontoblastic layer of the dental papilla and has also been reported to be present in differentiating odontoblasts. Glycogen remains absent from the dental papilla though it is evident in the surrounding dental follicle. RNA is evenly distributed throughout the dental papilla and will later become concentrated in the odontoblast layer.

Intercellular glycosaminoglycans can be demonstrated in the stellate reticulum, in the central zones of the dental papilla and at the future amelodentinal junction.

Though the above substances can be demonstrated, their precise functions remain unknown; alkaline phosphatase has been implicated in matrix formation and calcification (Book 1), glycogen with the synthesis of proteoglycans, and proteoglycans with calcification and morphogenesis.

FORMATION OF THE VESTIBULE
(Fig. 8.11)

The vestibular lamina lies labially and buccally to

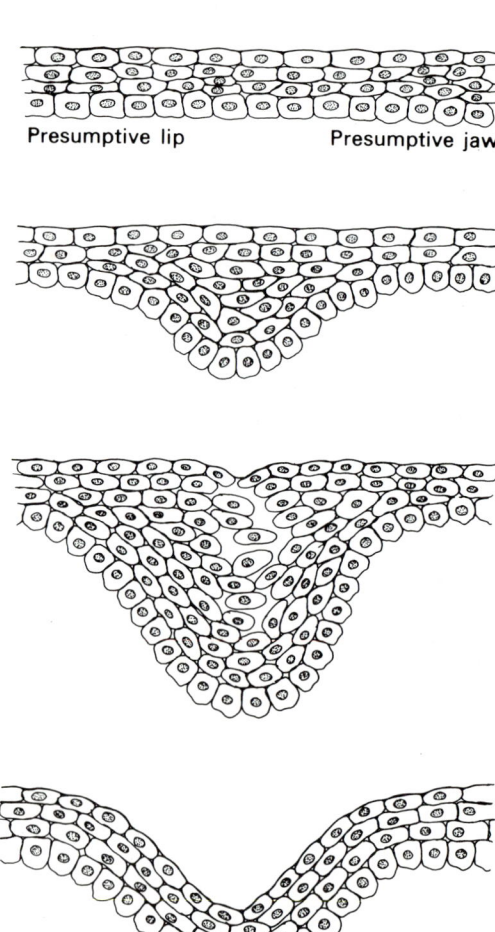

**Fig. 8.11.** Diagrams showing the development of the vestibule.

the dental lamina (Fig. 8.2a). The cells of the vestibular lamina proliferate, thereby increasing its bulk. Degeneration of the central epithelial cells of the vestibular lamina results in the formation of a sulcus, the vestibule, separating the lips and cheeks from the tooth-bearing jaw region (Fig. 1.31).

### THE FATE OF THE DENTAL LAMINA

The dental lamina grows downwards and backwards from the second deciduous molar into the posterior region of the developing jaw where it successively gives rise to the permanent molar teeth. The permanent molar teeth, therefore, do not appear to have a direct independent connection to the oral epithelium. Following tooth development, the dental lamina degenerates (Fig. 8.9). Some of the lamina remnants are capable of proliferating and produce small epithelial masses, the so-called 'glands' of Serres.

## Epithelial/mesenchymal interactions during odontogenesis

The fundamental processes in tooth development involve actions and reactions between the epithelial enamel organ and the mesenchymal dental papilla. Indeed, the developing tooth germ is often used as a model for the study of epithelial/mesenchymal interactions, interactions which are common to many other developing systems such as hair follicles and salivary glands. Before describing such interactions, mention should be made of the origin of the mesenchymal tissue.

It seems probable that ectomesenchymal cells from the neural crest (Figs. 1.14 and 4.4) migrate to the developing jaws and contribute to the formation of the dental papilla and to the induction of the enamel organ. The dentine-forming cells (odontoblasts) in amphibians can be shown to be derived from neural crest cells. The essential role played by neural crest in the development of amphibian teeth has been shown by experiments involving either removal of neural crest cells (in which case teeth do not form in the jaws) or transplanting them to different sites (inducing tooth formation at these different sites). In mammalian embryos, however, though neural crest cells have been traced migrating towards the developing jaws (they can be recognized because of their characteristically high RNA, alkaline phosphatase and glycogen content), their subsequent behaviour has yet to be established though it is presumed that they play a role in tooth development.

The interdependence of the epithelium and mesenchyme of the developing tooth is well illustrated by the fact that, should the enamel organ be separated from the dental papilla (by bathing a dissected tooth germ in trypsin) at an early stage in development and each cultured separately, further differentiation ceases. If, however, the components are recombined in tissue culture they develop and differentiate further.

The question arises as to the relative importance of each component during the various stages of tooth development. At present, because of experimental limitations, little information about this is available for stages earlier than the cap stage. The contributions of the enamel organ and dental papilla to the control of crown form have been investigated in the following way. The enamel organs and dental papillae of mouse tooth germs are separated by trypsinization before the teeth have appeared to take on their distinctive morphologies. Should a molar dental papilla be recombined in culture with an incisor enamel organ, a molar-shaped tooth develops. Conversely, should an incisor dental papilla be recombined in culture with a molar enamel organ, an incisor-shaped tooth develops. These results are taken to indicate that the dental papilla controls the shape of the tooth germ. (N.B. an isolated dental papilla can only produce a ball of cells).

The relative importance of the developing dental tissues in histogenesis has been determined by experiments which, though similar to those described above, are designed to discover whether only the presumptive odontogenic epithelium is competent (p. 3) to form enamel organs or whether epithelium from non-odontogenic sites can be induced to form enamel organs when combined with dental papillae. When epithelia from the vestibular band or from the diastema region of the oral cavity were combined with mouse molar dental papillae, enamel organs formed in culture. Conversely, when molar enamel organs were cultured with diastema mesoderm, the enamel organ regressed. The inductive capacity of the dental papilla was shown even more dramatically when epithelium from the plantar surfaces of the feet was combined with mouse molar dental papillae. In these transplants, enamel organs developed from the non-odontogenic epithelium.

In another experiment, only the cervical loop tissues of a developing tooth germ were explanted. It was observed that this cervical loop region, inclusive of both epithelial and adjacent mesenchymal components, was able to differentiate into a complete, but smaller, tooth.

Though the above experiments suggest that the dental papilla is important in the induction of the enamel organ and in the determination of crown form, the nature of the induction process itself remains obscure (p. 2). Earlier work in which successful development was obtained in systems where the epithelium and mesenchyme were separated by a Millipore filter was interpreted as indicating that, since the cells of each layer were not in contact, induction was mediated by chemical substances which passed through the filter from one cell to another. However, recent work has shown that, in many instances, cells can send long cytoplasmic processes through membrane filters which may therefore not necessarily prevent contact between interacting cells. Thus, problems relating to the role of cell contacts and/or chemical inducers remain unresolved.

Immediately prior to the onset of hard tissue formation the internal enamel epithelium and dental papilla are separated by an extracellular organic matrix, approximately 3–20 $\mu$m in thickness. This matrix is a complex structure consisting of collagen, glycoproteins, glycosaminoglycans and membrane-limited, spherical bodies (matrix vesicles) of varying size (50–100 nm), density and shape, some of which contain RNA. When isolated, this extracellular matrix has the ability of inducing some degree of differentiation into isolated dental epithelial or dental papilla cells. Though this differentiation may be a result of the physical properties of the extracellular matrix, RNA in this matrix may be the transmitter of inductive information. The source of this RNA is not known, though both the adjacent epithelial and mesenchymal cells may be involved. There is some evidence showing that during morphogenesis collagen within the extracellular matrix may have a stabilizing influence, for, should a substance which inhibits cross-linking in collagen (i.e. lathyrogens such as $\beta$-aminopropionitrile) be administered to a developing tooth in culture, morphogenesis is suppressed.

If dental papilla cells are grown in monolayer culture, they lose their cytological characteristics and appear to become primitive mesenchyme cells (i.e. the cells seem to have 'de-differentiated'). However, these cells do not lose their ability to direct the histogenesis of teeth, for, when mixed with freshly dissociated epithelium, tooth germs can be developed in culture.

Experiments have been undertaken to assess the role of local factors such as 'morphogenetic fields' and the positions of nerve fibres and blood vessels in determining the shape, positions and numbers of teeth during development. In these experiments, developing first molar tooth germs of mice were cultured as intraocular grafts. In some cases, a graft produced all three molar teeth in their normal sequence and with approximately correct individual shapes and proportions. These data suggest that the whole molar dentition develops out of a single cell mass whose growth is initiated and whose ultimate size is determined by the initial induction of the first molar. Recent studies have highlighted the possible influence of the innervation on the initiation and patterning of tooth germs.

An hypothesis concerned with the mechanism of morphogenesis of the crown likens the developing tooth germ to a fluid-filled sphere partitioned across the middle by the internal enamel epithelium; the stellate reticulum is on one side of the partition and the dental papilla the other. The pressures are thought to be balanced on either side of the internal enamel epithelium which increases its surface area by mitosis. Because it is somewhat restricted at its margins in the cervical loop region, the proliferating internal enamel epithelium buckles to form the primary cusp. Cell division continues at the sides of the primary cusp so that its height is increased by a deepening of its flanks down into the dental papilla rather than further growth up into the stellate reticulum. Additional cusps may form in the same manner. If the shape into which the internal enamel epithelium buckles is determined by its pattern of cell division, then previous work already referred to would suggest that this pattern is controlled by the dental papilla.

CLINICAL CONSIDERATIONS

Disturbances in the development of the dentition may give rise to the following congenital abnormalities.

*Anodontia*
The total absence of teeth (complete anodontia) is a rare condition and in most cases is associated with other forms of ectodermal dysplasias. Of more common occurrence is partial anodontia (hypodontia), permanent teeth being more frequently absent than deciduous. The permanent teeth most frequently absent are third molars, upper lateral incisors and lower second premolars.

*Supernumerary teeth*
Extra teeth may be present within the dentition and may or may not have a recognizable tooth form. They may arise separately from the dental lamina or result from complete division of an early developing tooth bud. The most common site for a

supernumerary tooth is between the upper central incisors and such teeth (mesiodens) may prevent eruption of the incisors.

*Abnormalities of size and shape*
Teeth may be unusually large (macrodontism) or small (microdontism). This condition may be generalized, as in certain hormonal disturbances, or localized. There may be changes in the shape of teeth and the addition or loss of roots or cusps.

A geminated tooth is one in which an enamel organ has incompletely divided into two, resulting in a bifid crown with a single root. A similar clinical appearance may arise where two separate tooth germs become fused together during development (fused teeth). When the teeth fuse late in development they are joined by cement. This is referred to as concrescence.

There may be an invagination during development involving either the crown or root with resultant formation of internal ridges and folding of the dental tissues.

*Odontogenic cysts*
These cysts are formed in the jaws by odontogenic epithelium. The dental epithelium may form a cyst instead of a tooth, or a cyst may develop from the epithelial remnants between teeth. Alternatively, a cyst may form from remnants of the dental lamina overlying a developing tooth.

*Tumours*
Instead of forming a normal tooth, the various cellular constituents may give rise to tumours involving both hard and/or soft tissues. Thus, there may be tumours of ectodermal origin (e.g. ameloblastomas), mesenchymal origin (e.g. cementomas) and mixed origin (e.g. odontomas).

## DEVELOPMENTAL CONTROLS

### Tooth succession

Nearly all non-mammalian vertebrates continue to replace their teeth throughout life, the condition of polyphyodonty. Multiple tooth replacements may be required to compensate for wear and accidental loss of teeth. However, there is a further and more probable explanation. Because these animals grow throughout their lives it may be necessary to replace small teeth by larger teeth which are more commensurate with the size of the growing animal.

The great majority of polyphyodont animals replace their teeth in a sequence which is referred to as the wave replacement of alternate teeth (Fig. 8.12). This pattern of tooth replacement is presumably retained because it is more efficient than other possible patterns, amongst which would be random replacement. The pattern may be efficient because it ensures that any resorbing or erupting tooth is always flanked, and therefore protected, by firmly attached teeth; and no gap in the dentition is ever longer than a single tooth position.

Mammalian teeth are never replaced more than once and their pattern of replacement appears to be very irregular (e.g. man). However, within a species there is remarkable consistency in the timing and sequence of tooth replacement. In order to understand the units from which the complex dentitions of mammals are constructed it is helpful to trace, as far as is possible, their evolution from the dentition of reptiles which due to their simplicity are easier to analyze.

Obviously the tooth is a unit of the dentition but if we are to be able to account for the wave replacement of alternate teeth found in most non-mammalian dentitions it is natural to look for some unit larger than the tooth and smaller than the whole dentition. Three such units have been proposed; odontostichos (Greek: tooth row); Zahnreihe (German: tooth row); and clones.

THE ODONTOSTICHOS MODEL

In 1919, Bolk proposed that the odontostichos (Fig. 8.13a) is a biological unit of reptilian dentitions: an odontostichos consists of a row of alternate teeth. Therefore, it can be seen that

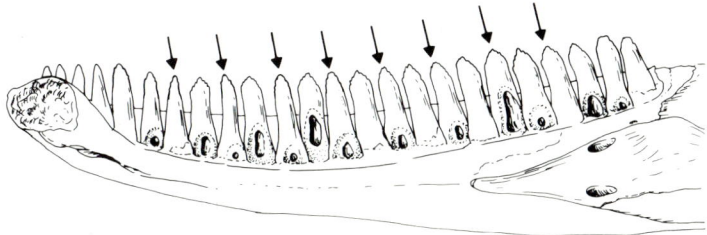

**Fig. 8.12.** Teeth are replaced in waves that sweep from the back to the front of the jaw through alternate tooth positions. The size of the hole beneath each tooth is equivalent to the size of its replacement. Arrows point to a replacement wave.

256    Chapter 8

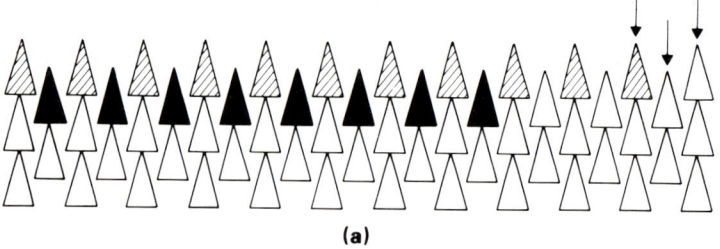

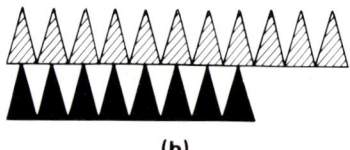

**Fig. 8.13.** Bolk's odontostichi theory.

Bolk's model requires two types of odontostichi; one type which fills and replaces odd-numbered positions and another type related to even-numbered positions. The wave replacement of alternate teeth is initiated and maintained by alternating the contributions of odd- and even-numbered odontostichi to the functioning dentition.

For this model it is suggested that mammalian dentitions maintain only the first of the odd- and even-numbered *odontostichi* (Fig. 8.13b). One has been pushed together to become the deciduous dentition together with the permanent molars—the other has been pushed together to become the replacement teeth.

### THE ZAHNREIHE MODEL

In 1960, Edmund proposed that the Zahnreihe is a biological unit of vertebrate dentitions: a Zahnreihe consists of a row of consecutive teeth (cf. an odontostichos which is a row of alternating teeth). The teeth which constitute a Zahnreihe develop in sequence from the front to the back of the jaw (Fig. 8.14a). New Zahnreihen continue to be initiated at the front of the jaw throughout life. The surprising feature of the Zahnreihe model is that, provided the time interval between the initiation of new Zahnreihen is within certain limits, alternate teeth are replaced in sequence from back to front despite the fact that con-

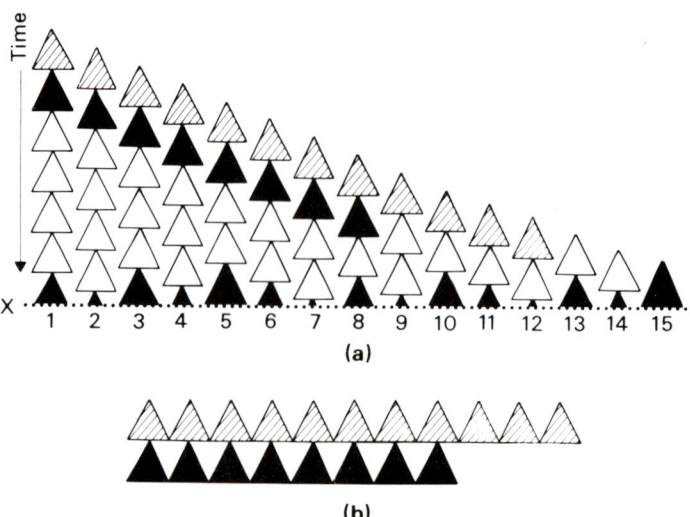

**Fig. 8.14.** Edmund's Zahnreihe theory. (After Osborn J. W. (1973))

secutive teeth are being initiated from front to back.

In terms of this model, the dentitions of mammals contain two Zahnreihen (Fig. 8.14b): one contributes the deciduous teeth and permanent molars; the other contributes the replacement teeth.

CLONE MODEL

For homodont (non-mammalian) dentitions the clone model recognizes only two dental units; the tooth and the dentition. The jaws of these animals develop from two homogeneous populations of mesenchymal cells; the dental clone produces the teeth and their supporting tissues; the basal clone produces the remaining bone of the jaw.

The dental clone induces the development of the dental lamina and together they become competent to initiate new teeth whenever space is available. This vigour is tempered because each newly initiated tooth is surrounded by a region in which the initiation of a new tooth is temporarily inhibited. It will be noted that this type of control inexorably drives the dentition into the wave replacement of alternate teeth (Fig. 8.15). Waves of tooth replacement sweep regularly through the clone throughout life.

In the upper jaw of reptiles, the replacement waves are broken at the premaxillary-maxillary suture. This suggests that the upper jaw contains two dental clones. In many cotylosaurs the premaxillary clone contains larger teeth than the maxillary clone (Fig. 8.16a). In the later pelycosaurs a third 'canine' clone was added (Fig. 8.16b). Later still, in cynodonts, heterodonty appeared in the maxillary clone (Fig. 8.16c).

Mammals retain three dental clones in each quadrant. The incisor clone grows posteriorly; the canine clone generates only the canines; and the molar clone grows forwards early in development to produce the deciduous molars and backwards to produce the permanent molars (Fig. 8.17). In some animals, such as man, the molar clone only grows posteriorly; the most anterior molar, the first deciduous molar, is the first to develop and the remaining molars develop in sequence posteriorly.

**Tooth shapes**

In all mammalian dentitions the teeth within a particular class, incisor or molar, have graded shapes and sizes (e.g. Fig. 8.18). Two models have been proposed in order to account for these gradients; a field model and the above clone model.

MORPHOGENIC FIELDS

This model proposes that all tooth primordia are equivalent. The shapes into which they develop are controlled by substances (or signals), generated elsewhere in the jaws, which perfuse the primordia and activate certain 'receptors'. All primordia contain the same 'receptors', which might be thought of as the sites for potential cusps; the differences between teeth are due to differences between the nature and concentration of the different field substances which perfused the original tooth buds thereby activating the development of different cusps.

The ancestral eutherian mammal possessed eleven tooth primordia (of which the anterior eight were replaced). Three types of field substance are produced, each generating a different morphogenetic field. The anterior substance spreads back, successively perfusing the three most anterior primordia and fades away in the region of the fourth primordium. The posterior substance perfuses the seven posterior primordia; the middle substance perfuses the fourth primordium. The three morphogenetic fields overlap to a greater or lesser extent. The largest and most complex tooth within each field develops from the primordium which is influenced by the maximum concentration of the relevant field substance; the position of maximum effect. During evolution a particular field substance can spread to influence more teeth. For example, the incisor morphogenetic field of artiodactyls spreads to influence the fouth primordium (the ancestral canine) inducing it to become incisiform (Fig. 10.1j). In a similar way, the substance corresponding with the molar morphogenetic field may have its greatest concentration anywhere from Pm4 to M3, resulting in the largest and most complex tooth being at any of these four positions; but it is generally at the same position for any particular species. For example, in man the maximum effect is at M1 while in the gorilla it can be at M3.

If the concentration of field substances is low a tooth is very small and, with even lower concentrations, the tooth is lost from the dentition.

CLONE MODEL AND SHAPE

It will be recalled that each clone can grow either anteriorly or posteriorly, or both, to generate a tooth class. Each newly initiated primordium is surrounded by a zone of tissue in which the initiation of a new primordium is temporarily inhibited. When the growing border of the clone has escaped from the inhibitory zone, a new

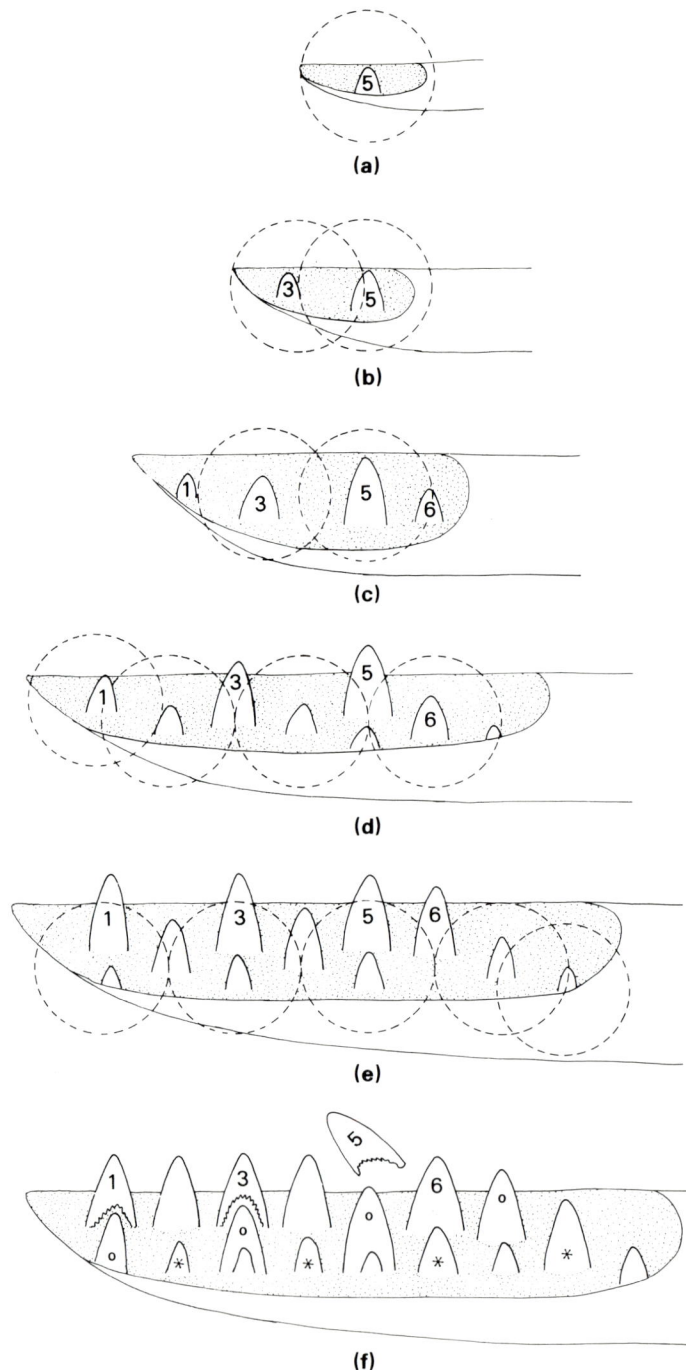

**Fig. 8.15.** Clone model. The stippled clone (and dental lamina) grows anteriorly and posteriorly from position 5. In this example, teeth 5, 3 and 1 become separated by interstitial growth. Each newly initiated tooth is surrounded by a region (interrupted circle) in which the initiation of a new tooth is temporarily inhibited. (After Osborn J. W. (1973))

primordium is initiated. In the clone model it is suggested that gradients in tooth shape are related to the sequences in which teeth are initiated.

A concept of shape competence is introduced here. The shape of a tooth is determined from the moment its primordium has been initiated (cf. a field model in which all primordia are equivalent). All the cells in a clone are potentially capable of generating tooth primordia but the zones in which the initiation of primordia is inhibited become the

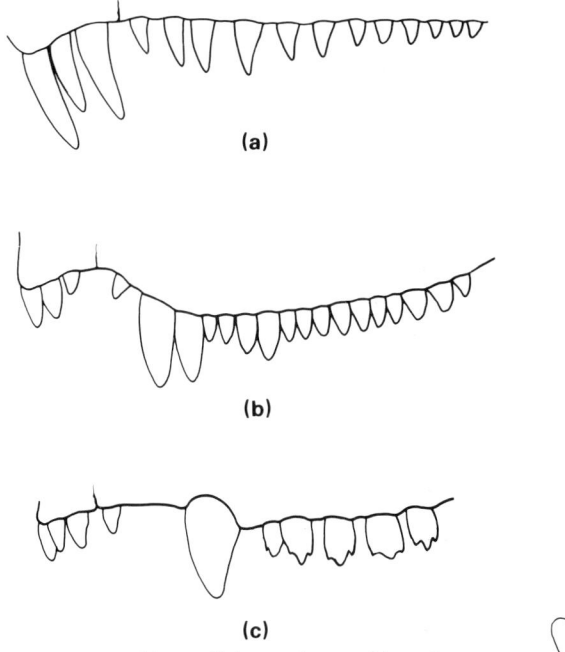

**Fig. 8.16.** Dentitions of (a) a cotylosaur, (b) a pelycosaur and (c) a cynodont.

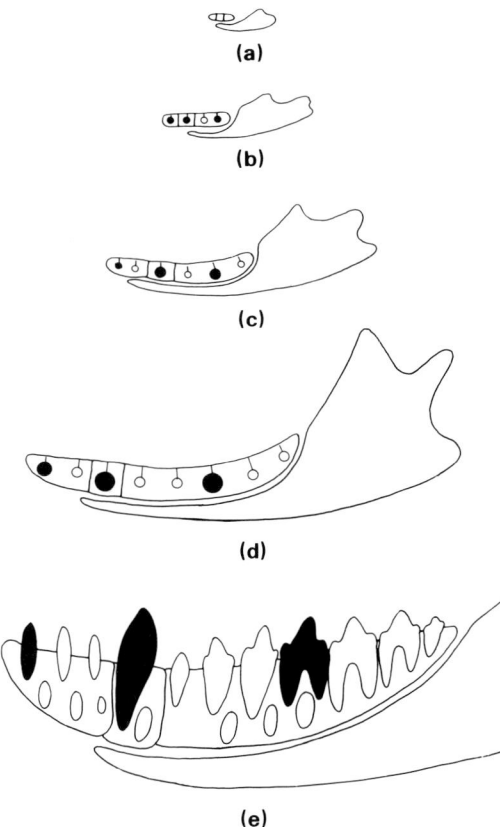

**Fig. 8.17.** The growth of three dental clones in a mammal. The first bud in each clone is black.

tissues between teeth. Shape competence, a theoretical concept, refers to the competence of clone cells, whether or not they actually develop into primordia, to develop a complex tooth shape. While the clone enlarges, the shape competence of the cells at its growing border may fall, or rise and fall, but it cannot fall and rise again (cf. embryonic competence to react to an inducing stimulus: p. 3). It will be appreciated that gradients in tooth complexity must follow the sequences in which tooth primordia are initiated, these sequences matching the directions in which the clone grows.

DISCUSSION

There is very little evidence which can be used to distinguish between the above models. The evidence from embryo lizards (and crocodiles) and mammals, suggests that teeth are very rarely, if ever, developed in sequence from the front of the jaw (the sequence backed by the Zahnreihe model). But it could be that undetected, or unrecognizably small, primordia are developed in all these animals.

With one possible exception no field substances have been discovered anywhere in any animals. They remain as concepts.

Perhaps the most important data come from observations that any mammalian tooth primordium, isolated and cultured *in vitro*, continues to develop its correct shape, provided the culture conditions are good enough. This suggests, in accordance with the clone model, that all primordia are different. But a protagonist of the field

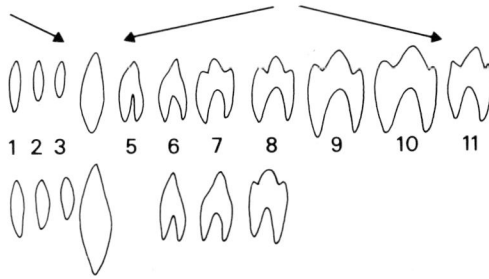

**Fig. 8.18.** The full eutherian dentition. Incisors develop in sequence posteriorly. Deciduous molars develop in sequence anteriorly and permanent molars in sequence posteriorly.

model can argue that field effects have penetrated the dental lamina before primordia are initiated.

This latter explanation focuses attention on a very important defect of field models. The field is like an ace of trumps which can be played to account for any card of variation. If a tooth has a very unusual shape, if it is very large, if it erupts early or late, if it is absent from the dentition, and so on, it can always seem to be accounted for by saying that there has been a change in the field.

## DENTINE AND PULP FORMATION

### Morphogenesis

In the early bell stage of tooth development the tooth germ consists of three components: the enamel organ, the dental papilla and the dental follicle. This section is concerned mainly with the dental papilla which gives rise to the dentine and pulp, but the enamel organ and its derivative, Hertwig's sheath, also play a part in the formation of the dentine.

At the early bell stage the dental papilla consists of a mass of mesenchymal cells. Those on the surface of the papilla are induced by the inner enamel epithelium to differentiate into the odontoblasts which are responsible for laying down dentine; experiments in tissue culture show that without the presence of internal enamel epithelium odontoblasts cannot differentiate in the papilla. It has been shown that, in amphibians, the odontoblasts are derived directly from neural crest cells. The neural crest probably contributes to the dental papilla in all vertebrates but so far this has not been proved experimentally.

The dental papilla, besides its function as a formative tissue, appears to control the shape of the tooth germ. The shape of the enamel–dentine junction, which is essentially the same as that of the completed crown, is determined by the shape of the boundary between the papilla and the inner dental epithelium. This boundary folds before the dentine is formed. If the dental papilla from a molar tooth is cultured with the enamel organ from an incisor tooth, the interface between the two folds into the shape of a molar tooth. Thus, the dental papilla seems to control the shape. An important factor in the shape-determining function of the papilla seems to be the collagenous connective tissue in which the mesenchymal cells lie; if, in the above experiment, the formation of collagen is inhibited, the internal enamel epithelium does not fold.

It is during the bell stage of development that the smoothly curved interface between the enamel organ and the dental papilla folds into the pattern which determines the ultimate shape of the crown. First, cells in the region which will become the primary cusp stop dividing. This is followed by a buckling upwards of the internal enamel epithelium. Further cell divisions on the flanks of this lead to further elevation of the cusp. If another cusp is to be developed, cells stop dividing on the flank of the primary elevation to be followed by a buckling of the interface in this new region. The cells between the two elevations continue dividing (Fig. 8.19). These dividing cells in the valleys between the cusps not only push the cusps further apart but also increase their height by deepening the valleys. Away from the areas mentioned, cell division slows down and ultimately ceases before the cells differentiate. The superficial cells of the papilla develop into odontoblasts and begin to lay down dentine matrix against the basement membrane. Some component in this matrix induces the cells of the inner enamel epithelium to differentiate into ameloblasts (cells which secrete enamel matrix on to the surface of the dentine).

Dentinogenesis begins shortly after the epithelium has buckled (Fig. 8.19). In incisors and canines, dentine is first laid down at the tip of the dental papilla, at the site of the future incisal surface, and then extends laterally to cover the walls of the crown. In molars and premolars, dentinogenesis begins at the site of the 'primary' cusp. Formation of hard tissue in the remaining cusps begins some time later (Fig. 8.19). The mineralization of the cusps in the cheek teeth follows a sequence and time course which is characteristic for each tooth type. With time, hard tissue formation extends into the valleys thereby uniting the developing cusps. This stabilizes the shape of the crown and prevents further separation and growth of the cusps by cell division. The external shape and relationships of the cusps are modified during later development by variation in the thickness of enamel laid down in different regions of the crown. For example, more enamel is laid down over the tips of cusps than along the sides of teeth.

After the shape of the crown has been established, the dental epithelium and papilla continue to grow downwards to form the root portion of the tooth. The dental epithelium in the root region, the epithelial root sheath of Hertwig, is a downward growth of the cervical loop. Its functions are to outline the shape of the root(s) and to induce the differentiation of odontoblasts. It differs from the coronal enamel organ, being composed solely of the inner and outer epithelial

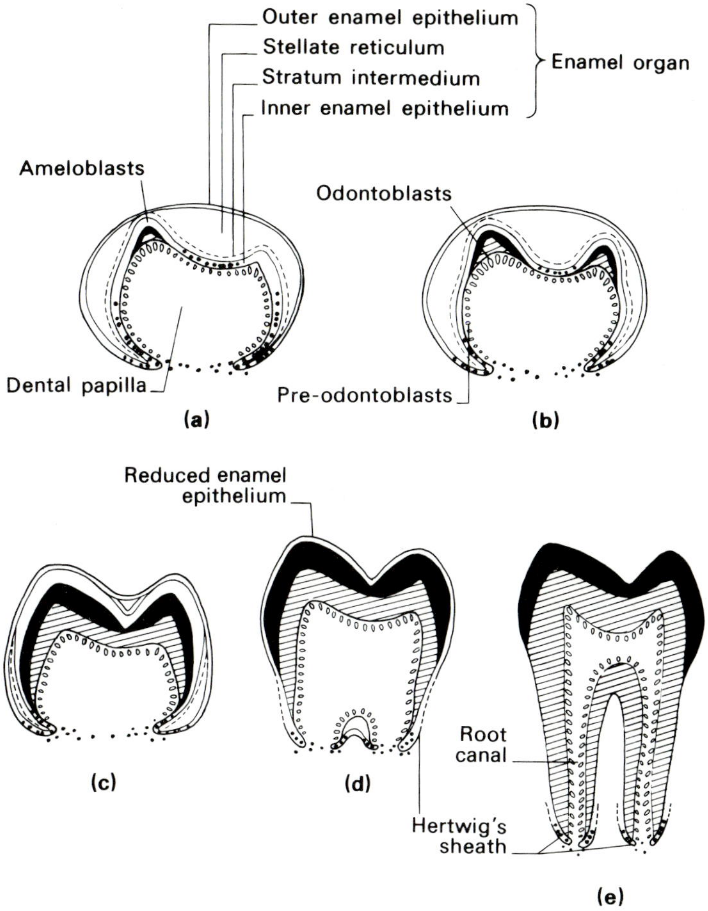

**Fig. 8.19.** Stages in the morphogenesis of a molar: (a) bell stage, showing initial deposition of hard tissues in the principal cusp; (b) later bell stage, with formation of hard tissues in the secondary cusps and extension of the initial mineralisation; (c) crown well formed; (d) early root development; (e) late stage of root development in an erupted tooth. ■, Enamel, ▨, dentine; ∴, cell division.

layers without the intervening stellate reticulum and stratum intermedium (Fig. 8.20). Furthermore, Hertwig's sheath does not maintain its integrity throughout tooth development. Soon after the first deposition of dentine near its advancing edge it breaks up into small islands of epithelial tissue which persist in the periodontium of the mature tooth as the epithelial rests of Malassez (Fig. 8.20). These are especially common in the apical region and a role in the pathogenesis of certain dental cysts has been ascribed to them. The breakup of Hertwig's sheath allows access to the dentine surface of follicular cells involved in the formation of cement and the periodontal ligament.

In incisors and canines, Hertwig's sheath forms a simple tube but in premolars and molars it becomes divided into two or more tubes corresponding to the number of roots in the mature tooth. The subdivision of the sheath is accomplished as in Fig. 8.21. After the establishment of the crown form, tongues of epithelium grow

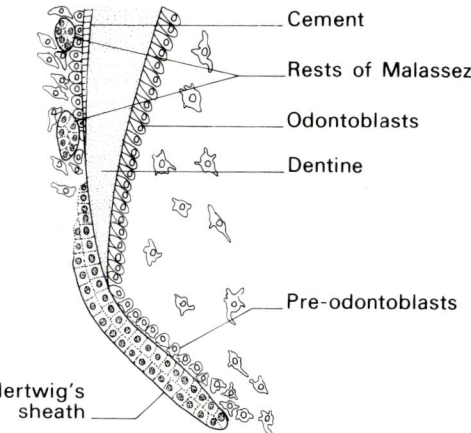

**Fig. 8.20.** Apical tip of growing root, showing the structure of Hertwig's sheath, the formation of rests of Malassez by degeneration of the sheath and differentiation of odontoblasts and cementoblasts.

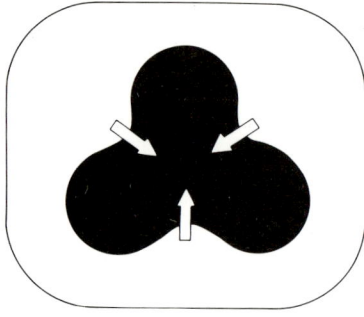

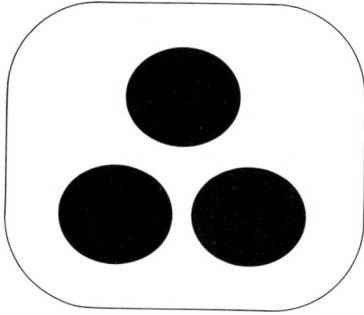

**Fig. 8.21.** Tooth germs viewed from below to show the mode of subdivision of the root sheath.

inwards from the base of the enamel organ under, but in contact with, the dental papilla and fuse in the centre, forming a perforated epithelial floor to the coronal region. The epithelium surrounding these large perforations then grows downwards as separate tubular root sheaths. During the mapping out of the roots, blood vessels are present, running into the pulp from below, and Hertwig's sheath grows downwards to enclose them.

Dentine is laid down a short distance behind the advancing edge of Hertwig's sheath (Fig. 8.20). The initiation and subsequent thickening of the dentine in a lengthening (developing) root maintains a knife-edge of dentine at the growing margin of the root; this is easily observed in the apices of young teeth extracted before the roots have formed completely.

As the developing root nears its full size the diameter of Hertwig's sheath progressively decreases, giving the root its characteristic taper. The roots are completed by thickening of dentine to the point where each root is penetrated only by a narrow root canal containing pulpal elements, blood vessels and nerves. The neurovascular bundle enters the roots by way of one or more apical foramina. Where there are multiple foramina the root canal is branched in the apical region. This may lead to complications in endodontic procedures. The roots are not completed until 2 or 3 years after eruption.

The bulk of dentine laid down before eruption and up to the time of root closure is often referred to as the primary dentine, to distinguish it from the secondary dentine which is formed more slowly during the later life of the tooth (see below).

In places, dentine may fail to form and this leads to the production of narrow subsidiary lateral root canals which may perforate the side of the root. Their occurrence is unpredictable (they probably develop around aberrant blood vessels supplying the growing pulp), but they tend to be more frequent in the region of the bifurcation of the roots, particularly in deciduous molars. Lateral root canals can lead to clinical problems and provide a potential path for infection to travel from the pulp into the periodontal ligament.

**Dentine formation**

In the account that follows, the formation of mantle and circumpulpal dentine will be considered first, followed by a discussion of the other tissues.

MANTLE DENTINE MATRIX

This is formed by odontoblasts which have just begun to differentiate. Before the start of dentine formation the cells of the dental papilla are small, irregular in shape and possess little cytoplasm. The superficial cells then differentiate, first into pre-odontoblasts (Fig. 8.22a), then into odontoblasts (Fig. 8.22b). The main features of this process are as follows. The volume of cytoplasm in the distal region (towards the enamel organ) increases, causing the nucleus to lie at the proximal pole. The distal cytoplasm becomes much richer in organelles, especially those associated with protein synthesis and secretion, namely the rough endoplasmic reticulum and the Golgi apparatus. During mantle dentine formation the odontoblasts have not yet reached their full size. The odontoblasts initially possess a variable number of small processes at the distal pole but during mantle dentine formation these join to become larger, single odontoblast processes. At the same time the odontoblasts start to develop desmosomes and tight junctions which join them together.

The first stage in the formation of mantle dentine is the deposition of matrix which contains collagen fibres embedded in a ground substance

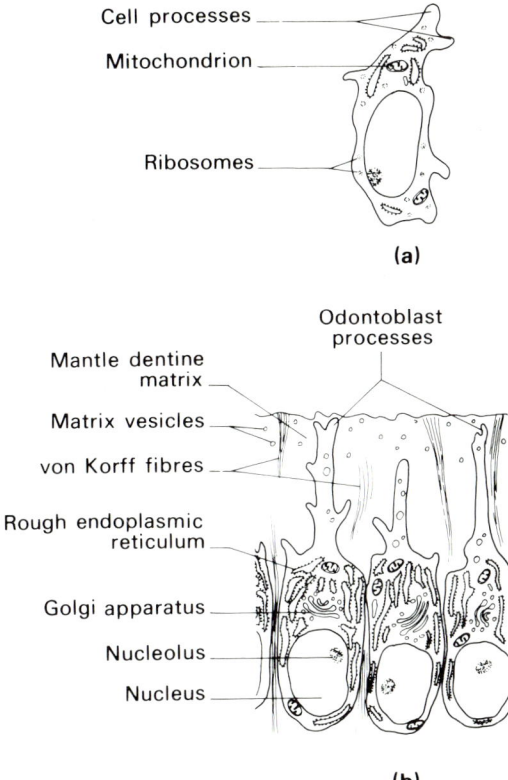

Fig. 8.22. (a) Pre-odontoblast. Note the small size of the cell and the small number of organelles. (b) Young odontoblasts involved in the formation of mantle dentine. Note the increase in rough endoplasmic reticulum and the large Golgi apparatus, together with the formation of a true odontoblast process (branched at this stage). In the matrix, only the von Korff fibres and matrix vesicles are depicted.

rich in glycosaminoglycans and also the cytoplasmic processes that are trailed out by the odontoblasts as they move away from the growing matrix. The collagen fibres are arranged in a complex network, with a large proportion (von Korff fibres) standing perpendicular to the basement membrane under the dental epithelium (Fig. 8.22b). Under the light microscope these fibres are demonstrated by the use of silver impregnation techniques and appear as coarse black fibres passing from the subodontoblast region between the odontoblasts and fanning out before terminating at the basement membrane. With some techniques they appear to have a spiral course and have been called 'corkscrew fibres'. Although, in the light microscope, von Korff fibres appear to make up a large part of the the matrix of mantle dentine, electron microscopical studies do not bear this out. At the ultrastructural level, bundles of collagen fibres, together with fibres which may consist of elastin, are observed between the odontoblasts but these fibre bundles are much finer than the coarse, silver-stained (argyrophilic) structures of light microscopy. The best explanation for this discrepancy seems to be that, during silver impregnation, the fibres are apparently thickened by heavy deposits of silver around them. The great affinity for silver may be due to the presence of reducing sugars in the ground substance; reticulin fibres, which consist of fine collagen fibres associated with large quantities of carbohydrate, are also argyrophilic.

It has been claimed that the primary source of the mantle dentine matrix is not the odontoblasts but the layer of pulp cells immediately underneath them. This was suggested mainly by an observation that, during the earliest stages of dentine formation, the subodontoblastic cells are rich in alkaline phosphatase which appears to be absent from the odontoblasts themselves; this distribution is reversed during the formation of circumpulpal dentine. The exchange in the roles of odontoblasts and subodontoblast cells is suggested because alkaline phosphatase has been implicated in protein secretion in other tissues. However, electron microscope studies suggest that the odontoblasts secrete more protein than the subodontoblastic cells, so it seems likely that the odontoblasts produce the bulk of mantle dentine matrix. The subodontoblastic cells clearly contribute to the formation of von Korff fibres which ultimately become part of the matrix but, as noted above, these fibres are not the major component of the matrix.

CIRCUMPULPAL DENTINE

After the formation of mantle dentine the odontoblasts continue to 'mature' and begin to lay down the matrix of circumpulpal dentine. During the formation of this tissue, the cells are larger and therefore more crowded together with very narrow intercellular spaces; this crowding eventually leads to the formation of a pseudostratified layer of columnar odontoblasts several cells deep. Each cell now possesses only one well-developed odontoblast process but may continue developing short lateral processes. The main process is separated from the cell body by a sheet of microfilaments which stretch into the cytoplasm from a ring of desmosomes. As more and more dentine is laid down the cell bodies retreat inwards towards the pulp trailing their lengthening pro-

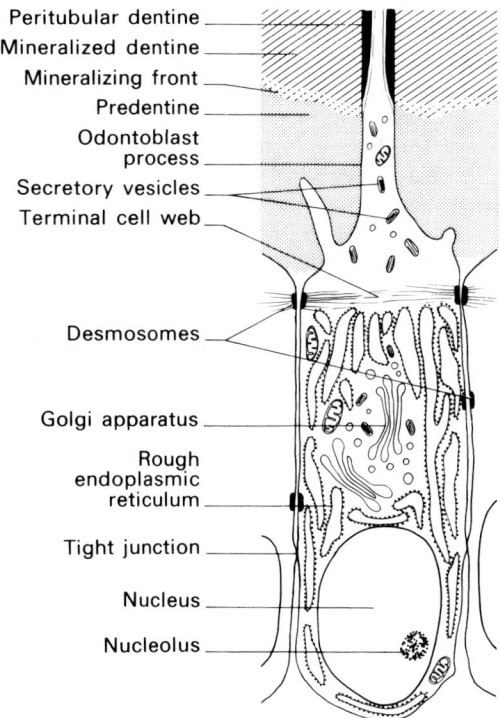

**Fig. 8.23.** Odontoblast involved in circumpulpal dentine formation. The cell is larger and richer in organelles than in mantle dentine formation (see Fig. 8.21) and shows new features, such as the terminal web of microfilaments. The formation of peritubular dentine is shown in relation to the mineralizing front.

cesses, around which matrix is deposited, and thereby producing tubules. The small lateral processes become trapped in the dentine like the main processes and appear as branches of the tubules in the mature tissue. The odontoblast process only occupies the full length of the dentinal tubule during the earlier part of dentine formation; thereafter, the tip of the process appears to be either withdrawn or broken down.

The cytoplasm of the odontoblast process contains microfilaments, microtubules and vesicles; other organelles, such as mitochondria, are only rarely present (Fig. 8.23). The body of the odontoblast, on the other hand, contains mitochondria, large quantities of rough endoplasmic reticulum and a very active Golgi apparatus. The role of these structures in collagen synthesis is described in Book 1.

### MINERALIZATION

Mineralization begins at the presumptive enamel–dentine junction and spreads inwards in the wake of matrix formation. Thus a layer of unmineralized matrix (predentine) is always present between the odontoblasts and the mineralized part of the dentine (Fig. 8.23).

The first sign of mineralization is the appearance in the mantle dentine of very small clusters of crystals visible only with the electron microscope. Reasonable evidence has accumulated to suggest that these first crystals are initiated within small extracellular vesicles which bud from the odontoblasts and enter the matrix (Fig. 8.22b). It is suggested that as the crystals enlarge they perforate the membranes of the vesicles and grow into the matrix (Book 1). During formation of circumpulpal dentine, matrix vesicles have not been identified and mineralization advances along a front into the predentine. At the mineralizing front, apatite crystals appear to form mainly in relation to the matrix collagen fibres. In the superficial layers of the dentine, mineralization progresses more rapidly along the von Korff fibres than on the other matrix fibres. The mineralization of collagen involves the formation of nuclei (small clusters of solid mineral) at sites both within the fibres and at their surface. Then by taking up ions from solution in the tissue fluid bathing the matrix, the nuclei grow to become recognizable crystals. In dentine, as in bone, the crystals grow to a much smaller size ($3 \times 20$–$100$ nm) than those of enamel. The restraining factor appears to be the presence of strong covalent cross-links between the collagen molecules making up the fibres, which limit the space available for crystal growth. At the mineralizing front complex reactions involving proteoglycans and glycosaminoglycans lead to change in histochemical reactions and histological staining properties in a region which histologists often refer to as intermediate dentine.

In circumpulpal dentine formation a large proportion of the mineral is laid down in advance of the mineralizing front in the form of calcospherites within the predentine (Fig. 8.24); this is an important feature distinguishing dentine from bone. The crystals within them have two orientations. Some crystals form in association with collagen fibres, as above, while others radiate from the centre of the calcospherite. Normally, the calcospherites grow by addition of mineral at the outer surfaces until this ceases as the mineralizing front first contacts and then surrounds them. The calcospherites can still be recognized in mature dentine by using the polarizing microscope, which can detect the radially-arranged clusters of crystals (Fig. 6.12). The distribution of

# Development of Dentition

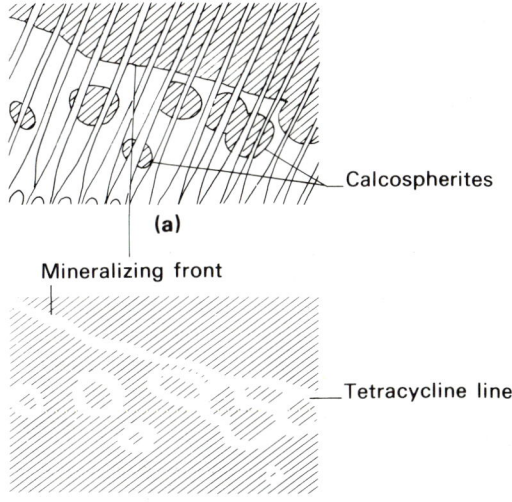

**Fig. 8.24.** (a) Showing the dual process of dentine mineralization; as a mineralizing front and as calcospherites. (b) The fluorescent line which would be formed by administration of the drug tetracycline, which binds to sites of mineralization, at the stage shown in (a).

Peritubular dentine appears to be absent from mantle dentine and the timing and extent of its development in the circumpulpal dentine are variable. In the rat and in the deciduous teeth of the cat, for example, it appears to be lacking. In many ungulates it begins to form level with the mineralizing front of the intertubular dentine but in the elephant it forms in advance of the mineralizing front. In man, although the amount of peritubular dentine increases with age, the formation of the tissue is not uniform: in dentine from teeth of people at all ages, even over 70 years, some tubules are ringed with peritubular dentine, some lack a hypermineralized wall altogether and others are completely occluded. Occlusion of tubules is considered below. Peritubular dentine does not form within interglobular regions.

calcospherites and interglobular dentine is described on p. 168. After injection of tetracycline, which is fluorescent and is deposited at sites of mineralization, linear bands are observed under ultraviolet light in the mantle dentine and a mixture of linear, globular and linear/globular bands in the circumpulpal dentine (Fig. 8.24b). A study of interglobular regions in deciduous teeth suggests that they may be produced in areas where matrix formation is more rapid than mineralization, so that the latter process is not completed. Intergobular regions are absent from dentine formed *in utero* and from the slowly-formed regular secondary dentine. In the deciduous dentition, interglobular regions are very common in the thick coronal dentine of the molars, less common in the canines and absent from the incisors.

It seems likely that peritubular dentine formation (p. 170) is under the control of the odontoblast process. Autoradiographic evidence indicates that protein is transported along the processes and deposited on the walls of the tubules. However, the details of secretion of the organic and mineral components of the peritubular dentine are not known. The matrix of peritubular dentine is not collagenous but its composition has not yet been identified. In the electron microscope it appears in demineralized sections as an amorphous material.

## CURVATURE OF DENTINAL TUBULES

The odontoblasts do not follow a straight course during their centripetal migration in advance of the forming dentine. This is shown by the sweeping S-shaped primary curvature (Fig. 6.11). These deviations from a straight line are the result of directions in which the odontoblasts move as they migrate inwards. The movement is probably caused by pressures between the cells set up as a result of the odontoblasts being increasingly more crowded together as the pulp becomes smaller. It has been suggested that the length of an odontoblast process formed in a given time may be greater than the distance travelled by the cell in the same time; this could result in a buckling of the process within the predentine to accommodate the excess, thus accounting for the secondary curvatures.

## INCREMENTAL LINES

The von Ebner lines, about 5 $\mu$m apart, separate regions containing slightly differently orientated fibres but nothing is known about the control of this orientation. The control is almost certainly local rather than systemic. Clearly, the neonatal line develops as a result of the immediate postnatal systemic disturbance which, more importantly, leads to a loss in the weight of the baby. The contour lines of Owen are the result of a similar and simultaneous change in the directions in which the adjacent odontoblasts are moving. The origin of the forces inducing this change in direction are disputed and unclear: they are almost certainly local. The lines due to variations in mineralization which are seen in microradiographs could be the result of either local or systemic factors.

ROOT DENTINE

The bulk of the root is made up of circumpulpal dentine which forms as described above. The formation of the outer layers, however, appears to differ and is not very clear, despite numerous studies.

The granular layer of Tomes is less well mineralized than the circumpulpal dentine, for which several explanations exist. It may be that mineralization of the matrix, which is said to be coarsely fibrous, is incomplete thereby producing minute interglobular spaces. Alternatively, the dark appearance of the layer might be caused by scattering of light from air trapped in dilatations or loops of the terminal parts of the dentinal tubules.

The outermost hyaline layer of tissue, superficial to the granular layer, poses numerous problems. Its thickness and structure vary between different animals. It is often difficult to distinguish from the adjoining layer of acellular cement because it contains few tubules although in some species, such as the dog, the outermost layer does contain tubules and resembles mantle dentine. Recent studies on the dog provide some evidence that the hyaline layer mineralizes centrifugally rather than centripetally and that the outermost layer, which does not mineralize, forms a basis for the attachment of the fibres of the developing periodontal ligament (temporarily taking on the role of cement).

**Development of the pulp**

As the superficial cells of the dental papilla differentiate into odontoblasts and begin to lay down dentine the central region of the papilla begins to differentiate into pulp tissue. The cells, initially small and undifferentiated, become more widely dispersed and the great majority develop into active fibroblasts. The cytoplasm increases in amount and organelles associated with protein synthesis and secretion, the rough endoplasmic reticulum and Golgi apparatus, become more abundant. The fibroblasts secrete collagen into the intercellular space throughout development of the tooth. In the young pulp the collagen is dispersed evenly in the form of fine fibre bundles. Coarse fibre bundles appear only at about the time that the tooth reaches maturity and in the pulp of the adult tooth there is a tendency for the collagen to become increasingly concentrated in such fibres with age. Also present in the extracellular space is a ground substance rich in proteoglycans, the most abundant glycosaminoglycans of which are hyaluronic acid and chondroitin sulphate. These increase in amount until the time of eruption and then decrease.

Towards the time of eruption a cell-rich zone forms underneath the odontoblast layer. The formation of this zone seems to be accomplished by cell migration; studies with tritiated thymidine show that its formation is not due to increased cell division. In man and some other species, such as the Rhesus monkey, but not in others such as the rat, the cell-rich zone is separated from the odontoblasts by a layer in which cells are scanty. This layer is known as the basal or cell-free zone of Weil which takes the place of the subodontoblast cells in the developing tooth.

Vascularization of the developing pulp starts during the bell stage, with small branches from the principal vascular trunks of the jaws entering the base of the papilla (Fig. 8.25). Of these small pioneer vessels, a few become the principal pulpal vessels. These enlarge and run through the pulp towards the cuspal regions. Here, they give off numerous small branches which form a bed of venules, arterioles and capillaries in the subodontoblastic and odontoblastic layers. The vascularity of the odontoblast layer increases as dentine is progressively laid down, probably as the result of the odontoblasts retreating inwards through the vascular bed. Eventually, some capillaries are found immediately next to the predentine surface. As the dentine thickens and grows inwards, these capillaries are closed off but occasionally a capillary loop may become trapped in the dentine. During the apposition of dentine, subsidiary vessels enter the pulp alongside the principal vessels and give off lateral branches supplying the walls of the tooth. The time and pattern of appearance of lymphatics in the pulp has not yet been established. The mature pulp contains macrophages, pericytes and lymphoid cells in addition to fibroblasts. These probably enter the pulp with the invading blood vessels but the defence cell population of the developing tooth has not been studied.

The first nerve fibres to enter the pulp accompany the blood vessels. They are non-myelinated and are presumed to be autonomic. Much later, when root formation is well advanced and the time of eruption is approaching, sensory branches grow out from the dental nerves supplying the jaws, unite and enter the root canals as pulpal nerves (Fig. 8.26). These course towards the cuspal regions and give off branches to the subodontoblastic region. Lateral branches to the walls of the tooth are also formed. In man, the principal network of nerve fibres in the subodontoblastic region occupies the cell-free zone of Weil and is

# Development of Dentition

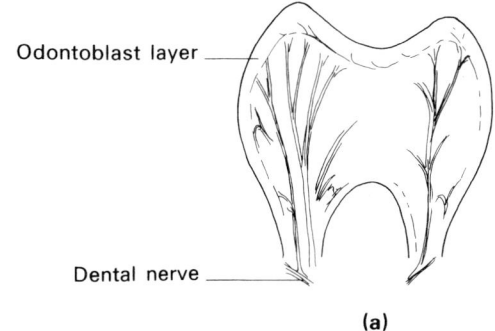

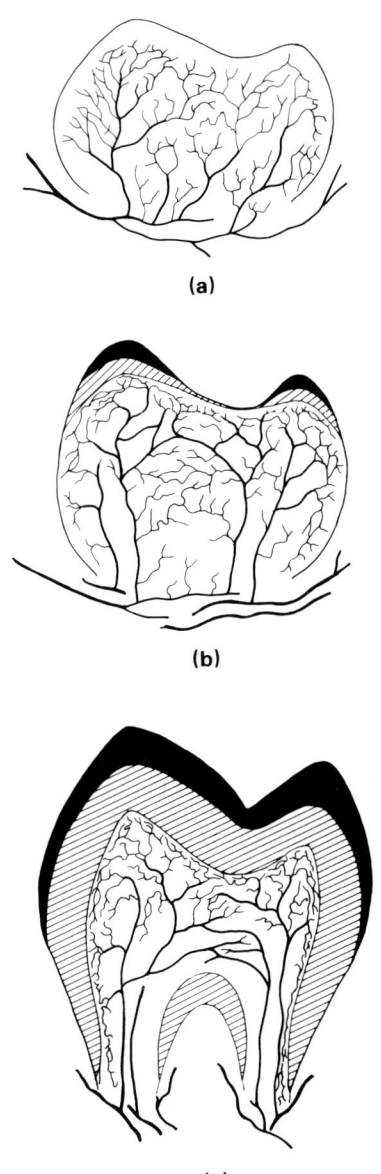

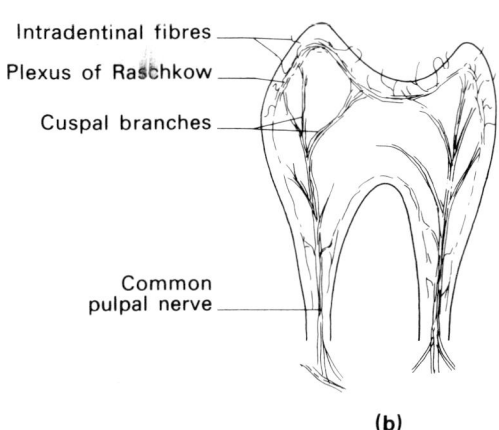

**Fig. 8.26.** The innervation of the pulp: (a) before eruption, during root formation; (b) after eruption. Note the appearance of fine nerves within the odontoblast layer and within the dentine.

**Fig. 8.25.** The distribution of pulpal blood vessels during: (a) bell stage; (b) crown formation, (c) root formation.

known as the plexus of Raschkow. It is not established until root formation is nearly complete. Nerve fibres cross the layer of odontoblasts and form a subsidiary marginal plexus next to the predentine. A few extend into dentinal tubules for a short distance, lying alongside the odontoblast process. With continuing formation of dentine some nerve fibres become trapped in predentine or dentine as loops which double back and re-enter the pulp.

## ENAMEL DEVELOPMENT

The enameloid of fishes and amphibians is a mixture of the secretions of odontoblasts and the internal enamel epithelium (Fig. 6.2). In reptiles and mammals the odontoblasts secrete and mineralize a narrow strip of dentine before the cells of the internal enamel epithelium begin to secrete their contribution. This mineralized layer separates the products of the enamel organ from those of the odontoblasts with the result that a new pure tissue, enamel, formed entirely from ectodermal (or endodermal) cells, is developed.

### The functions of the enamel organ

The enamel organ has the following functions:

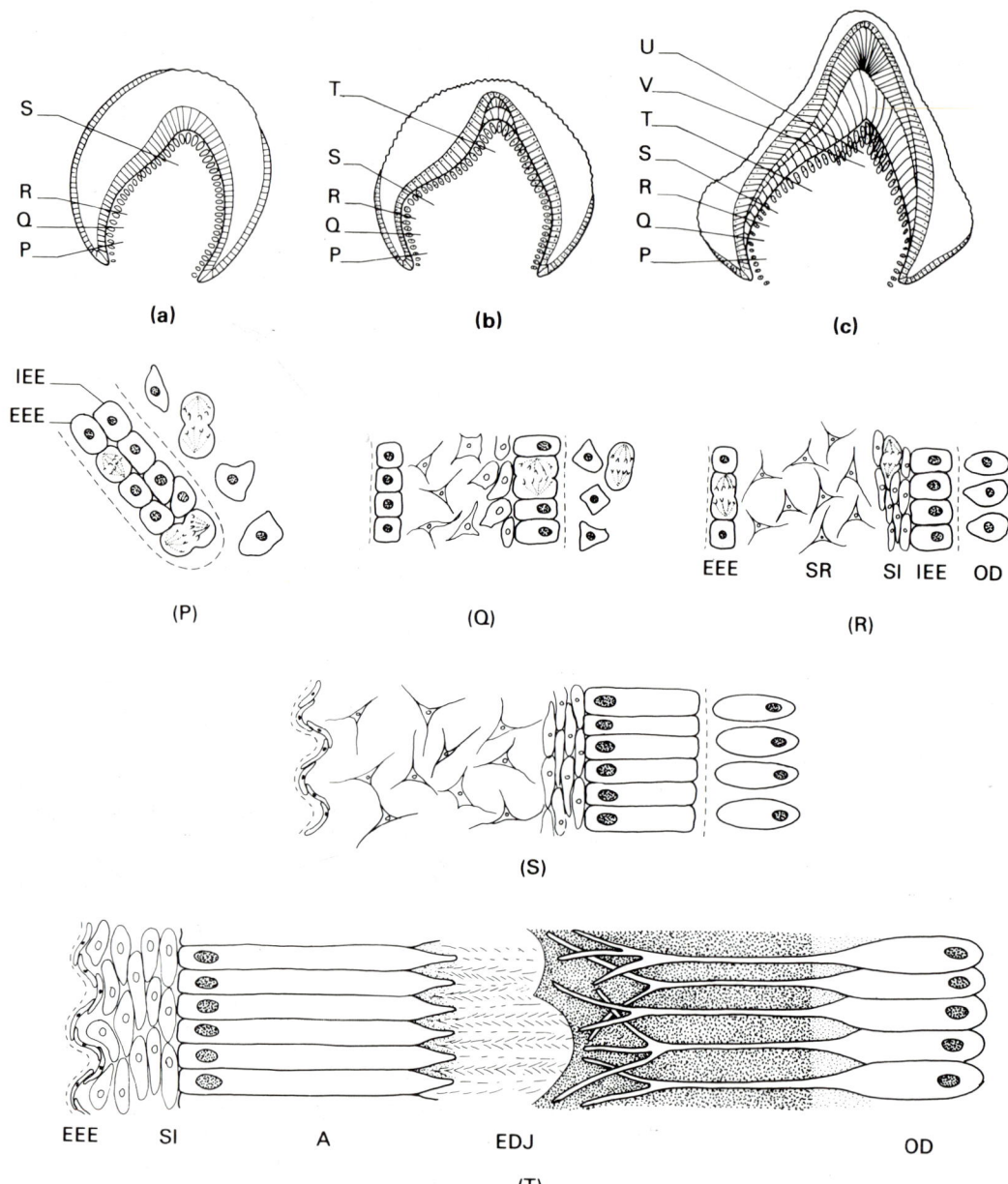

Fig. 8.27. Three stages in growth and differentiation of the enamel organ (a, b, c). The histological appearances of different sections are shown in P, Q, R, S and T. The dotted line is basement membrane. OD, odontoblasts; IEE, internal enamel epithelium; SI, stratum intermedium; SR, stellate reticulum; EEE, external enamel epithelium; EDJ, enamel–dentine junction; A, ameloblasts.

1  Together with the dental papilla it outlines the shape and regulates the size of the tooth.
2  It induces the differentiation of odontoblasts.
3  It makes the enamel prisms.
4  Its cervical loop continues to grow as Hertwig's root sheath which, together with the dental papilla, outlines the shape and regulates the size of the root.
5  It may form an enamel cuticle or cuticles.
6  Together with the oral epithelium it generates junctional epithelium and its related epithelial attachment.

## The structure of the enamel organ

Three stages in the life of an enamel organ are shown in Fig. 8.27. The previous chapter described how dentine formation starts at what is later the tip of the dentine cusp and spreads down the sides of the crown. Enamel formation follows the same course.

The changes which lead to prism formation start in the oldest part of the enamel organ (near the centre of the internal enamel epithelium in a single cusped tooth) and spread down the sides of the tooth. Before the full crown has been mapped out by the growing cervical loop, all stages in amelogenesis can be found in a single enamel organ (Fig. 8.27c).

### PREPARATION FOR AMELOGENESIS

During the cap and bell stages of the tooth germ a stellate reticulum and later a stratum intermedium greatly increase the bulk of the growing enamel organ (Fig. 8.3). At its growing rim (the cervical loop) an outer layer of cuboidal cells, the external enamel epithelium (EEE), is continued inwards as an inner layer of cuboidal cells, the internal enamel epithelium (IEE) (P, Fig. 8.27). The IEE lengthens not only by mitoses at the cervical loop but also over its whole span. Behind the growing edge of the cervical loop increasing numbers of a new population of cells separate the EEE from the IEE (Q, Fig. 8.27). These cells become the stellate cells of the stellate reticulum (SR). Soon after the SR appears, the stratum intermedium (SI) is differentiated against the elongating cells of the IEE (R, Fig. 8.27). Despite the fact that the SR is the first to appear, the SI later acts as a source of new cells for the thickening SR.

Although the stellate cells of the SR have a quite different shape from the flattened cells of the SI they contain similar organelles; amongst these are a Golgi apparatus, a sparse rough endoplasmic reticulum, mitochondria and several types of vesicle. The cells of the EEE contain even fewer of these organelles. All the cells of the enamel organ are connected by desmosomes.

After the appearance of the SI the cells of the EEE flatten from cuboidal to squamous (S, Fig. 8.27). It seems possible that the cells of the EEE are 'stretched' from cuboidal to squamous by expansion of the SR. However, this cannot be the whole explanation because the EEE is now thrown into minute folds greatly increasing its surface area. At the same time a rich capillary bed proliferates in the adjacent mesoderm. These events are usually interpreted as manoeuvres to increase the efficiency with which the enamel organ absorbs nutrients from the tooth follicle in preparation for amelogenesis.

The differentiation of odontoblasts can now occur at the tip of what will later be the dentine cusp. The odontoblasts retreat and deposit dentine matrix which is then mineralized. Coinciding with these events the immediately adjacent IEE cells stop dividing and become differentiated into ameloblasts which lay down the enamel (T, Fig. 8.27). The actual process of amelogenesis will be described in detail later.

### TIMING

The earliest dentine is laid down at the tip of the dental papilla and a wafer-thin edge of developing dentine subsequently spreads down the sides of the crown (Fig. 8.19). Because the formation of dentine appears to be the final stimulus for the differentiation of ameloblasts, it is clear that the advancing edge of enamel formation follows behind the equivalent dentine edge down the sides of the crown (Fig. 8.27b, c). From this it can be visualized that the developing prisms are longer and more mature over the cusps than they are at the sides of the crown (U and V, Fig. 8.27c). In the same way enamel formation ends over the cusps earlier than it ends at the sides of teeth. This can also be appreciated by studying the brown striae of Retzius (Fig. 6.24).

### NUTRITION

Prior to making enamel prisms the IEE cells might derive their nutrition from the dental papilla, but as soon as a layer of mineralized dentine has been deposited on the surface of the papilla this source is cut off. The newly differentiated ameloblasts now depend on a lengthy supply line running through the full thickness of the enamel organ. In preparation for this 'blockade' the cells of the IEE have earlier accumulated glycogen in their cytoplasm: the ameloblasts call upon this store of energy during the first stage of prism formation. While the ameloblasts are spending this reserve, their supply route is dramatically shortened by the mysterious 'disappearance' of the adjacent stellate reticulum (Fig. 8.27b, c). Whether the cells of the stellate reticulum die or whether they become displaced down the sides of the enamel organ is not known. In any event their 'disappearance' brings the ameloblasts much closer to their blood supply.

The above series of events itself unfolds in sequence opposite each of the cells of the IEE from the tip of what will be the tooth cusp down the sides of the enamel organ ending at what will be the cervical margin, the limit of the anatomical crown (Fig. 8.27c).

THE 'RESPONSIBILITIES' OF CELLS

Presumably each cellular layer in the enamel organ fulfils a particular set of functions. Clearly the layers work together, with the ameloblasts 'at the business end'.

*The external enamel epithelium*
The EEE is a 'containing' layer of cells: it is the outer limit of the enamel organ with a basement membrane separating it from the surrounding mesoderm. Being the outer layer, the EEE transfers materials to and from the remainder of the enamel organ. Its alkaline phosphatase may be required in the process of transporting glycogen in a phosphorylated form.

*The stellate reticulum*
This layer is very thin, even unrecognizable, in the enamel organs of all non-mammalian vertebrates. It is reduced to almost nothing as soon as amelogenesis starts in mammals. This obviously suggests that it may serve its purpose before amelogenesis starts. One argument proposes that a hydrostatic pressure generated in the stellate reticulum, due to the absorption of water by the hydrophilic proteoglycans (p. 254) which the cells secrete, balances the pressure produced by the growing dental papilla. The shape of the internal enamel epithelium is stabilized by the equal pressure on each of its sides and, in some way, permits it to fold without any undue interference from the two cell masses between which it is sandwiched.

Another argument proposes that the glycosaminoglycans in the spaces between the stellate cells are rapidly passed through the stellate reticulum on to the ameloblasts and out into the first developed enamel.

*The stratum intermedium*
This cell layer seems to be active throughout amelogenesis. It is usually thought to prepare materials acquired from the external enamel epithelium before passing them on to the ameloblasts. It is interesting that the stratum intermedium contains alkaline phosphate, an enzyme which, with the notable exception of ameloblasts, is found in all cells which form calcified tissues. However, it should be remembered that this enzyme is also found in the external enamel epithelium and in the stellate reticulum.

The stratum intermedium is connected to the ameloblasts by desmosomes, structures which are thought to facilitate intercellular transport.

*The ameloblasts*
These are the cells which actually secrete the enamel matrix and control the development of enamel.

## The development of an idealized prism

DIFFERENTIATION

During the bell stage of development the low columnar cells of the inner enamel epithelium (IEE) begin lengthening towards the cells at the surface of the dental papilla, later inducing them to differentiate into odontoblasts (Fig. 8.28a–d).

*Reversal of polarity*
Due to some undiscovered interaction the polarity of the IEE cells is now reversed, the nuclei moving towards the ends of the cells furthest from the dental papilla. This reversal in polarity is a very unusual event. It is the nature of nearly all basal epidermal cells and their derivatives such as glands, hair follicles, feathers and so on, to push their products (e.g. saliva) or daughter cells (e.g. prickle cells) towards the surface. The early change in polarity of the IEE cells later allows them to secrete their product in the opposite direction; away from the surface of the oral cavity.

*Induction*
From the time at which they start lengthening and reverse their polarity the cells of the IEE begin to construct and arrange an elaborate machinery of intracellular organelles. It seems probable that these first stages in differentiation are induced by the ectomesenchymal cells of the dental papilla. The centrioles move towards the proximal end of the IEE, the end farthest from the odontoblasts. Many mitochondria, which are self-generating organelles proliferate and fill the cytoplasm on the proximal side of the nucleus. The cisternae of an extensive network of rough endoplasmic reticulum and Golgi apparatus are contructed to fill the cytoplasm on the distal side (towards the odontoblasts) of the nucleus, the Golgi apparatus lying in the middle with endoplasmic reticulum at the ends and sides. Most of the cisternae are aligned parallel to the long axis of the cell.

A disc of microfilaments is stretched across the cytoplasm between the mitochondria and the proximal end of the cell: this so-called terminal

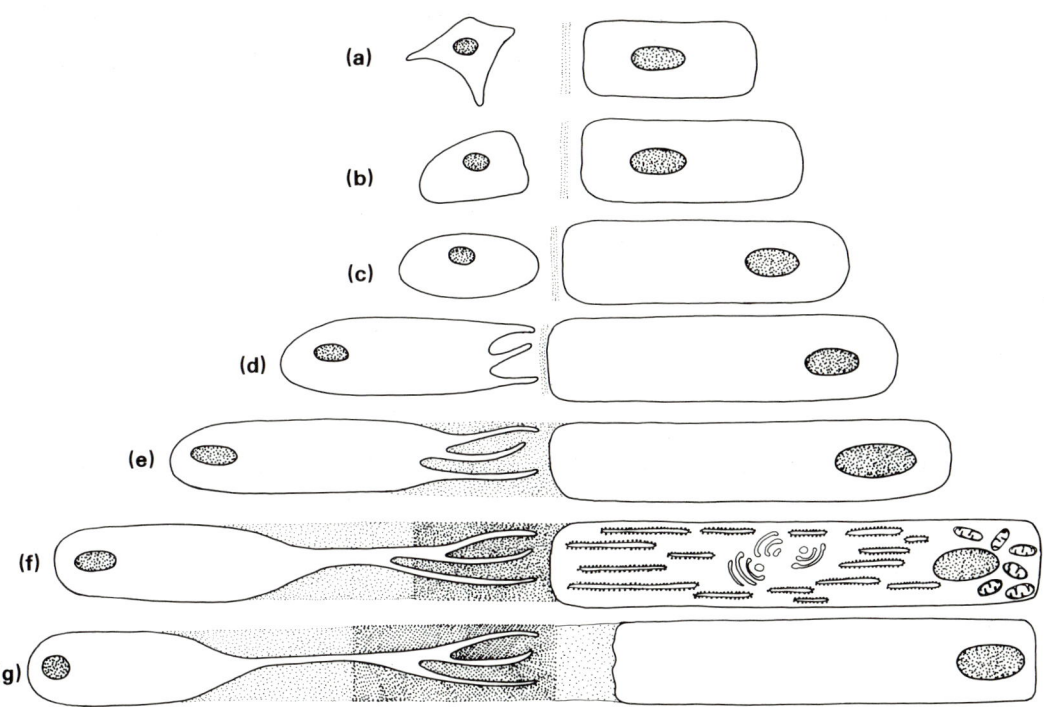

**Fig. 8.28.** Stages in the differentiation of odontoblasts (left) and ameloblasts (right).

web is continuous at its periphery with a circle of junctional complexes (Book 1) connecting adjacent cells. The sides of the cells are joined intermittently along their whole length by tight junctions and by desmosomes.

While the IEE cells are lengthening the odontoblasts begin to lay down matrix and the basal lamina which separated the ectodermal and mesodermal cells disappears (Fig. 8.28e). The odontoblasts move away from the IEE mineralizing the old matrix and continuing to secrete new matrix. The distal ends of the IEE cells, which are now about 40 μm long and 5 μm wide (in man), are separated from mineralized dentine by a few unmineralized tags of collagen in dentine matrix that has escaped the attention of the odontoblasts. This mineralized dentine induces the final differentiation of the IEE.

SECRETION

Once the cells of IEE begin to secrete material they are called ameloblasts: their secretion may be called amelogenin, although this term has been used to describe only part of the ameloblast secretions.

*Tomes' process*

When amelogenin is first secreted onto the surface of the mineralized dentine the ameloblasts shorten instead of moving (Fig. 8.28g). In electron micrographs amelogenin looks stippled when it is secreted. Almost immediately very narrow crystals, about 1.5 nm wide, start to grow outwards from the surface of the mineralized dentine into the amelogenin (Fig. 8.29a). The distal end of the ameloblast now changes shape: its originally flat secreting cell membrane is distorted into a conical process known as Tomes' process of the ameloblast (Fig. 8.29b). A row of these conical processes is described as producing a 'picket fence' appearance (Fig. 8.29c). Sectioned transverse to its long axis each ameloblast is hexagonal: the appearance of a cross-sectioned layer of ameloblasts close to their Tomes' processes gave rise to the 'honeycomb layer' (Fig. 8.29d).

After a brief period, during which they shorten, the ameloblasts move away from the dentine surface secreting amelogenin through their conical Tomes' processes. The cytoplasm of the Tomes' process is partly separated from the body of the cell by the distal terminal web (see above).

# Chapter 8

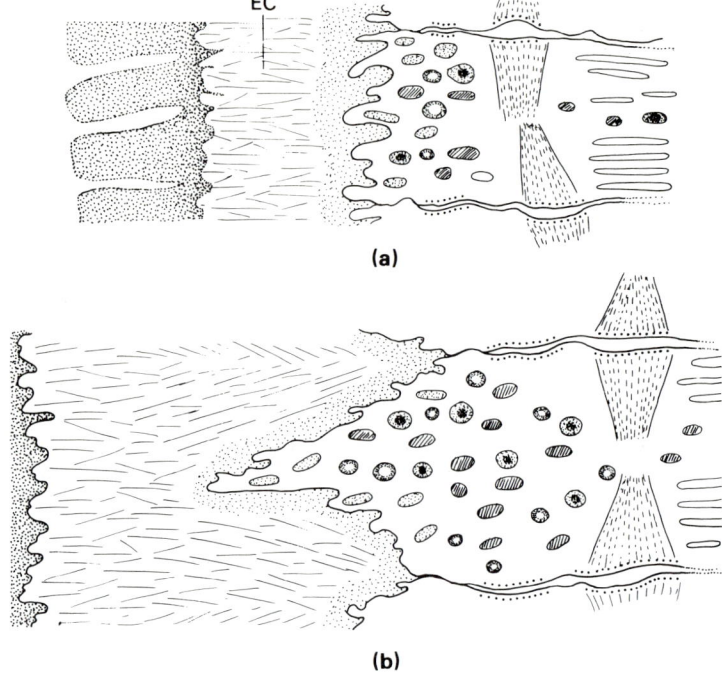

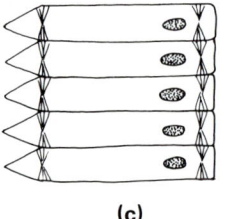
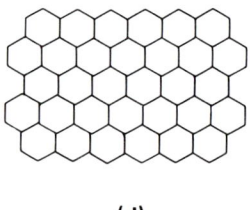

**Fig. 8.29.** (a) The first enamel crystallites (EC) are more randomly orientated. (b) Later they develop the preferred orientations which correspond with prisms. (c) The ends of the ameloblasts present a 'picket fence' appearance. (d) Viewed in cross-section the ameloblasts are hexagonal.

The process has an irregularly folded surface (Fig. 8.29b) and it contains several types of vesicle, some containing stippled material similar in appearance to the amelogenin just outside the Tomes' process.

*Amelogenin*
Because of the small quantities which can be purified, and the difficulties of purification, the exact structure and composition of amelogenin is not known. It contains water, probably at least three different proteins, glycoproteins, proteoglycans, citrate and lipids. The nature of amelogenin will be discussed in more detail when the 'maturation' of the enamel is considered. The term 'amelogenin' is necessary to distinguish it from the matrix of fully developed enamel.

*The developing enamel*
Almost as soon as amelogenin is secreted it becomes invaded by tape-like crystals spreading into it from the surface of the mineralized dentine. As the ameloblasts move away so the ends of the lengthening crystals follow them with the result that only a very thin layer of mineral-free (stippled) amelogenin, about 100 nm wide, separates the ends of the crystals from the folded surface of the Tomes' process. Matrix vesicles have not been seen inside the developing enamel.

*Crystal orientation*
For the idealized, hexagonal-shaped prisms under consideration, all the crystals lengthen out towards the edges of the Tomes' process and colonize the newly secreted (stippled) material (Fig. 8.30). Thus, new crystals are constantly being developed in the middle of the prism, lengthening out towards its edges, and then ending where they abut the ends of similar crystals in an adjacent prism. A prism sheath develops along the boundary between differently orientated crystals.

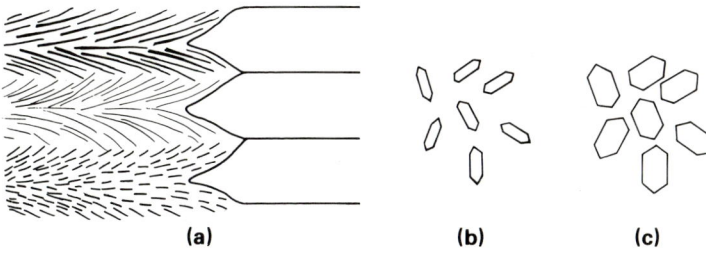

Fig. 8.30. (a) Crystals diverge away from the Tomes' process of the ameloblast towards the centre of the prism. A prism sheath develops in the region where there is a sudden change in crystal orientation. In cross-section the crystals are narrow when first developed (b), and thicken as they grow (c).

An alternative, more generally accepted, view is that the crystals are much shorter; only a few hundred instead of a thousand nanometres long (bottom and top of Fig. 8.30a). It has so far been impossible to prove which view is correct because the fragile crystals are shattered when an ultrathin section, cut by a diamond knife, is prepared for electron microscopy.

MATURATION

Although when first developed the crystals are very thin, they are so numerous that they occupy about 27% of the volume of the developing prism (Fig. 8.30b). By thickening at their sides they subsequently grow to occupy about 88% of the volume (96% by weight). In cross-section each crystal is a slightly flattened hexagon, about 40 nm at its widest. It is interesting and probably significant that randomly arranged hexagons packed into an area would theoretically occupy 88% of that area (Fig. 8.30c); the same as the percentage actually occupied by crystals in enamel.

It will be appreciated that if, from occupying 27% of the developing enamel, the crystals eventually fill 88% of the volume, then an equivalent volume of amelogenin must be removed. This dramatic change in the composition of developing enamel is referred to as the 'maturation' of enamel, a process in which enamel attains its full volume of hydroxyapatite and loses an equivalent volume of protein and water.

*Crystal growth*
The calcium and phosphate ions required for crystal nucleation and growth all pass through the ameloblasts: none comes from the dentine. Presumably amelogenin contains a high concentration of these ions.

The cross-striations of enamel prisms, thought to be the effect of a diurnal rate of secretion, are about 4 $\mu$m apart (Fig. 6.20). Therefore it takes about one year to secrete a 1.5 mm long prism. It will be appreciated that the crystals initiated at the beginning of the year are fully grown when those formed at the end of the year are being initiated. However, the width of a crystal does not increase at a uniform speed: it starts slowly and after some time accelerates very rapidly (Fig. 8.31a). This can be deduced from microradiographs in which an apparently sharp border separates very radiodense older enamel from much more radiolucent younger enamel (Fig. 8.31b). If crystals grew at a uniform rate microradiographs of developing enamel would show an equivalent uniform change in radiodensity. It is because of the sudden change in composition of developing enamel that the concept of enamel maturation was originally proposed.

In order to reach the older regions of a maturing prism, calcium and phosphate ions must pass through the younger region nearer its ameloblast. In autoradiographic studies labelled amino acids have been shown to travel through ameloblasts and deep into the developing enamel. It is reasonable to assume that calcium and phosphate ions are carried with the amelogenin. Presumably the slowly widening crystals in the younger enamel extract only a small proportion of these ions from the amelogenin leaving sufficient for the widening crystals in the rapidly maturing enamel.

*Enamel matrix*
The majority of enamel matrix consists of water and proteins: the remaining fraction contains glycoproteins, proteoglycans, citrate and lipids. Little is known about the citrate and lipids and they probably have little effect on the development, structure and properties of enamel matrix.

*Glycoproteins.* Some vesicles containing protein, newly synthesized by the adjacent rough endoplasmic reticulum, probably pass to the region of the Golgi apparatus. Within the Golgi apparatus hexosamines are added to the protein to produce a glycoprotein (Book 1). The glycoprotein is transported down the ameloblasts as a secretory granule, into the Tomes' process and then out to the amelogenin.

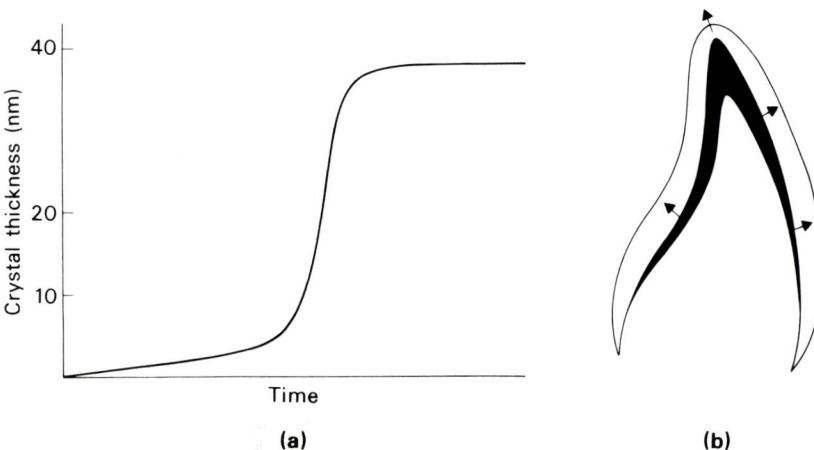

**Fig. 8.31.** (a) There is a sudden increase in crystal thickness associated with the maturation of enamel. (b) Arrows show direction of maturation.

*Glycosaminoglycans.* The long chains of repeating disaccharide units which characterize glycosaminoglycans are probably linked together in the Golgi region. They are also sulphated here and then passed down into the amelogenin in one of the forms known as chondroitin sulphate.

*Proteins.* The different proteins in enamel are studied by separating them out of solutions of demineralized enamel, purifying them and then measuring the proportions of amino acids which each contains. Unfortunately different techniques yield different numbers of proteins. The most conservative estimate is three different proteins. Because they are very alike, the first two can be lumped together as proteins X (Fig. 8.32X). The third protein, protein Y, is very different (Fig. 8.32Y): in particular, proline and glutamic acid account for nearly half its amino acids. Because protein Y accounts for over half the developing enamel proteins it is clear that developing enamel contains a large amount of proline and glutamic acid.

In contrast, mature enamel protein consists largely of proteins X. Much of this protein is insoluble in acids and is concentrated in the tufts. However, small quantities are spread throughout the enamel, some being soluble and some insoluble.

Such analyses also show that enamel contains almost no cystine or hydroxyproline. This indicates that enamel protein is probably not a keratin (keratins contain cystine) nor collagen (collagen is almost the only protein containing hydroxyproline in the body). However, there is some resemblance between the proportions of the remaining amino acids in tuft protein and in keratin, a similarity which is not so surprising because both are products of epidermal cells.

From observations of developing enamel it has been argued persuasively that amelogenin is a gel rather than a fibrous matrix such as is found in all the remaining mineralized tissues. This would account for the mobility of enamel proteins which are transported deep into the enamel and then back to the ameloblasts. The argument continues; if the protein were not a gel which can easily be removed, space could not be created for the crystals to grow to the huge size which typifies those in enamel when compared with other mineralized tissues. However, other observations have suggested that some of the protein is fibrous and that the fibres form a scaffold on which, or in which, the crystals of hydroxyapatite grow.

TERMINATION

When the full length of the prism has been developed the ameloblasts stop retreating and no longer secrete amelogenin. The cells now shorten considerably and lose the majority of the organelles which have been manufacturing secretions (Fig. 8.33). The mitochondria change ends, being mostly on the enamel side of the ameloblast against a cell membrane which loses its Tomes' process and becomes deeply infolded. This arrangement indicates that the ameloblasts are now preoccupied with absorption rather than

# Development of Dentition

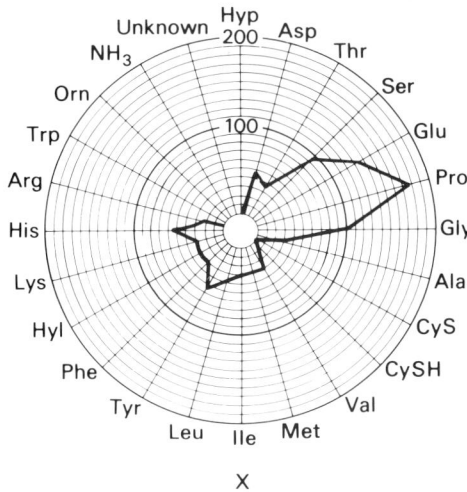

X

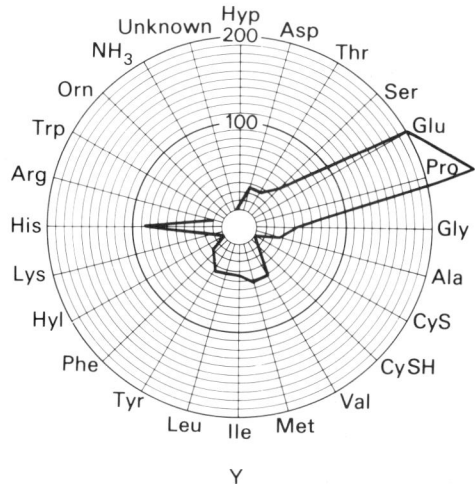

Y

**Fig. 8.32.** A 'rose diagram' showing the amino acid proportions in two different types of enamel protein. (After J. A. Weatherall and C. A. Robinson.)

secretion. For example, autoradiographic data show that labelled sulphur previously deposited in the enamel is now returned to the ameloblasts. Resorption continues until the whole length of the prism is fully mineralized, hydroxyapatite replacing amelogenin.

The ameloblasts are now further reduced to cuboidal cells, the inner layer of the reduced enamel epithelium (Fig. 8.42). During these final stages the ameloblasts may be responsible for developing enamel cuticles.

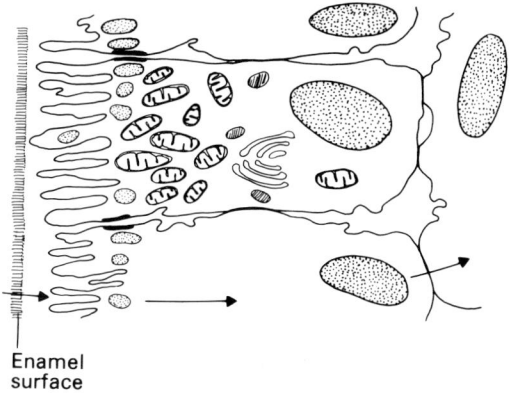

**Fig. 8.33.** At the end of amelogenesis the ameloblasts shorten and change their appearance.

### The development of the interprismatic region

The description given above is simplified in only one important way; the interprismatic region has been ignored. Unfortunately, this complicates the relationship between ameloblasts and prisms.

OBSERVATIONS

The following descriptions are based on appearances seen with the electron microscope.

*In the transverse plane (battlements)*
Sectioned roughly transverse to the long axis of the tooth but along their length, prisms and ameloblasts have the appearance shown in Fig. 8.34a. This plane of section shows each apparently flattened Tomes' process as a 'battlement'. The interprismatic regions extend between the battlements with the prisms forming opposite the battlements. The prism sheath separates the prism and interprismatic region.

The crystals point away from the Tomes' process towards the centre of the prism. An equivalent orientation is repeated in the much narrower interprismatic region.

*In the longitudinal plane (picket-fence)*
Although it has long been recognized, the most surprising aspect of this view of amelogenesis is that the long axis of the ameloblast is sharply angled to the long axis of the prism (Fig. 8.34b). The prism points upwards and outwards, the long axis of the ameloblast points downwards and outwards. Despite the direction of its long axis, it is clear that the ameloblast must move in the direction of the prism it is secreting; that is, it makes a crab-like movement.

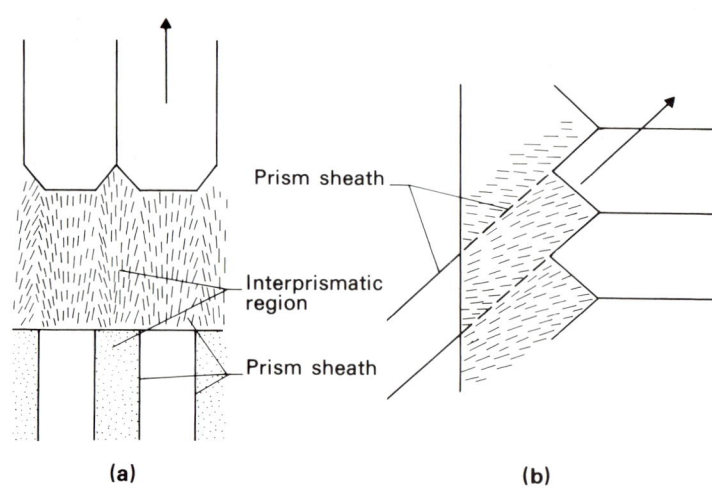

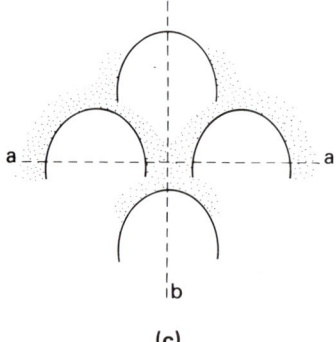

**Fig. 8.34.** (a) The appearance of the ameloblasts and crystals in the transverse plane of the tooth and (b) in the longitudinal plane of the tooth. The planes of section are indicated in (c).

In this plane, the prism sheath is lined up with the tip of the Tomes' process. All the crystals are directed away from the Tomes' process towards a point near the cuspal border; from a direction nearly parallel to the axis of the prism at the cuspal edge they deviate progressively more upwards and inwards as they approach the cervical edge of the prism.

IN THREE DIMENSIONS

The third dimension has been introduced in Fig. 8.35. One diagram (Fig. 8.35a) illustrates the origin of roughly circular prisms surrounded by an interprismatic region, the other (Fig. 8.35b) illustrates keyhole-shaped prisms. It must be emphasized that in each case the structures represented are, in every way, identical; it is merely the terminology, the technique for describing the raw structure, which is different.

In order to understand some of the problems imagine looking down through prisms at the 'honeycomb' arrangement of the ameloblasts (Fig. 8.36a). The tips of the Tomes' processes protrude out of the page towards the viewer (Fig. 8.36b, c).

A section along line P produces the appearance already shown in Fig. 8.34b. This is the most commonly described plane of section, the picket-fence plane. A section along line Q produces the appearance in Fig. 8.34a. This is the more rarely described battlements plane. A section along line R produces the very rarely described appearance in Fig. 8.36e.

A change in plane of section between P and R produces very different appearances, in particular a dramatic change in the dimension of the interprismatic region. In both planes of section the interprismatic region cannot be distinguished from the cuspally adjacent prism because there is no abrupt change in crystal orientation: the c-shapes open into the interprismatic region cervically.

# Development of Dentition

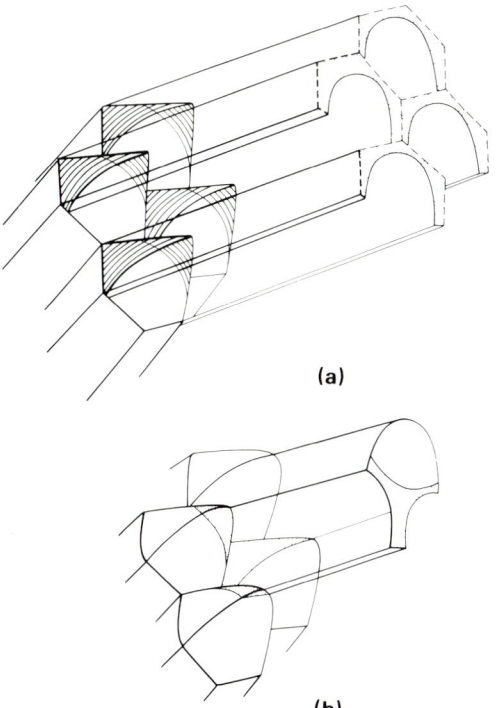

**Fig. 8.35.** Ameloblasts and prisms in three dimensions: (a) circular prisms and interprismatic region; (b) keyhole-shaped prisms. In (a) the (stippled) interprismatic region corresponds with the shaded surfaces of Tomes' processes. In (b) the (stippled) tail corresponds with the stippled surfaces of Tomes' processes.

## Hypotheses

None of the following hypotheses has been tested, and indeed it is very difficult to know how they could be tested. However, they do make it easier to understand what is actually known about amelogenesis.

### MOVEMENT OF AMELOBLASTS

It is obvious that some mechanism is needed to move the ameloblasts from the enamel–dentine junction out to the enamel surface, let alone to form prisms. The ameloblasts contain none of the structures associated with motile cells such as flagellae, pseudopodia or ruffled membranes. It has been suggested that the aggregation of mitochondria at the proximal end of the cell pumps material from the stratum intermedium down the ameloblast (Fig. 8.37a). This raises the intracellular pressure compressing the ameloblasts into their hexagonal cross-section (Fig. 8.37b). When the intracellular pressure exceeds the extracellular pressure at the distal end, material is secreted (Fig. 8.37c). This secreted material initially gathers in a region enclosed on one side by the ameloblasts and on the other side by the mineralized dentine. As more material is secreted the hydrostatic pressure within this region increases. When this pressure exceeds that outside the other end of the ameloblasts, it pushes the cells backwards (Fig. 8.37d). So long as the hydrostatic pressure in the newly secreted matrix is greater than the restraint that can be exerted by the remainder of the enamel organ, the ameloblasts continue to move.

### TOMES' PROCESS

1  One view suggests that the Tomes' process is, in some direct way, genetically determined.

2  The alternative is that the Tomes' process results from a mechanical distortion of the cell membrane by the material it is secreting. Material flowing along a tube moves most rapidly down its centre and is almost stationary at its sides. The initially flat, secreting end of the ameloblast is distorted into a conical extension because the centre receives the greatest outward push while the sides are not pushed out at all.

### CROSSING OF AMELOBLASTS

1  One view suggests that in some genetically determined way the cellular layers of the enamel organ cooperate to induce the crossing of ameloblasts.

2  Another view looks to the developing prisms themselves as the source of a force pushing the secreting ends of the ameloblasts across each other. Each Tomes' process occupies a depression in the developing enamel. If the left side of this depression grows more rapidly than the right side, the process which occupies this depression is pushed over to the right.

3  The final view suggests that the ameloblasts are distorted between a pressure developed in the matrix on their distal sides and forces which restrain their backward movement (the cellular layers in the enamel organ and tooth follicle). A mechanical analogue suggests that such opposing forces would initially distort the long axes of ameloblasts as in Fig. 8.38. As an ameloblast pushes out material its secreting end oscillates from side to side due to analogous forces (the force of reaction to that of secretion). Because it is also moving back, the side to side oscillations are represented by the sinuous courses of the prisms.

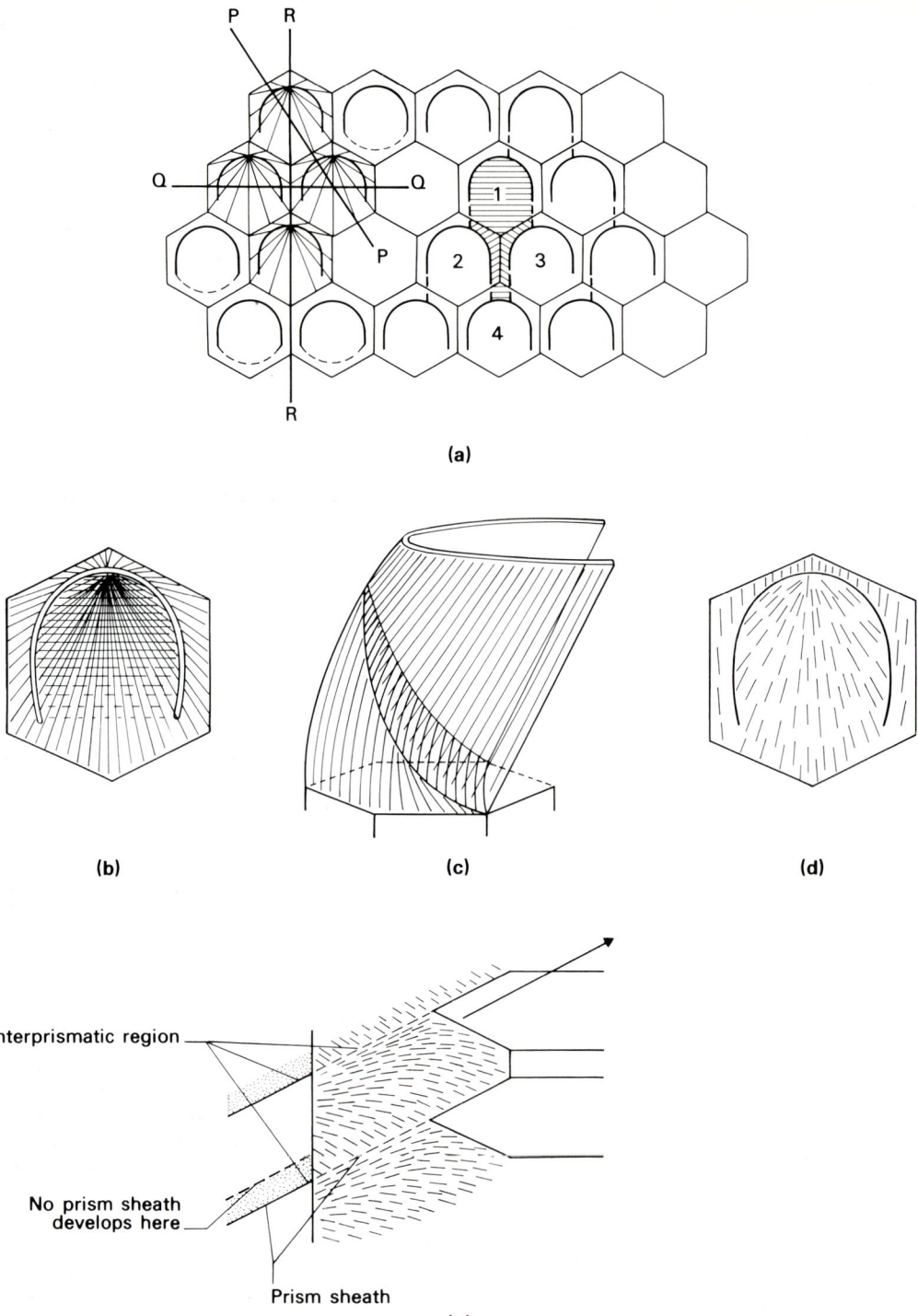

**Fig. 8.36.** (a) Hexagonal appearance of cross-sectioned Tomes' processes. (b) A single Tomes' process and its relation to a prism sheath, and (c) the same process seen from the side. (d) The orientation of crystals in view (b). Four Tomes' processes and their prisms are indicated in the top left of (a). A section P–P would produce the appearance shown in Fig. 8.34(b); along Q–Q, the appearance in Fig. 8.34(a); and along R–R, the appearance in Fig. 8.34b(e). Also shown in (a) is the interpretation that four ameloblasts produce one keyhole-shaped prism.

278

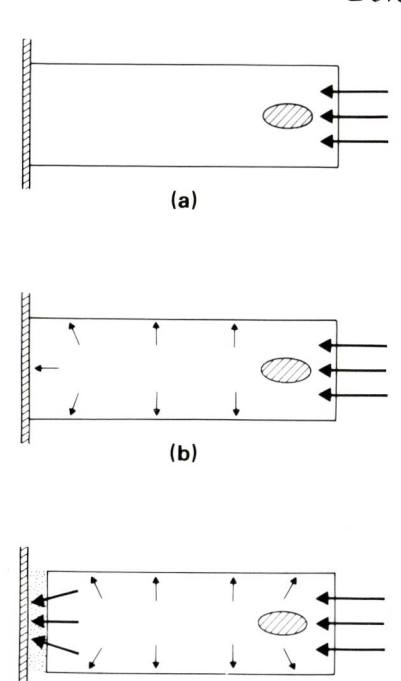

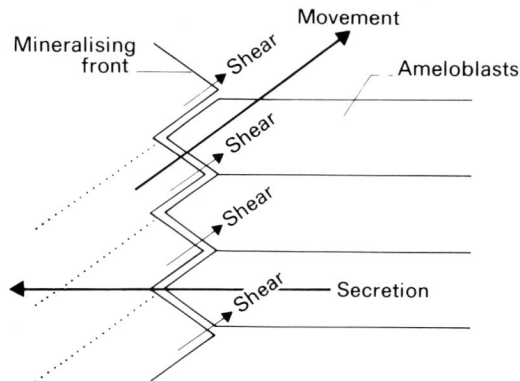

Fig. 8.39. As the ameloblasts move at an angle, they shear across the developing crystals on the cuspal side of each depression occupied by a Tomes' process.

CRYSTAL ORIENTATION

1  Although in itself it does not provide an explanation, one view suggests that protein fibrils in the matrix form a scaffold on which or in which the crystals grow. In other words proteins control the crystal orientation.

2  The most commonly accepted explanation is that some physical property of the crystals or their environment causes them to lengthen at right angles to the mineralizing front. It is then necessary to account for the deviations from this right angle (Fig. 8.34b). The hypothesis draws attention to the fact that the ameloblasts 'shear' across the mineralizing front (Fig. 8.39). The cuspal surface of the Tomes' process moves in a direction which 'shears' its adjacent crystals away from the right angle.

3  The final view suggests that the secretions of the ameloblasts are reflected back by the mineralizing enamel (Fig. 8.40a). The pattern of flow suggested in this figure has been demonstrated in an analogue. The explanation continues by suggesting that the reflected material is absorbed by the ameloblasts; and that the crystals lengthen parallel to the flow lines in the same way that a weather vane is stabilized when parallel to the wind (cf. Figs. 8.40a, b).

In the longitudinal plane, because of the angle at which the ameloblasts move, the flow lines are sheared into the pattern illustrated in Fig. 8.40b. This part of the explanation has only been partially tested with an analogue.

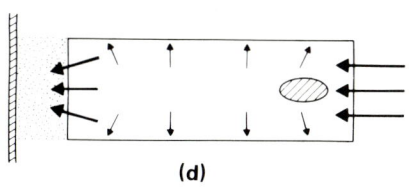

Fig. 8.37. Material sucked in from the right (a) raises the pressure inside the cell (b). When this gets too high material is secreted on the left (c). Secreted material moves the cell.

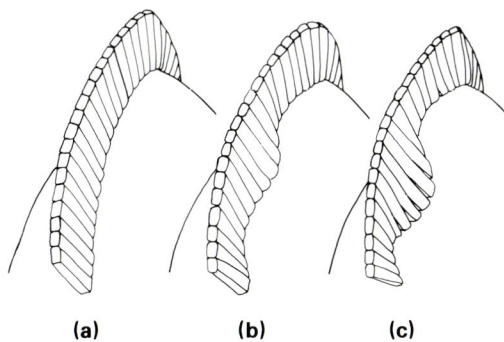

Fig. 8.38. A vertical row of ameloblasts passing over the tip of a cusp (a) is distorted (b) in such a way that their secreting ends cross (c).

REMOVAL OF THE PROLINE-RICH PROTEIN

1  Either the ameloblasts can select the proteins

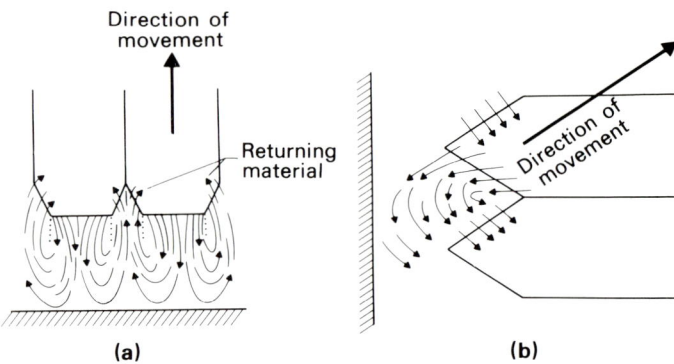

**Fig. 8.40.** Material is reflected back towards the ameloblasts (a) in the transverse plane of the tooth where ameloblasts move roughly parallel to the direction in which they secrete; and (b) in the longitudinal plane where the directions are not parallel. It must be remembered that much of the secreted material moves deep into the developing enamel.

they absorb or the proline-rich protein is more mobile than the others.

2 As the crystals in the maturing enamel grow they compress the matrix between them. This matrix is thixotropic; that is, it flows when compressed. In this way the proline-rich protein is squeezed back towards the ameloblasts.

However, an opposite view points out that the crystals are denser than the matrix in which they crystallize. Therefore, as the crystals grow there is a net contraction of the enamel which tends to 'suck' in matrix from the ameloblasts. This is the opposite movement to that suggested above. Neither hypothesis has been tested.

3 The flow theory (crystal orientation, 3) predicts that the material reflected back towards the ameloblasts is absorbed. This suggests, for example, that the cuspal surface of a Tomes' process only absorbs material and its cervical surface only secretes material (Fig. 8.40b). This strict patterning of flow in enamel should be compared with the more generally believed view that any part of a Tomes' process can either absorb or secrete material.

THE 'MEANING' OF A PRISM

1 Four ameloblasts contribute to each keyhole-shaped prism. This can be visualized by studying Fig. 8.36a. A prism body is contributed by a single ameloblast throughout amelogenesis. Its tail is contributed by the three cervically adjacent ameloblasts. Because prisms cross each other the tail is contributed by different ameloblasts at different times (Fig. 6.23). And at other times the ameloblasts 'secrete' an interprismatic region (Fig. 6.23e).

2 A prism forms in material flowing out of the ameloblast. The interprismatic region develops in material flowing back to the ameloblast. Each ameloblast forms the same prism and its surrounding interprismatic region throughout amelogenesis (Fig. 8.36a and Fig. 6.23). The prism sheath develops between the outflow and the backflow.

## CUTICLES

From the stage at which its development has been completed and throughout its life the enamel surface is either patchily or completely covered by thin layers of organic material referred to collectively as cuticles. Some are developmental, others are acquired.

### Nasmyth's membrane

Over 100 years ago Nasmyth discovered an enamel cuticle. When a newly erupted tooth was placed in acid, he noted that a thin cuticle floated off the enamel surface. The cuticle consisted of two layers, an outer cellular layer, three or four cells thick, and a very thin structureless, inner layer (Fig. 8.41). The two-layered structure came to be

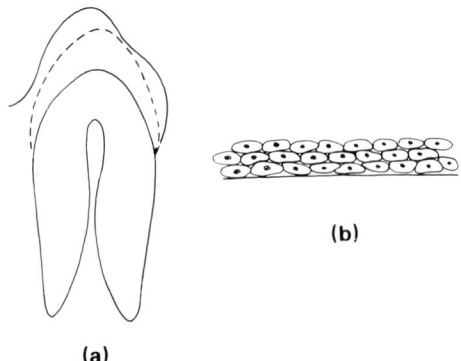

**Fig. 8.41.** (a) Nasmyth's membrane can be floated off a newly erupted tooth dissolved in acid. (b) It consists of an outer cellular layer and a variable inner structureless layer.

# Development of Dentition

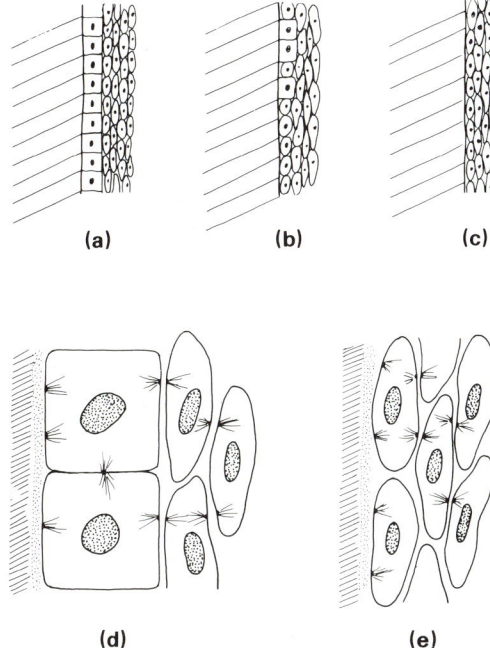

**Fig. 8.42.** (a) Initially the reduced enamel epithelium consists of an inner cuboidal layer of reduced ameloblasts and two or three layers of flattened cells from the remainder of the enamel organ. (b, c) By the time the tooth has erupted the cuboidal cells are gone. (d, e) At all times the reduced enamel epithelium is connected to a basal lamina by hemidesmosomes.

known as Nasmyth's membrane. The existence of the outer, cellular layer has never been questioned: it consists of the remnants of the enamel organ, the reduced enamel epithelium. The inner, structureless layer, which is about 1 μm thick, is called the primary enamel cuticle; its development has never really been understood and it is possible that it does not even exist, at least in the form described by Nasmyth.

At the end of amelogenesis the enamel is covered by shortened, now cuboidal, effete ameloblasts together with a two- or three-cell layer of squamous cells (Fig. 8.42). During the time prior to the eruption of the tooth, which may be up to three or four years, the inner cuboidal cells become replaced by squamous cells that blend indistinguishably with the other cells of the reduced enamel epithelium; perhaps the reduced ameloblasts die and are replaced by other cells, or perhaps they themselves become flattened. All the cells are connected by desmosomes, just as they were in the enamel organ. The inner surface of the reduced enamel epithelium is separated from the enamel by the ubiquitous basal lamina to which it is 'connected' by hemidesmosomes.

The primary cuticle (1 μm thick) is not always seen. Gottlieb (1947) suggested that the thin outer layer of enamel matrix does not normally mature (a view with which most workers would now disagree) and becomes the primary cuticle. If the outer layer mineralizes it cannot be distinguished from the remaining enamel and therefore a cuticle cannot be seen.

In a more recent study, sections from a tooth were viewed with the light and electron microscopes. The cuticle appeared as a 1 μm thick refractile layer under the light microscope: however it could not be seen under the electron microscope. It was suggested that the primary enamel cuticle is an artefact although the source of the artefact has not been traced. However, this same study revealed a thin layer of mineralized tissue lying on the neck of the enamel, next to the root cement (Fig. 8.43). This tissue differed from normal cement because it did not contain collagen fibrils. It was called 'afibrillar coronal cement' and its origin (but not its structure) may be similar to that of ordinary coronal cement (see later).

## Dental cuticle(s)

Sometimes a much thicker (about 4 μm), readily stained, structureless cuticle separates the reduced enamel epithelium, and later the junctional epithelium, from the surface of the tooth. This cuticle was once known as the secondary enamel cuticle but the name has now been abandoned because the structure is not confined to the enamel. It could have three possible sources:

1 Gottlieb suggested it was the keratinized inner layer of the epithelium adjacent to the tooth surface.

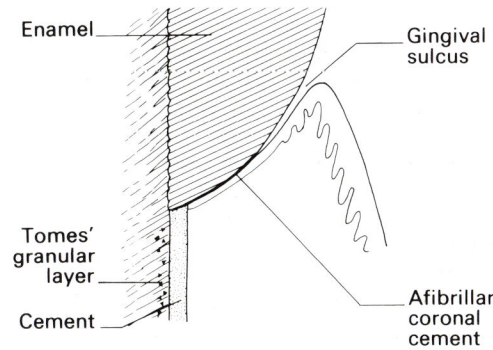

**Fig. 8.43.** Afibrillar coronal cement is sometimes present at the neck of the tooth.

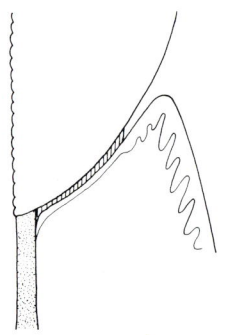

**Fig. 8.44.** A thick secondary enamel cuticle may be an excess of basal lamina material.

2 It may be due to degenerated red blood cells which have leaked into the space between the tooth and epithelium.

3 It may be an excessive thickness of basal lamina material secreted by the adjacent epithelial cells which have a rapid turnover rate (p. 283) as they creep up the surface of the enamel to be shed into the gingival sulcus (Fig. 8.44).

Three further points can be made: (a) many teeth do not have a dental cuticle; (b) the above differences of opinion indicate that there might be more than one form of dental cuticle; (c) when present, the dental cuticle(s) must lie between the epithelium and the primary cuticle (if it exists) because the primary cuticle is part of the enamel.

### Coronal cement

In many animals the reduced enamel epithelium breaks down long before the tooth erupts, allowing the mesoderm of the tooth follicle to come into contact with the enamel. This is followed by the differentiation of cementoblasts and the deposition of coronal cement. It may be noted that, in the same way, root cement is laid down following the breakdown of Hertwig's root sheath.

Occasionally the reduced enamel epithelium in man breaks down in places before the tooth erupts. Patches of coronal cement are laid down. Over the bulk of the crown this cement contains collagen fibrils. However, at the neck of the tooth afribrillar coronal cement is laid down. The absence of collagen fibrils in this cement seems to suggest that it might have a different origin; perhaps from the (ectodermal) enamel organ rather than from (mesodermal) cells of the tooth follicle.

### Acquired pellicle

Glycoproteins from the saliva are probably precipitated onto the surface of all erupted teeth producing an acquired pellicle which cannot readily be removed by brushing.

### Plaque

If the acquired pellicle and other organic debris and bacteria are allowed to remain on the surface of a tooth for some time, they mould into a very adherent plaque. In plaque on the surface of the enamel, the (acidic) by-products of bacterial metabolism probably initiate caries. Around the neck of the tooth minerals may be precipitated in the plaque to produce calculus (tartar). The mineralized (or unmineralized) plaque around the necks of teeth initiates most gingival and periodontal disease. Plaque is probably the most important cause of dental disease.

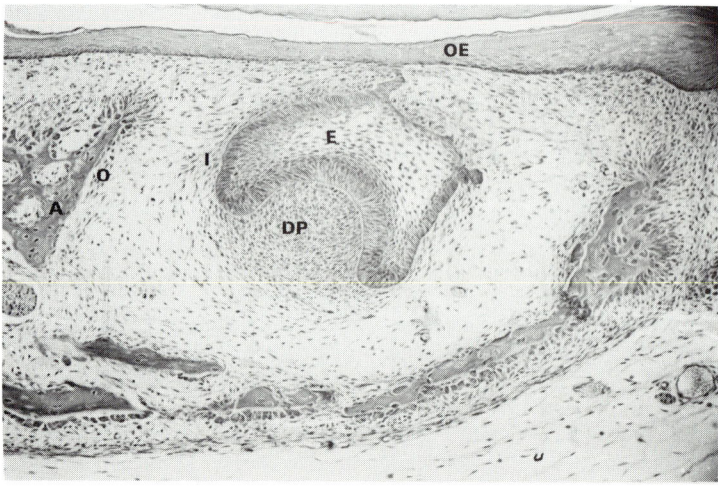

**Fig. 8.45.** Tooth germ at the early bell stage of development. The dental follicle separates the tooth germ from the wall of the developing alveolus (A) and can be divided into layers; an inner layer (I), three to four cells thick which closely invests the tooth germ and has a relatively high cell density; an outer layer (O) lines the developing alveolus. Loose connective tissue lies between the two layers. E, enamel organ; DP, dental papilla; OE, oral epithelium.

## Fates of the cuticles

The reduced enamel epithelium and primary cuticle (if it exists) are worn away rapidly from the surface of a newly erupted tooth apart from the region of the gingiva. From now on, the bulk of the enamel can only be covered by an acquired pellicle or by plaque.

The enamel facing the gingival sulcus also attracts pellicle and plaque but remnants of primary cuticle, afribrillar coronal cement or dental cuticle(s) may still persist.

The junctional epithelium together with its basal lamina may be separated from the enamel by primary cuticle, afibrillar coronal cement or dental cuticle(s).

When the junctional epithelium has grown on to the root of the tooth, it may be separated from the root cement by dental cuticle. The primary enamel cuticle can only lie on enamel but, until the origin of afibrillar 'coronal' cement is discovered it cannot be known for certain whether or not it normally extends onto the root of the tooth (cf. afibrillar cement: p. 198).

## DEVELOPMENT OF THE PERIODONTIUM

With the onset of morphogenesis and cytodifferentiation the enamel organ partially surrounds the tissues of the dental papilla. Between the enamel organ and the wall of the developing bony crypt is the mesenchymal tissue of the dental follicle which generally seems to have three layers. The inner layer is a vascular, fibrocellular condensation, three to four cells thick, immediately surrounding the tooth germ; the nuclei of the cells are generally elongated circumferentially (Fig. 8.45). There is some evidence to suggest that the cells of this layer may be derived from the neural crest. The outer layer, which lines the developing alveolus, is vascular mesenchyme. Between the two layers is loose connective tissue with no marked concentration of blood vessels. The existence of a real structural separation between the inner and outer layers of the dental follicle, the loose connective tissue layer, is indicated by the finding that tooth germs removed from the jaw are surrounded by the inner, but not the outer, layer of the dental follicle. There is no apparent fibre continuity between the inner layer of the dental follicle and the bony crypt. The majority of cells of the dental follicle at this stage contain few cytoplasmic organelles and the extracellular compartment is largely structureless.

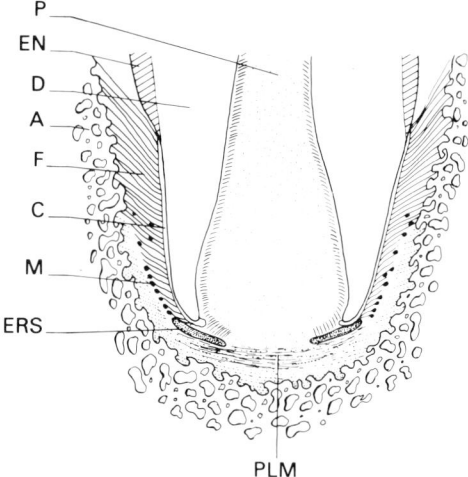

**Fig. 8.46.** Diagram to show principal features of root and periodontal ligament formation. The epithelial root sheath (ERS) induces the adjacent cells of the developing pulp (P) to differentiate into odontoblasts and commence dentinogenesis. The epithelial sheath loses its continuity and its remnants contribute the rests of Malassez (M) in the adult periodontal ligament. Cells of the inner layer of the dental follicle become apposed to the dentine surface, differentiate into cementoblasts and commence cementogenesis. There is an associated organization of the periodontal ligament and principal fibre groups (F) are seen passing from the alveolar bone (A) to cement (C). The change from the unorganized dental follicle to the organized periodontal ligament is relatively abrupt. At the apical end of the growing root, fibres of the dental follicle pass beneath the pulp opening forming a pulp-limiting membrane (PLM) and merge at the sides with the fibres of the developing ligament. These fibres are not attached directly to alveolar bone. EN, enamel; D, dentine.

The root starts to form shortly after the appearance of the epithelial root sheath which induces the adjacent cells of the dental papilla to differentiate into odontoblasts and form root dentine. The epithelial cells of the root sheath lose their continuity, separate from the surface of the forming root dentine, and later become the epithelial rests of Malassez seen in the adult periodontium. Mesenchymal cells of the dental follicle adjacent to the root dentine differentiate into cementoblasts which lay down cement (Fig. 8.46). There appears to be a species difference in the fate of some of the epithelial cells of Hertwig's root sheath; for example, in the mouse molar (unlike man), some of these cells become trapped between forming cement and dentine.

Following the onset of root formation, changes become apparent within the dental follicle associated with the development of the principal fibre groups of the periodontium. Differences in subsequent development may be encountered depending on the species and, perhaps more importantly, on whether the tooth has a predecessor. Cells of the dental follicle, especially from the inner layer, become obliquely orientated along the root surface. They now have an increased number of intracellular organelles and differentiate into fibroblasts which secrete collagen into the extracellular compartment. In monkeys the first organized fibres are short, closely-spaced and attached to the forming cement surface. Shortly after this, fibres, which appear thicker and more widely-spaced than those on the cement side, are seen attached to the forming alveolar wall. In the rat molar, however, the fibres attached to the alveolar bone appear shortly before those related to the cement surface. At this early stage the central portion of the developing periodontium, the original loose connective tissue layer, remains relatively unorganized. In molar teeth, which have no predecessors, this central region now becomes rapidly organized by forming bundles of fibres which link those of the inner and outer layers thereby making the principal dento-alveolar fibres: even at this early stage, the fibres are obliquely orientated. In addition, the future dentogingival fibres are represented by a bundle of fibres passing from the cement outwards and occlusally along the side of the crown (Fig. 8.47). The mechanism responsible for the orientation of the fibres of the periodontium is not clear, but it has been suggested that it may be related to lines of stress set up at the growing end of the root and/or to the orientation of the pulp-limiting membrane.

As more of the root is formed, so the amount of organized periodontal ligament increases. There is an abrupt transition from a loose connective tissue containing young fibroblasts and minimal extracellular collagen at the growing end of the root to a highly organized connective tissue consisting of active fibroblasts separated by dense bundles of collagen fibres more coronally (Fig. 8.46). The loose proliferative connective tissue of the dental follicle passes beneath the growing root apex to form a pulp-limiting 'membrane' (Fig. 8.46). This

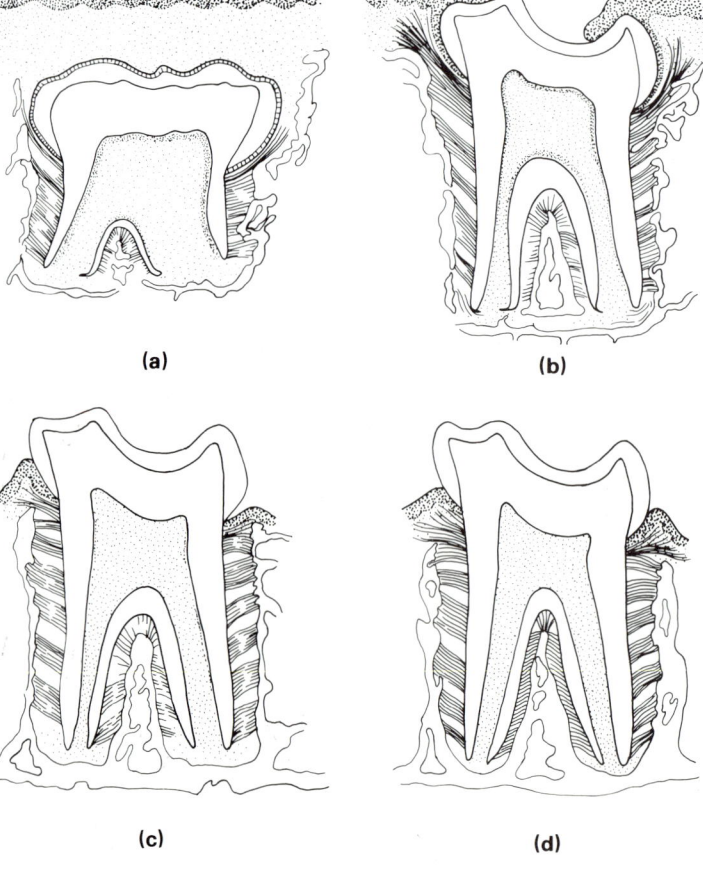

**Fig. 8.47.** Diagram to show the development of the principal fibres of the periodontal ligament in the permanent molar of a marmoset. (a) With root formation well advanced, but prior to eruption, dentogingival and oblique dento-alveolar fibres are evident. (b) Upon emergence into the oral cavity the periodontal ligament is well differentiated with obliquely orientated dento-alveolar fibres forming the main component. (c) With occlusal function changes in orientation of fibres result in further groups of fibres becoming evident in the cervical region of the tooth. (d) With continued function the fibres become even more clearly grouped and, perhaps, thicken. [After Grant D. A., Bernick S., Levy B. M. & Dreizen S. (1972) A comparative study of periodontal ligament development in teeth with and without predecessors in Marmosets. *Journal of Periodontology* **43**: 162.]

structure has erroneously been described as being attached at its margins to the wall of the bony alveolar crypt, forming the so-called 'cushioned hammock ligament' which was thought to play a role in the process of tooth eruption.

At the time the tooth penetrates the oral mucosa, about two-thirds of the root has formed. As the crown continues to erupt into the oral cavity past the alveolar crest, there is a change in the orientation of the adjacent fibres which become the alveolar crest and cervical group of fibres (Fig. 8.47). There is also some evidence that the oblique fibres become less obliquely orientated after the tooth has erupted. Transseptal fibres are usually apparent before the tooth penetrates the oral mucosa but their orientation and stage of development varies with the stage of development of the adjacent teeth. Following completion of the root the apical fibres develop. It has been suggested that the periodontal fibres become thicker once the tooth is functioning. Throughout these stages of development there is a continual turnover of the connective tissue elements of the periodontium, involving both cells and extracellular material.

An indication of the important role played by the inner layer of the dental follicle in the formation of the periodontium can be deduced from experiments in which developing tooth germs, surrounded only by the inner layer of the dental follicle (it will be recalled that the middle layer is a natural plane of cleavage), are removed from the jaws and transplanted to other sites. These tooth germs continue developing in ectopic sites to produce a root, periodontal ligament and alveolar bone. Using techniques which allow the transplanted cells to be recognized (such as initially labelling mitotic cells with tritiated thymidine), there is evidence to show that the inner layer of cells of the dental follicle gives origin to cementoblasts, fibroblasts and the osteoblasts associated with alveolar bone. The periodontium of such transplants shows organization of the principal fibre groups, illustrating adaptation to later function. Such experiments, however, do not preclude a major contribution from the outer layers of the dental follicle to the periodontium and alveolar bone during normal development.

The above description refers to the development of the periodontium in teeth without predecessors. In the case of teeth with predecessors, the permanent incisors, canines and premolars, some fundamental differences have been reported in monkeys. In these teeth during the pre-eruptive stage, few periodontal fibres are visible, most of the dental follicle being occupied by loose collagenous elements. As the tooth penetrates the oral mucosa the future dentogingival, transseptal and alveolar crest fibres are evident. At this stage the remainder of the developing periodontium is still unorganized and fibres extend on either side from the alveolar bone and cement towards the central area of the periodontium. This central area contains loosely structured collagenous elements forming an intermediate zone or plexus. By the time the first occlusal contact is made the principal oblique dento-alveolar fibres become apparent cervically but fibre formation is still progressing in the apical third of the root which exhibits an intermediate zone. With continued function and further development of the oblique dento-alveolar fibres, the intermediate plexus disappears. These features are summarized in Fig. 8.48. Thus, compared with teeth without predecessors, the principal fibre groups in teeth with predecessors develop more slowly, resulting in the presence of an intermediate zone. The lack of a well organized periodontium during the main eruptive phase may be relevant when considering the possible role of this structure in the process of tooth eruption. The problems relating to the presence of an intermediate zone or plexus are discussed elsewhere (p. 221).

Recent evidence suggests that periodontal ligament fibres may pass straight through the alveolar bone to merge with the dento-alveolar fibres of adjacent teeth. The development of these transalveolar fibres has not been elucidated.

Little is known concerning the development of oxytalan fibres (p. 223). These fibres develop after collagen and its surrounding extracellular substance have been formed. As the epithelial root sheath breaks apart oxytalan fibres are incorporated into cement, initially at the cervical margin of the tooth, and later progressing apically. The major oxytalan fibres extend for varying distances into the periodontium and may follow the course of the major groups of collagen fibres. They appear to have an important association with blood vessels, perhaps maintaining the patency of vessels if they become compressed during mastication.

Little information is available concerning the development of the nervous and vascular supply to the periodontium. In the teeth of the marmoset, and also the rat molar, no sensory innervation is established until the periodontium becomes functionally organized at the time of tooth eruption. In the early phases of human tooth development there is a particularly rich nervous innervation, presumably autonomic, associated with the inner layer of the dental follicle.

286  Chapter 8

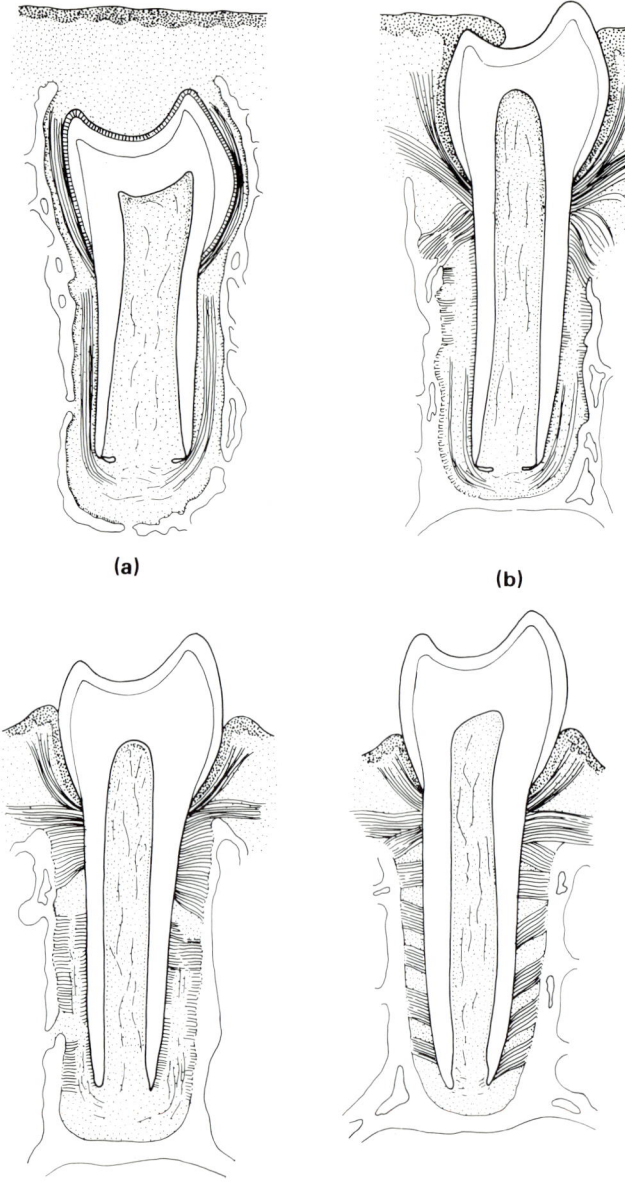

**Fig. 8.48.** Diagram to illustrate the development of a permanent premolar tooth in a squirrel monkey. (a) With root formation well advanced, but prior to eruption, only the dentogingival fibres are demonstrable as an organized entity. The developing periodontal ligament is composed of loosely structured collagenous elements. (b) Upon emergence into the oral cavity, dentogingival, transseptal and alveolar crest fibre groups become evident. More apically, however, organized fibre groups are not demonstrable. (c) With occlusal function the fibre groups in the cervical third of the root become demonstrable. Apically the fibres become progressively less mature. (d) With continued function, the fibre bundles become thicker and show classical organization. [After Grant D. & Bernick S. (1972) The formation of the periodontal ligament. *Journal of Periodontology* **43**; 17.]

Little is also known about changes in the ground substance during development. Studying bovine periodontal ligament from molars at varying stages of development, it has been reported that the content of insoluble non-collagenous glycoproteins and collagen hexoses was higher in developing than in mature ligament and that hyaluronic acid progressively decreased relative to chondroitin sulphate on eruption.

## CEMENT

### The epithelial root sheath of Hertwig: differentiation of cementoblasts

Root formation begins after the basic form of the crown has been outlined by the inner enamel epithelium of the enamel organ and dentine has extended to cover all of the future enamel–dentine junction. Two of the layers of the enamel organ, the inner and outer dental epithelia, continue to proliferate at the cervical loop and form a cellular cuff which maps out the future position of the cement–dentine junction of the root. The epithelial cells lie on a basal lamina which is continuous around the outside of the epithelium. There are minimal spaces between the cells and junctional complexes occur between them.

The surface cells of the dental papilla next to the inner cells of Hertwig's root epithelial sheath differentiate to form odontoblasts (Fig. 8.20). These cells are polarized, with many small cell processes that extend towards the basal lamina of the root sheath. As they elongate they begin to lay down predentine which forms a template upon which the initial cement is to be deposited. Lagging slightly behind the odontoblasts, cells of the dental follicle adjacent to the outer cells of the root sheath also differentiate into specialized cells, the cementoblasts. Both cell types are of similar origin, arising from condensations of mesodermal (probably ectomesenchymal) cells associated with invaginations of the dental lamina.

The basal lamina encasing the epithelial cells begins to disintegrate as the odontoblasts and cementoblasts differentiate. Cell processes from the precementoblasts penetrate between the epithelial cells and breach the continuity of the root sheath. The epithelial cells reorient themselves so that they lie with their long axes at right angles to the predentine surface and then migrate towards the dental follicle. Both the precementoblasts and the epithelial cells seem to participate actively in this exchange of position. Some of the epithelial cells, encased once more by a basal lamina, remain as the epithelial rests of Malassez. It is not known if they ever contribute to the cement once they have left the root surface (Fig. 8.49).

The epithelial cells of the root sheath on the lingual surfaces of rodent and lagomorph incisors produce enamel protein prior to, and possibly after, their migration from the dentine surface. It is debated whether the matrix of afibrillar cement and the ground substance of extrinsic fibre cement may be wholly or partly formed by the epithelial cells in other teeth, including human ones. As yet, there is no firm evidence that this is so.

If the epithelial cells fail to migrate, they become included within the cement matrix close to the dentine. The resultant intermediate cement (p. 202) only commonly develops in the premolars and permanent molars of human teeth, and primarily in the apical one third or so of their roots; this is a consequence of the very rapid root growth and cement deposition in this region.

### The cement–dentine junction

Precement is generally deposited directly on the predentine. Mineralization initiated in the latter tissue spreads back to and across the interface. As both tissues mineralize, the junction between them

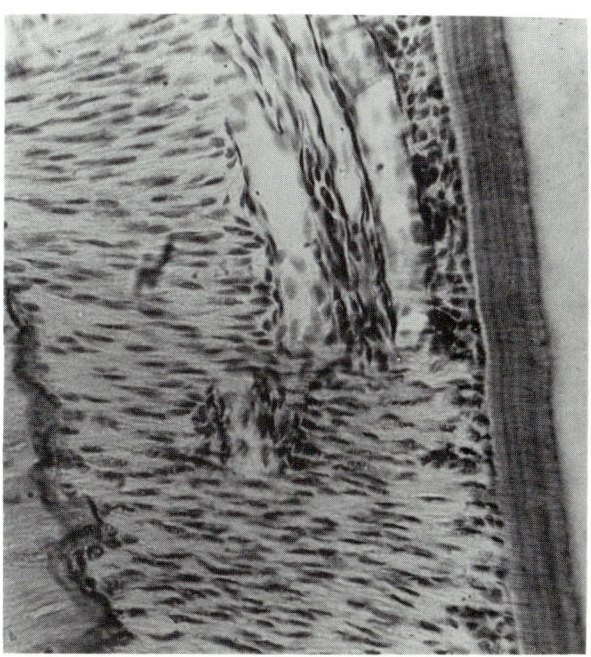

**Fig. 8.49.** Epithelial rests lie close to the cement surface, which has a light border of precement. Cementoblasts lie between the fibres of the periodontal ligament whose long axes can be deduced from the direction of the fibroblast nuclei. Alveolar bone at lower left. Incremental lines mark the cement lengthwise; the extrinsic fibres mark it crosswise. Decalcified longitudinal section. LM, field width 450 μm.

becomes obscure. It is agreed from microradiographic, TEM and SEM evidence that a narrow, more highly mineralized zone exists at the cement–dentine junction but whether this zone lies in dentine or cement, or spans the two tissues, is disputed. It probably represents an abundance of mineralized ground substance in the region which calcifies to a greater degree than the adjacent, more collagenous tissue; not unlike, for example, resting lines, peritubular dentine and perilacunar bone. It is tempting to indict afibrillar cement for the radiodensity but more information on the origin, organic constitution and thickness of this layer must be gained. It is possible that more than one cell type contributes to it.

## Formation of cement

Cementogenesis varies according to the constitution of the cement; afibrillar, extrinsic fibre, mixed fibre or intrinsic fibre.

### AFIBRILLAR CEMENT

A small amount of cement is deposited on the dentine template before the inclusion of extrinsic fibres. This early deposit may be afibrillar or fibrillar, the former being more common cervically and the latter apically. Little is known of the origin or development of afibrillar cement. It may constitute the earliest secretion of cementoblasts during the formation of the root in the prefunctional phase of the tooth. However, it is thought that the epithelial cells may contribute to the matrix of this layer.

### EXTRINSIC FIBRE CEMENT

*Matrix formation*

This cement contains extrinsic fibres embedded in ground substance. The extrinsic fibres originate in the periodontal ligament where they are formed by fibroblasts. They are composed of fibrils up to 150 nm in diameter that exhibit the characteristic 64 nm cross-banding of collagen when demineralized sections are examined by transmission electron microscopy (Fig. 8.50). The fibrils are grouped into parallel fibres which vary from about 3 to 12 $\mu$m in cross-sectional diameter and are very closely packed.

Cementoblasts lie close to the cement surface in the periodontal ligament, lodged between the perforating extrinsic fibres. They are distinguished from fibroblasts by several features. The fibroblasts are irregular cells with stellate extensions of the cytosol. Each lies with its long axis, often discernable only from that of its nucleus, parallel to the major axis of the adjoining collagen fibres. The cementoblasts are more regular, oval cells which lie parallel to the cement surface during matrix production, although they may assume a more vertical orientation when quiescent, accommodating themselves to the orientation of the surrounding fibres.

Cementoblasts have cell processes, mostly directed towards the cement surface, but these are not numerous in this type of cementogenesis. As the incremental rate is so slow and the contribution of the cementoblasts to the tissue is probably limited to the ground substance, the cementoblasts do not

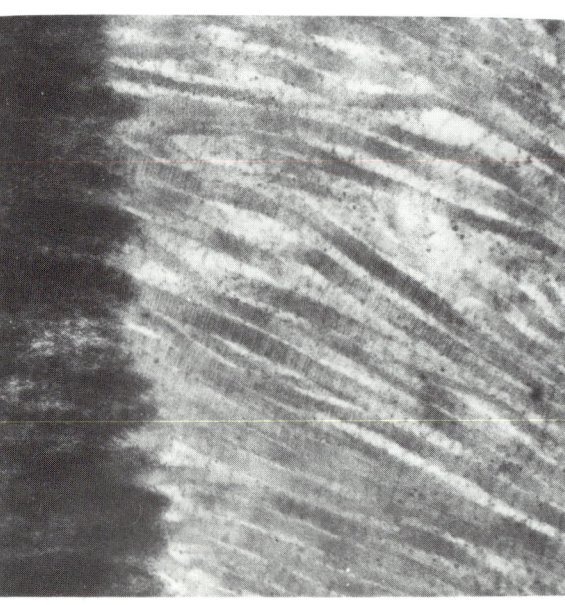

**Fig. 8.50.** The mineralizing border of human deciduous cement containing only extrinsic fibres. The collagen 64 nm cross-banding can also be seen in the partly demineralized cement (left). Mineralization is spreading along the collagen fibrils. TEM, field width 3.4 $\mu$m.

# Development of Dentition

have the cytological features of highly productive cells. Thus their rough endoplasmic reticulum, Golgi apparatus and secretory vesicles are relatively modest. Cementoblasts never become incorporated in extrinsic fibre cement.

*Mineralization pattern*
A thin layer of unmineralized tissue, precement, borders the mineralized cement while matrix is being deposited. The precement is mineralized first by a slow extension of crystal formation along the individual collagen fibrils (Fig. 8.50). The contribution of the ground substance to the mineralization process is not well understood: the role of the cementoblasts is probably limited to providing the medium for mineralization rather than the mineral ions.

The mineral surface usually appears flat when viewed by light microscopy. Ultrastructurally, it may have very shallow, clearly demarcated mounds (Fig. 8.51). These presumably represent individual extrinsic fibres in which the level of mineralization slightly exceeds that of the interfibrillar space and is more advanced in the centre. All parts of the extrinsic fibres mineralize in this slowly forming cement. The density of the mineral through the thickness of this cement is much more even than in mixed fibre cement but hypercalcified layers are produced if matrix formation ceases.

## MIXED FIBRE CEMENT

*Matrix formation*
The extrinsic fibres are again incorporated from the periodontal ligament where they are formed by fibroblasts but constitute a smaller and variable proportion of the tissue (Figs. 8.52 to 8.54).

The cementoblasts forming mixed fibre cement secrete not only the ground substance but also intrinsic collagen fibres that are oriented within the plane of the developing surface. The cells are plumper and larger during matrix production, with a well-developed granular endoplasmic reticulum, Golgi apparatus and secretory vesicles, and plentiful mitochondria. Resting cementoblasts have reduced organelles and are thinner and more extended so that they resemble fibrocytes. They may align parallel to either the intrinsic or extrinsic fibre component.

The forces which organize the arrangement of the intrinsic fibres are unknown but it is thought that the movement of the cells with respect to the surface they are forming may be responsible. Collagen fibres tend to be random in tissues in which a lateral translatory movement of the cells is unlikely to occur, whilst oriented fibres occur where cellular movement is relatively unrestricted.

Precement is a more obvious layer at the surface of developing mixed fibre cement, often reaching 5 $\mu$m thick. The depth of the unmineralized layer is reduced as the appositional rate decreases and the mineralizing front approaches the matrix surface. When matrix formation ceases, the mineral front may reach the level of the matrix surface, eliminating the precement zone.

*Mineralization patterns*
The gross pattern of mineralization in mixed fibre cement is complex. Mineralization proceeds relatively independently in extrinsic fibres, intrinsic fibres and the ground substance. The spread of mineral is preferentially along the length of collagen fibres: hence that in the intrinsic fibres is approximately at right angles to the spread in the extrinsic fibres (Fig. 8.54). If the latter are angled

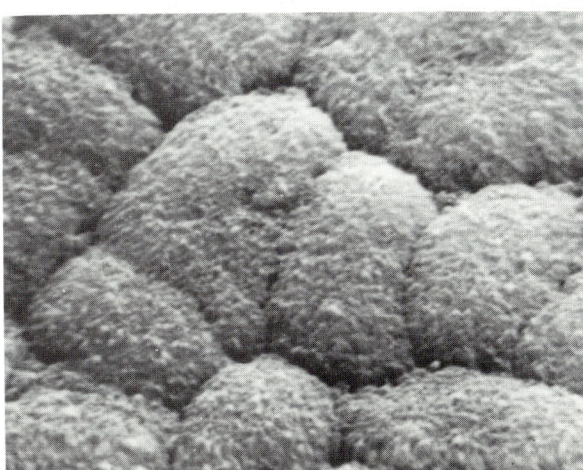

**Fig. 8.51.** The mineral front of extrinsic fibre cement. Each fibre is represented by a hump in the surface. Cervical region of root of permanent lower first molar of 14-year-old child. SEM, field width 16 $\mu$m.

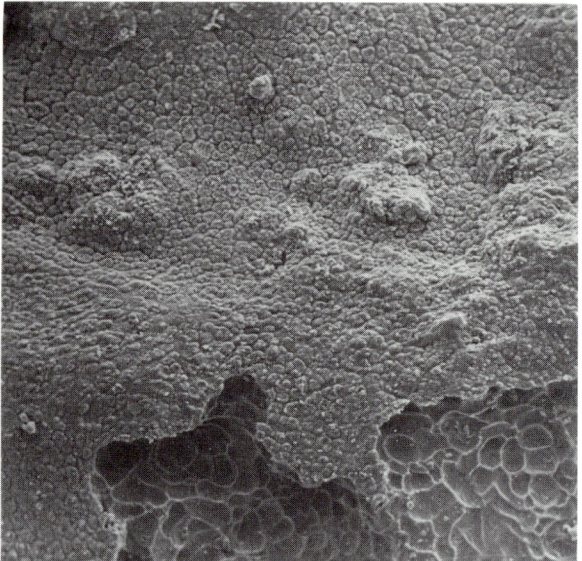

**Fig. 8.52.** The peripheries of the extrinsic fibres, seen as small projections, are mineralized to a more superficial level than the centres. Intrinsic fibres separate the extrinsic ones. A large resorption bay (bottom right) undermines the cement surface and extends into dentine. Anorganic preparation, human lower third molar. SEM, field width 450 μm.

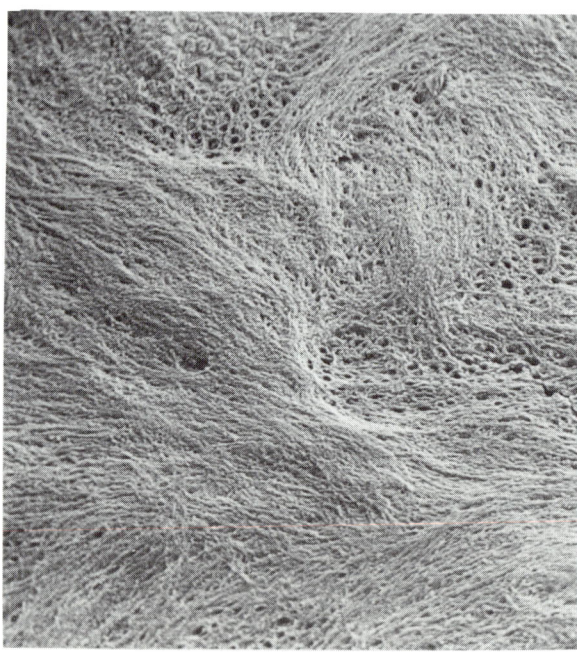

**Fig. 8.53.** Extensive fields of parallel bundles of collagen fibres of the intrinsic matrix resemble lamellar bone in appearance. Patches of mixed fibre cement can be recognized by the sites of extrinsic fibres seen as holes or projections. Human permanent upper second molar root apex. Anorganic preparation. SEM, field width 500 μm.

obliquely to the cement surface the mineral level within them tends to be normal to the long axis of the fibre, and hence at an angle to the part of the surface formed by the intrinsic fibres: this results in a stepped mineral surface during both formative and resting phases. Moreover, the intrinsic fibres that closely wrap the obliquely inclined extrinsic fibres tend to lie normal to the latter.

The degree of mineralization attained by the tissue is, to a large extent, dependent upon its rate of formation. Centres of mineralization appear within the intrinsic matrix fibres and extend lengthwise along the fibres to become spindle-shaped. These mineral nodules coalesce end to end and finally the fibres may become completely mineralized. The initiation of new centres of mineralization can proceed over all the advancing front simultaneously (Fig. 8.55) and as the intrinsic fibres are relatively thin they commonly mineralize throughout their thickness in human

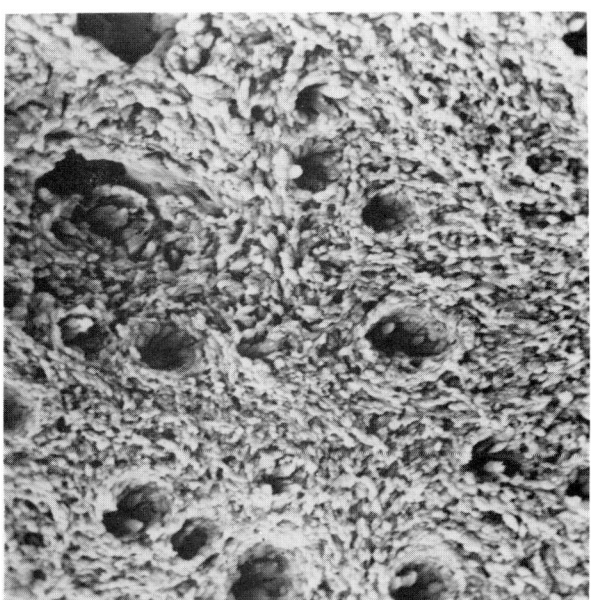

**Fig. 8.54.** The orientation of the mineral particles in the extrinsic fibres that were sited at the holes in the surface is different from those in the intrinsic fibres. Two cementocyte lacunae were developing in the mineral surface (upper left); note the irregular shape of the lower one. Forming mixed fibre cement of permanent lower first molar of 8-year-old child. Anorganic preparation. SEM, field width 80 μm.

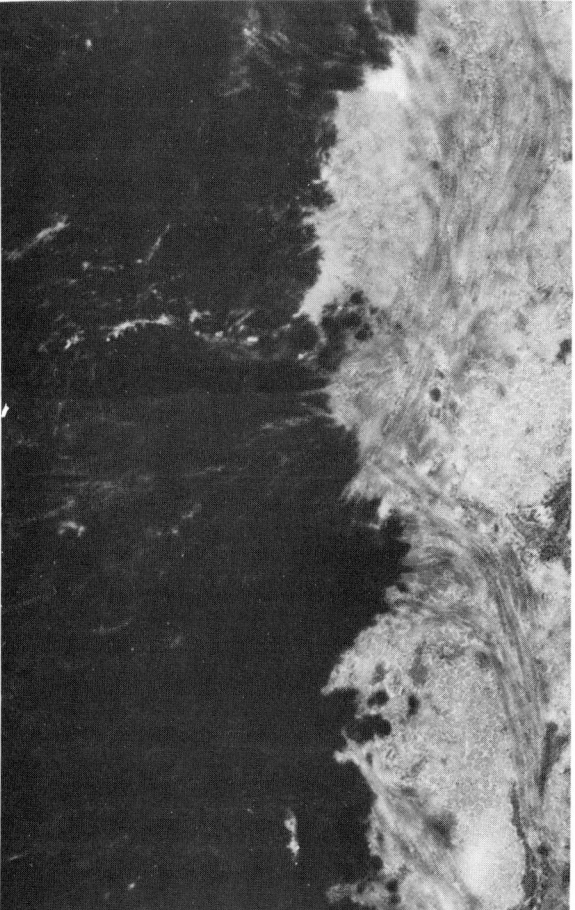

**Fig. 8.55.** Mineralizing front of forming human deciduous mixed-fibre cement. Note the separate mineral clusters, the extension of mineral along the collagen fibrils, and the varying orientations of the collagen fibres within the cement (left) and precement. TEM, field width 7.3 μm.

cement. The progress of mineralization in the extrinsic fibres is much slower and generally begins in the outer regions of these thick fibres first. The mineral surface of developing mixed fibre cement therefore contains holes which mark the sites of the extrinsic fibres (Fig. 8.54).

As the rate of formation of the intrinsic matrix slows, so the discrepancy between the levels of mineral in the two sets of fibres diminishes. If the matrix formation ceases, mineralization still continues until all the surface fibres of the intrinsic component of the matrix are fully mineralized, and the level of mineralization in the extrinsic fibres reaches the true surface of the tissue, or may in time exceed it slightly (Fig. 8.52). In this situation the sites of the extrinsic fibres would be represented as projections in the mineral surface of the cement which would be coincident with the matrix surface.

The areas of projections and depressions of the cement surface, caused by different levels of mineralization in the two sets of fibres, provide a sensitive method of studying the dynamics of cement formation (Figs. 8.53, 8.56). Projections and depressions occur in unmixed fields of varying extent and indicate that apposition occurs in patches rather than in continuous layers, particularly in apical cement. Depressions are rare in the coronal part of a root, confirming that a slow rate of apposition of cement is the norm there except in the furcation areas and regions where repair of resorption is occurring.

In mixed fibre cement an extrinsic fibre may show several degrees of mineralization along its length, providing a permanent record of formative rates at different levels of its inclusion into the tissue. The intrinsic fibres may also fail to mineralize fully, but this is not as prominent a feature of human cement as it is in some large mammals such as elephants and sperm whales.

Mineralization of the ground substance occurs after that of the collagen fibres and is particularly evident when matrix formation has ceased for some time. Then the extension of mineralization into the ground substance obscures the intrinsic fibre pattern at the surface, and may eventually be evident as a resting line in the tissue.

It follows that, in general, the more slowly the tissue forms the more highly mineralized it is likely to be. Thus, cellular cement is usually less well mineralized than acellular cement and contains more prominent radiodense resting lines.

INTRINSIC FIBRE CEMENT

The formation and mineralization of intrinsic fibre cement is the same as that of the intrinsic component of mixed fibre cement (Fig. 8.57). Matrix vesicles of cementoblastic origin have not been described to date in precement, in association with its mineralization. It is quite possible, however, that such cellular particles would be developed during very rapid formation of intrinsic fibre cement (and cellular mixed fibre cement). Whether matrix vesicles would be significant in the calcification of the tissue is another matter: the pattern of mineralization is generally not spheritic but collagen-dependent.

**Resorption and repair**

Cement is resorbed intermittently as a physiological process during the shedding of the deciduous teeth. When resorption ceases, the surface may be repaired with cement and the periodontal ligament reattached. Most children recognize that even once a tooth has been quite wobbly it may later become firm to the inquiring finger, often for a considerable period.

Resorption of deciduous teeth unassociated

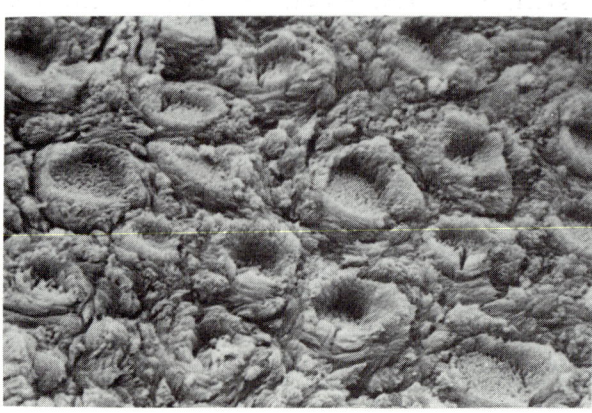

Fig. 8.56. There is an abrupt change in the extent of the mineral within the fibrils from the periphery to the centre of these extrinsic fibres. The intrinsic fibre component is about 40%. Anorganic cement surface of permanent lower first molar of a 14-year old child. SEM, field width 50 μm.

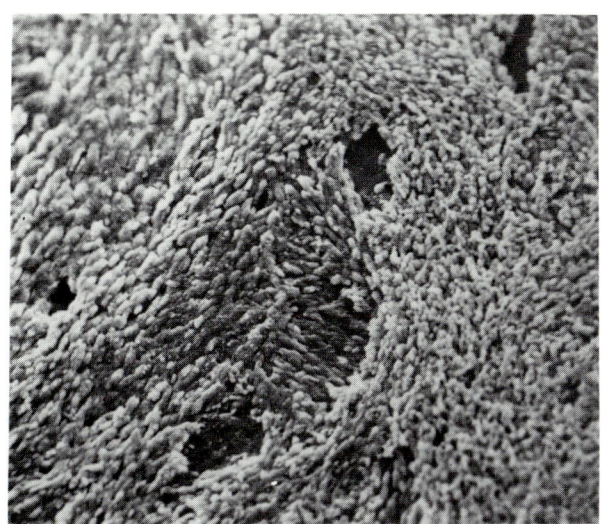

Fig. 8.57. Intrinsic fibre cement showing intrinsic fibres lying in domains of parallel fibres with lamellar formation. The smaller size of the mineral particles at the right indicates a more rapid formation of the tissue there. Several lacunae are at various stages of inclusion into the mineralized cement. Anorganic preparation of human upper third molar. SEM, field width 175 μm.

with their shedding and of permanent teeth is not at all uncommon (Fig. 8.52). The resorption may be limited to the activity of a single resorptive cell (Fig. 8.58) or be quite extensive and deep. It is associated with an increase or change in the stress placed upon the tooth and commonly accompanies orthodontic manoeuvres. If resorption occurs where cement is thin it often continues into the dentine (Fig. 8.59). However, resorption of the cement of permanent teeth is commonly limited to the thicker apical region where it further increases the irregularity of the root surface. Resorption often undermines cement and may then proceed back towards the periodontal ligament.

Both cement and precement are resorbed. It is a fallacy that unmineralized matrix is not resorbed; however resorption is more likely to follow a resting phase rather than a forming phase. Highly mineralized zones are more resistant to resorption and remain slightly proud on the resorbed surface.

The cells that resorb cement (and other hard dental tissues) are indistinguishable from osteoclasts. The observation that the individual resorption lacunae on teeth, particularly in dentine, are small and deep has led to the opinion that some mononucleate osteoclasts, or very small multinucleate ones, may be responsible but the various textures and contents of the dental tissues may influence the resorption patterns.

One of the explanations offered for the generally readier resorption of alveolar bone than of cement, particularly in cervical and midroot regions, is the greater ease with which osteoclasts can approach the bone surface. This may be due both to the proximity of the blood vessels and to the different density and distribution of the extrinsic fibres at either side of the periodontal ligament. Direct access to the apical cement is easier: osteoclasts may replace quiescent cementoblasts over intrinsic fibres even before the disruption of extrinsic fibres.

Evidence of past root resorption is retained in the cement and dentine as reversal lines. These have a characteristic scalloped appearance and

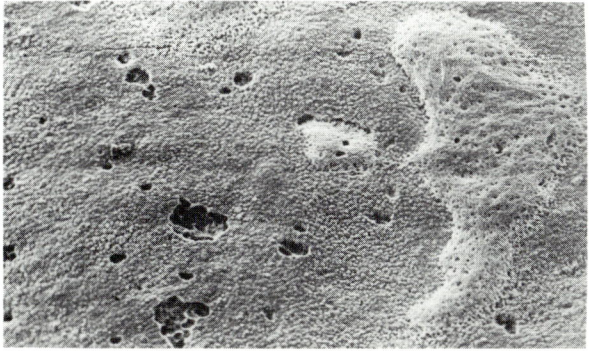

Fig. 8.58. One (close to centre) of the many small resorption bays in the cement was being repaired by cellular mixed fibre cement which has extended over the unresorbed surface. Forming cementocyte lacunae (the larger holes) can be seen in the mineral surface of the forming mixed fibre cement. SEM of anorganic preparation of lower third molar of 21-year-old person. Field width 900 μm.

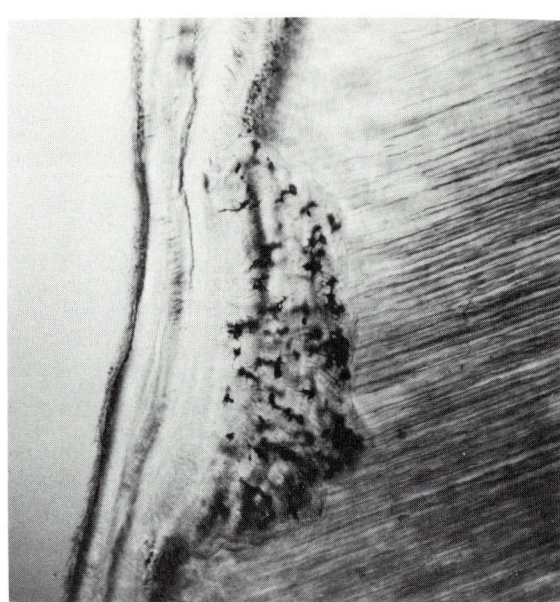

**Fig. 8.59.** This deep resorption bay into dentine (right) was repaired with cellular cement which was then covered by acellular cement. Longitudinal ground section of human permanent canine. LM, field width 450 μm.

mark the furthermost position of the resorption lacunae. A very thin, more highly mineralized layer, rich in ground substance, coats the resorbed surface. The repair tissue is fibrillar and is most commonly, but not always, cellular.

The pattern of mineralization in the first repair tissue deposited may mimic that of woven bone, with spheres of mineral extending simultaneously into both the collagenous and non-collagenous compartments of the matrix. The intrinsic fibre orientation in this early tissue tends to be random. As extrinsic fibres are incorporated, the repair fabric becomes mixed fibre cement. The resorbed space is often refilled before the rate of formation drops to the general level and the inclusion of cells stops. The stimulus for an increased appositional rate may extend to involve the cells just peripheral to the resorbed area, so that an appearance of overflowing is produced on the root surface. A compensatory hyperplasia may be present near extensive resorbing sites.

Repair tissue is more likely to be acellular in those regions of the root that normally have only slowly forming cement. Here a depression in the root surface may persist for a long period, as the character and deposition rate of the new cement lining the resorption cavity equal that of the general, unresorbed root surface.

Successive periods of resorption and repair occur on older teeth apically. The tooth may become ankylosed to the surrounding alveolar bone if the repair is too exuberant. Deciduous teeth in the process of shedding may also become ankylosed and consequently submerged because they fail to maintain their position at the occlusal plane as the height of the alveolar bone increases.

## DEVELOPMENTAL ANOMALIES

### Normal development

Because teeth start to calcify along the amelo-dentinal junction of their occlusal surfaces, their crowns are only a little smaller at this stage than their final size. The thickness of the enamel is added outside this line to achieve their full size. At birth, all the temporary teeth and the first permanent molars have started to calcify and the tooth crypts occupy up to a half or two-thirds of the depth of the bone of the maxilla and the body of the mandible (Fig. 8.60).

By about 8 months of age, the temporary incisors are usually erupting and this dentition is complete by $2\frac{1}{2}$ years. By 5 years, the roots of the temporary incisors and molars begin to be resorbed as the permanent incisor and premolar crypts with their developing crowns move towards their functioning position in the mouth. The developing crypts are surrounded by complete rings of lamina dura (Fig. 8.61). These rings become interrupted when the crypt reaches the bone surface or if it approaches the resorbing roots of predecessors.

By 7 years, the body and alveolar process of the mandible are much deeper, the ramus is longer and

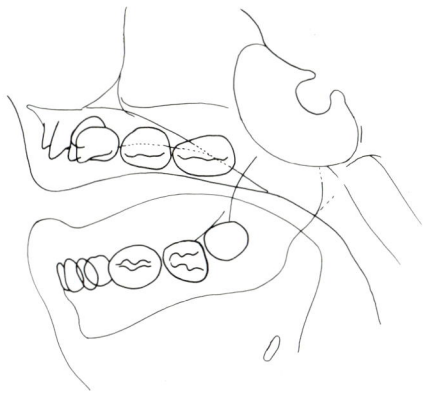

**Fig. 8.60.** Lateral projection of the jaws at birth. There is some calcification of the teeth in their crypts and the outline of the crypts is incomplete where these have reached the bone surface.

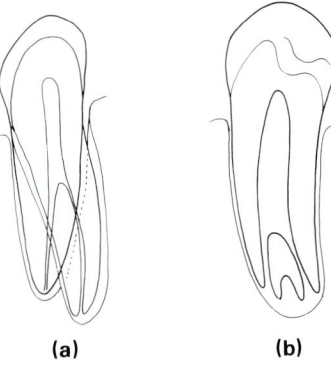

**Fig. 8.62.** (a) Taurodont lower right canine with its roots completely formed showing the long pulp chamber bifurcating low down. (b) Taurodont lower left first premolar at 12 years with its root apices still incomplete. The root canals become narrower as the tooth grows older and the taurodont form is more easily overlooked then.

the angle is less shallow than in infancy. The mandibular cortex is well defined but not as thick as in the adult jaw and it is also less dense and more vascular than in adults. The alveolar process of the maxilla becomes deeper and both jaws grow steadily larger in depth as well as in the other dimensions. In the adult, the maxillary antra extend below the level of the nasal floor towards the alveolar process on each side (Fig. 7.8).

## Developmental irregularities

### TAURODONTISM

This is a primitive tooth form (p. 390) which crops up in molars in patients with partial anodontia and sporadically in lower premolars (occasionally in lower canines or upper premolars) in patients with normal dentitions. The pulp chamber is long and bifurcates near the apical third of the tooth into two short root canals (Fig. 8.62).

### ENAMEL HYPOPLASIA

This may occur as a line of pits across permanent incisor and first molar crowns as a result of early childhood fevers like measles where the exanthema has a toxic effect on the ameloblasts. The result is usually more striking clinically than radiologically.

### AMELOGENESIS IMPERFECTA OR HEREDITARY ENAMEL HYPOPLASIA

In this there is generalized enamel deficiency in both dentitions. The enamel may be extremely thin but even in distribution over the tooth crowns or of irregular thickness though still thinner than normal (Fig. 8.63). Its irregular distribution is accentuated by caries which readily attacks the rough tooth surface.

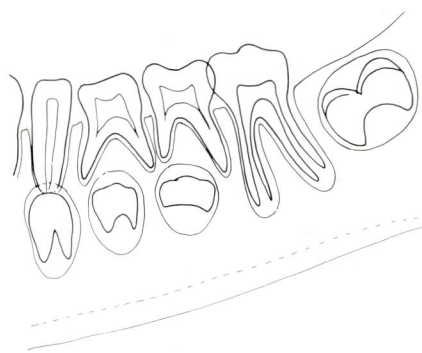

**Fig. 8.61.** Part of a bimolar projection of the left teeth in a boy of 7 years. The first molar has erupted but its roots are incomplete. The other permanent teeth have little or no root formed yet and their crypts are contained in a ring of lamina dura.

### DENTINOGENESIS IMPERFECTA OR HEREDITARY OPALESCENT DENTINE

This is a developmental abnormality of the dentine which is greyish or brownish in colour. The teeth are smaller than normal and the discoloured dentine shows through the translucent but normal enamel. The anchorage of the enamel to the abnormal dentine is poor and enamel frequently flakes off leaving the dentine

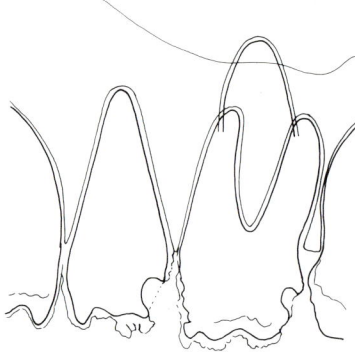

Fig. 8.63. Amelogenisis imperfecta in a boy of 11 years. The enamel layer of all these teeth was thin and irregular in thickness, and the irregularity of the crowns was aggravated by caries. The pulp outlines have been omitted.

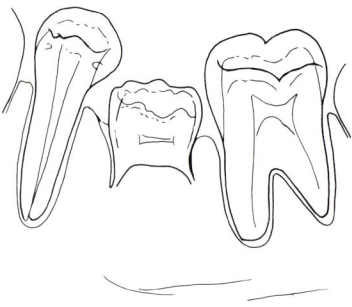

Fig. 8.65. A submerged second temporary molar with no successor in a youth of 15 years. Sometimes the dark line of the peridontal membrane looks to be largely intact but sometimes it appears to be deficient in the film. There is little doubt that the root of such a tooth is ankylosed to the bone at some point of their contact and this effect usually happens when the roots have been partly resorbed.

exposed to caries. Radiologically, the dentine tends to obliterate the pulp space which becomes narrowed and reduced in length even before a tooth erupts (Fig. 8.64). After eruption the pulp spaces are almost completely eliminated though the last molar pulps may remain fairly large.

The condition occurs in some subjects with osteogenesis imperfecta but rather more often in otherwise normal patients.

MISPLACED TEETH

The lower third molar is displaced frequently but, even when in correct relation to the other teeth, it commonly fails to erupt clear of the gum because the modern jaw is short for the size of teeth. There then occurs stagnation under this gum flap and pericoronitis (inflammation around the crown) is a very common and painful condition associated with the wisdom tooth.

The upper canine is the other most commonly displaced tooth in the arch.

SUBMERGED TEETH

Second deciduous molars having reached occlusion may become ankylosed to the alveolar bone and so fail to continue erupting with the other teeth as the jaws continue to grow. They thus become submerged below the occlusal plane and may become covered with gingiva, sometimes even with a filling in the crown acquired when the tooth was in occlusion. This state of affairs more

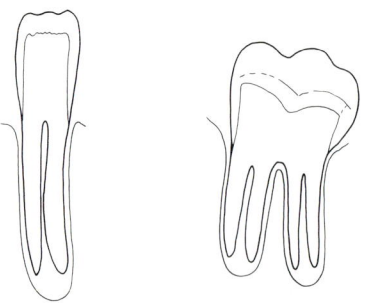

Fig. 8.64. Dentinogenisis imperfecta in a girl of 6½ years. The lower right central had just erupted and still had its three tubercles along the incisive edge. The lower first molar also had just erupted but, although their roots were still incomplete, the pulps were already receding from the crowns and even the root canals were narrowed.

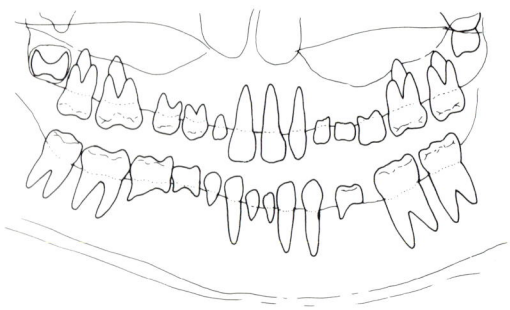

Fig. 8.66. A Panelipse film showing partial anodontia in a girl of 10 years. Many permanent teeth are missing—all the premolars, three canines, three incisors and the lower third molars though these latter could still develop.

often arises when the successor is absent (Fig. 8.65).

MISSING TEETH

Sometimes all or some of the third molars are absent and this can avoid their peculiar trouble although the third molar may become a useful member of the dentition when other teeth have been lost.

The upper lateral incisor and the lower second premolar are examples of isolated teeth which may be absent and this can be symmetrical. When several permanent teeth fail to develop, the condition is called partial anodontia and, even then, the temporary dentition is usually complete. When temporary teeth are late being shed this condition may be suspected (Fig. 8.66).

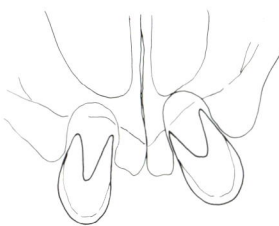

**Fig. 8.67.** An upper occlusal film showing severe partial anodontia in a boy of 7 years. He had ectodermal dysplasia and only two teeth, apparently permanent canines, were developing in his undersized jaws.

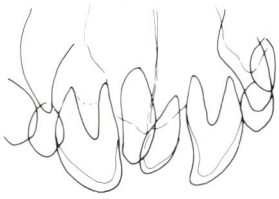

**Fig. 8.68.** Two mesiodentes, one facing forwards and the other back, deflecting but not delaying both centrals in a girl of $6\frac{1}{2}$ years. Their roots are already complete although the central roots are little formed yet.

In severe partial anodontia, both dentitions are depleted and there can be very few permanent teeth (Fig. 8.67). There is usually ectodermal dysplasia in these patients with deficiency of hair, lashes, eyebrows and sweat glands.

SUPERNUMERARY TEETH

Third premolars and fourth molars occasionally develop but supernumeraries are most common in the upper incisor region. The mesiodens forms in the midline between the two dentitions in time and size. It is usually a conical tooth, may point forwards or backwards and there may be a second mesiodens just across the midline (Fig. 8.68). Other developmental abnormalities of the teeth and jaws are described in Volume III.

## FURTHER READING

APPLETON J. & WILLIAMS M.J.R. (1973) Ultrastructural observations on the calcification of human dental pulp. *Calcified Tissue Research* **11**, 222.

ATKINSON M.E. (1972) The development of the mouse molar periodontium. *Journal of Periodontal Research* **3**, 255.

BARTON J.M. & KEENAN R.M. (1967) The formation of Sharpey's fibres in the hamster under non-functional conditions. *Archives of Oral Biology* **12**, 1331.

BERKOVITZ B.K.B. (1967) An account of the enamel cord in *Setonix brachyurus* and on the presence of an enamel knot in *Trichosurus vulpecula*. *Archives of Oral Biology* **12**, 49.

BUTLER P.M. (1956) The ontogeny of molar pattern. *Biology Reviews* **31**, 30.

DECKER J.D. (1963) A light and electron microscope study of the rat molar enamel organ. *Archives of Oral Biology* **8**, 301.

EISENMANN D.R. & GLICK P.L. (1972) Ultrastructure of initial crystal formation in dentin. *Journal of Ultrastructural Research* **41**, 18.

FINN S.B. ed. (1968) *Biology of the Dental Pulp Organ.* Alabama, University of Alabama Press.

FREEMAN E. & TEN CATE A.R. (1971) Development of the periodontium: An electron microscope study. *Journal of Periodontology* **42**, 387.

FREEMAN E., TEN CATE A.R. & DICKINSON J. (1975) Development of a gomphosis by tooth germ implants in the parietal bone of the mouse. *Archives of Oral Biology* **20**, 139.

FURSETH R. (1968) The resorption process of human deciduous teeth studied by light microscopy, microradiography and electron microscopy. *Archives of Oral Biology* **13**, 417.

GAUNT W.A. & MILES A.E.W. (1967). Fundamental aspects of tooth morphogenesis. In *Structural and Chemical Organization of Teeth*, Vol. 1, p. 151, Miles, A.E.W., ed. London: Academic Press.

GLASSTONE S. (1952) The development of halved tooth germs. A study in experimental embryology. *Journal of Anatomy (London)* **86**, 12.

GRANT D.A., BERNICK S. LEVY B.M. & DREIZEN S. (1972) A comparative study of periodontal ligament development in teeth with and without predecessors in Marmosets. *Journal of Periodontology* **43**, 162.

HODGES G.M. (1969) Stromal-epithelial interactions. In *Biology of the Periodontium*, p. 27, Melcher A.H. & Bowen W.H., eds. London: Academic Press.

ISOKAWA S., KOSAKAI T. & KAJIYAMA S. (1963) Interglobular dentine in the deciduous tooth. *Journal of Dental Research* **42**, 831.

JONES S.J. & BOYDE A. (1972) A study of human root cementum surfaces as prepared for and examined in the scanning electron microscope. *Zeitschrift für Zellforschung* **130**, 318.

KAWASAKI K. & FEARNHEAD R.W. (1975) On the relationship between tetracycline and the incremental lines in dentine. *Journal of Anatomy* **119**, 49.

KOLLAR E.J. (1972) Histogenic aspects of dermal-epidermal interactions. In *Developmental Aspects of Oral Biology*, p. 125, Slavkin H.C. & Bavetta L.A., eds. London: Academic Press.

LESTER K.S. (1969) The incorporation of epithelial cells by cementum. *Journal of Ultrastructure Research* **27**, 63.

LESTER K.S. & BOYDE A. (1970) Scanning electron microscopy of developing roots of molar teeth of the laboratory rat. *Journal of Ultrastructure Research* **33**, 80.

LISTGARTEN M.A. (1975) Afibrillar dental cementum in the rat and hamster. *Journal of Periodontal Research* **10**, 158.

LISTGARTEN M.A. (1976) Structure of surface coatings on teeth. *Journal of Periodontology* **47**, 139.

MAIN J.H.P. (1965) A histologic survey of the hammock ligament. *Archives of Oral Biology* **10**, 343.

MILES A.E.W. ed. (1967) *Structural and Chemical Organization of Teeth*, 2 vols. New York: Academic Press.

MOSS M.L. (1974) Studies on dentine. I. Mantle dentine. *Acta Anatomica* **87**, 481.

OSBORN J.W. (1973) Variations in structure and development of enamel. In *Dental Enamel* Oral Science Reviews, Volume 3, p. 3. Copenhagen: Munksgaard.

OWENS P.D.A. (1974) A light microscope study of the development of the roots of premolar teeth in dogs. *Archives of Oral Biology* **19**, 525.

PANNESE E. (1960) Observations on the ultrastructure of the enamel organ. 1. Stellate reticulum and stratum intermedium. *Journal of Ultrastructural Research* **4**, 372.

PANNESE E. (1962) Observations on the ultrastructure of the enamel organ. III. Internal and external enamel epithelia. *Journal of Ultrastructural Research* **6**, 186.

PORTOIS M. (1961) Contribution a l'etude des bourgeons dentaire chez la Souris. Periodes d'induction et de morphodifferentiation. *Archives of Biology (Liege)* **72**, 17.

REITH E.J. (1970) The stages of amelogenesis as observed in the molar teeth of young rats. *Journal of Ultrastructural Research* **30**, 111.

ROBINSON C., LOWE N.R. and WEATHERALL P. (1977) Changes in amino acid composition of developing rat incisor enamel. *Calcified Tissue Research* **23**, 19.

SCHONFIELD S.E. & SLAVKIN H.D. (1977) Demonstration of enamel matrix proteins on root-analogue surfaces of rabbit permanent incisor teeth. *Calcified Tissue Research* **24**, 223.

SELVIG K.A. (1964) An ultrastructural study of cementum formation. *Acta Odontologica Scandinavica* **22**, 105.

SILVA D.G. & KAILIS D.G. (1972) Ultrastructural studies on the cervical loop and the development of the amelo-dentinal junction in the cat. *Archives or Oral Biology* **17**, 279.

SISCA R.F. & PROVENZA D.V. (1972) Initial dentine formation in human deciduous teeth. An electron microscope study. *Calcified Tissue Research* **9**, 1.

SLAVKIN H.C. (1970) Epithelial–mesenchymal interactions related to periodontal disease. *Journal of Periodontology* **41**, 373.

SLAVKIN H.C. (1974) Towards a cellular and molecular understanding of periodontics. Cementongenesis revisited. *Journal of Periodontology* **47**, 249.

SLAVKIN, H.C. (1974) Embryonic tooth formation: a tool for developmental biology. *Oral Sciences Reviews* No. 4. Copenhagen, Munksgaard.

SYMONS N.B.B. ed. (1968) *Dentine and Pulp*, Edinburgh: Livingstone.

TAKUMA S. & NAGAI N. (1971) Ultrastructure of rat odontoblasts in various stages of their development and maturation. *Archives of Oral Biology* **16**, 993.

TEN CATE A.R. (1969) The development of the periodontium. In *Biology of the periodontium*, p. 53., Melcher A.H. & Bowen, W.H., eds. London: Academic Press.

TEN CATE A.R. (1972) Developmental aspects of the periodontium. In *Developmental aspects of oral biology*, p. 309. Slavkin H.E. & Bavetta L.A., eds. London: Academic Press.

TEN CATE A.R., MILLS C. & SOLOMON G. (1970) The development of the periodontium. A transplantation and autoradiographic study. *Anatomical Record* **170**, 365.

TONGE C.H. (1963) The development and arrangement of the dental follicle. *Transactions of the European Orthodontic Society* p. 118.

TROTT J.R. (1962) The development of the periodontal attachment in the rat. *Acta anatomica* **51**, 313.

# CHAPTER 9
# Development and Maintenance of Occlusion

## EVOLUTION

It will be recalled that the upper and lower teeth of most reptiles cannot be brought together because the lowers are placed well inside the uppers and the lower jaw cannot be swung laterally to bring the teeth into occlusion. However, when viewed from the side of the jaw, the cusps of the lower teeth are often positioned between the cusps of the upper teeth. Because the ankylosed teeth of reptiles cannot be displaced after they have erupted it seems that this 'interdigitation' must be the outcome of some developmental control rather than of tooth movement in response to the environment.

In the lineage(s) which finally produced the mammals, well differentiated heterodonty evolved before the jaw could be swung laterally and the upper and lower teeth be brought together. For example, in the cynodont (Fig. 10.6), *Thrinaxodon*, the anterior postcanines are simple conical teeth while the posterior postcanines possess four mesiodistally arranged cusps surrounded by an array of cingulum cusps. The relationship between upper and lower postcanines is variable: in some animals they are in line and in others they are not. In *Thrinaxodon*, the teeth are gomphosed and it is therefore possible that they could have been moved into their most efficient positions by forces generated during 'mastication'. The number of replacement teeth has been reduced to three presumably because the teeth remained efficient for a longer time than those of the ancestors of *Thrinaxodon*: it can be assumed that the frequency of tooth replacement was related to the time for which teeth remained efficient.

By the time the earliest known mammal, *Eozostrodon*, had evolved the dentition was diphyodont and the upper and lower teeth could be occluded, features which are characteristic of nearly all mammals. The oval-shaped (in cross-section) upper molars of *Eozostrodon* always lie just behind the equivalent lower molars in all specimens studied. The development and maintenance of this precise relationship between upper and lower molars, which is typical of nearly every mammal, was important because it enabled efficient, matched surfaces with shearing edges to be gouged into opposing teeth (Fig. 10.8b). The newly erupted, unworn, upper and lower teeth did not accurately fit together; from which it can be understood that, with use and wear, the dentition became increasing efficient. It seems probable that this is the reason why mammals evolved diphyodonty. If the animals had remained polyphyodont, every newly erupted molar would, because of its high unworn cusps, have disrupted the smoothly efficient shearing edges which had previously been created by attrition. However, it was still necessary to develop a deciduous dentition of small teeth to be accommodated in the small jaws of the infants.

It is possible for a gomphosed tooth to be moved into a new position after it has erupted; but only within narrow limits. Therefore, in order to establish the most efficient relationship between upper and lower dentitions, it is necessary for the jaws and the teeth within the jaws to develop in the correct relationship. Although the controls are difficult to visualize, a study of the cat dentition has shown that the upper and lower molars develop and maintain their correct relationships from the time they are initiated until they erupt. When they erupt each tooth can be twisted and turned, in response to masticatory and other muscular forces, in order to effect the minor adjustments necessary to move it into its most efficient position. Environmental forces provide a fine adjustment for development controls.

## OCCLUSION

Occlusion of the teeth means the meeting together of upper and lower teeth. Although human teeth can, with some effort, be made to meet in a variety of different positions, there are certain occlusal relations which are inherent and natural and which play an important part in the function of the teeth, especially in mastication and chewing.

**The intercuspal position**

This is one of the names given to the situation when the teeth are closed together naturally in the most comfortable position. There are a variety of other names given to this, including 'centric occlusion' and 'the position of maximum cuspal interdigitation'. Although it is important to understand this relationship between the teeth, it is in fact a relationship which is comparatively seldom employed. At rest the teeth are slightly apart in which is called the rest position with a gap of some 2 or 3 mm between the molar teeth. In chewing the lower teeth normally move across the upper teeth and pass through the intercuspal position without stopping. The only time the intercuspal position is achieved is during swallowing (and not always then) and during the deliberate clenching of the teeth.

The intercuspal position is usually coincident with centric jaw relationship. This latter exists when the mandible is in a bilaterally symmetrical position, with the condyles as fully retruded in the glenoid fossae as is comfortably possible. Centric jaw relation exists at any stage in jaw opening from the occlusal position to a wide gape. It is possible in most adults to retract the mandible slightly from the intercuspal position, although this involves some effort and is often termed 'forced retrusion'. In the child it seems probable that the intercuspal position coincides with full retrusion.

Abnormally, in cases of malocclusion, the intercuspal position may be displaced from centric jaw relation. It is therefore less confusing to avoid the term 'centric occlusion' as a synonym for intercuspal position.

The condition which it is now proposed to describe is sometimes called ideal occlusion. Like most ideals it is seldom achieved in life. In civilized man the result of genetic crossing, together with an absence of Darwinian natural selection, means that almost all individuals have some departures from the ideal occlusion and in many cases these departures are so great that the condition could reasonably be described as a malocclusion. In primitive communities, malocclusion is by no means unknown but nevertheless quite a large proportion of such populations have nearly ideal occlusions. The main departure is due to wear of the teeth with the first molars often being quite severely worn before the last molars have erupted. Something close to ideal occlusion is shown in the skull which forms the subject of Fig. 9.1. It will be noted that the upper incisors overlap the lowers slightly, giving a slight positive overjet and overbite. (Overjet is the horizontal overlap of the incisal edge of the upper incisor over the lower; overbite is the vertical overlap). In ideal occlusion this is transformed gradually to an edge-to-edge relationship because of two factors. In the first place, the incisal edges of the teeth wear away thus eliminating the overbite; and second, there is, probably throughout life, a tendency for the lower dentition to move forward slightly relative to the upper dentition and this helps to achieve the edge-to-edge position. In civilized man, the overbite is maintained throughout life and indeed is often rather greater than shown in this skull. Upper and lower incisors oppose each other and their chisel-shaped edges enable them to be used, as their name suggests for incising or cutting food into pieces large enough for chewing. It will be noted that the upper incisors are wider than the lower incisors and consequently the canine teeth do not directly oppose each other, but the upper canine has its cusp occluding between the cusp of the lower canine and that of the first premolar. This alternation of the buccal cusps is a feature of normal occlusion, with each cusp in one jaw apparently fitting between two cusps in the opposing jaw. Fig. 9.1b shows that the same is true for the lingual cusps. This alternation of cusps is not confined to the anteroposterior plane. Fig. 9.2b shows a cross-section through the jaws in the region of the first permanent molar; each lower buccal cusp occludes in the groove or valley between an upper buccal and palatal cusp, while each lower lingual cusp occludes on the lingual side of the row of upper palatal cusps.

In fact, the above description is somewhat oversimplified. Fig. 9.1c shows an occlusal view of the lower posterior teeth superimposed upon the corresponding upper ones. Perhaps the key to this occlusion can be seen in the largest cusp of each upper molar, its mesiopalatal cusp. This occludes in the centre of a basin in the corresponding lower molar. It lies at the buccal end of a groove between the two lingual cusps of the tooth. Superficially, the distolingual upper cusp appears to occlude between the two corresponding lower molars. If it did occlude precisely over the contact point it would have the effect of forcing the food down between these two teeth. In fact it occludes slightly mesially to the contact point. The buccal cusps of the upper molars lie on the buccal side of corresponding grooves in the lower molars, that is between the lower molar cusps. To this rather precise relationship there is a reciprocal relation-

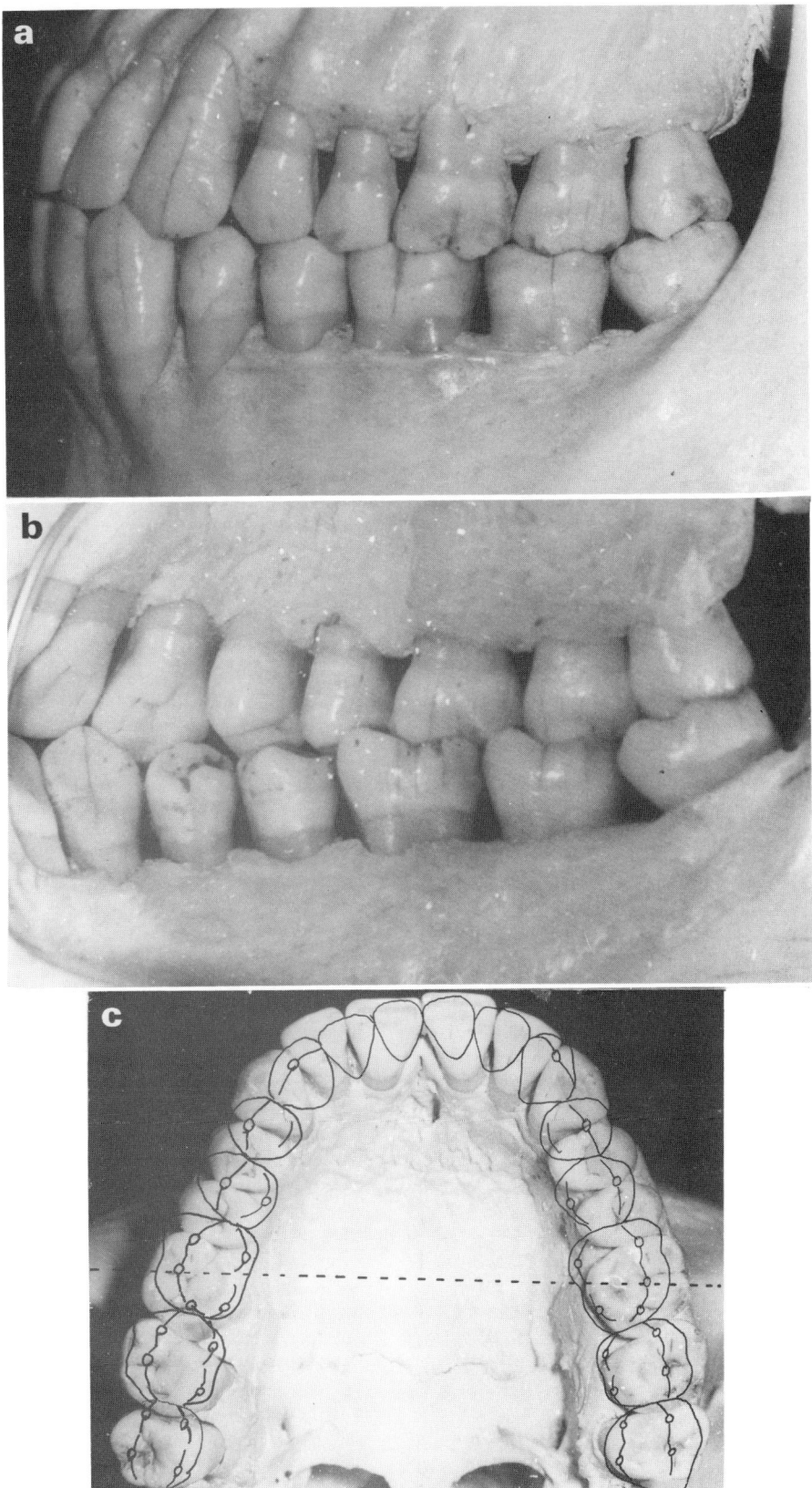

**Fig. 9.1.** A normal occlusion viewed (a) bucally, (b) lingually and (c) occlusally. In (c) drawings of the lower teeth have been superimposed on a photograph of the upper teeth.

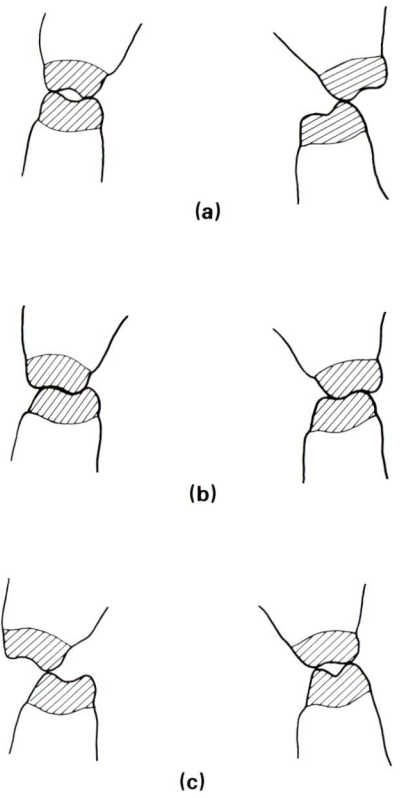

**Fig. 9.2.** The relationship between upper and lower molars in the coronal plane during a chewing movement on the left side (viewed from behind) and passing from the buccal phase (a), to centric (b), to the lingual phase (c), on the left side.

ship of the lower cusps. The distobuccal cusp of the lower molar occludes in the centre of a basin which lies at the lingual end of a groove between the buccal cusps of the upper molar. The mesiobuccal cusps of the lower molar again appear at first sight to occlude on the contact point between the upper molars but in fact occlude somewhat distally to this in a small basin. Where a distal cusp is present on a lower molar it occludes in a basin in the distal part of the upper molar. The lower lingual cusps again lie to the lingual side of the corresponding upper cusps and between them.

The premolars have a basically similar relationship except that the distal parts of both upper and lower teeth have been 'eliminated' so that occlusion is confined to the more mesial parts of these teeth.

The above relations are constant in animals with similar teeth to those of man: indeed, it can be found with variations throughout the mammals.

### Dynamic occlusion (Articulation)

The intercuspal position attracts considerable attention in the study of the individual human dentition. It is a position in which the orthodontist normally examines the teeth either in the mouth or in the form of plaster models. It is a position in which all too often teeth are set in dentures. If the teeth occlude well in the intercuspal position it is quite likely that they will function well during dynamic occlusion but this is not always the case. It may be satisfying to clench our teeth in moments of stress but apart from this and the transient closure in swallowing, the intercuspal position is one we very seldom adopt in life.

In the act of chewing, a morsel of food is placed between upper and lower posterior teeth by the tongue and cheeks. It is initially pounded by a vertical action of the jaw and assuming that the food is reasonably tough, the teeth do not come really close to each other until a certain amount of initial comminution has taken place. This has been called puncture-crushing activity. It is succeeded by chewing proper. The puncture-crushing period would probably suffice alone in the case of soft, prepared foods, where chewing could be unnecessary. Chewing is normally carried out on one side of the mouth at a time although the bolus of food may be moved from one side to the other; some authors believe that ideally the individual should chew on both sides simultaneously. Let us suppose that the individual is chewing on the right side of the mouth. He starts the chewing stroke by displacing the mandible to the right and to some extent downwards; the food is placed on the table of the mandibular posterior teeth. The lower teeth then sweep across the upper teeth from buccal to lingual as shown in Figs. 9.2, 9.3 and 9.4a,b. To achieve this each lower buccal cusp slides down between two corresponding upper buccal cusps until the intercuspal position is reached. The crests which run lingually from the tips of these cusps slide down the opposing grooves and to some extent guide the occlusion during this movement. The crests which run mesially and distally act as cutting blades to shred the food in much the same way as a domestic vegetable shredder. The lingual cusps act in a similar way, with the lower lingual cusps sliding down the grooves between the upper palatal cusps.

It is noticeable that a cusp does not slide across the contact point between two opposing teeth but down a groove which is separated from the contact point by a marginal ridge thereby preventing the food being packed down between the teeth. This protection of the contact point is a feature which is

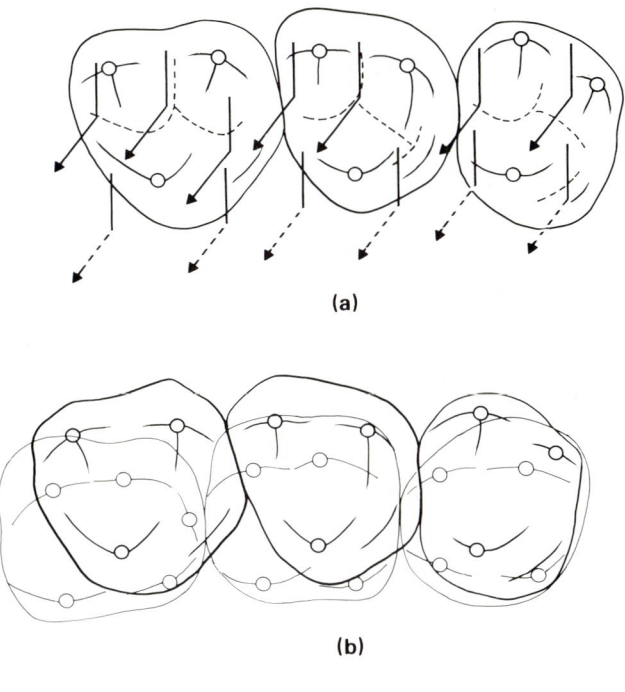

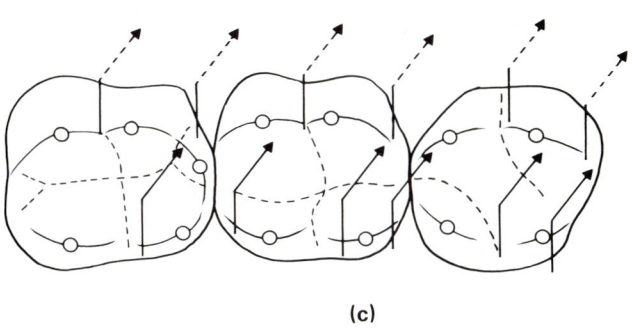

**Fig. 9.3.** Centric relation in (b). During a chewing movement the cusps of the lower teeth move in the directions of the arrows in (a). The cusps of the upper teeth, relative to the lower ones, move in the directions of the arrows in (c).

seen in all those animals which are able to chew their food.

Movement from the closing stroke (Book 1) to the intercuspal position has been called the buccal phase of chewing. During this phase the mandible rotates about the right condylar head with the left condyle being drawn upwards and backwards from the articular eminence. The late Sir Norman Bennett once suggested that rotation was not the only movement taking place, but that simultaneously there was a very small sideways movement of both condyles. The existence of this so-called Bennett movement has been a matter of controversy ever since. It may be that there is some individual variation in this matter but recent research would seem to show that Bennett movement does exist, at least in some individuals, although it is very small.

When the teeth have reached the intercuspal position, they continue without pause into the lingual phase of chewing (Fig. 9.2, 9.3 and 9.4b,c). In this phase the lower lingual and upper buccal cusps lose contact with their opponents but the lower buccal cusps slide across the upper lingual cusps in a rather different manner from that seen previously. Instead of ridges sliding down grooves, the flat occlusal surface of the lower buccal cusps slides across the corresponding occlusal surface of the upper palatal cusps. This is brought about by the mandible rotating about the balancing side condyle—in this case the left one—while the working side condyle moves forward

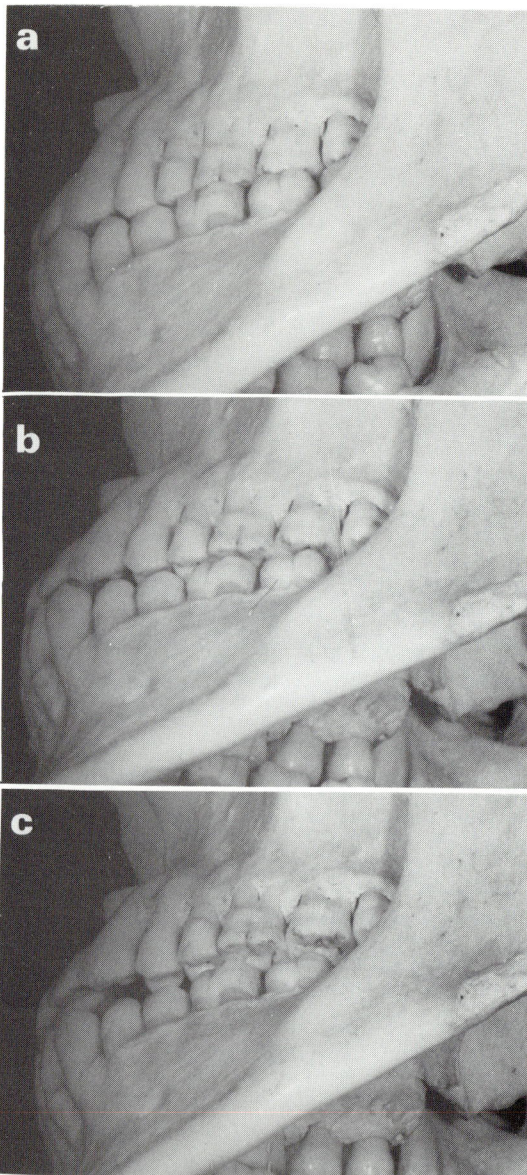

**Fig. 9.4.** The relationship between upper and lower teeth during the buccal phase (a) and the lingual phase (c) of a chewing movement on the left side.

down the articular eminence. There is a change of direction of any point on a lower tooth at this stage and those cusps which have to cross an opposing contact point do so at an angle, thus avoiding food impaction. Suppose we examine the slightly worn teeth of a skull such as that shown in Figs. 9.1 and 9.3. If we move the teeth on the right side of the jaw as described above, it would be seen that while the teeth on the right side are moving through the buccal phase of occlusion, those on the left are following the lingual phase, but of course in the reverse direction. As those on the right continue into the lingual phase the teeth on the left follow the reversed buccal phase. This is shown diagrammatically in Fig. 9.2a, c and has given rise to the concept of balanced occlusion which is widely used in prosthetic dentistry. It is nice to believe that as the teeth are functioning on one side of the mouth, they are equally in contact on the opposite side, thus preventing trauma to the joint where natural teeth are present, or tilting of artificial dentures. Unfortunately there are certain snags in this theory.

First there is considerable doubt whether the

teeth do come into contact during chewing. This point will be considered in some detail but certainly if they do so this must be very transient. Once the posterior teeth are in contact, there is no longer food between them and they are clearly serving no useful purpose so that the automatic reaction would be to take another bite of food and start again. Second if there is food between the teeth on the right side of the mouth there is unlikely to be food on the left side, and even if there were, it is unlikely to be of precisely the same consistency on both sides of the mouth. Third, although balanced occlusion can be easily demonstrated in unworn teeth of a dried skull, there is some controversy as to whether such balance exists in life. A more accurate description would probably be as follows:

In the young adult dentition, a balanced occlusion such as described above is perfectly possible, but the dentition would only be balanced if there were no food between the teeth. The shapes of wear facets suggest teeth are balanced in this way. All teeth exhibit two types of wear (Fig. 10.5). Abrasion is a generalized, rounded wear which is produced by chewing food between the teeth. Attrition is the wear of tooth against tooth and produces flat wear facets. These facets on upper and lower teeth correspond to each other and are either flat, or curved in one plane only. Superficially they appear almost mirror-flat although on higher magnification under the microscope they are seen to be covered by fine scratch marks. These marks are parallel, indicating that they develop due to movement along a single line. Those facets produced during the buccal phase on one side of the mouth appear to be parallel to a set of facets produced during the lingual phase on the other side. It is difficult to understand how these could be produced during chewing. It could only be assumed that following the complete comminution of the food or at some other time, the individual continues to chew apparently purposelessly, perhaps as a self-sharpening mechanism thus producing the wear facets on the teeth (Fig. 10.5). This attritional wear does however have the effect of reducing the height of the upper lingual and lower buccal cusps, so that in a moderately or severely worn occlusion the cusps responsible for the balancing occlusion are no longer high enough to meet, and balancing occlusion therefore disappears fairly early in the human dentition. Wear of the affected cusps (upper palatal and lower buccal) continues in the buccal phase.

In more civilized communities the edge-to-edge incisor occlusion is no longer seen, man being left with an overbite, often quite a deep one, which affects not only the incisors but also the canines. As a result of this, lateral excursions from the centric relationship take the posterior teeth out of occlusion; it has been suggested that this so called 'canine rise' (the rise is necessary to 'unlock' the canines in a lateral movement) is a mechanism to protect the posterior teeth from trauma. The canine rise is not however found in primitive man, from which it would seem to be one of the unfortunate by-products of civilization without any great advantage.

To summarize, in the ideal occlusion which is seen in primitive races, there is probably a balancing occlusion shortly after the teeth erupt. Those cusps which function in the lingual phase of occlusion, that is the upper lingual and lower buccal cusps, are rather rapidly reduced in height, so that they no longer contact in this phase but pass each other a short distance apart. Therefore, during the buccal phase on the working side there is no balancing occlusion on the opposite side. In civilized man where a positive overbite has developed, the posterior teeth may be taken out of contact shortly after they leave the intercuspal position by virtue of the overbite of the canines. It is difficult to believe that this serves any useful purpose.

Some authors describe a condition of protrusive occlusion. As the mandible is protruded from the intercuspal position, the condylar head slides down the articular eminence, while the mesial slopes of the lower cusps slide down the distal slopes of the more anterior upper cusps (Fig. 9.5). It is suggested, in the concept of protrusive occlusion, that the lower incisors should simultaneously slide down the lingual slopes of the upper incisors, so that an edge-to-edge relation of the incisors is achieved simultaneously with the cusp-to-cusp relation of the posterior teeth. This arrangement may be useful in dentures to prevent their displacement on incision, but is seldom achieved in the natural dentition, and would seem to serve no useful purpose there. It does not occur in the skull shown in Fig. 9.5.

**Axial inclination of the teeth**

In 1890 Ferdinand Graf Spee suggested that, when viewed laterally, the tips of the lower teeth lay on the arc of a circle 6.5 to 7 cm in radius. If this arc was continued it touched the anterior surface of the condyle. Monson (1920) took the theory further and suggested that the cusps of the lower teeth, together with the incisal edges of the incisors, touched the surface of an imaginary

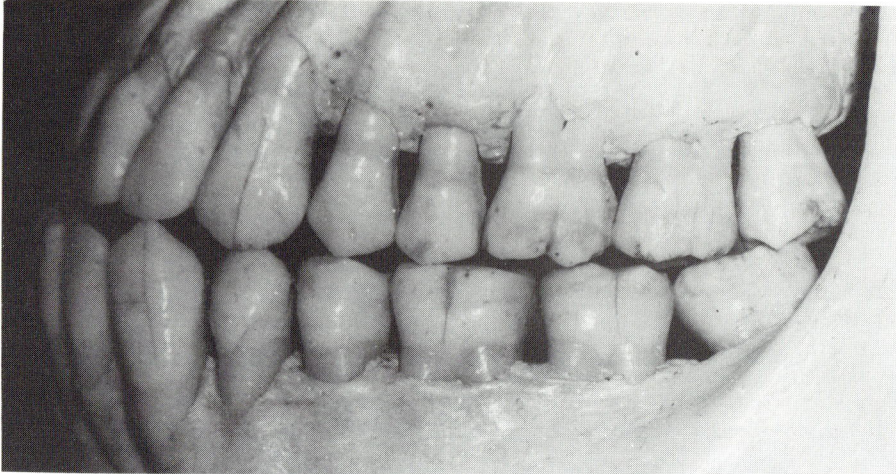

**Fig. 9.5.** During a protrusive movement the incisal tips are separated in this dentition (with a deep overbite, the molar cusps are separated in a protrusive movement).

sphere of 4 in (10 cm) radius. That is, he extended the idea of Spee to the third dimension. This almost metaphysical concept did not stand up to close investigation and has been abandoned. Nevertheless, it is true the tips of the cusps of the lower arch when seen laterally do lie on a curve (although not usually an exact arc of a circle) and it is customary to speak of this as the curve of Spee. Equally the lower molars are inclined lingually to an increasing extent as one passes backwards in the mouth, so that in coronal view their cusps lie on another curve which is often referred to as the curve of Monson, although strictly Monson's concept was three-dimensional.

If the cusps and fossae of teeth are to remain in contact, not only in the intercuspal position, but during the whole of the two phases of dynamic occlusion, it is obvious that the relation of the teeth to the temporomandibular joint must be quite precise. If upper and lower teeth were simply arranged on a flat plane it would be quite easy to arrange for them to occlude in the intercuspal position, but they would not all remain in contact during the wide range of occlusal movements. This can easily be demonstrated using artificial teeth on an anatomical articulator. The curve of Spee and to a lesser extent, the curve of Monson, are therefore necessary for the teeth to remain in contact during all aspects of dynamic occlusion.

There are, however, other reasons for the angulation of the teeth. The maxilla is somewhat narrower than the mandible and this discrepancy in width increases as one passes backwards in the mouth. In order that the teeth can meet it is necessary for the upper molars to lean buccally while the lower molars lean lingually, and as the discrepancy increases so does the angulation of the teeth increase as one passes backwards. The premolars are probably the only teeth whose long axes are more or less at right angles to the occlusal plane.

The upper and lower incisors are both somewhat proclined. That is, they lean labially. This enables the lower incisal edge to impinge on the cingulum of the upper incisor. All teeth have some potential to erupt for a short distance beyond the occlusal position. This is probably a mechanism to compensate for the wear which occurs in more primitive dentitions. In the premolar and molar teeth it is prevented by the occlusal surfaces of these teeth but if the upper and lower incisors were parallel there would be nothing to prevent this over-eruption. Since they are proclined, the cingulum of the upper incisor prevents further eruption of the lower incisor and a reciprocal effect is also present to control the upper incisor. Where the angle between the long axes of upper and lower incisors is abnormally high, this is almost invariably associated with an increase in overbite.

A great deal has been made in the past of the angulation of the teeth, both individually, and in the form of the curves of Spee and Monson. It should be kept in mind that teeth are only of value as individual units of the dentition. It is the dentition which is the functional organ and not the individual tooth. The curves of Monson and Spee are not always of the same diameter but are adapted to the needs of the individual to produce a functioning machine.

## Occlusion in the deciduous dentition

The development of the dentition will be dealt with in detail in the next section and here it is only proposed to consider the relationship of the teeth in occlusion. The condition in the newly erupted deciduous dentition, (Fig. 9.6a), largely mirrors that in the permanent dentition. At this stage in an ideal occlusion there is an overbite with a corresponding overjet and it is interesting to note that the deciduous canines often have an interlocking relationship similar to that seen in our closest relatives, the great apes; that is, the upper canine occludes in a small space between the lower deciduous canine and first deciduous molar, while the lower canine occludes between the lateral incisor and canine in the upper arch, where there is a small space to accommodate its tip. This interlocking relationship has been lost in the permanent dentition of man where the canine has become effectively a third incisor, while in the permanent dentition of the great apes it is exaggerated (Fig. 12.29).

The arch of deciduous teeth is considerably shorter than the final permanent arrangement. The deciduous molars lie behind the canines in the position where the elevator muscles of the mandible produce their maximum force. Their occlusion at this stage would seem to be similar to that seen later in the permanent molars with both buccal and lingual phases active. As the child grows and the jaws lengthen, the axis about which the mandible rotates moves further away from the deciduous molars with the result that the path of the lower cusps over the upper teeth gradually changes. Possibly to accommodate these changes the cusps of the deciduous molars are comparatively low and wear away rather rapidly in the short period during which they function. It is probable that the premolars which replace them when the jaws have lengthened have shapes which are more suitable for the lengthened arc of movement.

Some changes take place in the static occlusal relations of the deciduous teeth during their lifetime. Throughout the development of the dentition there is, in most individuals, a gradual forward movement of the lower dental arch relative to the upper. This may be seen in Fig. 9.6; the models in Fig. 9.6a show the condition immediately after the eruption of the second deciduous molars. The incisor teeth have an overbite and overjet similar to that seen in the permanent dentition, while the lower molar teeth appear to occlude somewhat too far distally for a normal relation with the uppers. The distal surfaces of the lower and upper molars are in a straight line. The models of the same child shown in Fig. 9.6a were taken as the first permanent molar was erupting. It will be noted that the lower dental arch has moved anteriorly relative to the upper so that the permanent molars are erupting into normal occlusion. At the same time the lower incisors have moved into an edge-to-edge position; whereas an incisal edge-to-edge relationship is rare in modern civilized man in the permanent teeth, it is still common in the deciduous dentition. The tips of the deciduous canines similarly wear

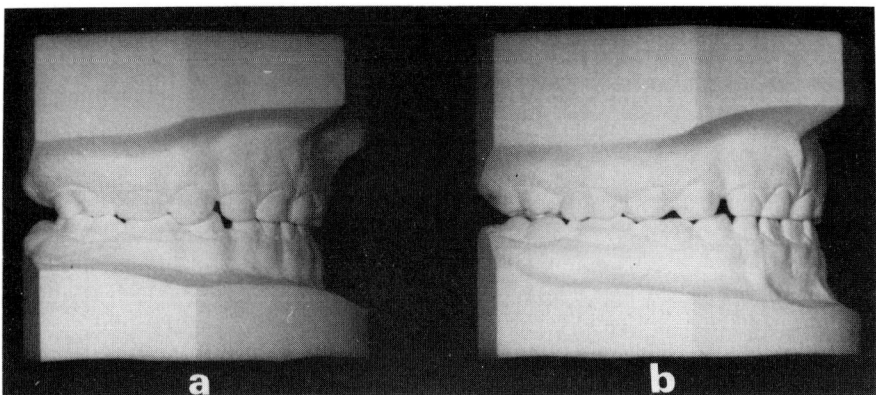

**Fig. 9.6.** Occlusal relations in a deciduous dentition where (a) the second deciduous molars have just erupted, and (b) the first permanent molars have just erupted.

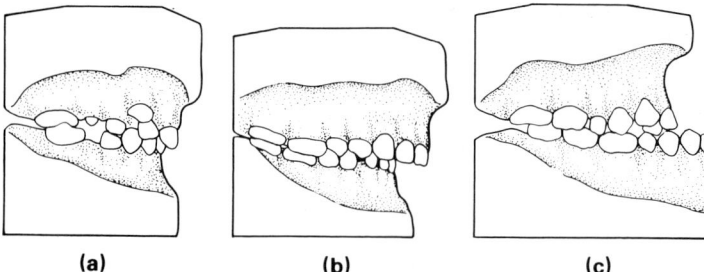

**Fig. 9.7.** (a) A crowded dentition with an Angle's Class I relation, (b) an Angle's Class II relation, and (c) an Angle's Class III relation.

flat and the interlocking relationship disappears, the deciduous canine becoming essentially a third incisor. As the dental arches increase in length with the eruption of permanent molars, the attachment of elevator muscles of the mandible migrates backwards so that their point of maximum activity lies opposite the new major chewing area. In the condition shown in Fig. 9.6b this is the second deciduous and first permanent molars; gradually the deciduous molars cease to be important chewing units and become in the nature of 'pre-molars'. Eventually of course they are replaced by premolars. These are smaller teeth more suited to the diminished muscle force available in this region.

**Malocclusion**

Malocclusion is the term used to describe states in which the occlusion departs from the normal. If we were to accept the normal as being synonymous with the ideal condition described above, it is probable that almost every individual in European populations would have a malocclusion. It is therefore customary to regard normal occlusion as including minor variants from the ideal. Assessments of the incidence of malocclusion vary considerably depending on how wide one sets the range of normal occlusion. A reasonable estimate is that in the United Kingdom between one quarter and one half of the child population have a malocclusion sufficiently severe to warrant orthodontic treatment. It is not proposed to consider this subject in great depth here since it will be dealt with more fully in a later volume of the work.

In general, malocclusion of the dental arches may occur in any one or more of three planes of space. The best known classification is that evolved by Angle and refers only to the anteroposterior dimension (Fig. 9.7). It is based on the relationship of the first permanent molars, although if the first molars are missing or are unrepresentative due to local drifting of these teeth, it is customary to extend it by consideration of other teeth. Class I malocclusion involves those cases where the occlusion of the molar teeth is normal. Class II malocclusion involves those cases where the lower first molar is distally placed relative to its opposite number. Although the discrepancy may occur due to an abnormality in either arch, it is conventional to describe the position of the lower teeth relative to the upper and the Class II malocclusion is therefore sometimes called distocclusion or post-normal occlusion. Class III malocclusion involves those cases where the lower first molar is mesial to its correct relation. There is a natural tendency for the newly erupted teeth to adjust until cusps occlude in opposing grooves and fossae, so that in a typical Class II malocclusion the mesiobuccal cusp of the lower first molar occludes between the two buccal cusps of the opposing upper molar, and similarly in a Class III malocclusion it occludes between the buccal cusps of the two upper premolars. Nevertheless, this cusp-in-groove relationship is not always present and intermediate positions are not uncommon.

Similarly if the relationship of teeth in the coronal plane is examined a malocclusion may be present; here it is usual for the cusp-in-groove relationship to be maintained. It may be that the upper buccal cusps occlude in the central groove of the lower teeth with the upper arch narrower than the lower; alternatively and rather more rarely, the lower arch may be narrower that the upper, so that the lower teeth occlude completely lingually to the upper teeth. Both these conditions are referred to as crossbites and the first is sometimes called a buccal and the second a lingual crossbite. Either of these may be unilateral or bilateral. Third, there may be a malocclusion in the vertical dimension such that the overbite of the anterior teeth is increased or decreased. Where the upper incisor teeth fail to meet the lowers altogether, the condition is often referred to as an open bite. These three types of malocclusion may be combined in the same individual, they may be unilateral or bilateral, and they may involve any number of teeth.

Although malocclusion traditionally refers to

departures from the normal intercuspal position, increasing attention is now being given to what has been called dynamic malocclusion; that is, an occlusal position which is abnormal during the chewing actions which have been described above. It may or may not be combined with a malocclusion in the intercuspal position although this is usually the case. This again will be dealt with in detail in a later volume of the work.

Without an occlusion most teeth are useless (tusks do no occlude). A careful study would seem to show that each structure on the crown of the molar teeth, even the smallest cusp or ridge, has an occlusal function. With a modern civilized diet man can survive with a very indifferent occlusion, or even with no occlusion, but living under more natural conditions even a moderate malocclusion could shorten life.

## TOOTH ERUPTION

### Movements

Eruption is the term used primarily to denote the movement which results in the crown of a tooth being carried from its developmental position within the alveolar crypt of the jaw into a functional position within the oral cavity. Thus, the main component of movement is axial in direction. Since a tooth also moves after it has attained its functional position, though at a greatly reduced rate, eruption can be regarded as a lifelong process. Teeth move in planes other than those of their long axes; by drifting (bodily movement in the mesial, distal, buccal or lingual planes), rotating (movement around the longitudinal axis) and tilting (movement around a transverse axis).

The stages of tooth development leading up to root formation result in the determination of crown form and subsequent deposition of dentine and enamel. During these early stages of development, tooth germs may be crowded together. The lateral incisor, for example, is lingually positioned between the central incisor and the canine (Fig. 8.8). Accompanying this early phase of development there is associated resorption of the internal wall of the enlarging alveolar crypt. Though lack of suitable fixed reference points at this early stage of development makes it difficult to interpret in which direction a tooth is moving, the evidence suggests that there is little axial movement of the developing crown. However, movement in other planes does occur. Thus, the teeth may be moved outwards and forwards or backwards, depending on their position within the jaw. Such movements can be deduced by observing the pattern of bone activity in histological sections. For example, deposition of bone on the posterior wall and resorption on the anterior wall of the crypt indicates anterior (mesial) drift. Whether such bone activity is a cause or an effect of tooth movement has not been established. Radiographic study shows that the inclination of human permanent maxillary incisors changes during development.

The main phase of axial movement of the tooth starts shortly after the onset of root development and ends when the tooth reaches its appropriate functional position. During this phase the tooth penetrates the oral mucosa. Initially there is a period of slow eruption when the crown is carried towards the oral mucosa; for permanent teeth this period may take between 2–4 years depending on the particular tooth involved. A tooth erupts more rapidly as its crown enters the oral cavity, at which time the length of its root is about two-thirds complete; it now slows down again as the crown approaches the occlusal plane. The clinical crown may take between 1–2 years to reach the occlusal plane. The emergence of the clinical crown is partly due to axial movement of the tooth (active eruption) and partly due to retraction of the adjacent soft tissues (passive eruption).

For human maxillary incisor teeth the maximum eruption rate of the clinical crown is about 1 mm/month and occurs at the time of crown emergence; for maxillary third molars the maximum rates are seen in spaced dentitions and are less than half that recorded for incisors, while in crowded dentitions the rates are even lower (less than 1 mm/6 months).

The teeth are believed to occupy a position of equilibrium between the soft tissues of the cheeks and lips externally and the tongue internally. In support of this hypothesis it has been shown that if the buccal surface of a tooth is thickened by an overlay, the tooth moves lingually. In other words it seems that the thickened tooth is pushed lingually by the cheek. Nevertheless, the opposing forces between which an equilibrium position is reached are seldom equal; in general the labial forces are greater than the force from the tongue. The developing crowns of the mandibular molars face mesially and upwards and those of the maxillary molars distally and downwards. The crowns of the lower incisors are frequently rotated around their longitudinal axis. The teeth twist and turn into these planes during the establishment of a 'normal' occlusion.

Once a tooth is in occlusion, tooth substance is lost following attrition both on the occlusal and interproximal surfaces. Since there is often no apparent loss of facial height, nor do interdental spaces appear, it is assumed that the teeth continue to move both axially and mesially. This situation is best visualized in the dentition of primitive peoples. Thus, in the lower jaw of Stone Age man before the eruption of the third permanent molars, interproximal wear and associated mesial drift reduced the length of the dental arch on both sides by approximately 7 mm, incidentally providing more room for the third molar (Fig. 3.26). In a sample of a modern population with a 'normal' occlusion, the maxillary permanent first molar drifted a distance of approximately 4 mm in a mesial direction between the time it emerged into the oral cavity and 18 years of age, and for the maxillary permanent canine this distance was 3 mm; there was little associated interproximal wear (presumably 1 mm between the canine and first molar). (N.B. lower premolars are about 3 mm narrower mesiodistally than their deciduous predecessors, p. 325.) It has been suggested that lack of attrition in civilized man is responsible for the high incidence of malocclusions.

The axial movement which can take place after a tooth reaches the occlusal plane is often seen when, following extraction of the opposing teeth, the tooth over-erupts. Though increased cement formation has been observed in this situation, the small amount of movement involved and the difficulty in separating cause and effect have precluded identification of the mechanism(s) responsible for the movement. Animal experiments have demonstrated an 'over-eruption' rate of 70 $\mu$m/week: they indicated that the amount of over-eruption depended on the position of the tooth with respect to the missing opposing teeth, the degree of masticatory stress and the length of time the tooth remained unopposed.

**Mechanisms**

Many experiments have been designed in attempts to determine the mechanism(s) responsible for generating the force which results in tooth eruption. The majority of works have investigated axial movement in the continuously growing incisors of rodents (Fig. 12.31), since these teeth in normal occlusion erupt at rates sufficiently fast (approximately 400 $\mu$m/day) to be measured daily either directly by using a binocular microscope incorporating a calibrated eyepiece, or indirectly by using photographs or radiographs. More recent technical advances have made it possible to record eruption continuously in anaesthetized animals (Fig. 9.8). Eruption rates can be significantly increased to about 1 mm/day simply by cutting the tooth free from occlusion, producing 'unimpeded' eruption (as opposed to 'impeded' eruption when occlusion is maintained).

One method of testing whether a particular biological force causes tooth eruption is either to reduce or to increase the activity of the factor under study and then to observe whether eruption rates are correspondingly altered. Thus, suppose it is thought that cellular proliferation of the pulp produces the eruptive force. The hypothesis can be tested by surgically removing the pulp or by administering antimitotic drugs, when eruption rates would be expected to fall. However, is it reasonable to suggest that conclusions based on experiments on the rodent incisor can be applied to the human situation; and is the eruptive mechanism the same throughout all phases of tooth eruption? These are two questions to which, as yet, there are no answers.

During eruption tooth movement may be resisted by the overlying soft tissues and alveolar bone, by the viscosity of the surrounding periodontal ligament and by occlusal forces. Therefore at any given moment a tooth moves at a rate which represents a balance between, on the one hand forces tending to move the tooth (eruptive force) and on the other forces tending to prevent movement (resistive force) (Fig. 9.9). It is clear, for example, that an increased eruption rate could result from a decrease in the resistive force, the eruption force remaining unaltered. Thus, natural or experimental changes in eruption rate are generally not as informative as one would like because it is not known which of the forces has been affected.

In common with many other systems, it is difficult to separate cause and effect in the eruptive process. For example, it has been established that when eruption rates are increased there is a corresponding increase in cell proliferation; but it is not known whether the increased cell proliferation is a cause of the increase eruption rate or an effect of it. Also it is difficult to isolate parts of the eruption system and to interpret results obtained following drug injection since the inability to localize drug activity means many other body systems may be affected.

Little is at present known for certain about the eruptive force. Studies bearing on the problem have shown the force necessary to oppose the movement of continuously growing incisors by placing elastic bands of varying tension over these teeth. A force of 5 g and 7 g is required to stop eruption of the rat and rabbit incisor respectively.

# Development and Maintenance of Occlusion

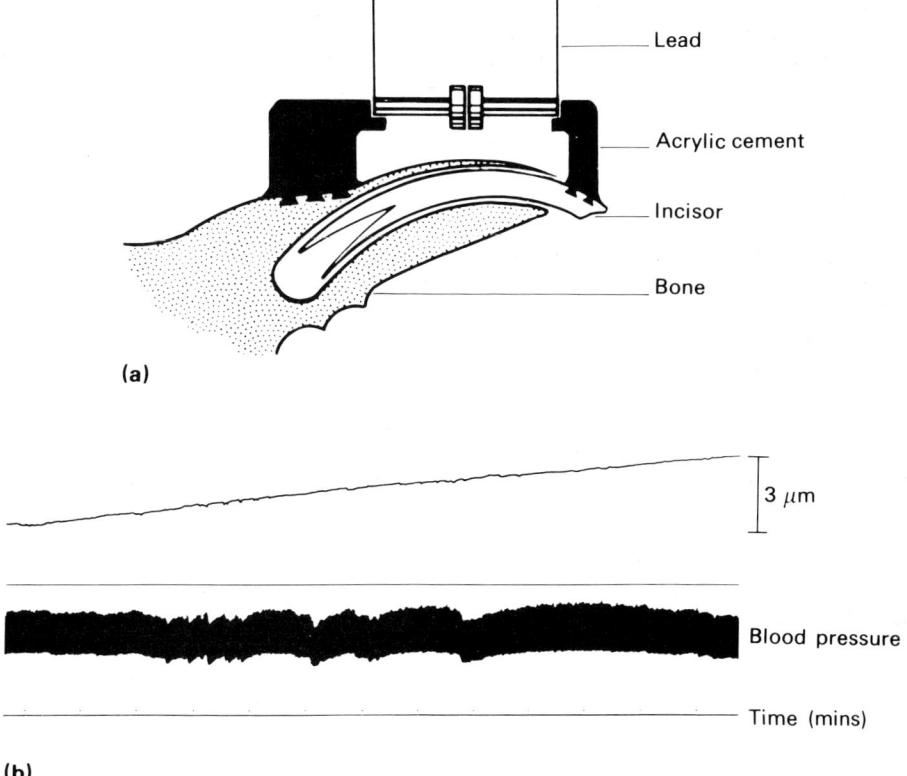

**Fig. 9.8.** (a) Diagram showing method for monitoring continuous tooth movement. One plate of a movement transducer is attached to bone by acrylic cement and acts as a reference plate. The other plate is cemented to a rabbit lower incisor tooth. Leads pass to a movement transducer. Movement of the tooth results in separation of the plates which can be displayed as a linear deflection on a pen recorder. (Modified from Matthews B. & Berkovitz B. K. B. (1972) *Archives of Oral Biology* **17**, 817.) (b) Portion of a trace obtained from movement transducer. The tooth has moved 3 μm in 12 min. A blood pressure recording is also displayed. Time scale is in min.

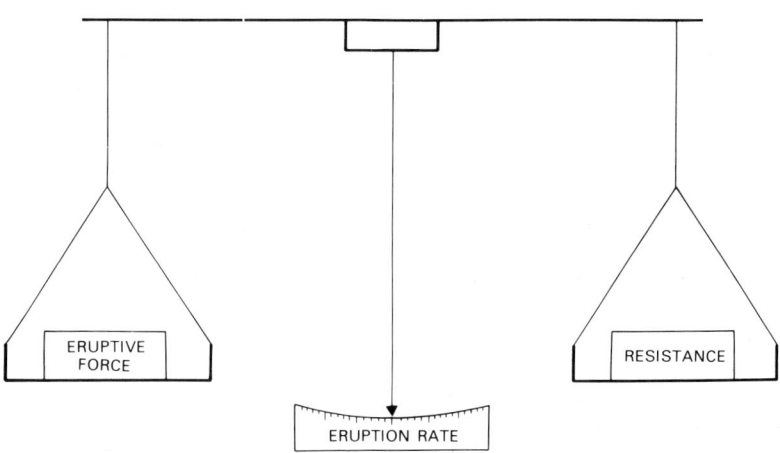

**Fig. 9.9.** Schematic diagram to illustrate that the observed eruption rate represents the resultant between the eruptive and resistive forces. An increase in the observed eruption rate could be due to an increased eruptive force or a decrease in the resistance to eruption.

This force cannot represent the total eruptive force but must be the difference between the sum of the eruptive forces and the sum of the resistive forces. It is not known whether the eruptive force is continuous or intermittent in nature.

The theories put forward to explain the mechanism responsible for axial movement during tooth eruption suggest that the force is generated by (a) alveolar bone deposition, (b) cellular proliferation (especially in the basal region of the pulp), (c) root growth, (d) tissue-fluid pressure or (e) tension generated within the periodontal ligament. The majority of authors implicate only one of these systems as being primarily responsible for eruption—the prime mover.

It has been suggested that gubernacular cords, strands of fibrous tissue and remnants of dental lamina connecting the follicles of permanent teeth to the oral mucous membrane, influence the movements of these teeth through the growing jaws, perhaps by providing a duct, a path of least resistance or even by actively pulling up the tooth. The gubernacular cord lies in a bony canal, the gubernacular canal. These canals are clearly visible in the skulls of children (Fig. 9.20). Whatever its role, if any, during this phase of eruption, the gubernacular cord cannot be implicated in the process of eruption once the tooth has breached the oral mucosa.

Though changes in the connective tissue overlying erupting teeth do not appear to contribute actively to the eruptive process, they may affect the resistive force. Abnormal changes within this tissue could increase the resistive force sufficiently to prevent a tooth from erupting. This view accounts for the fact that human upper incisors and canines exhibiting delayed eruption can usually be induced to erupt by surgically removing the overlying oral mucosa.

ALVEOLAR BONE DEPOSITION

Bone formation at the alveolar crest, and also at the interradicular septum of multi-rooted teeth, is a conspicuous feature during tooth eruption. It has been suggested that alveolar bone deposition, especially in the region of the fundus beneath the tooth, may be the source of the eruptive force. This theory relied heavily upon the observation that bone was deposited in the alveolus of some erupting teeth. However, no evidence has been offered to show that such bone deposition is a cause rather than an effect of eruption (i.e. infilling behind the erupting tooth). It must surely be obvious that alveolar bone deposition alone could not account for tooth eruption because the total distance of axial eruptive movement is equal to the thickness of alveolar bone formed beneath the tooth plus the length of root formed.

Other work does not support the view that bone deposition is directly related to tooth eruption. Most important, eruption of the continuously growing rodent incisor cannot be explained by fundic bone deposition; no bone is deposited in this situation. A study on postnatal growth of the mandible of the rat, guinea-pig and cat using tetracycline as a bone marker, indicates that throughout the period of root formation in all three species the predominant activity in the fundus of the molar crypts is one of bone resorption, coupled with bone deposition at the lower border of the mandible. Occasional bone deposition in the canine crypt of the cat is interpreted as being related to relocation of the crypt within the growing mandible rather than with tooth eruption.

PULP CELL PROLIFERATION
AND ROOT GROWTH

During eruption considerable mitotic activity is evident in the basal tissues of the growing root. Such activity is related to the production of root tissue, but it has been suggested that these proliferating tissues could also generate a force sufficient to cause the tooth to erupt. Though the epithelial root sheath and the developing periodontal ligament may be implicated, the greatest mitotic activity is associated with the base of the pulp. It is presumed that any force generated by growing and dividing cells would not be immediately dissipated. If this cellular activity increases pressure beneath the tooth, the problem arises as to why the tooth should move rather than the adjacent alveolar bone be resorbed. An early explanation concerned the presence of a 'cushioned hammock ligament' which was described as consisting of a fibrous network with fluid-filled interstices passing beneath the tooth and being attached at its margins to the alveolar bone; it was thought to provide a resistant cushion against which the growing root could push. However, more recent histological evidence suggests that such a structure does not exist. This evidence does not necessary invalidate pressure theories of eruption since, even in the absence of a cushion, fundic bone may be able to withstand pressures without undergoing resorption.

Some evidence which may possibly indicate that the basal proliferative tissues are capable of generating a force concerns the finding that, if eruption is prevented, the root continues to be formed at the expense of the adjacent bone. Thus,

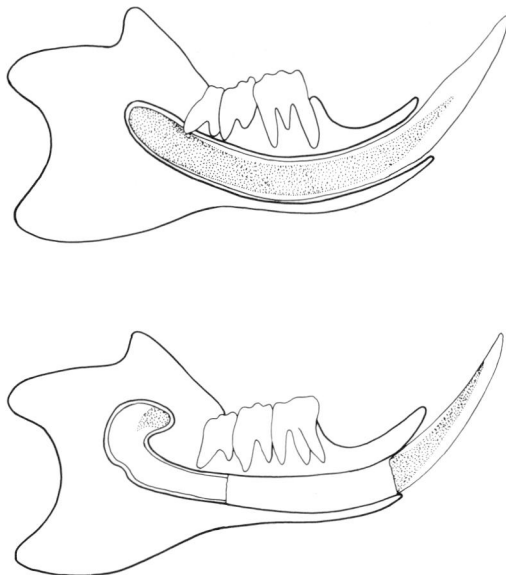

**Fig. 9.10.** Diagram to illustrate proliferative activity of the basal tissues of the rat incisor. The upper drawing shows the outline of the normal dental tissues. In the lower drawing the incisor has been surgically divided into two parts by a dental bur. The distal segment continues to erupt and is eventually exfoliated. The proximal segment, however, fails to erupt, but the basal tissues continue to proliferate and become re-curved. Hatched areas represent pulp. (Modified from Berkovitz B. K. B. (1972) *Archives of Oral Biology* **17**, 1279.)

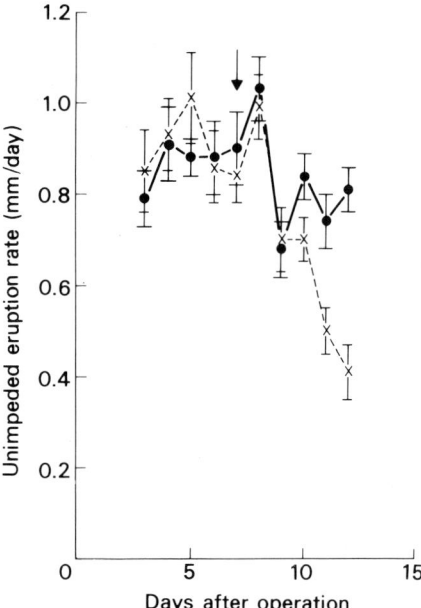

**Fig. 9.11.** Graph showing the effects of the cytotoxic agent triethanome lamine on unimpeded eruption rates in rat incisors. Points indicate group mean daily eruption rates and the bars denote ± 1 standard error of the mean. The first five readings shown are control figures for both groups. Then on day 7 (arrowed) 0.6 mg/kg body weight triethanomelamine (TEM) was injected into the experimental group daily for the remaining 5 days. This drug produced a significant retardation in eruption rates on the last 2 days.
●——●, Normal control; × --- ×, normal + TEM. (Modified from Berkovitz B. K. B. (1972) *Archives of Oral Biology* **17**, 937.)

human teeth which have failed to erupt still develop roots while if rat incisors are prevented from erupting the roots may grow back into the jaws (Fig. 9.10).

One experiment designed to assess the role of cell proliferation in the eruptive process involves the administration of drugs which stop cell proliferation. The daily administration of the drugs demecolcine (antimitotic) or triethanomelamine (cytotoxic) significantly retards the eruption rate of rat incisors, demecolcine having an almost immediate action while the affects of triethanomelamine become apparent only after a few days (Fig. 9.11). Though these results would appear to provide evidence in support of the cell proliferation theory, drug activity, as previously mentioned, cannot be localized to the dental tissues. Drugs like demecolcine interfere with cell division in other body tissues, increase the viscosity of hyaluronic acid, affect the contractility of granulation tissue, reduce collagen synthesis and increase blood pressure. Thus, a simple interpretation of the results is not possible. Also, as has previously been stated, when the eruption rate is altered, it is not possible to determine whether the eruptive or retarding forces have been affected. The retardation in eruption rate following administration of antimitotic and cytotoxic agents may not be due solely to the effect on basal cell proliferation; this is evident from the finding that drug administration produces a similar retardation in the eruption rate of teeth whose proliferating pulp tissues have been surgically removed (Fig. 9.12).

When the proliferative basal tissues of the rat incisor are surgically removed (root resection) the tooth continues to erupt at the same rate as controls (Figs. 9.13, 9.14). An alternative surgical approach is to leave the proliferative basal tissues intact but to divide the tooth transversely (root transection), if necessary pinning the proximal segment; the distal segment continues to erupt (Fig. 9.15). These experiments indicate that eruption can proceed in the absence of the proliferative basal tissues.

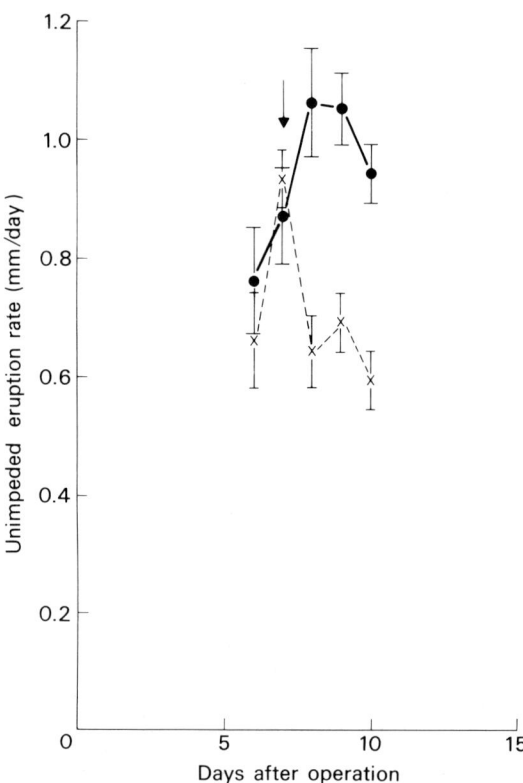

**Fig. 9.12.** Graph to illustrate that the effects of antimitotic drugs on eruption rates in rat incisors are not due simply to the effects on pulp cell proliferation. Both control and experimental groups had the proliferative pulpal zones surgically removed (i.e. root resection) on day 0. Points indicate the group mean unimpeded eruption rates and the vertical bars denote $\pm 1$ standard error of the mean. From day 7 (arrowed) the experimental group received daily two successive injections, separated by a 4 hour interval, of 2 mg/kg body weight demecolcine. The three subsequent readings were all significantly lower than controls. ●——●, control root resection; ×---×, root resection + demecoline. Modified from Berkovitz B. K. B. (1972) *Archives of Oral Biology* **17**, 937.

When eruption rate is doubled by cutting a rodent incisor tooth free of occlusion, the amount of proliferative basal activity is increased correspondingly. It has yet to be established whether the increased proliferation in any way causes the increased eruption or is an effect of it. Human unerupted incisor or canine teeth which have fully formed roots, and therefore have little proliferative basal activity, can erupt to reach the occlusal plane following suitable surgical treatment.

It has been suggested that eruption is caused by root growth and the arguments for and against

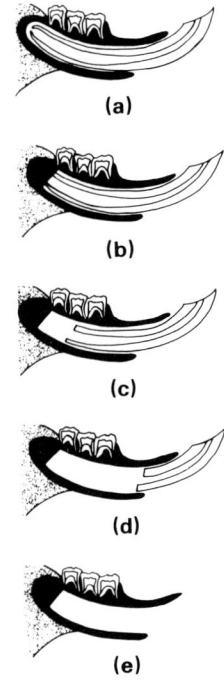

**Fig. 9.13.** Diagrammatic representation of the eruption of a rat incisor following surgical removal of the proliferative basal tissues (i.e. root resection). (a) Normal. (b) Proliferative basal tissues removed and the wound filled with a blood clot. (c) Tooth continues to erupt. (d) Base of tooth near the level of the alveolar crest. (e) Tooth has been exfoliated from socket.

this view are similar to those discussed with respect to cellular proliferation. X-irradiation of a developing tooth may prevent root development yet the resulting 'rootless' teeth have been observed to erupt into the oral cavity though the rates of eruption, which appear to be retarded, have not been measured. Occasionally lower incisors are erupted in newborn babies: these also have no roots, but if they are not extracted roots later develop.

TISSUE FLUID PRESSURE

It has been postulated that the force of eruption is derived from pressure generated by tissue fluid beneath and/or around the erupting tooth. In support of this theory measurements have shown that tissue fluid pressures within the vicinity of the tooth are unusually high when compared with most other connective tissues. For the dental pulp a tissue fluid pressure of about 25 mm Hg above atmospheric has been recorded (though the range of values of 0–65 mm Hg reported in the literature are probably indicative of the difficult technical

# Development and Maintenance of Occlusion

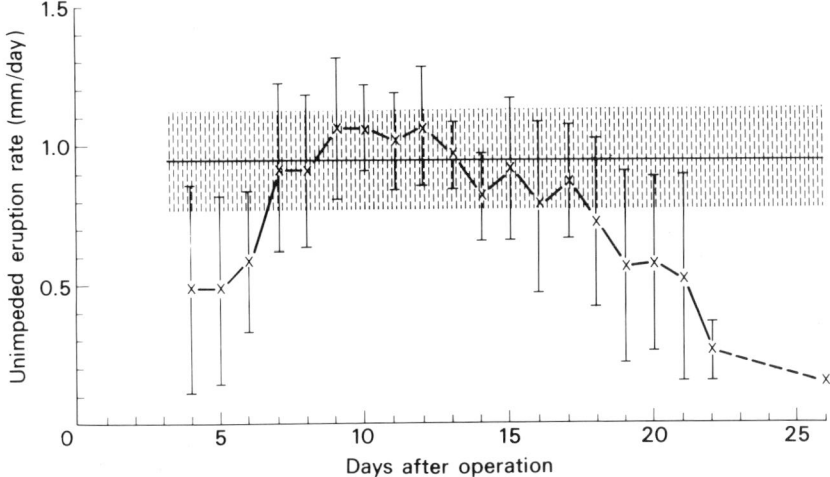

**Fig. 9.14.** Graph showing the effects of removing the basal proliferative tissues of the rat incisor on unimpeded eruption rates. The upper solid line and associated hatched area indicate overall mean control eruption rate ± 1 standard deviation. Points represent group mean eruption rates and vertical bars ± 1 standard deviation. Immediately following root resection ( ×——× ) there is a decreased eruption rate, but this value soon reaches control levels which are maintained until the tooth reaches the edge of the socket when, prior to eventual exfoliation, eruption rates are again decreased. (Modified from Berkovitz B. K. B. & Thomas N. R. (1969) *Archives of Oral Biology* **14**, 771.)

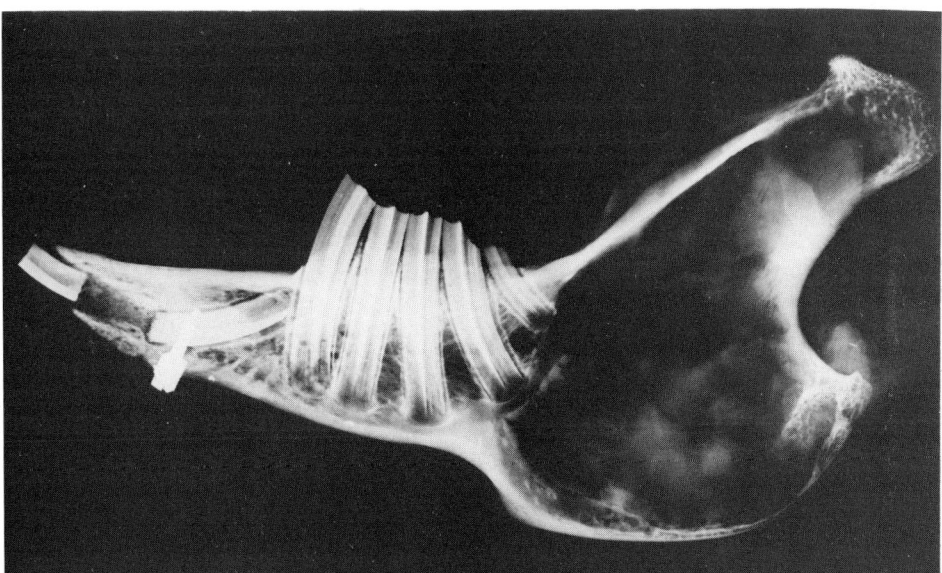

**Fig. 9.15.** Diagram to show that when a rabbit incisor is surgically divided transversely into two segments, and the proximal segment is prevented from erupting forwards by a pin, the distal segment continues to erupt without any contribution from the proliferative basal tissues. (From Moxham B. J. & Berkovitz B. K. B. (1974) *Archives of Oral Biology* **19**, 903.)

procedures involved), while the value in the periodontal ligament of an erupted tooth is about 10 mm Hg. In most other connective tissues the pressure is 1–3 mm Hg above atmospheric. Once a tooth has erupted into the oral cavity any pressure around the root which is greater than atmospheric could be envisaged as promoting eruption. However, for this theory to be tenable a pressure gradient must be present prior to the appearance of the tooth within the oral cavity; the tissue fluid

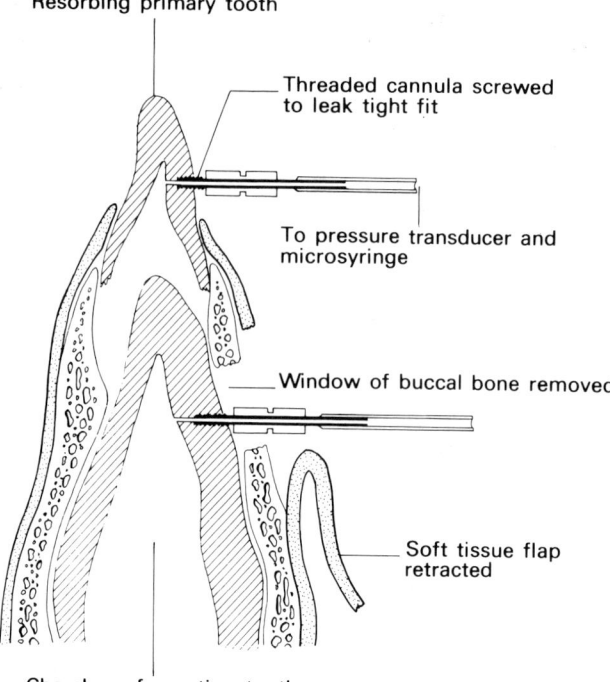

**Fig. 9.16.** Diagram to show experimental set-up for measuring pulp pressures in deciduous and corresponding permanent teeth of the dog. In all instances a pressure differential favouring eruption has been recorded. (From Van Hassel H. J. & McMinn R. G. (1972) *Archives of Oral Biology* **17**, 183.)

pressure beneath and around the tooth must be greater than that above it. A pressure gradient of this nature has been shown to exist (Fig. 9.16). In the case of erupting but still buried permanent canine teeth in dogs, the average tissue fluid pressure above the crown was $10 \pm 5$ mm Hg, while intrapulpal tissue fluid pressure monitored within the upper portion of the crown was $23 \pm 6$ mm Hg. From these figures it has been calculated that an average force of 15 g could be generated by tissue fluid. It is not clear how such pressure differentials are maintained.

That the vascular system is capable of causing movement of teeth is seen in human incisors which, at rest, undergo pulsatile movements synchronous with the arterial pulse. Each pulse shifts the tooth from the neutral position towards the labial side, the displacement being of the order of 0.4 $\mu$m, with a very much smaller axial movement.

Although relative to adjacent tissues there may be a high tissue fluid pressure associated with the erupting tooth, it is still necessary to prove that this produces the eruptive force. The obvious approach is either to increase or decrease the tissue fluid pressure and observe whether a corresponding change in eruption rate occurs. Experiments designed towards increasing tissue fluid pressure have involved sympathectomy and inferior dental nerve section (since this nerve is also thought to contain vasoconstrictor fibres). The results of such studies have been conflicting, some authors reporting an increased eruption rate, others observing no change. In no study was fluid pressure monitored. Recently, using a continuous recording technique to monitor tooth movements following the injection of various vasoactive drugs, eruption could be increased or decreased in a manner consistent with a tissue fluid pressure hypothesis. One should also consider other factors such as the accompanying changes in metabolism and tooth support, before interpreting the results in favour of the tissue fluid pressure hypothesis.

### TENSION WITHIN THE PERIODONTAL LIGAMENT

The continued eruption of rat and rabbit incisor teeth following various surgical procedures (Figs. 9.13, 9.15, 9.17), by a process of elimination, implicates the periodontal ligament as the source of the eruptive force. Some evidence suggests that the eruptive mechanism in these surgically produced situations resembles that of the normal tooth. For example, it has been found that drugs which retard eruption in a normal tooth produce a similar effect in root-resected teeth (Fig. 9.12). The

# Development and Maintenance of Occlusion

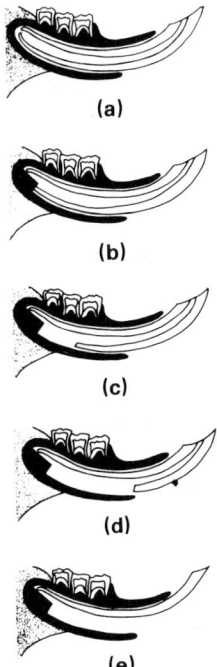

Fig. 9.17. Diagrammatic representation of the effects of partial root resection on eruption which implicate the periodontal ligament in the eruptive process. (a) Normal. (b) The buccal region containing the enamel organ has been removed from the proliferative basal region and is replaced by a blood clot. (c) Only Hertwig's epithelial root sheath continues to produce new dental tissue in the proliferative basal region and eruption carries the remaining enamel-covered portion of the tooth away from the base. (d) Continued eruption carries the enamel-covered portion of the tooth to the alveolar crest. (e) The original enamel-covered part of the tooth has been lost but the lingual element consisting of dentine, cement and the periodontal ligament has continued to erupt. (Modified from Berkovitz (1971) *Archives of Oral Biology* **16**, 1033.)

force produced within the periodontal ligament could be one involving pressure or tension. Thus, the ligament could either push or pull a tooth out of its socket. Pressure forces (cell proliferation and tissue fluid) have already been considered. It has been postulated that a tensional force could be generated by contraction of collagen fibres or contraction/motility of fibroblasts.

Concerning the collagen contraction theory, it has been suggested that tractional forces are set up within the oblique fibres of the periodontium due to the cross-linking and aggregation that occurs during collagen maturation; a 10% contraction in the length of the collagen fibre during its maturation is postulated. As yet, however, there is no evidence that such a contraction occurs *in vivo*. Once it had contracted, a collagen fibre could not contract again and therefore to keep a tooth erupting such a theory implies that there must be a continuous turnover of collagen within the periodontium; and this is indeed the case. Using tritiated glycine and proline, the turnover rate of collagen in the periodontal ligament is only of the order of a few days. However, there is no evidence to indicate that this turnover is a cause rather than effect. One method of assessing the relationship between cross-linking of collagen and eruption is to administer drugs which inhibit cross-linking. The administration of one such drug, the lathyritic agent aminoacetonitrile, results in the impeded eruption rate (of a functioning lower incisor) being significantly retarded and it would appear to provide evidence to support the collagen contraction theory. However, arguing against the theory is the finding that, in the same animals, the unimpeded eruption rate of the other lower incisor (kept short so that it did not meet the upper incisor) is unaffected. These results indicate the importance of occlusal loads on eruption rates; in the lathyritic animal the impeded teeth are functioning with a greatly weakened periodontal ligament with the result that biting forces may continually push the erupting tooth back into its socket. Thus, studies need to be undertaken on both impeded and unimpeded teeth. There is evidence which indicates that the periodontium of succedaneous teeth is only poorly organized during the main eruptive phase (p. 286) and this would also argue against collagen contraction pulling such teeth out of the bone.

Concerning the fibroblast contraction theory, the process may be analogous to the contraction produced during wound healing although even here the mechanism is not fully understood. However, there is no evidence that periodontal fibroblasts possess the necessary contractile characteristics. With respect to the fibroblast motility theory, though there is some evidence that fibroblasts in the tooth-related part of the periodontal ligament move with the erupting tooth, there is no evidence to separate cause and effect. Furthermore, such possible functions are not reflected in any morphological specializations of the periodontal fibroblasts which closely resemble fibroblasts in other sites.

In summary, no one theory of eruption is yet supported by sufficient experimental evidence for it to be identified as the prime mover. The overall process of eruption probably requires the integrated activity of all the biological systems within the periodontal ligament.

CLINICAL FEATURES

Sometimes a tooth, generally of the permanent dentition, fails to erupt. The simplest causes of this condition are the presence of a supernumerary tooth blocking the eruptive path (esp. upper central incisors), impaction due to the crowding of teeth (esp. lower third molars) or malpositioning where the tooth seems to have lost its way (esp. upper canines). Occasionally upper incisor teeth may remain immediately beneath the oral mucosa and fail to erupt. Surgical exposure of such teeth is generally followed by their eruption. Early loss of a deciduous tooth may result in early eruption of the permanent tooth; equally, drift of adjacent teeth into the extraction site in a crowded dentition may delay permanent tooth eruption. Delayed eruption of many teeth in a dentition may be symptomatic of a more generalized condition (e.g. hypothyroidism or cleidocranial dysostosis). Abnormal soft tissue relationships, in association with skeletal imbalance, will influence the position of teeth. Thus, incompetent lips in conjunction with thumb-sucking and tongue-thrusting, are frequently associated with protruding upper anterior teeth (Angles Class II, malocclusions).

The fact that teeth can be moved with relative safety following the application of carefully controlled forces forms the basis of orthodontics. Examples of such forces are (a) for tipping, 20–50 g; (b) for bodily movement, 100–150 g; (c) for intrusion or extrusion, 10–30 g.

**Establishment of the dentition**

Before giving a detailed account of the way in which the human teeth erupt into function several general biological considerations will be discussed. The completion of the deciduous dentition is not, in itself, a primary objective in dental development but should be considered merely a stage in the gradual progression of events which equip a growing individual for changing functional requirements. The biological problem is to provide a child with the most effective masticatory apparatus appropriate to his needs at that time, consistent with the space available in the jaws. The possession of two series of teeth in mammals imparts the advantages of equipping the young, in a short time, with teeth capable of cutting, crushing and grinding while the much larger and more durable, but therefore more slowly formed, permanent teeth are being constructed and erupted. The potential functional weakness of the transition period is minimized by the sequence of events. When the central incisors are lost the deciduous lateral incisors and canines can be used to incise food, while loss of the deciduous molars does not prevent crushing and grinding because the first permanent molars are already in place.

The normal positions which the teeth come to occupy in the jaw and their relationship to other teeth depend on the following factors:
1   Heredity.   The shape of the dental arches and the alignment of teeth tend to be inherited in the same manner as other more obvious morphological features.
2   Available space.   The position of the teeth when they erupt is influenced by the space available for their development: if there is inadequate room the final alignment is prejudiced.
3   Relationship between the dental arches.   Although the growth of one jaw is related to growth of the other they are not perfectly synchronized: a minor disturbance in the amount of growth of one jaw does not necessarily affect the interrelationships between the teeth it contains but it can affect the relationship of these teeth to their opponents.
4   Muscle forces.   The precise part played by the tongue, the lips and cheeks on the positions of the teeth in the horizontal plane is not fully understood although it is likely that the teeth come to occupy a position of balance between the forces generated by these opposing muscle masses. The magnitude of peak forces on the teeth is probably less important than the average force during the 24 hours. The position of a tooth in the vertical plane is determined similarly by a balance between extruding forces tending to cause it to continue erupting and intruding forces of mastication, swallowing etc. The existence of extrusive forces is demonstrated by active eruption following attrition, for example, but a tooth can be intruded if prolonged occlusal contact is created by a high filling or an orthodontic appliance.
5   Space in the arch.   The correct alignment of a tooth as it erupts depends on there being adequate space: the proximal surface of an adjacent erupted tooth may act as a guide for the path of eruption.
6   The presence of opposing cusps.   The position of the tooth as it erupts is finally modulated by opposing cusps which tend to interdigitate.
7   The existence of habits.   Prolonged thumb sucking, for example, may have profound effects on the vertical and horizontal position of teeth, arch shape and on arch growth, largely due to disturbing the balance of forces acting on the teeth (see **4**).
8   Stabilizing factors.   As the position of the teeth in the arches becomes settled, an increasingly dense mat of supracrestal collagen fibres sur-

rounds and restrains the teeth from being moved by horizontal displacing forces.

**9** The degree of use. Extensive use results in loss of occlusal and proximal tooth substance. This wear (attrition and abrasion) is compensated by activities in the supporting tissues which tend to induce teeth to drift in an occlusal and mesial direction.

**10** Tooth loss. The loss of a tooth disturbs the positions of neighbouring teeth because the normal compensatory mechanisms (in **9**) overcorrect often with profound and adverse clinical consequences.

From this sequence of factors it is apparent that tooth positions can be, and often are, modified throughout life. For the individual living on a soft Western diet little change may be seen for several decades after the teeth have erupted, but in the heavily stressed dentition of the Aborigines, substantial amounts of occlusal and proximal enamel and dentine may be lost even prior to the eruption of the third molars. The horizontal and vertical position of each tooth is adjusted to meet the changing forces imposed upon it.

ESTABLISHMENT OF THE
DECIDUOUS DENTITION

Bearing in mind the continuous changes in occlusion throughout life, it is convenient to consider as the first milestone the events leading up to the completion of the deciduous dentition. The faster it is completed the sooner the child is able to consume enough nutritionally rich food for optimal general growth and development. To this end the deciduous teeth begin to develop well before birth so that they are sufficiently well formed to erupt only a few months after birth.

At birth the cerebral development of the infant needs to be as great as possible but against this the skull, including the jaws, must be small enough to permit the head to pass down the birth canal. As a result the developing teeth are cramped within the jaws: the lateral incisors develop lingual to the central incisors and canines, while the latter develop in a more apical position (Fig. 9.18). More space is available posteriorly so that the forming deciduous molars and first permanent molars lie in a straight line viewed from above. When the molars start to mineralize the cusps are much closer together than in the formed tooth: when calcification spreads from the tip of the cusps the intervening tissues in the valley expand pushing them apart. Little or no space is needed for the successional teeth at this stage as mineralization does not start until several months after birth.

The relationship of the jaws during the weeks before birth is post-normal, that is, the mandible is in a retruded position relative to the maxilla, but soon after birth and for several months the lower jaw grows more rapidly in an anterior direction so that it comes to occupy a more prominent relationship to the maxilla. The outward manifestation of this change is that the gumpads (the thickened oral tissue covering the underlying tooth germs) are directly opposite each other during the first few months after birth. Whether the gumpads 'occlude' in the infant is not clear but observations suggest that the tongue normally occupies the space between the opposing arches.

*Phase of eruption of the deciduous teeth*

The order in which the deciduous teeth erupt corresponds with the order in which mineralization beings. The incisors start to calcify rather earlier than the molars or even the canines. In consequence they are ready to erupt sooner than the more posterior teeth, the first to appear being the mandibular central incisors. In spite of the short distance through which the teeth migrate to reach the mouth and the lack of overlying bone considerable local discomfort and systemic upset is often produced, i.e. teething. This may be due to the density of the fibrous tissue of the gumpads through which the teeth must pass by dissolution of the collagen network.

The sequence of eruption is usually:

$$\frac{A \quad B D C E}{A \quad B \quad D C E}$$

When they first appear in the mouth the incisors and first molars are well spaced from their neighbours but gradually the spaces are reduced as the canines and second molars emerge. For many children spaces remain between the anterior teeth while occasionally a well-marked space mesial to the maxillary canine recalls to mind the diastema of closely related primates.

Although the incisors may be brought together as soon as they are sufficiently erupted the young infant has not yet learnt to coordinate any mandibular movements beyond simple opening and closing. Only when the first molar teeth erupt into the region between the tongue and cheeks does contact between opposing teeth become more frequent and purposeful occlusion of the deciduous dentition, as yet incomplete, can now be said to be present. The remaining teeth gradually enter into the mouth during a period in which coordination of the masticatory muscles is increasing with the result that chewing is learnt and becomes an automatic process. During this period the articular fossa is deepening due to growth of the articular eminence anteriorly. It could be suggested that once the first deciduous molars have erupted the infant can begin to masticate hard food and be successfully weaned. In most primitive communities, however, the child continues to be suckled many months after the deciduous teeth have erupted and become fully functional. The relationships of the teeth in the arches and the way they occlude with their opponents is described earlier.

*Formation of junctional epithelium (epithelial cuff)*

One of the most remarkable protective mechanisms in the mouth which, because it is so successful, passes almost unnoticed even at the time of eruption is the union of the oral epithelium with the enamel. If these tissues were not united before the crown emerged into the mouth, the mesenchyme would be exposed to the flora of the mouth with all the possible consequences of infection and bleeding that this would bring. This potential hazard is avoided because the epithelial cells of the germinal layer of the oral epithelium meet and blend with the reduced enamel epithelium which closely envelops the underlying crown: both layers proliferate to form a protective plug of epithelium through which the tooth erupts. While the tooth migrates towards the mouth the intervening connective tissue almost imperceptably disintegrates so that the two epithelial layers approach each other and finally merge. (Fig. 9.18: 4 and 6 months: 5 and 6 years). As the tooth continues to erupt the overlying

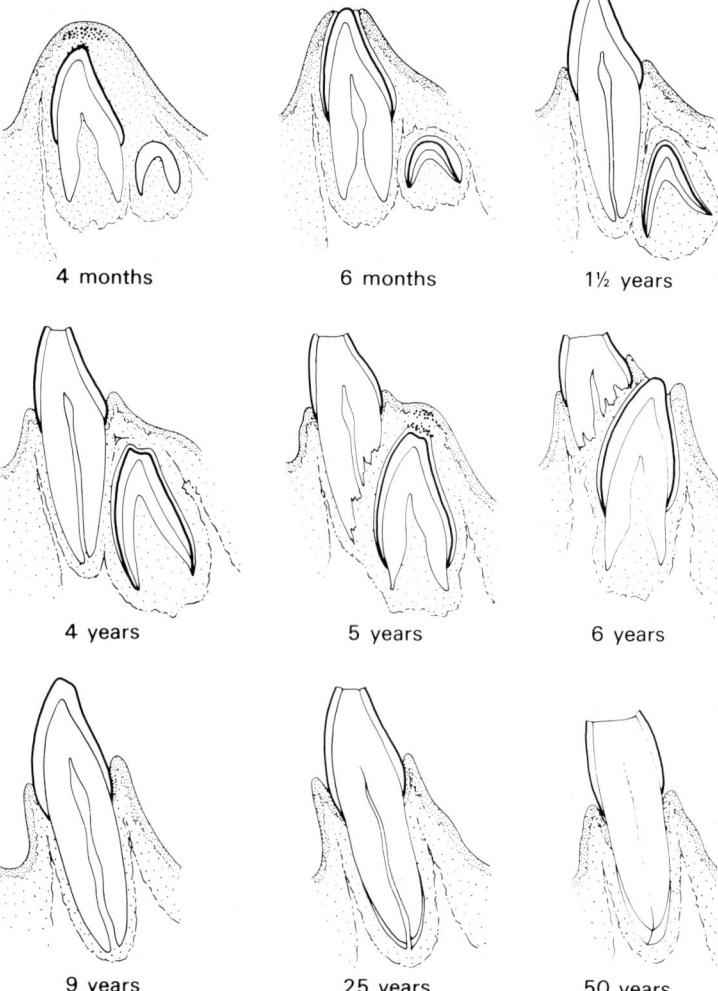

Fig. 9.18. Diagramatic representation of the sequence of changes in the lower incisor region. As the deciduous tooth erupts so the epithelial cuff is established by union of the reduced enamel epithelium covering the crown with the overlying oral epithelium. Gradually the latter replaces the former as the method of union of tooth and epithelial cells (4–18 months). The steady expansion and eruption of the permanent tooth on the lingual aspect of the deciduous incisor causes the intervening alveolar wall and then the root to be resorbed. The successional tooth appears in the mouth lingual to its predecessor ($1\frac{1}{2}$ years–6 years). The stages in the functional tooth are shown at the bottom in which occlusal wear, apical cement formation and migration of the epithelial cuff on to the root are of importance.

epithelial cells become reduced in number until the cusps (or incisive edges) are exposed to the mouth. A thin non-cellular layer, the primary enamel cuticle (Fig. 8.41) may cover the enamel together with a few residual epithelial cells. The crown steadily moves into the mouth through the mucosa so that the oral epithelium appears to slide slowly towards the neck of the tooth. Because the reduced enamel epithelium covers the whole crown, epithelium extends in continuity to the enamel–cement junction; that part in contact with the tooth has the shape of a collar known as the epithelial attachment or cuff, or junctional epithelium (Fig. 9.19). For the first few weeks after

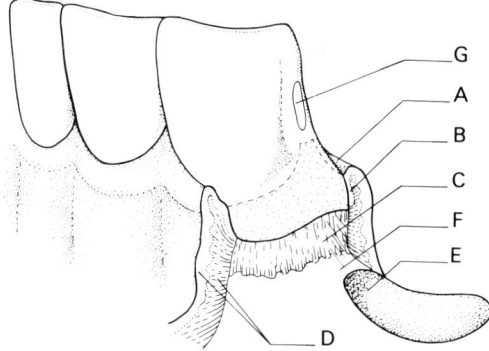

Fig. 9.19. Three-dimensional diagramatic representation of incisors and overlying tissues. The gingiva has been cut away from the proximal surface of an incisor and the adjacent tooth has been removed. A, Gingival crevice; B, epithelial cuff or junctional epithelium attached to the enamel (the stippled area indicates the area of enamel from which the epithelial cells have been stripped away); C, cervical region of the root covered with alveolar crest fibres and some transseptal fibres severed from the adjacent tooth; D, masticatory mucosa, here the attached gingiva; E, socket; F, interdental crest of bone; G, contact point.

the tooth appears in the mouth the gingiva is loose and can easily be lifted away from the crown without damage; but gradually the soft tissues become firmly applied to the enamel, due in part to the development of a well-organized system of collagen fibres within the gingiva.

The origin of the cells forming the epithelial cuff is twofold. When the crown first enters the mouth the cells in contact with the enamel are probably derived from the enamel organ but they are almost certainly replaced from the oral mucosa by cells which migrate over the reduced enamel thereby becoming the basal, proliferating, layer of the junctional and sulcular epithelium. Some years after eruption the junctional epithelium migrates on to cement but it can only do this if the collagen fibres attached to the neck of the tooth break down. As the junctional epithelium migrates so the gingiva peels down the crown and after many years it is located on the cement. The figurative description of becoming 'long in the tooth' is justified anatomically on this basis.

*Phase of the complete deciduous dentition*
During this period, which usually extends from $2\frac{1}{2}$ to $5\frac{1}{2}$ or 6 years of age, several changes in the form and arrangement of the teeth and their occlusion can be observed while important alterations are also occurring to the roots. In the first 12–18 months after a tooth appears in the mouth the apical third of the root is completed gradually, the larger the root (e.g. the canine or second molar) the longer is this period. The increased surface area, which is being provided for the attachment of the principal fibres while the roots are being completed, prepares the ligament for the higher masticatory loads developed by the growing muscles of the growing child.

A further process is at work, however, in response to expansion of the developing permanent teeth. In the labial segment the permanent incisors and canine lie close and lingual to the roots of their predecessors (Fig. 9.20), while the premolar germs develop between the divergent roots of the deciduous molars. As each germ expands, the wall of its crypt is resorbed and where this lies next to the deciduous tooth there comes a time when the wall disappears and the follicle is in direct contact with the periodontal ligament of the functioning tooth. So early is the onset of this process that the roots of the second deciduous molar are completed almost at the same time as resorption of the central deciduous incisor begins, i.e. at about $3\frac{1}{2}$ years. Further expansion of the permanent germ is now associated with resorption of the cement and dentine of the deciduous root. This process starts at about 4 years of age for incisors and 8 years of age for canines and molars, and continues in an irregular manner until the tooth is finally exfoliated. As its root is shortened so a tooth becomes more mobile but, because phases of resorption alternate with phases of repair during which principal fibres are reattached by cement deposition, the tooth becomes firm again for limited periods. In this way a tooth can be used in normal function to within a few weeks of its loss with very little discomfort to the child even when practically all the root has been removed (Fig. 9.21).

It is usually thought that the osteoclasts which resorb the roots of the deciduous teeth

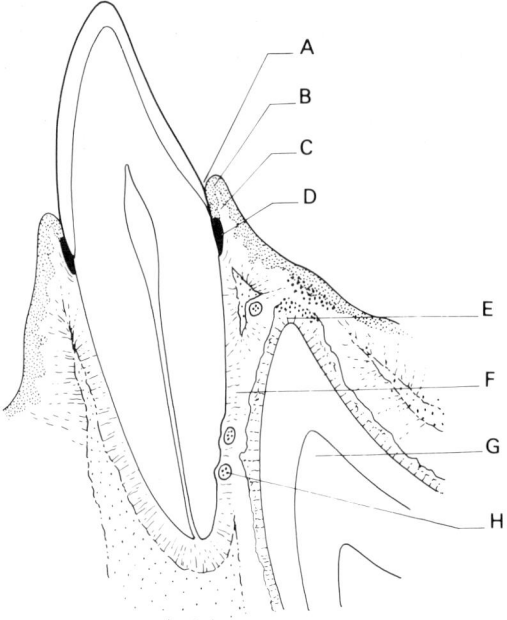

**Fig. 9.20.** Diagram of the incisor region at 4 years of age. The developing crown of the permanent tooth is approaching the root of the deciduous incisor. A, Gingival crevice; B, gingival crest; C, junctional epithelium or epithelial cuff cells of gingival origin gradually replacing the epithelial cuff cells derived from the reduced enamel epithelium of the deciduous tooth (D); at E, reduced enamel epithelial cells cover the enamel of the crown of the permanent tooth as it erupts towards the overlying oral mucosa through the gubernacular canal; F, area of union of periodontal ligament and cells of the follicle around the successional tooth (the alveous has been resorbed here); G, dentine of the permanent tooth. H, multinucleated giant cells, or osteoclasts, beginning to resorb the root of the deciduous tooth.

differentiate in response to pressure generated by the erupting permanent tooth. The enamel of the permanent tooth is protected from resorption by its covering of reduced enamel epithelium.

During the change from a deciduous to a permanent dentition the height of the alveolar bone (defined as the bone containing the tooth) is greatly increased (Fig. 3.16). Externally, this is seen as an increase in the height of the face (Fig. 3.10). At the same time the jaws also increase in diameter but to a smaller extent (Fig. 9.22). Probably as a result of pressure from the expanding tongue the deciduous teeth are pressed outwards and, associated with this, new bone is laid down on the external surface of the alveolar processes. As a consequence of this centrifugal drift spaces may either appear or widen between adjacent teeth. This spacing is enhanced by wear at the proximal surfaces which is often severe and may extend into the dentine even in children who eat a Western diet. Since the incisors are somewhat fan-shaped, loss of the incisive edges results in a gradual reduction in mesiodistal widths. Spaces between the incisors therefore increase with heavy function.

The crown of a tooth becomes shorter due to attrition; this shortening is compensated by further eruption to meet its opponent with the result that the clinical crown (that part exposed to the oral environment) extends towards the enamel–cement junction, (Fig. 9.18). The rate of occlusal wear seems to be greater than the progressive exposure of the crown due to the combined effects of passive eruption and active eruption so that in heavily worn dentitions the clinical crown becomes noticeably reduced in height. When the teeth of the 5-year-old are brought into occlusion the overbite and overjet are seen to be reduced and, for many children, the anterior teeth meet in an edge-to-edge position by the time the central incisors are being lost.

ESTABLISHMENT OF THE PERMANENT DENTITION

*The phase of the mixed dentition*
The exfoliation and replacement of the lower central deciduous incisors or the eruption of the lower first permanent molars heralds the onset of the so-called mixed dentition which usually lasts from about 6 years until the early teens when all the deciduous teeth have been lost. Developing as they do lingual to their predecessors it is to be expected that the lower central incisors often erupt lingual to the deciduous teeth. From this position the permanent incisors migrate labially, probably because the sum of the forces from the tongue exceeds the forces from the lips; in this process the deciduous teeth are shed ('pushed out').

The forces and histological changes involved in the process of erupting teeth into the mouth and establishing the epithelial attachment are the same for permanent teeth as for primary teeth, except that far more remodelling of bone is needed around the migrating crown of a permanent tooth; also its root is so incompletely formed when it erupts that it begins to function 2 years or so before its apex is fully formed.

The eruption of the first permanent molar, at about 6 years, brings a marked change to the occlusion. In addition to substantially increasing the masticatory area there is a change in the plane of contact of the opposing teeth. The occlusal surfaces are not on the same flat horizontal line as the occlusal surfaces of the deciduous molars but are set at a slight angle to it. Thus the lower tooth is inclined mesially while the upper molar is inclined distally: in this way the first contribution is made to the formation of the curve of Spee of the adult dentition. For most children the mandibular first molar occludes slightly in front of its maxillary equivalent, the mesial surface of the upper tooth occluding just behind the mesial surface of the lower molar. For other children, however, the

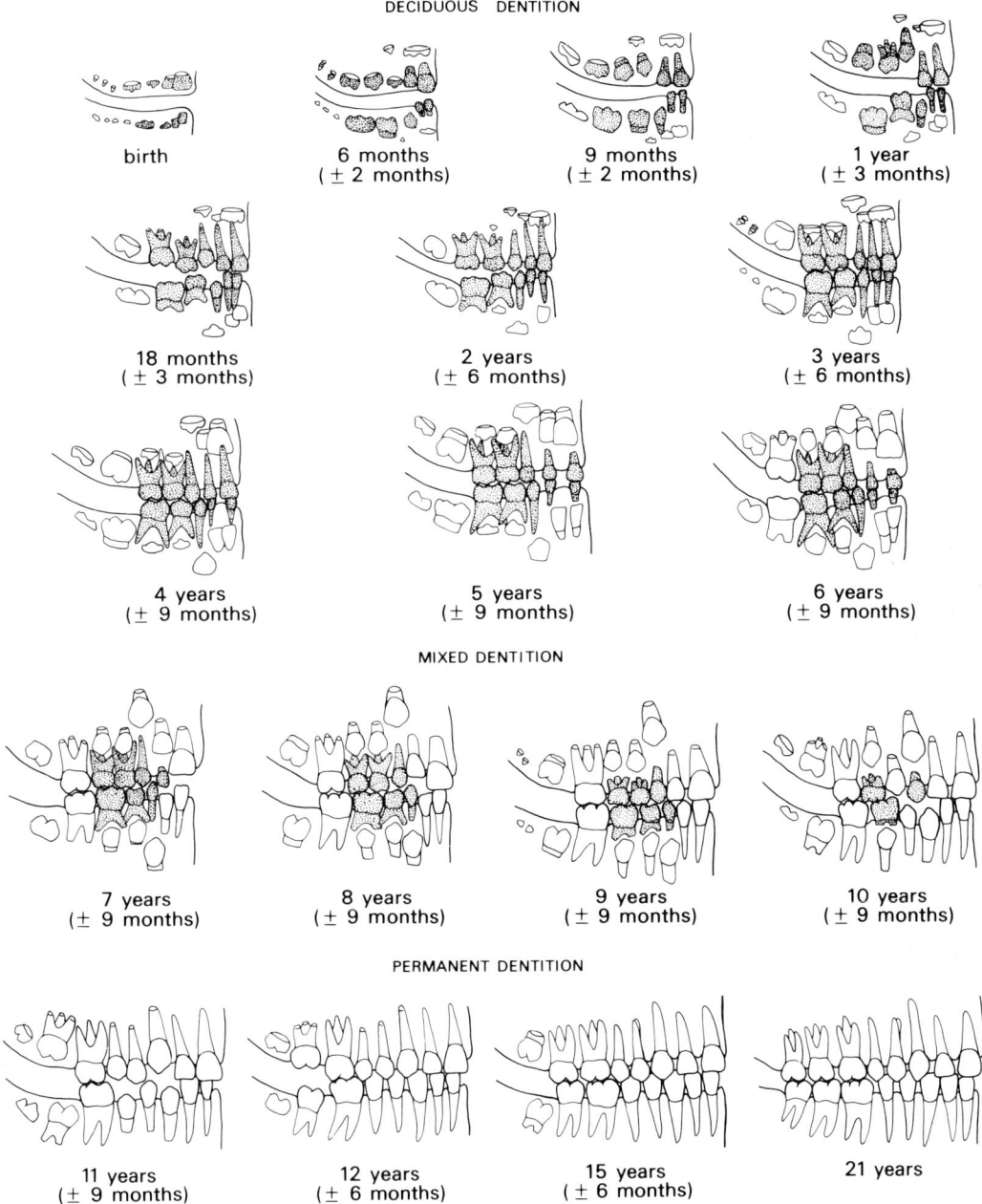

Fig. 9.21. Development of human dentition. (From Schour I. & Massler M. (1941) *Journal of American Dental Association* **28**, 1153.)

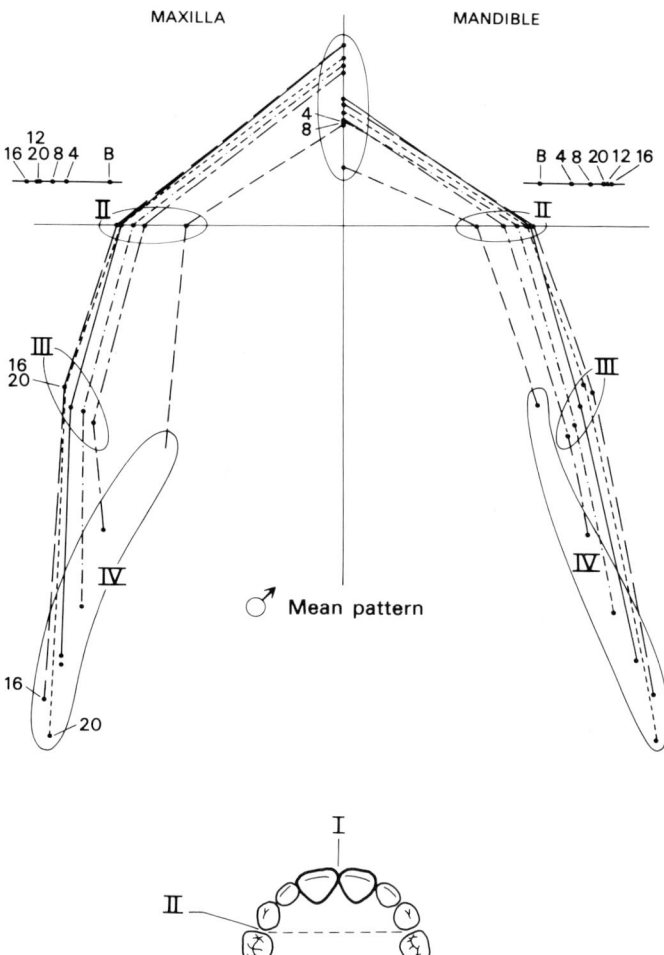

**Fig. 9.22.** Composite pattern of expansion of the dental arches of boys from birth to 20 years of age: ---, birth; ----, 4 years; ----, 8 years; ----, 12 years; ----, 16 years; -----, 20 years. The reference points were measured from a series of plaster casts of each individual. I, Crest of the interdental septum between the central incisors; II, distal wall of the canine alveolus or midpoint on the distal surface of the canine; III, distal wall of $TM_2$ alveolus or midpoint on the distal surface of $TM_2$ or $PM_2$ (not present at birth); IV, distal aspect of alveolus of $M_2$. (From Sillman J. H. (1964) *American Journal of Orthodontics* **50**, 824.)

deciduous lower second molar may not have assumed the more usual occlusion with the upper deciduous molars so that the distal surfaces of both second molars may be flush. It follows that when the lower permanent molar erupts it is distally placed with respect to the equivalent upper tooth. The full occlusion may later be normal, however, for these children because the lower molar migrates mesially when the deciduous cheek teeth are lost (Fig. 9.23).

The sequence in which the permanent teeth erupt is 1, 6:2:4:3, 5:7:8. It should be stressed that the sequence is slightly variable, but more important, the dates of eruption are very variable. In addition to genetic and physiological factors other influences, such as enforced extraction of the overlying deciduous tooth, may also affect the time at which a permanent successor erupts by removing the obstruction to its movements: in this instance it may erupt several months or even 1 or 2 years earlier than normal. If the deciduous tooth is lost some months before its successor is due to emerge the adjacent teeth may be drawn together thereby becoming tilted and so obstructing or displacing the successor.

One of the obvious differences between the two series is the size of the teeth. The permanent incisors and canines are all wider mesiodistally but the premolars are narrower than their predecessors. Since the permanent dentition is (usually)

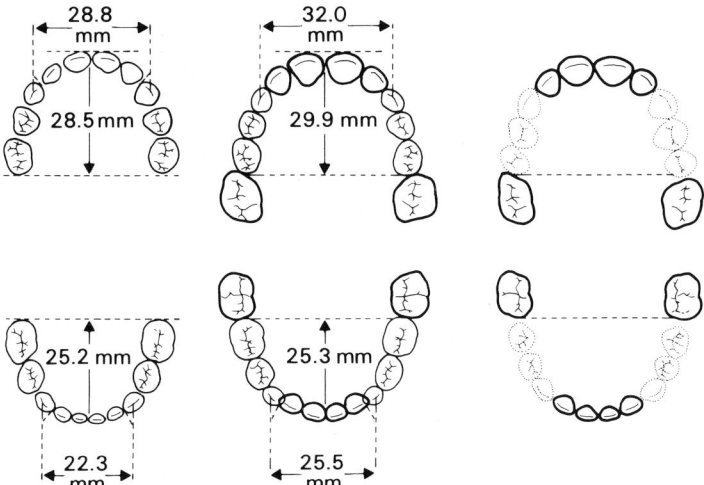

**Fig. 9.23.** (left) The deciduous maxillary and mandibular dentitions of the average male child, drawn to scale for all measurements of available space in the incisor, canine and premolar segments; arch lengths, the intercanine distances as well as mesiodistal crown diameters of the teeth. (centre) The transitional dentition of the average male child after eruption of all permanent incisors (note differences in size of permanent and deciduous incisors, crowding of mandibular incisors, increments in the maxillary and mandibular intercanine distances and increase only in the maxillary arch length). (right) The transitional dentition of the average male child at an imaginary phase where all deciduous posterior teeth are shed, just prior to the emergence of their permanent successors (note so-called leeway space). (From Moorrees C. F. A. & Chadha J. M. (1965) Available space for the incisors during dental development. *Angle Orthodont.* **35**, 12.)

lengthened by three large molars in each quadrant, the question of how the permanent teeth become accommodated in the jaws is an intriguing one. By comparing the alignment of the teeth in the labial segment it can be seen that while the long axes of the deciduous incisors are nearly vertical, the permanent successors erupt into a wider arc and are tilted outwards at a greater angle to the vertical. Due to this tilt the mesiodistal lengths of the permanent teeth (about 10.7 mm greater than the deciduous teeth in the maxilla and 7.3 mm in the mandible for boys) can be accommodated on the same amount of basal bone as the deciduous teeth. The permanent maxillary anterior teeth, unlike the mandibular incisors, may erupt labial to their predecessors; the central incisors and canines tend to do this most frequently.

For the premolars there is no problem, at least in Western children, as these teeth require less space than the deciduous molars: for boys, Moorrees found maxillary premolars to be 2.37 mm and mandibular premolars to be 3.27 mm narrower; for girls these differences were smaller. The necessity for the larger mesiodistal length of the deciduous molars may be understood from studies of the heavily worn dentition of the Aborigine, whose premolars would not find room to erupt unless the deciduous molars were large enough mesiodistally to allow for the very considerable proximal wear.

The manner in which the jaws grow and remodel to accommodate the permanent molars is described in Chapter 3. The most obvious dimensional change in the dental arcade during the period of the mixed dentition is a lengthening which allows the eruption of the permanent molars behind the deciduous teeth. However, there is also a small increase in its width during the transition (Fig. 9.22). The angulation of teeth and the mesiodistal length of the dental arcade changes within the next few years but largely as a result of the gradual loss of tooth substance due to wear.

Throughout this phase the temporomandibular joint continues to enlarge and change shape as the depth of the articular fossa increases. As a result when the mandible slides forwards during opening the mouth or lateral excursions the downward component of movement at the joint increases.

PHASE OF CONTINUING
FUNCTIONAL ADJUSTMENT

After the deciduous teeth have been replaced there are no further obvious short-term changes in the occlusion. Nevertheless, it is important to appreciate that the established occlusion is not a final and settled state but rather that it undergoes small but continual changes. The magnitude of these changes is directly related to the amount of use to which the teeth are subjected; in essence the changes compensate for loss of tooth substance on the occlusal and proximal surfaces.

*Occlusal wear—attrition*
The gradual loss of enamel from the incisive edges and tips of cusps produces little obvious change in the occlusion but once dentine is exposed tissue is lost at an appreciably greater rate. These occlusal facets are shallow hollows in which the more slowly worn enamel remains as a raised rim surrounding the softer dentine (Fig. 10.5). In the mandible the buccal cusps are lost at a greater rate than the lingual cusps, while this is reversed in the maxilla. The reason for this effect is said to be that a moving unit, whatever it may be, tends to become convex while the stationary unit against which it is rubbed becomes concave. In the present context the mandibular teeth are the moving unit and, as a result, the curve of Monson which is concave above, first changes to a horizontal plane and, later, to a convex curve known as the reverse curve of Monson. Since the amount of wear is greater for those teeth which are used for the longest time, it follows that the effect is most noticeable in the plane of the first molars and least obvious for the third molars.

As the anatomical crown of a tooth becomes shortened it tends to drift in an occlusal direction. The force causing occlusal drift is not clear but it may be a continuation of that causing active eruption, becoming effective only when the forces opposing it have been reduced. Loss of the incisive edges of anterior teeth reduces the overbite: when combined with a tendency for the lower incisors to tilt forwards, and edge-to-edge bite develops in the heavily used dentition.

*Proximal wear*
During chewing the teeth are displaced vertically into their sockets and horizontally. If this displacement is greater for one tooth than its neighbours then the proximal surfaces rub against each other. The greater the biting forces the faster is tooth substance abraded and the larger become the facets of wear (the contact areas). In the extreme case of Australian Aborigine skulls Begg found that approximately 3 mm of tooth substance were lost in each quadrant before the third molars had even erupted. In heavily worn dentitions, such as the Saxons of the Dark Ages, large areas of dentine were exposed by middle life but on present-day Western diets the wear is slight and rarely exposes dentine. If no other process occurred spaces would gradually develop between adjacent teeth with the result that food could become impacted on the interdental gingiva. However, for many years at least, horizontal migration of the teeth compensates for this loss of substance. In man, the process is known as mesial drift but it is part of a more general phenomenon in mammals called approximal drift in which groups of teeth migrate towards a common centre. The effect of this in man is that the teeth remain in contact as they drift towards the centre of the arch.

The principal cause of mesial drift appears to be contraction of tissue elements in the transseptal fibre system which links the proximal surfaces of adjacent teeth. It seems likely that this tissue by its strapping effect tends to stabilize the positions of the teeth in the arch and also accounts for the approximation of adjacent teeth after the accidental loss of a tooth. When a tooth has been removed fibres grow across the healing socket and contraction of this tissue causes the neighbouring teeth to tilt towards each other over the socket. Horizontal migration of teeth in the intact dentition may be hindered by the presence of opposing cusps. However, if proximal wear is heavy so also is occlusal wear with the result that cusps which might have interfered with mesial drift become flattened.

In the intact dentition the long axes of the teeth in man are inclined mesially. Thus during mastication there is a tendency for the teeth to be tilted forward under load in addition to being intruded into the sockets. The larger the food bolus the greater is the horizontal component of biting force. Biting on a hard fragment of food at the back of the arch causes more anterior teeth to be tilted mesially because neighbouring teeth are in contact. Most teeth are inclined buccally or lingually in addition to a mesial direction. Thus the maxillary incisors, for example, are tilted labially during incision as they are inclined labially. It seems probable that the collagen fibre network which extends round the arch in the attached gingiva on the labial side of these teeth together with the transseptal fibres come under tension at this time and resist labial tilting of the incisors. The first symptoms of disease of these tissues due to chronic marginal periodontitis may be labial drifting of the incisors with separation of adjacent teeth.

*Histology of mesial drift.* The mechanism causing teeth to migrate in response to small continuous or frequent intermittent forces is the same whether the force is applied by the orthodontist or is the result of an imbalance of biological forces. For mesial drift the force displaces the tooth across the periodontal soft tissues with the result that the principal fibres, ground substance, cells and blood vessels are under slight compression on the mesial side but are more extended than normal on the distal side (Fig. 9.24). The precise mechanism is not clear but, possibly due to a slight increase in tissue pressure, osteoclasts begin to appear in small numbers on the periodontal surface of the alveolar bone mesially. Due to their action small areas of bone are resorbed; principal fibres may be reattached to the freshly exposed surface or bone while osteoclasts appear at other sites causing gradual removal of the mesial surface of the alveolus. In this way the width of the periodontal ligament, which is determined by functional influences, is restored on the mesial side of the root.

On the distal side the ligament increases in width and the fibres are less relaxed than normal. It seems unlikely that they are actually under tension but mastication causes greater tension in the fibres than normal with an increased distortion of the distal wall of the socket under load. The result is that osteoblasts begin to lay down new bone between the principal fibres where they are attached to the distal wall of bone and the previous width of the ligament is restored. The fibre bundles must also be remodelled in order to re-establish their previous lengths. Here too the exact mechanisms are not known but can be accounted for by the rapid turnover of collagen in response to small forces acting over a long period of time.

The magnitude of these changes corresponds with the rate of drift. Thus for an adult living on a Western diet very little histological evidence is apparent, but for a heavily used dentition, there are extensive cellular changes around the first molar following loss of the deciduous second molar and around a tooth distal to an extraction site.

PHASE OF FUNCTIONAL SENILITY

If heavy function continues for many years, as in the Eskimo of bygone years, occlusal wear may extend as far as secondary dentine and finally the whole anatomical crown may be lost down to the furcation of multirooted teeth. It appears that active eruption does not sufficiently compensate for this extensive destruction of teeth because the space between the alveolar processes becomes severely reduced and the flattened 'occlusal' surfaces of the tooth fragments barely protrude into

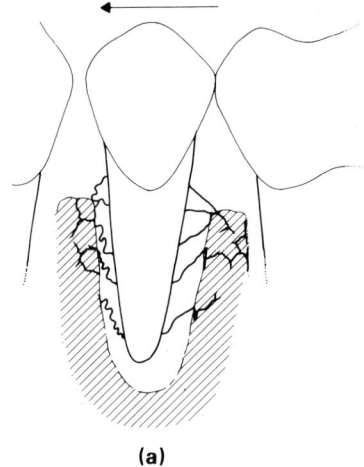

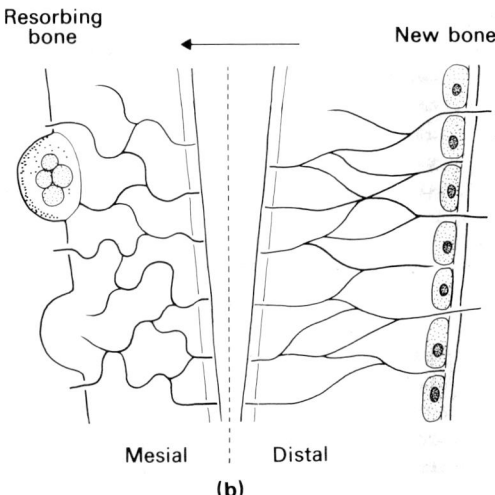

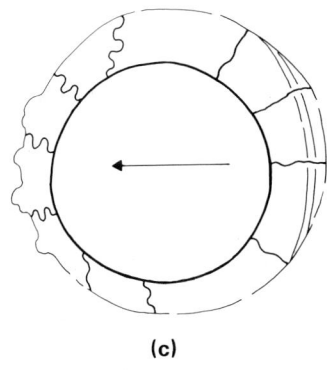

Fig. 9.24. Schematic representation of the structural changes associated with mesial drift of a premolar. (a) Longitudinal section; (c) transverse section.

the oral cavity. At the same time the considerable reduction in the mesiodistal lengths of the teeth cannot be adequately compensated by mesial drift so that large spaces appear between the adjacent tooth fragments. Loss of the incisive edges of anterior teeth combined with forward migration of mandibular teeth results in total loss of overbite and overjet. The resulting drop in the efficiency of the heavily worn dentition is more likely to affect incision rather than crushing. Although the shearing properties of cusps are lost it has been observed that maximal biting force from people with well-worn teeth (e.g. Eskimo) are substantially greater than in Europeans with relative unworn teeth.

## FURTHER READING

BEERTSEN W. (1973) Tissue dynamics in the periodontal ligament of the mandibular incisor of the mouse: a preliminary report. *Archives of Oral Biology* 16, 1033.

BERKOVITZ B.K.B. (1971) The effect of root transection and partial root resection on the unimpeded eruption rate of the rate incisor. *Archives of Oral Biology* 16, 1045.

BERKOVITZ B.K.B. (1972) The effect of demecolcine and of triethanomelamine on the unimpeded eruption rate of normal and root resected incisor teeth in rats. *Archives of Oral Biology* 17, 937.

BERKOVITZ B.K.B. (1975) Mechanisms of tooth eruption. In *Applied Physiology of the Mouth*, p. 93, ed. Lavelle C. L. B. Bristol: Wright & Sons.

BERKOVITZ B.K.B., MIGDALSKI A. & SOLOMON M. (1972) The effect of the lathyritic agent aminoacetoritrile on the unimpeded eruption rate in normal and root-resected rat lower incisors. *Archives of Oral Biology* 17, 1755.

GRABER T.M. (1972) *Orthodontics principles and practice*. Chapter 2. W. B. Saunders, Philadelphia.

GRON A.M. (1962) Prediction of tooth emergence. *Journal of Dental Research* 41, 573.

MANSON J.D. (1968) *A Comparative Study of the Postnatal Growth of the Mandible.*

MOORREES C.F.A., FANNING E.M. & HUNT E.E. (1963) Age variation of formation stages of ten permanent teeth. *Journal of Dental Research* 42, 1490.

MOORREES C.F.A., LEBRET L.M.L.S. & FROHLICH F.J. (1969) Growth studies of the dentition. A review. *American Journal of Orthodontics* 55, 600.

MURAI T., KIKUCHI A. & NAKAMURA T. (1958) The effect of irradiation on the developing permanent tooth of the young cat. *Bulletin of the Tokyo Medical and Dental University* 5, 81.

NESS A.R. (1964) Movement and forces in tooth eruption. In *Advances in Oral Biology* Vol. 1, p. 33, ed. Staple P. H. London: Academic Press.

OSBORN J.W. (1973) The evolution of dentitions. *American Scientist* 61, 548.

POOLE D.F.G. & STACK M.V. (eds.) (1976) *The eruption and occlusion of teeth* Colston Papers No. 27. London: Butterworths.

SCHOUR I. & MASSLER M. (1941) The development of the human dentition. *Journal of the American Dental Association* 28, 1153.

SILLMAN J.H. (1964) Dimensional changes of dental arches, longitudinal studies from birth to 25 years. *American Journal of Orthodontics* 50, 824.

TEN CATE A.R. (1972) Morphological studies of fibrocytes in connective tissue undergoing rapid remodelling. *Journal of Anatomy* 112, 401.

THOMAS N.R. (1967) The properties of collagen in the periodontium of an erupting tooth. In *The Mechanisms of Tooth Support* p. 102. Bristol: Wright & Sons.

VAN HASSELL H.J. & MCMINN R.G. (1972) Pressure differential favouring tooth eruption in the dog. *Archives of Oral Biology* 17, 183.

# CHAPTER 10

# Dentition in Function

## FUNCTIONS OF TEETH

Teeth are products of the skin, and they probably originated as part of the dermal exoskeleton which covers the body in primitive vertebrates (Fig. 4.2). With the evolution of jaws, scales at the edges of the mouth became modified to form teeth. The teeth have in the course of evolution developed a wide diversity of shapes in adaptation to the diversity of feeding habits of the vertebrates. Further information on this is given in Chapter 4; the present section deals particularly with the mammals.

### Functions not connected with feeding

Before discussing the functions of teeth in relation to feeding it is necessary to remember that in a variety of animals other functions are involved. The large incisors of rodents are used, for example, for gnawing inedible materials: rats and mice make holes in woodwork, and beavers cut down trees to construct their dams (Fig. 10.1). Teeth are also convenient for holding and carrying objects: familiar examples are gun-dogs carrying birds and mother cats carrying kittens. They are also widely used for fighting: the musk-deer (Fig. 12.15), which has no antlers, has large upper canines, absent in other deer; the canines of baboons are important in maintaining social status, as well as in defence against predators. Unusual uses of teeth are for burrowing, in the mole-rat, for climbing on ice, as the tusks in the walrus (Fig. 12.9), for biting breathing-holes in the ice, in the Weddell seal, and for combing the fur, in the lemurs (Fig. 12.21).

In humans the teeth have a wide variety of uses, from tailors biting thread to Eskimos softening seal skins by chewing them. Teeth are also often important in facial expressions.

### Obtaining food (Fig. 10.1)

One of the basic functions of vertebrate teeth is the prehension of food. In most vertebrates the jaws function like a pair of forceps, and the teeth are pointed structures that improve the grip. Some insectivores, such as the hedgehog, have enlarged incisors which enable them to pick up insects and worms: the anterior lower incisors are horizontal and their tips meet the more vertical upper incisors. In shrews (Fig. 12.1) the grip is improved by the development of a distal cusp on the upper incisor, followed by a row of small pointed teeth. When food is too large to be taken in whole, pieces are torn off by jerking the head and body; this is the mode of feeding of sharks and crocodiles, and even hedgehogs are known to eat mice and snakes in this way.

Herbivorous mammals have special adaptations for cropping grass and leaves. Thus the horse has very mobile lips, used to gather up a tuft of grass which is gripped by the incisors and torn off by a movement of the head. Ruminants like the cow and sheep have prehensile tongues which hold the grass tuft so that it can be cut off by the front mandibular teeth (three incisors and an incisiform canine); there are no opposing teeth in the upper jaw. The elephant's trunk, derived from a muscular upper lip, is extremely effective in putting food into the mouth. The tusks of elephants, which are enlarged upper incisors, are used in conjunction with the trunk for such purposes as tearing down branches on which the animal can feed. The tusks of pigs are canines; they project laterally and are used for rooting in the ground. A razor-sharp upper incisor is used by the vampire bat to remove a piece of its victim's skin.

The primates, including man, have prehensile hands used for collecting food, and their incisors are adapted for biting pieces out of fruit (or sandwiches). The use of the hands in feeding may also be seen in rodents, which hold the food object between their paws while nibbling it with their incisors.

In many animals the teeth are involved at an earlier stage in the obtaining of food. Thus the canines of carnivores are used for killing. The most

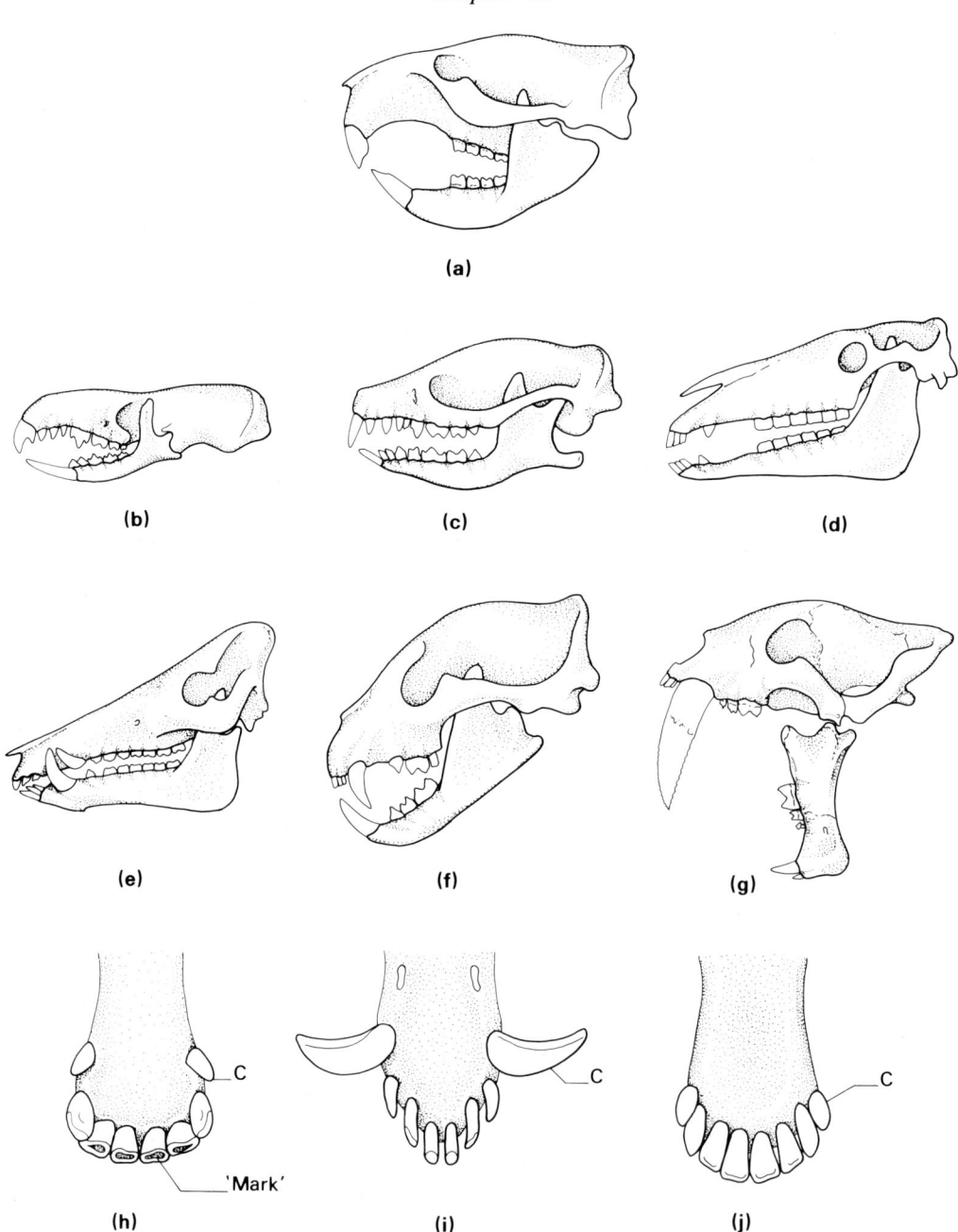

**Fig. 10.1.** Adaptive modifications of incisors and canines in various mammals: (a) beaver, (b) shrew, (c) hedgehog, (d) horse, (e) pig, (f) lion, (g) sabre-toothed tiger; anterior lower teeth of (h) horse, (i) pig, (j) cow (C, canine).

specialized carnivores, now extinct, were the sabre-toothed 'tigers' (not especially related to the living tiger, but belonging to the same cat family). They had huge dagger-like upper canines which were used to stab the large animals on which they preyed, perhaps even elephants. The mandibular joint was so constructed that the mouth could be opened very widely when the 'daggers' were used. The edges of the canines were sharp and serrated, and the wound would be enlarged by ripping.

## Manipulating food in the mouth

The teeth involved in getting food into the mouth are usually near the front, but rows of teeth normally extend well back in the mouth cavity, often in lower vertebrates on the palate as well as on the jaws (Fig. 10.2), and in some fish there are pharyngeal teeth on the gill-bars. These more deeply situated teeth are used to prepare the food for swallowing. Although most vertebrates swallow their food whole, it has to be oriented so that it can go down the throat: if sideways in the mouth it has to be turned round. Moreover the prey may well be still alive and struggling; backward pointing teeth help it on its way (Fig. 10.2) (p. 213). In other cases the back teeth are broad and flat, and the food is crushed; for example, in fish that feed on molluscs and in some plant-eating lizards (Fig. 10.2). Crushing teeth are more effective far back in the mouth near the jaw muscles, where more pressure can be applied. The function of chewing is developed only in the mammals.

## Toothless animals

When considering the functions of teeth it should be remembered that some vertebrates manage very well without them. All toothless animals have descended from ancestors that possessed teeth: in each case the loss of teeth has presumably benefited the group by improving the efficiency with which food can be ingested.

The jaws of birds are ensheathed with keratinous beaks that have become adapted for dealing with a very wide variety of foods (Fig. 10.2); the grinding function of the mammalian molars is performed by the gizzard, a muscular sac filled with grit. Chelonians (tortoises and turtles) also have horny jaw coverings (Fig. 10.2), sharp-edged anteriorly and broadened for crushing posteriorly.

Among mammals the duck-billed platypus (*Ornithorhynchus*) has teeth only in early life, replacing them by keratinous plates used for crushing aquatic insects, crustaceans and molluscs. Most toothless mammals eat ants, or more frequently termites: besides the anteaters of South America (Fig. 10.2) there are the pangolins of Africa and India, and the Australian echidna. All these have very long protrusible tongues, made sticky with saliva, by which they pick up termites and ants that do not need chewing.

The whalebone whales feed on planktonic crustacea; a mouthful of water is taken in, and by raising the tongue the water is forced out again through a sieve of whalebone plates that strains out the food (Fig. 10.2). Only rudimentary teeth develop in the embryo.

# CHEWING

It is a characteristic of mammals (except for the highly specialized ones just mentioned) that they retain the food for a time in the mouth, breaking it up by rhythmic movements of the jaws and tongue, and mixing it with saliva; that is to say, they chew. Chewing not only requires a complex jaw musculature and multicuspid molar teeth, it also requires the development of palatal folds which, by meeting and fusing in the midline to form a secondary palate, separate a dorsal respiratory passage from a ventral food passage (Fig. 1.28). Mammals also differ from lower vertebrates in that their saliva contains digestive enzymes that are mixed with the food being chewed, and thus the mouth has become the first part of the digestive system.

## The origin of chewing

Mammals are derived from the Synapsida, or mammal-like reptiles, which flourished during the Permian and Triassic Periods (Fig. 4.17). Some of these were herbivorous, others carnivorous, and it is believed that the most direct ancestors of mammals are carnivorous members of the group of synapsids known as Cynodontia. Cynodonts had enlarged canines, separating the small incisors anteriorly from the cheek teeth posteriorly. The cheek teeth were elongated mesiodistally, and additional cusps developed mesially and distally to the main cusps, forming a serrated cutting edge along the jaw that must have been used for chopping the food. A cingulum protected the gingival margin on the lingual side of the lower teeth and on both sides of the upper teeth. The upper teeth closed outside the lower teeth, but they did not come into contact with them (Fig. 10.4). No lateral movement of the jaw was possible.

The mandible of cynodonts (and of all non-mammalian vertebrates) was made up of several bones, of which only the dentary bore the teeth. It formed the lateral and anterior part of the jaw. Of a number of bones at the posterior end of the lower jaw one, the articular, formed a joint with the quadrate bone of the skull; this type of jaw joint is found in all vertebrates except the mammals (Fig. 10.3). In the earliest synapsids the jaw muscles were attached to the posterior bones of the lower jaw, but in the course of time they became larger and more complex, in association with the devel-

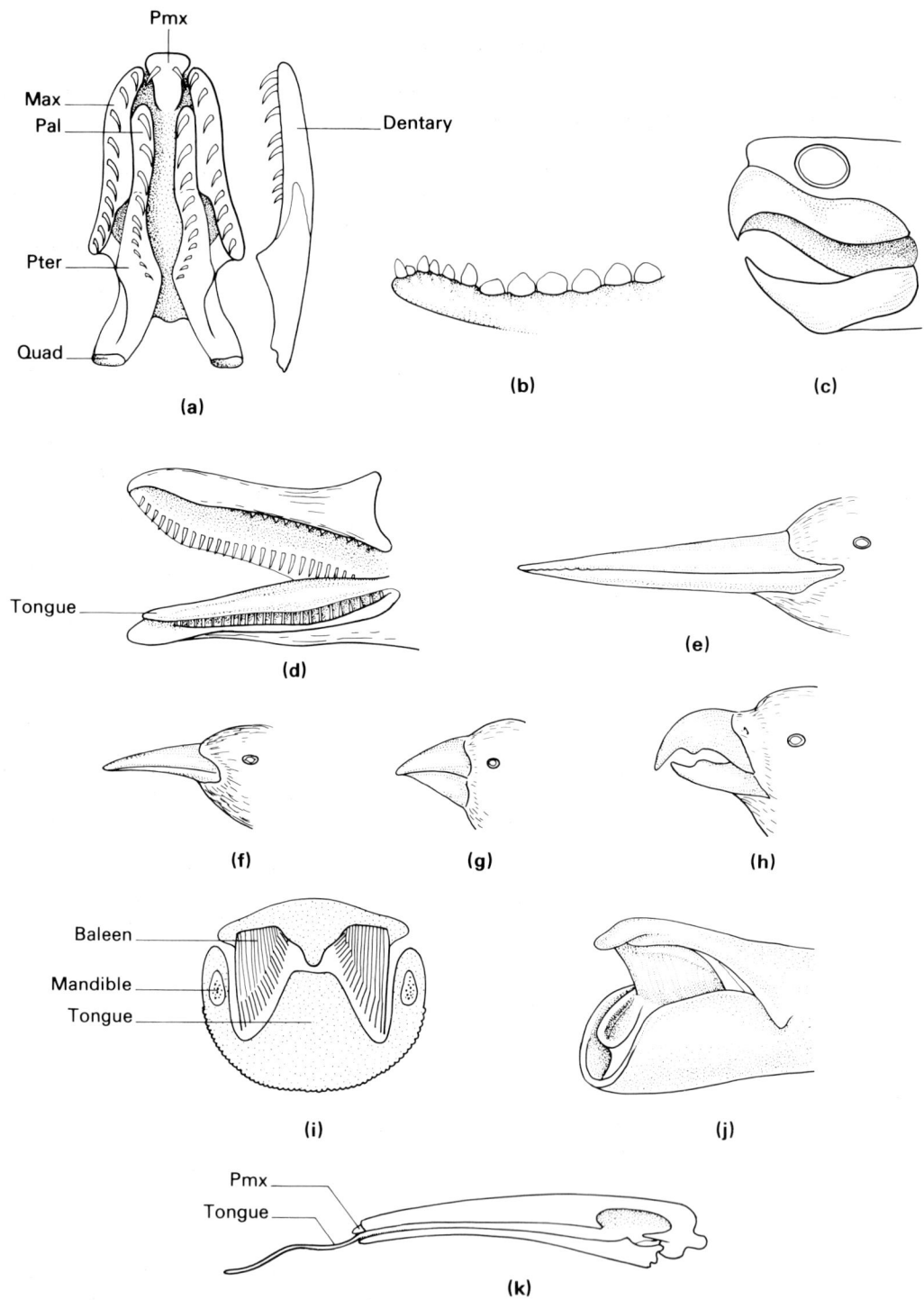

**Fig. 10.2.** (a) Python skull in palatal view, and lateral view of lower jaw. Teeth are borne on the maxilla (Max), premaxilla (Pmx), palatine (Pal), pterygoid (Pter) and dentary. All the teeth point backwards. The jaw articulates with the skull via the quadrate (Quad). (b) Crushing teeth of a herbivorous lizard, *Dracaena*; (c) Keratinous beak of a chelonian (alligator turtle). (d) Beak of a duck. By means of the lamellae it filters small objects from the water. (e–h) Some bird beaks adapted to different modes of feeding: (e) heron (spears fish); (f) tree-creeper (picks small insects from bark); (g) hawfinch (cracks seeds); (h) falcon (carnivorous). (i, j) Mouth of a whalebone whale: (i) is a cross-section; plates of baleen function as a sieve. (k) Skull of anteater, a toothless mammal that picks up food by a protrusible tongue.

opment of chewing. This set in motion the following changes, one of which resulted in the evolution of the middle ear of mammals.

As the jaw muscles enlarged they began to transfer their insertions on to the dentary (Fig. 10.3). This bone gradually enlarged; it developed a coronoid process for attachment of part of the musculature corresponding to the temporal muscle of mammals. Expansion of the dentary was accompanied by reduction of the remaining bones, until the dentary formed most of the lateral surface of the mandible, extending back almost to the joint. Eventually it came into contact with the squamosal bone of the skull and a new joint was formed between the two bones: the temporo-mandibular joint of mammals. This was situated immediately lateral to the articular–quadrate joint. For a time both joints worked together, but the dentary–squamosal joint became increasingly important and finally the articular bone was detached from the mandible, becoming, together with the quadrate, involved in the conduction of sound vibrations across the middle ear (Figs. 4.29–4.32).

Primitively the jaw muscles occupied a space at the side of the braincase, roofed over by bone (Fig. 4.32). With their enlargement, ossification of the roof was reduced until only the zygomatic arch was left. The part of the musculature which originated from the zygomatic arch became differentiated as the masseter. Being situated nearer to the cheek teeth its contraction is more effective in producing a powerful bite. It also reduces the force of reaction at the joint. In primitive synapsids, biting with the cheek teeth produced a force on the jaw at the joint, acting downwards and forwards. This force would have tended to dislocate the joint if the bite were too strong. With development of the masseter the joint reaction eventually falls almost to zero, freeing movements at the joint in the manner necessary for mammalian mastication (Fig. 10.3b). This applies only when the bite is on the cheek teeth; when force is exerted by the incisors or canines there is always a reaction at the joint, hence its strong construction in shrews and carnivores (Fig. 10.18).

## Occlusal relations

The earliest mammals, from the end of the Triassic—*Megazostrodon*, *Erythrotherium*, *Eozostrodon* (also called *Morganucodon*: there is disagreement about its correct name) and *Kuehneotherium*—had advanced beyond the cynodonts in two important respects: the jaw was capable of lateral movements, and opposing teeth came into occlusal relation. Chewing was no longer a simple opening and closing movement: it involved a lateral swing of the mandible, probably essentially like that of the opossum today (Fig. 10.4). Whereas in the cynodonts the lower teeth bit to the lingual side of the upper teeth without touching them, now the teeth came into contact, the lower teeth moving lingually and upwards as they crossed the uppers; then the mouth would open again and the jaw would swing laterally, ready for the next cycle. Thus the chewing cycle can be divided into three parts: (a) an opening stroke, in which the jaw is moving downwards and laterally, (b) a free closing stroke with the jaw still displaced in a lateral position and (c) an upward and lingual movement, called the power stroke guided by occlusal contact between the teeth. Studies of primitive living mammals such as the opossum show that chewing takes place only on one side of the mouth at a time; the teeth of the opposite side are out of contact, the lowers lingual to the uppers. The two halves of the mandible are connected at the symphysis only by ligaments, and move on each other during the chewing process.

Occlusal contact of the teeth, or near contact when there is a thin layer of food between them, results in attrition facets. These facets enable us to determine how the opposing cusps related to each other in occlusion (p. 335). The earliest mammals inherited their cusp patterns from cynodonts, with the result that the fit of the teeth was not exact: some grinding in was necessary. Moreover the upper and lower teeth fitted together in different ways in different genera, as if their occlusal relations have been acquired independently. Once it was established however, the relationship between upper and lower teeth in mammals has remained remarkably constant, so that the history of some attrition facets can be traced from *Kuehneotherium* right up to man.

## Tooth wear

Attrition implies close contact between the teeth, which is clearly impossible when they are separated by a bulky piece of food. The earliest mammals were very tiny, shrew-sized, and they no doubt ate insects, which in comparison to the mammals must have been quite large. Observations on living mammals shows that the first cycles in chewing are rapid closing strokes with little lateral movement, during which the food is punctured by the cusps and crushed between the teeth. This crushing-puncturing action, in which the teeth do not meet, may resemble the chewing process of cynodonts. However, as the food

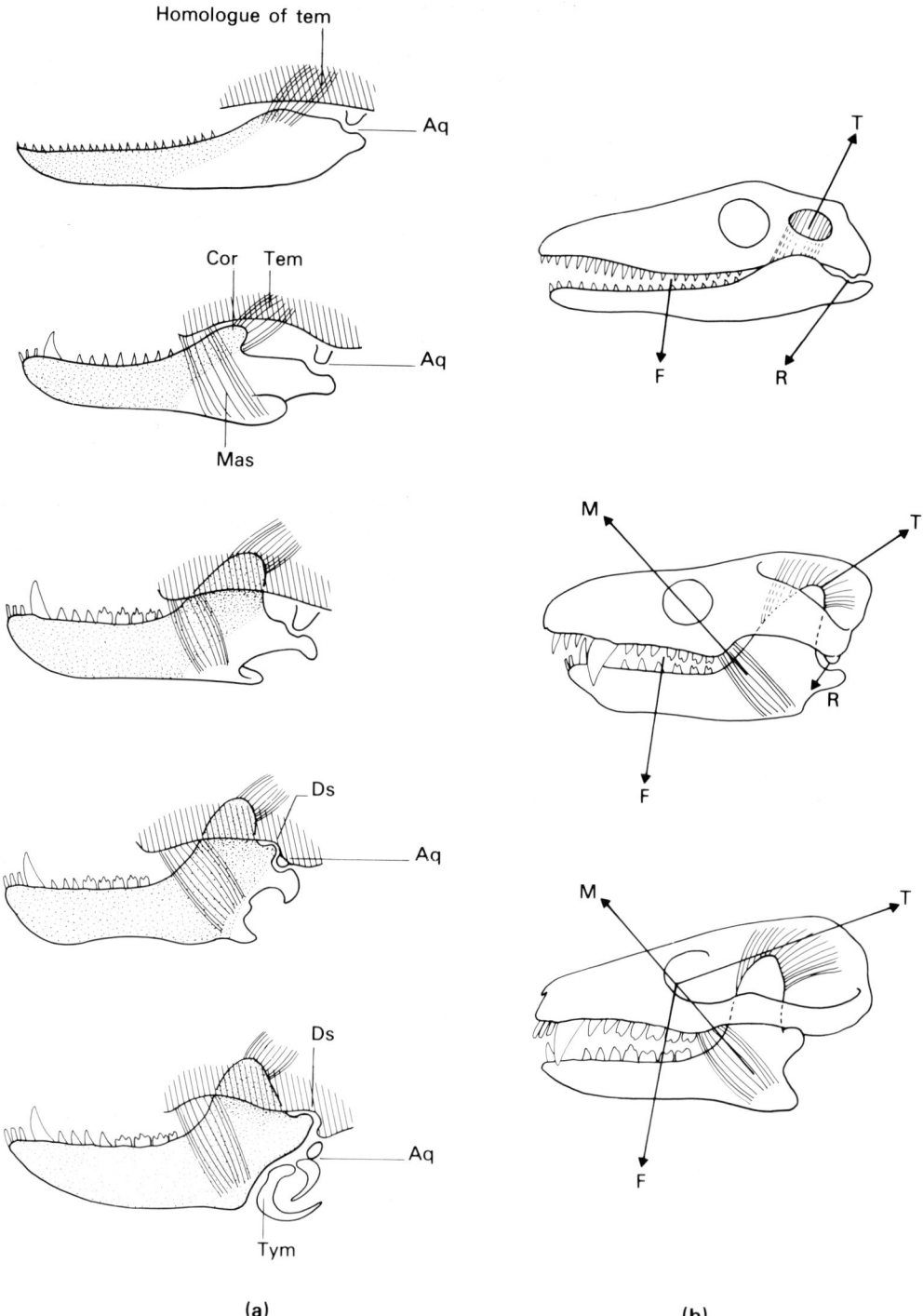

**Fig. 10.3.** (a) Stages in the evolution of the jaw in synapsids, leading to the mammal condition (bottom). The dentary is shaded. Tem, Temporal muscle; Mas, masseter muscles; Cor, coronoid process; Ds, dentary–squamosal joint; Aq, articular–quadrate joint; Tym, tympanic bone (originally part of the jaw). (b) Skulls of a primitive synapsid, an advanced synapsid (cynodont) and a mammal, to show the forces acting on the lower jaw when biting with the cheek teeth. T, Pull of temporal muscle; F, force due to food; R, reaction force at the joint. By the development of the masseter muscle (M) the force R is reduced. Finally in the mammal the lines of action of F, M and T meet at a point and R disappears.

334

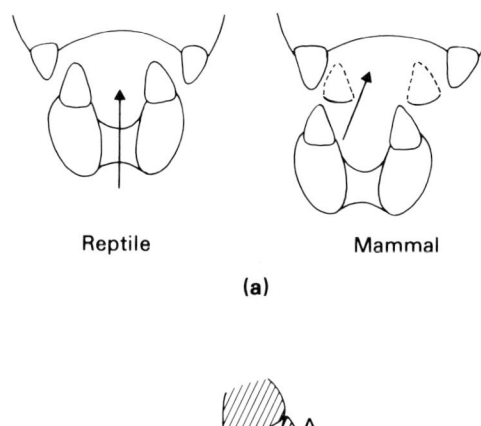

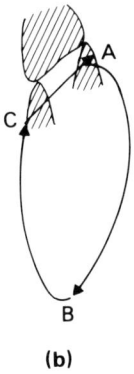

Fig. 10.4. (a) Relation of lower to upper teeth in a reptile and a mammal. In the reptile the jaw bites vertically and the teeth do not meet. In the mammal there is a transverse component and occlusion takes place. (b) The chewing cycle in a primitive mammal. AB, Opening stroke; BC, free closing stroke; CA, power stroke.

becomes reduced the teeth can meet through it, leading to the complete chewing cycle described above. Crushing-puncturing would be of considerable assistance to a small mammal dealing with cuticle-covered insects, and it probably explains the widespread presence of high, pointed cusps in the early mammals.

The wear produced by crushing-puncturing chewing is abrasion, as opposed to the attrition produced by occlusal contact (Fig. 10.5). Abrasion is a general removal of the tooth surface. It results in the rounding of cusp tips and crests and a smoothing of minor irregularities of the tooth surface. Where dentine becomes exposed by wearing away of the enamel, a pit develops because dentine is softer than enamel and abrades faster.

In contrast to abrasion, attrition produces flat, shiny facets where the tooth surface appears to be polished or filed. Attrition facets are often covered with fine parallel striations where the tooth has been scratched by particles of grit in the food. The striations show the direction of relative movement while the opposing teeth were in contact. The attrition facets of one tooth obviously correspond to those of its occluding tooth, and hence they show how the two opposing teeth fitted together. Abrasion, on the other hand, because it is so diffuse, can tell us very little about occlusal relations.

Attrition facets have been attributed to a process of thegosis (Every, R. G.), an activity different from chewing, having the function of sharpening the cutting edges of teeth which tend to

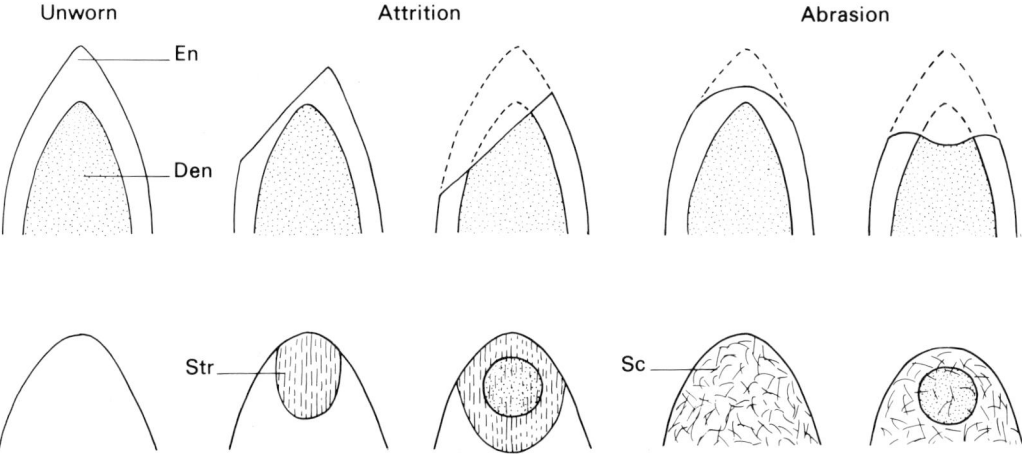

Fig. 10.5. Comparison of attrition and abrasion. Two stages of each process are shown, in section (above) and in surface view (below). En, enamel; Den, dentine; Str, parallel striations, characteristic of attrition; Sc, scratches in various directions in abrasion.

be blunted by use. According to Every, thegosis takes place when the mouth is empty; it prepares the teeth for chewing. Some animals do have what appears to be tooth-sharpening behaviour; for example baboons whet their upper canines against their lower premolars, which seem to be constructed for this function, and grinding the teeth as an expression of rage occurs in many mammals, including man. It is very doubtful however that molar facets should be explained in this way because they can be explained by normal chewing movements, and moreover because they are frequently marked with striations, implying that something was between the teeth when the facets were worn.

A third type of wear is produced where the tooth touches the neighbours in its own jaw. Slight relative movement of adjacent teeth results in contact facets. They never have striations, as would be predicted for purely tooth/tooth contact (see above). In old animals the mesiodistal length of the tooth may be reduced appreciably from this cause, but the gaps are kept closed by mesial drift (Fig. 9.24), so damage to the periodontium due to food being forced between the teeth is avoided.

# EVOLUTION OF MAMMALIAN MOLARS

## Molar shape in early mammals

After their first appearance at the end of the Trisassic Period the mammals branched out in several directions. Five orders can be distinguished in the Jurassic Period, differing in the structure of molars (Fig. 10.6). In the Triconodonta the molars were elongated mesiodistally and supported by two equal roots; there were three large cusps arranged in line, as well as some smaller cusps at the mesial and distal ends and a cingulum (buccal and lingual on the upper molar, lingual only on the lower). They were probably descended from Triassic morganucodonts. The triconodonts were the largest mammals of their time, reaching the size of a cat or fox, and they were probably carnivorous.

There were two orders of small, insectivorous mammals with triangular upper molars, the Symmetrodonta and the Pantotheria. In the Symmetrodonta there were still only two roots, but the distal root was broadened to support the lingual corner of the triangle as well as the distobuccal corner; in Pantotheria this upper root was doubled so that there were three roots. The lower molars of both orders had two roots, but their cusps were arranged in a triangle, known as the trigonid, that fitted between two upper molars, whose triangles were in reverse to those of the lowers. The Pantotheria differed from the Symmetrodonta in possessing additional cusps on the buccal side of the upper molar, and on the lower molar a distal heel, or talonid, which occluded with the most lingual of the upper cusps. The Pantotheria include the ancestors of modern mammals. Both Symmetrodonta and Pantotheria were probably derived from a Triassic mammal like *Kuehneotherium*.

In the order Docodonta the molars were broadened, with a crushing function; this group was probably of morganucodont origin. Finally there were the Multituberculata; probably herbivorous, rodent-like mammals with complex cheek teeth which functioned in a horizontal, mesiodistal grinding movement, quite unlike the chewing movements of their contemporaries. The relationship of multituberculates to other mammals is unknown; they might have a distant connection with morganucodonts.

## Shearing

Except in docodonts and multituberculates, the upper and lower cheek teeth of the earliest mammals did not directly oppose, but passed each other, the buccal surfaces of lower teeth moving up the lingual surfaces of upper teeth as the jaws closed. During this action the food was cut up by crests on the edges of the cusps. The process was like the action of scissors or shears, and is described as shearing.

For efficient shearing certain relationships between the blades are required. First, the blades should not be parallel, but should cross at an angle. Parallel blades meet along their whole length at the same time, and the force is dispersed along the whole length of the blade; if the blades cross, the force is concentrated at the crossing point, which travels along the blades as they come together (Fig. 10.7). With such a system the food would tend to be pushed towards the open end (e.g. buccally or lingually, if the blades are transversely arranged), but if the blades are notched food is pushed into the notch and cannot escape from between the teeth. Thus each cutting blade is usually supported between two cusps. A further requirement is that the blades should be pressed together, otherwise they are merely forced apart instead of cutting. The force that presses the blades together must come from contraction of the jaw muscles.

In addition to the scissor action of crests we also

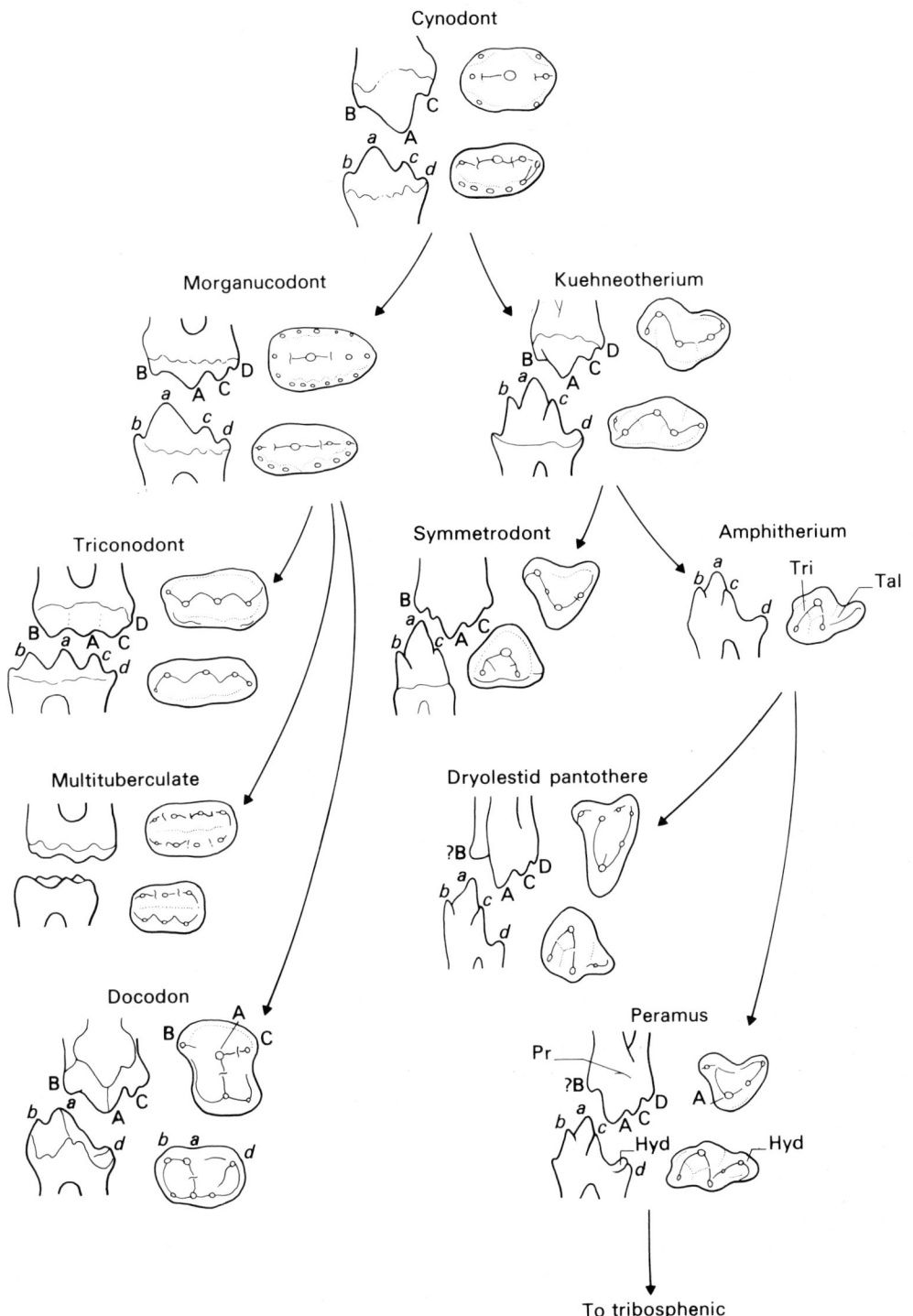

Fig. 10.6. The evolution of molar teeth before the establishment of the tribosphenic pattern. Upper and lower molars seen in lingual view and in crown view; mesial end to the left in each case. The upper molars of *Amphitherium* are unknown. In *Peramus*, Pr is the cingulum representing the first trace of a protocone, and Hyd is the rudimentary hypoconid. Most of the known pantotheres are dryolestids (e.g. *Melanodon*), but they are off the main line of mammalian evolution.

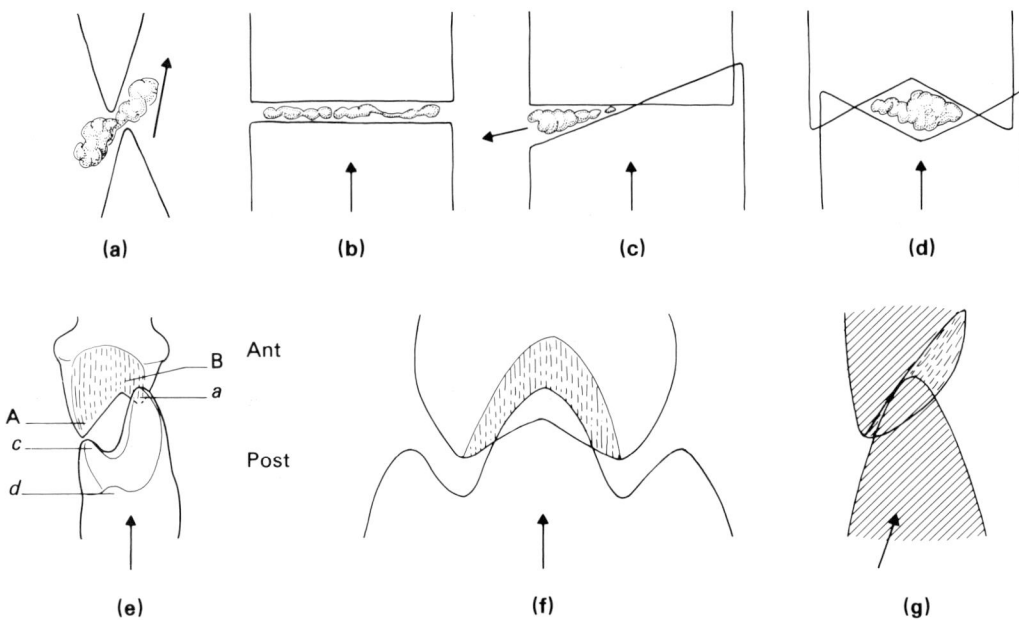

**Fig. 10.7.** Shearing. (a) Shearing crests in cross-section. (b) Crests parallel: cutting force weak. (c) Crossing crests: food pushed sideways. (d) Notched crests: food cannot escape, (provided that the blades are pressed together.) (e) An example of notched crests (*Kuehneotherium*); cusps labelled as in Fig. 10.8. (f) Cusp in groove action; (g) f in section.

have the motion of cusps up grooves, and of crests along surfaces. Although these are not cutting actions they assist in tearing apart the fibres of the food, and they are included under the general heading of shearing.

**Molar function in early mammals**

MORGANUCODONTS: SHEARING
SURFACES APPEAR

These have molar cusp patterns recognizably like those of cynodonts such as *Thrinaxodon* (Fig. 10.6, 10.8). On the upper molar of *Eozostrodon* there are three principal cusps arranged in a mesiodistal line. The central cusp (A) is the highest, (C) is on its distal side and (B), the smallest of the three, is mesial. At the distal end of the tooth is a smaller cusp (D), and the other minor cusps are arranged along the buccal and lingual edges, forming a cingulum. On the lower molar the cusps are arranged in a similar manner, and may be labelled *b, a, c* and *d*; however *a* is proportionately higher and *b* is lower than the corresponding upper cusps, and the cingulum cusps are confined to the lingual side. Because the large lower cusps *a* alternate along the jaw with the large upper cusps A the teeth wear into a slightly zig-zag pattern (Fig. 10.8) of shearing edges.

KUEHNEOTHERIUM: SHEARING
BETWEEN REVERSED TRIANGLES

In *Kuehneotherium* the three principal cusps have been rearranged so that the upper molar cusp B is displaced buccally and in the lower molar cusp *c* is displaced lingually. This is the beginning of the system of 'reversed triangles' that characterizes the occlusion of symmetrodonts and pantotheres. The two crests supported by the high cusp *a* shear down the widening embrasure between two upper teeth. In essence, *Kuehneotherium* evolved, by a process of tooth development, shearing surfaces which were similar to those which *Eozostrodon* developed by the process of wear.

PANTOTHERES: EVOLUTION OF
THE TALONID

The oldest pantothere is *Amphitherium* from the Middle Jurassic. This differs from *Kuehneotherium* in the development of a low ridge or heel (talonid) on the distal part of the lower molar. The trigonid triangle has closed up so that cusp *c* stands almost directly lingual to cusp *a* (Fig. 10.6, 10.9). In *Peramus*, from the Upper Jurassic, the talonid is still more enlarged. The effect of these changes is that the upper cusp A lost its distal relationship to the lower shearing crest *ab* of the

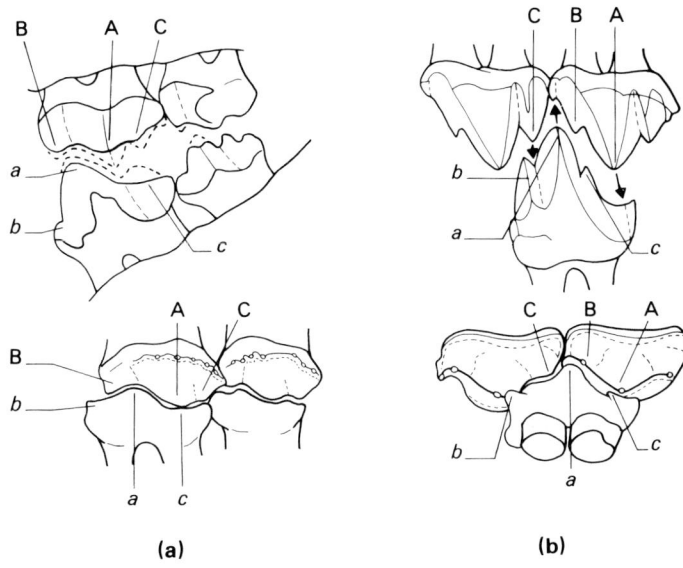

Fig. 10.8. Occlusal relations in two of the earliest mammals: (a) *Eozostrodon* and (b) *Kuehneotherium*. Occluding teeth are shown in lateral view (above), and as seen in the direction of the power stroke (below).

posteriorly adjacent tooth and concentrated on the surface of the trigonid (*ac*) on its mesial side. The shearing crest *ab* still sheared against cusp C and its distal crest (CD). As the talonid enlarged, cusps A and C moved farther apart and the talonid ridge bit between them. In *Peramus*, at the position opposite the groove between A and C a small cusp (hypoconid) began to develop, introducing an extra zig-zag into the definition.

TRIBOSPHENIC MOLARS: THE APPEARANCE OF THE PROTOCONE

On the palatal surface of the upper molars in *Peramus* there is a small cingulum bulge (arrowed in Fig. 10.9). It is now believed that this cingulum was enlarged in Cretaceous mammals descended from pantotheres (*Aegialodon* is the oldest known example), and a new cusp (protocone) developed

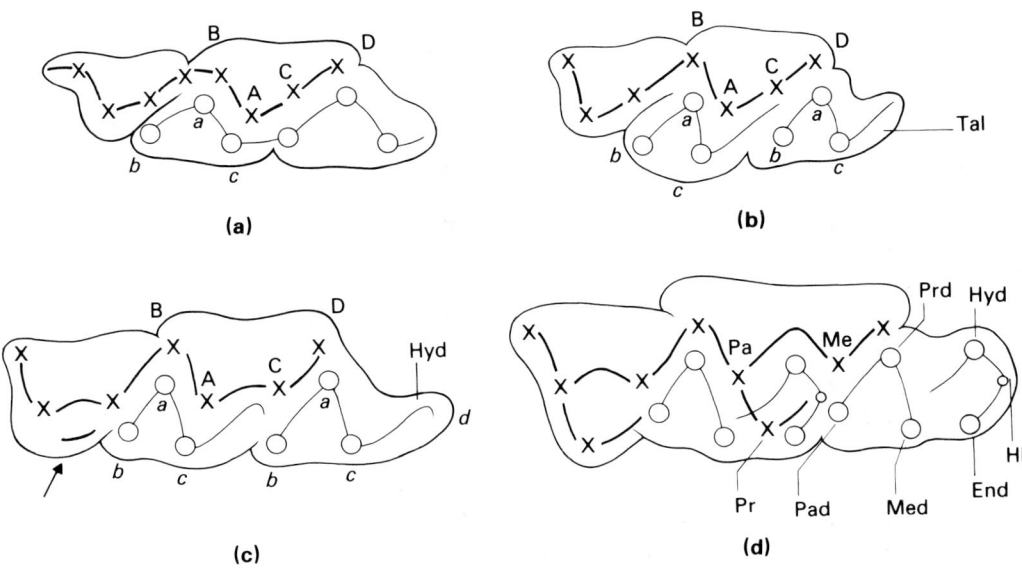

Fig. 10.9. Stages in the evolution of the talonid (Tal): (a) *kuehneotherium*; (b) a primitive pantothere, e.g. *Amphitherium*; (c) an advanced pantothere, e.g. *Peramus*; (d) a primitive tribosphenic form (Abbreviations as in Fig. 10.10.)

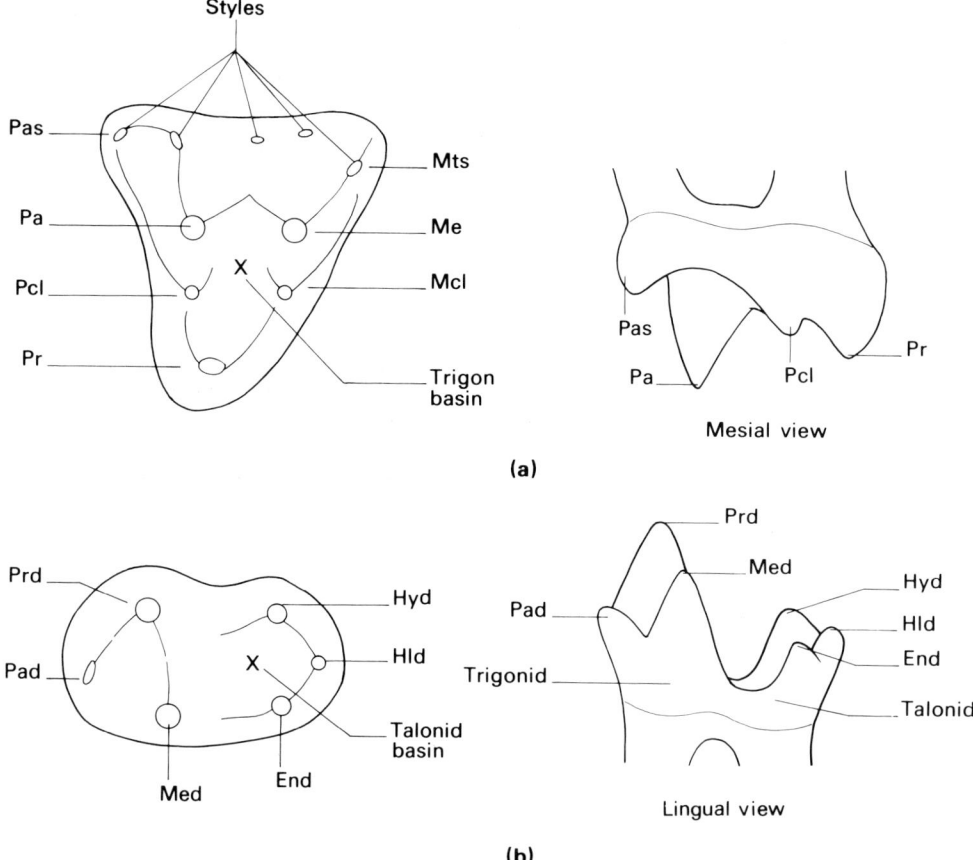

**Fig. 10.10.** Names of the cusps on tribosphenic molars. The following abbreviations are generally used: (a) Upper molar—Pa, paracone; Me, metacone; Pr, protocone; Pcl, paraconule; Mcl, metaconule; Pas, parastyle; Mts, metastyle. (b) Lower molar—Prd, protoconid; Pad, paraconid; Med, metaconid; Hyd, hypoconid; End, entoconid; Hld, hypoconulid.

from the cingulum. The protocone pounded into the surface of the talonid which had developed as a basin ringed by further cusps: the hypoconid buccally, the hypoconulid distally and the entoconid lingually (Fig. 10.10 gives the names of all the cusps: note that the names of lower cusps have the suffix -*id*).

The system of lettering cusps has been abandoned and they are now being given names. This is because from the Cretaceous onwards the homologies of the cusps of nearly all mammals are known with accuracy and the names have long been in use. The homologies of the cusps of pre-Cretaceous mammals with those of tribosphenic molars have only recently been cleared up, and some are still disputed. For the lower teeth it seems certain that cusp *a* is the protoconid, cusp *b* is the paraconid and cusp *c* is the metaconid. On the upper teeth cusp A is clearly the paracone, but there is not complete agreement over cusps B and C; it is assumed here that cusp B is the parastyle and cusp C is the metacone.

Cusp A (paracone) is the homologue of the single cusp of the ancestral conical tooth present in the earliest synapsids. This old reptilian cusp is not the homologue of the protocone, which in fact arose rather late in evolution. The inappropriate name of the protocone is derived from nineteenth-century studies based on an inadequate knowledge of the Jurassic and Cretaceous mammals. However, long usage has made it impossible (although there have been many attempts) to change the names of cusps from those given to them by H. F. Osborn. The theory of molar evolution on which he based the nomenclature (known as the Tritubercular theory) is depicted in Fig. 10.11.

The development of the protocone resulted in

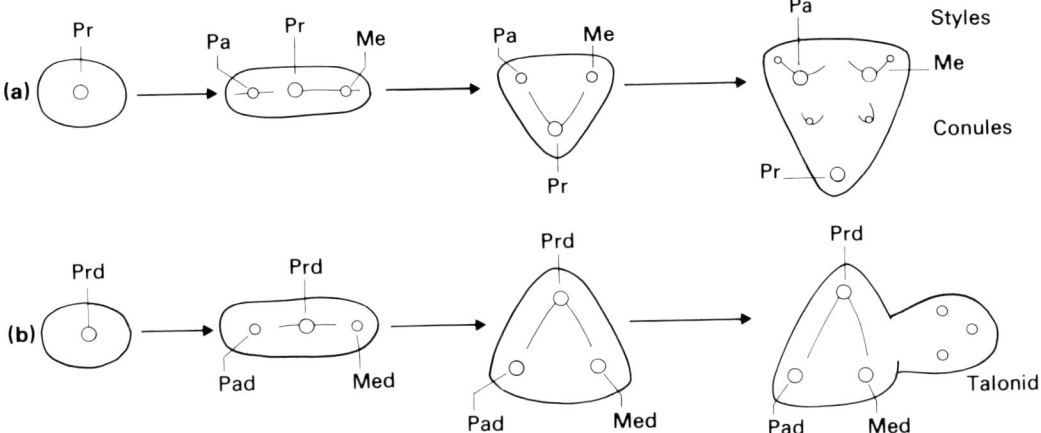

**Fig. 10.11.** The Cope–Osborn theory of molar evolution. Compare this with the modern view depicted in Fig. 10.9. Note that the theory was essentially correct as regards the lower molars (b), but not the upper molars (a). (Abbreviations as in Fig. 10.10.)

molars which combined the functions of shearing and crushing; hence the term tribosphenic (Greek *tribein*, to rub; *sphen*, a wedge). All living mammals, except the monotremes, have been derived from Cretaceous ancestors with tribosphenic molars.

During chewing, the protoconid bit into the wedge-shaped space (embrasure) between two upper molars, as in pantotheres (Fig. 10.9, 10.12). As the teeth closed the protoconid moved lingually and upwards into the embrasure. In doing this the mesial edge of the trigonid (protoconid–paraconid crest) sheared against the distal edge of the upper molar in front: first against the metacone–metastyle crest, and then against the metaconule crest. The distal edge of the trigonid (protoconid–metaconid crest) sheared against the mesial edge of the upper molar that bounds the embrasure distally. It sheared first against the paracone–parastyle crest, and then against the paraconule crest; meanwhile the metaconid sheared against the mesial crest of the protocone. The protocone cusp is ultimately driven into the talonid. At the start of occlusion the crests supported by the hypoconid sheared between the metacone and the paracone of the upper tooth, the hypoconid cusp itself ultimately occluding with the trigon basin (the low depression in the centre of the upper tooth). Thus the hypoconid/trigon and the protocone/talonid are reciprocal cusp/basin surfaces of interaction. The protocone shears against the entoconid on the lingual margin of the talonid before finally occluding in the talonid basin. Cusp and basin contact marks the limit of the power stroke and the beginning of the opening stroke of the next chewing cycle.

## DEVELOPMENTS FROM THE TRIBOSPHENIC PATTERN

Tribosphenic molars were more versatile than those of pantotheres and other early mammals; by emphasizing either shearing or crushing they could evolve in different directions in adaptation to different diet. Originally adapted for an insectivorous diet, tribosphenic molars enabled the mammals to take advantage of a much wider range of animal and plant food, and during the decline of the dinosaurs in the later Cretaceous a great evolutionary radiation of mammals began, leading to the diversity of Tertiary and modern forms. Only a sample of their dental adaptations can be discussed here.

### Carnivores: carnassials

Carnivorous animals do little chewing, compared with other groups, but they need teeth that can cut through the fibres of meat. One pair of cutting crests has been exaggerated: the mesial trigonid crest (protoconid–paraconid) on the lower teeth and the metacone–metastyle crest on the upper teeth (Fig. 10.13). With the enlargement of these features other elements of the pattern are reduced in importance: the metaconid, the talonid, and on the upper teeth the protocone. In carnivorous marsupials—the Tasmanian devil (*Sarcophilus*)

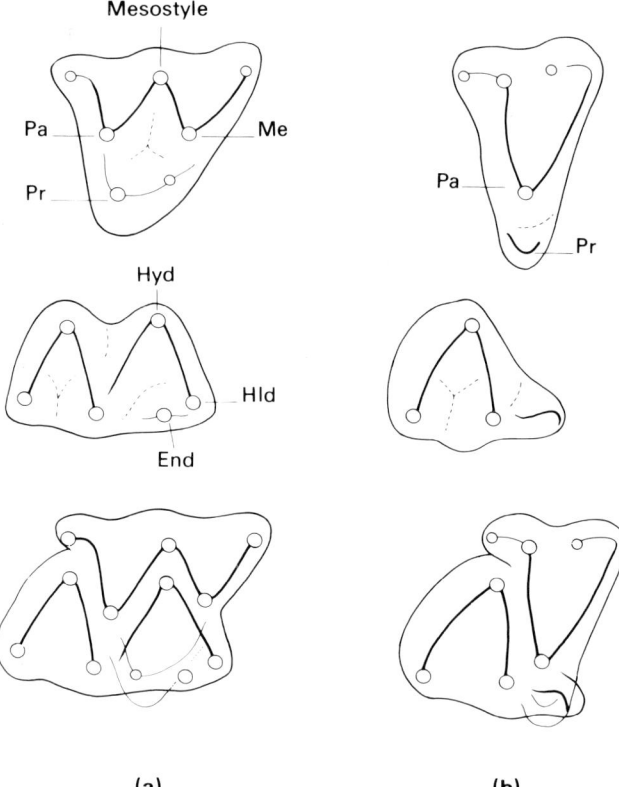

**Fig. 10.14.** Two types of molar in insectivorous mammals. (a) In dilambdadonts the hypoconid bites in a deep groove between paracone and metacone, bounded on the buccal side by a mesostyle cusp. (b) In zalambdadonts the protocone and talonid have been reduced, and the metacone has been lost.

and metacone. A deep groove between these cusps receives the Λ-shaped hypoconid (Fig. 10.14). The hypoconulid is displaced towards the lingual side of the talonid, near the entoconid, lengthening the hypoconid/metacone shear. Dilambdadont molars characterize the shrews, moles, insectivorous bats and *Tupaia*. A few insectivores, such as the tenrecs from Madagascar, have a much simpler tooth pattern formed of a single Λ, reminiscent of some pantotheres (dryolestids, Fig. 10.6). These are the zalambdadonts.

### The hypocone

In several evolutionary lines a cingulum ledge developed on the upper molar, distal to the protocone. When the jaws closed it met the edge of the paraconid. This was the beginning of a new area of opposition between the teeth, additional to the protocone–entoconid contact. A new cusp (hypocone) developed on the cingulum, biting against the top of the paraconid (Fig. 10.15). The hypocone increased in size and the paraconid correspondingly was reduced in height. Eventually the hypocone, in several lines of evolution, became as large as the protocone, the tooth became quadrangular instead of triangular, and the lingual root enlarged and often divided, so that there were four roots. The enlarging hypocone filled up the interdental embrasure into which the trigonid of the lower molar formerly passed. Now the trigonid met the hypocone, just as the talonid met the protocone, and the crushing area was doubled. A great many mammals are at some stage in this process (e.g. man), but it has reached its full development in herbivores.

### Herbivores

GRINDING

Ungulates and most primates move the jaw more horizontally when chewing than is the case with insectivores. The food, instead of being cut up by shearing crests, is ground as cusps travel along grooves in the opposing teeth. The cusps are low, with less steep sides. They are more equal in height; for example, the talonid is as high as the trigonid (Fig. 10.16). The chewing movement is still mainly transverse, but more complex forms of chewing,

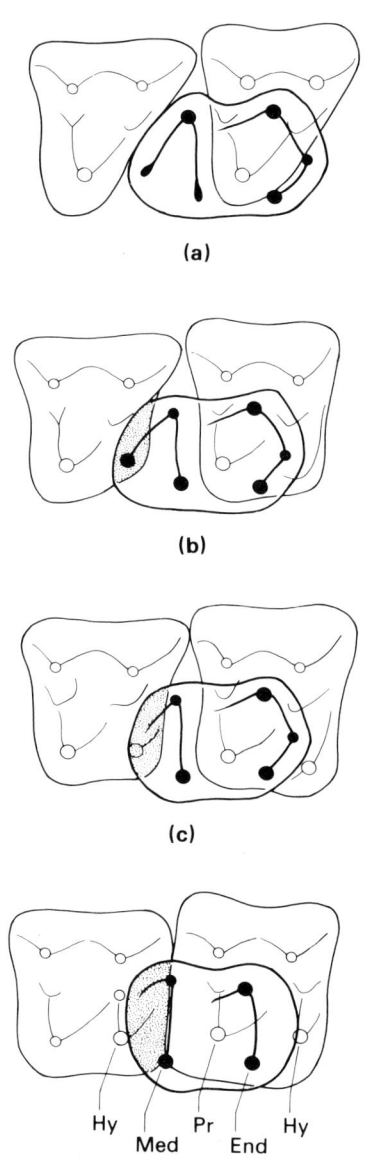

**Fig. 10.15.** Stages in the evolution of the hypocone (shaded): (a) tribosphenic; (b) distal angulum on upper molar meets the paraconid; (c) hypocone develops on the cingulum, paraconid reduced; (d) hypocone equal to protocone, occludes between entoconid (mesially) and metaconid (distally).

involving mesiolingual movements, have evolved in some groups (including primates), and in many rodents the chewing movement is almost directly mesial. Nevertheless, the cusps generally retain the same topographic relations to their opponents as in tribosphenic molars, and consequently their homologies can be recognized.

ENAMEL RIDGES (LOPHS)

The earliest fossil ungulates and rodents have molars with cusps like those of primates. Abrasion wears the cusps, exposing the dentine, and for much of its life the animal uses worn, more or less cuspless teeth. Because enamel is harder than dentine it wears more slowly, with the result that the cusp is replaced by a crater of dentine surrounded by a raised enamel rim. With horizontal chewing movements, ridges of enamel, called lophs, formed in this way can be made to cross one another and so act as shearing edges. Such teeth are called lophodont. The effect is similar to the ridges on a millstone. Herbivorous mammals have made use of this feature to produce very effective grinding dentitions. The enamel on the tips of their cusps is thin and therefore removed very soon after eruption, resulting in a pattern of enamel ridges on a more or less flattened crown surface. The grinding efficiency is improved if the lophs are approximately perpendicular to the direction of motion. Thus in ruminants the chewing movement is transverse, and the cusps wear into crescents pulled out mesiodistally (the molars are called selenodont). The horse also chews transversely, but its enamel pattern is very complex because of the development of numerous folds that increase the length of the cutting edge. The chewing efficiency of the horse is very high: by measuring grass fibres in horse droppings it has been found that their average length is only 3.7 mm; each mouthful of grass is chewed four to ten times to produce this amount of cutting.

Complex enamel patterns develop also in rodents, but here the ridges tend to run obliquely or transversely across the tooth, again perpendicular to the direction of movement. (The mesial movement of chewing in rodents must be distinguished from the protrusive movement that brings the lower incisors into contact with the upper incisors; when the incisors are in use the molars are out of contact.) In the mouse there are areas of the crown where enamel fails to develop, so speeding up the establishment of the ridge pattern. The elephant, which also chews from distal to mesial, likewise has transverse ridges on its molars (Fig. 10.16).

A special case of the use of the differential hardness of enamel and dentine is the rodent incisor. This has a band of enamel confined to the labial surface; elsewhere the dentine is covered with cement. Because the enamel wears more slowly it stands up as a chisel edge however much the tooth is worn.

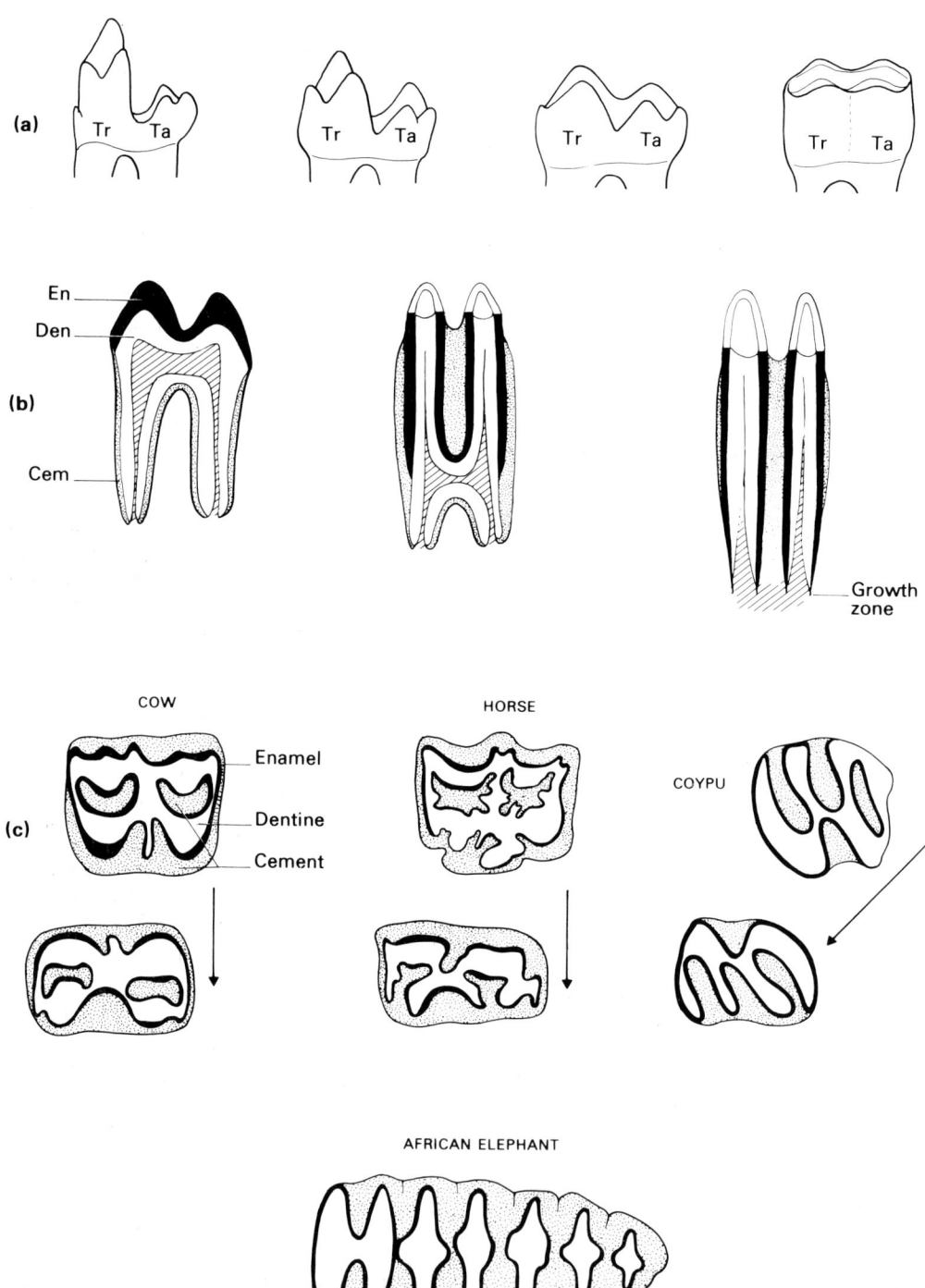

**Fig. 10.16.** (a) Evolutionary stages from tribosphenic to herbivorous lower molars. (b) Comparison of brachyodont and hypsodont teeth. (c) Enamel ridges on the molars of some herbivores. The arrows show the direction of the chewing movement.

## HYPSODONTY

The teeth of herbivores, especially those that eat grass, have to suffer much wear. Grass stems contain silica, a substance harder than enamel and therefore very abrasive. Grass-eating animals have compensated for this wear by evolving high-crowned, or hypsodont, teeth. The crowns of their teeth continue to grow for a long time before root formation begins, so that, in the molars of a horse or sheep for example, the tooth consists almost entirely of crown. Root formation may even be postponed indefinitely, and then we have 'open-rooted' teeth, as in the rabbit (Fig. 10.16). Such teeth can continue growing throughout life. The incisors of rodents are used widely in research on tooth development; they are continually being formed at one end while worn away at the other (Fig. 12.30).

The opposite of hypsodonty is brachyodonty, but no sharp line can be drawn: the molars of the cow are more high-crowned than those of the deer but less so than those of the sheep. The early fossil horses were brachyodont and they probably lived in woods and ate leaves; the height of their molar crowns increased rapidly when horses invaded the grasslands (Fig. 12.12).

As crown height increases the cusps become taller and the valleys deeper. Cement, normally developed only on the roots, extends to the crown, where it fills up the spaces between the cusps. Apart from giving support to cusps, the crown cement of hypsodont teeth is necessary in order to provide attachment for periodontal fibres.

## MOLARIZATION OF PREMOLARS

Some herbivores, notably the horse, tapir and rhinoceros, have increased their chewing efficiency by evolving complex premolars that resemble the molars; the process is called molarization of the premolars. More frequent is a tendency to enlarge the last molars. $M_3$ occludes with the whole of $M^3$ as well as with the distal part of $M^2$; it develops an additional distal structure (an enlarged hypoconulid) which takes the place of the trigonid of the missing $M_4$ (Fig. 10.17). This happens in a number of primates. Some of the pigs, such as the warthog, have still more complex last molars, $M^3$ being enlarged as well as $M_3$ (Fig. 10.17).

## DIASTEMATA

Another common feature of herbivores is a gap, or diastema, in the dentition between the anterior teeth used in taking food and the cheek teeth used

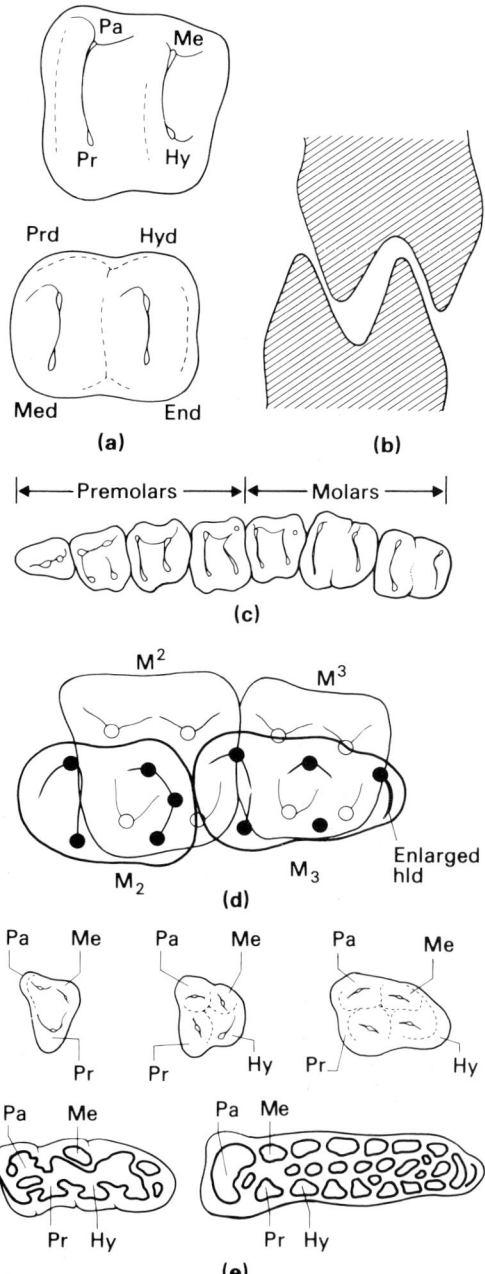

Fig. 10.17. Some herbivorous adaptations. (a) Bilophodont molars of a tapir. (b) Mesiodistal section of tapir molars in occlusion. (c) Upper dentition of a tapir to show molarized premolars. (d) To illustrate how an enlarged hypoconulid of $M_3$ occludes with the distal side of $M^3$, in a similar way to that in which the trigonid of $M_3$ occludes with $M^2$. (e) Stages in the evolution of the last upper molar of the warthog. Additional cusps have been added at the distal end. The elephant molar (Fig. 10.16) was produced by a similar process.

in chewing it (Figs. 10.1, 12.15). Not all herbivores have a diastema, and its significance is not always the same. In rodents it is occupied by a fold of skin that can close the mouth off when the incisors are used for gnawing. In the rabbit it is the region where grass blades are arranged lengthways to be fed back along the molar row; the food passes down a tunnel between the tongue and the cheek while it is being chopped up by the molars. In the horse the diastema may be merely a by-product of the lengthened face, enabling the long-legged animal to crop from the ground.

OTHER HERBIVOROUS ADAPTATIONS

There is a great variety of herbivorous mammals, and almost every statement about them must be qualified by exceptions. Thus the pig, which is omnivorous rather than strictly herbivorous, has brachyodont molars covered with extremely thick enamel. Its teeth are used for crushing rather than grinding, as there is only a little transverse movement in chewing. The tapir has shearing molars of a special type. The cusps are joined in pairs to form sharp, cutting crests lying transversely (Fig. 10.17).

## JAW MUSCLES

During occlusal contact, vertical, lingual and mesial movements are combined in different ways: in carnivores the power stroke is more vertical than in insectivores, in ungulates lingual (transverse) movement predominates, and in rodents there is an important mesial component. The jaw muscles that produce these movements are much the same in all mammals as in man, but there are differences in their proportionate development. Thus the temporalis is the largest in carnivores and the masseter and pterygoids in ungulates (Fig. 10.18), while in rodents the horizontal fibres of the masseter are particularly well developed. No doubt these differences are correlated with the different chewing movements, but it must be remembered that jaw movements are also involved in operating the incisors and canines: in carnivores the temporalis would be important for snapping with the canines, and in rodents the masseter would be required to protude the jaw to bring the incisors into use. The tongue, lips and cheeks are important in feeding the mastication.

The jaw muscles influence the form of the skull and mandible. In carnivores there is a large coronoid process on which the temporalis is inserted, and strong sagittal and nuchal crests for the origin of the muscle. Not only is the masseter smaller than the temporalis, but its principal line of action passes nearer to the jaw joint, so that its moment arm is shorter (Fig. 10.18). In ungulates on the other hand the masseter is larger than the temporalis, and its moment arm is longer because the condyle is so much higher than the occlusal plane. Their smaller temporalis is associated with a smaller coronoid process and an absence or weak development of the sagittal crest.

Carnivores resemble primitive mammals in that the angle of the jaw is produced to form an angular process (see shrew and hedgehog, Fig. 10.1). This provides insertion, laterally, for the superficial part of the masseter, and medially for the medial pterygoid. In ungulates, however, there is no angular process, but the angle of the jaw is broadly expanded for insertion of the large masseter. Internally, there is an equally large medial pterygoid; the jaw is suspended in a sling formed by the two muscles (cf. Fig. 3.20), which move it from side to side during chewing.

In rodents, the mesial chewing movement is brought about by the masseter which pulls forwards. The length of the muscle has been increased by a backward extension of the angle of the jaw, and also by a forward extension of the origin of the muscle on the skull, anterior to the orbit; in many rodents slips of the muscle pass through the infraorbital canal to be attached on the face (Fig. 10.18).

## JAW JOINTS

The temporomandibular joint is a remarkable structure. It is not simply a hinge, allowing opening and closing of the jaws; it also enables the mandible to slide on the skull. The synovial cavity is divided by a disc into an upper cavity, by which the disc slides against the squamosal bone, and a lower cavity, which is a hinge joint between the disc and the mandible. Sliding movements are brought about by the lateral pterygoid muscle which is inserted into the disc as well as into the head of the mandible. Primitively the joint cavity extended down the posterior side of the head of the mandible, on to the postglenoid process (Fig. 12.25).

In carnivores the joint acts mainly as a hinge: the condyle is cylindrical and transversely elongated (Fig. 10.18); it fits into a deep groove in the squamosal, bounded both anteriorly and posteriorly by bony flanges, These flanges together with strong ligaments make the joint very hard to dislocate. It has been shown that in

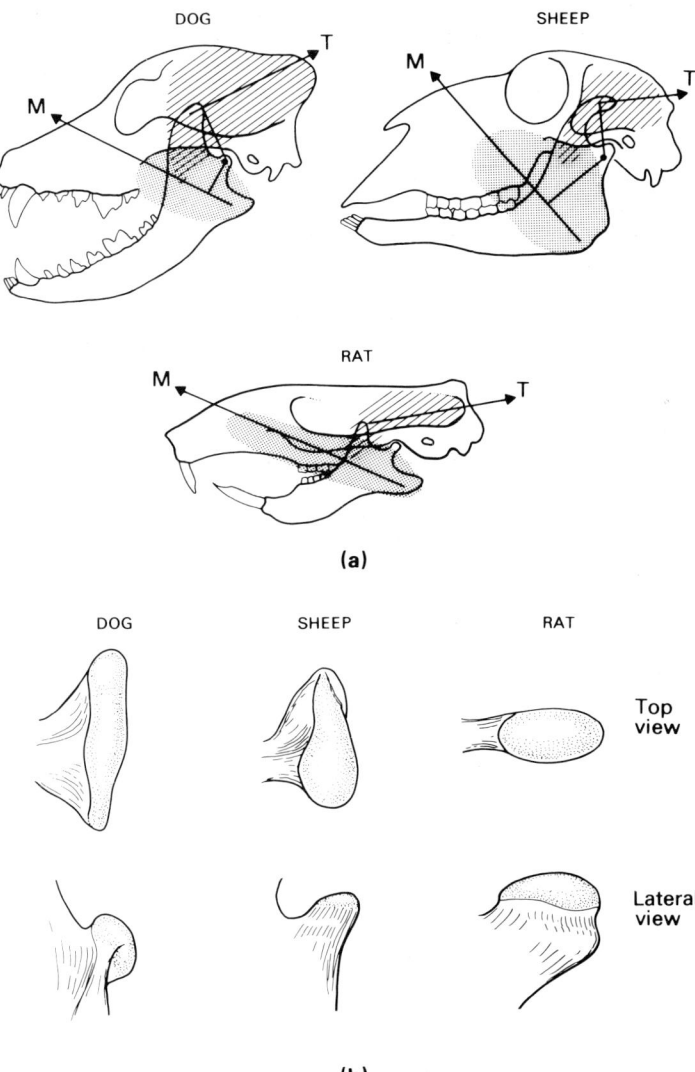

**Fig. 10.18.** Skulls of a carnivore (dog), an ungulate (sheep) and a rodent (rat), showing the spaces occupied by the temporal and masseter muscles. The main directions of pull are indicated. The temporal has a greater moment arm, in comparison with the masseter, in the carnivore than in the ungulate. In the rodent the muscles pull mainly in a fore and aft direction. (b) Condyles of the same animals, seen from above and laterally. Contrast the hinge of the dog with the freely sliding condyle of the sheep and the anteroposteriorly elongated condyle of the rat.

mammals the dislocating force produced when the cheek teeth are used is small, and this is true when the carnassials are in function. However, when a dog grips with its canines and tugs, often with considerable force, its jaw joints must be under much strain. Though the joint prohibits forward movement, it allows sufficient lateral movement for the carnassials on either side of the mouth to be brought into operation.

The jaw joints of ruminants on the contrary permit very free movement in all directions. The condyle slides against a flattened area of the skull and the joint is not constructed to withstand strains (Fig. 10.18). A small postglenoid process survives in the horse.

In rodents the condyle is elongated anteroposteriorly, and it slides anteroposteriorly in a longitudinal groove (Fig. 10.18).

From a functional point of view the teeth need to be seen not in isolation but as parts of a wider system. This includes besides muscles and bones the nervous system that controls feeding and chewing behaviour.

## FUNCTIONAL ASPECT OF DEVELOPMENT

### Morphology

It has already been mentioned that in the earliest

mammals the teeth had to be ground in before a good enough fit could be obtained to enable them to function efficiently. We have also seen that the use of enamel ridges for grinding presupposes an initial removal of the cusps. Clearly an animal would have a selective advantage if the development of teeth were controlled so that they fitted well even when newly erupted. It is especially so in primitive mammals with high cusps and sharp crests, where a poor fit would result in malfunction. It is not surprising therefore that there is a close correlation between the development of upper and lower teeth: teeth that are going to occlude grow at the same rate, they calcify and erupt together and have complementary shapes. Thus from a developmental as well as from a functional point of view the dentition behaves as a single organ; it is not just a collection of individual teeth.

### Replacement

In lower vertebrates the teeth are replaced continuously (polyphyodonty). At any given time the dentition is made up of teeth at all stages of development. Replacement takes place in waves, but only alternate teeth belong to one wave; thus numbers 1, 3, 5, 7 are replaced in order, and numbers 2, 4, 6, 8 are also replaced in order, but the even-numbered wave is completely out of phase with the odd-numbered wave (Fig. 8.12). This ensures that adjacent teeth are not replaced together: while number 5 is being replaced numbers 4 and 6 are firmly attached. Gaps are therefore avoided (Fig. 10.19a). The life of each tooth is short (about 4 months in a lizard), and an indefinite number of teeth is formed successively at each tooth location. Such teeth, that replace each other, form a tooth family. As the animal grows and the jaws lengthen, additional tooth families appear at the distal end.

This system is eminently suited to dentitions composed of numerous simple teeth that do not occlude, but would be unworkable in mammals. In mammals the teeth are complex and develop slowly; never more than two successive teeth are formed at a single location (diphyodonty) and in the molar region only one. Moreover, mammalian teeth have precise occlusal relations, such that each tooth occludes with two adjacent teeth in the opposite jaw; alternating replacement would make occlusion inefficient, for unworn teeth would have to occlude with worn teeth. In cynodonts like *Thrinaxodon*, where upper and lower postcanines do not meet, the teeth are still replaced alternately, but the number of replacements is reduced to at most three (Fig. 10.19b). In broad-toothed cynodonts in which occlusion has developed alternation is lost and the teeth are replaced in order. Cynodonts added new tooth families at the back of the jaw throughout life, at the same time losing teeth in the region immediately behind the

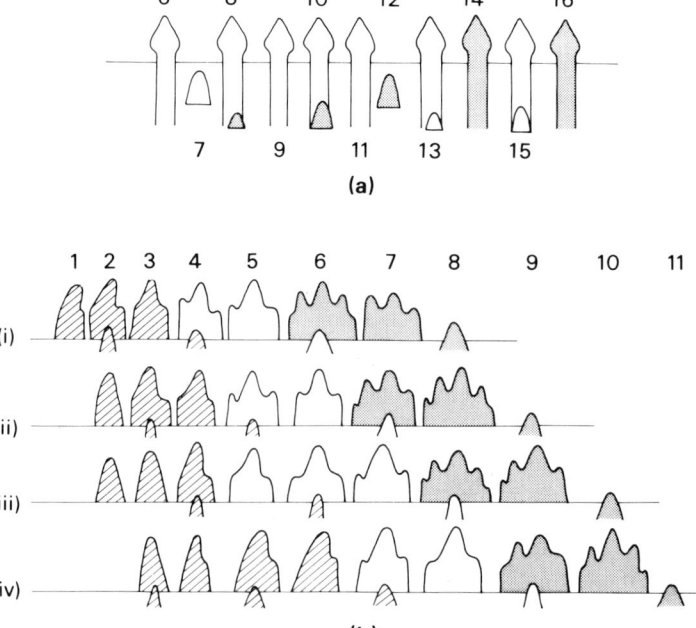

**Fig. 10.19.** (a) Part of the lower dentition of a lizard to show typical reptilian replacement. A wave of replacement can be seen in the even-numbered teeth (shaded), out of step with that of odd-numbered teeth. (b) Diagrammatic representation of replacement of the cheek teeth in a cynodont such as *Thrinaxodon*; (i)–(iv) are dentitions at different ages. Alternate teeth are replaced approximately together, and new tooth families are added at the back while the most mesial families are lost. The 'molars' are replaced by less complex 'premolars', so that the most complex teeth are always found near the posterior end of the dentition. To reach the mammalian condition, replacement must have become less frequent, so that the more mesial teeth (= deciduous teeth) were replaced once and the more distal ones (= permanent molars) not at all.

canine. Mammals cease to grow once they reach their adult size, and confine tooth eruption and replacement to the juvenile growing period.

**The deciduous dentition**

Most young vertebrates need teeth as soon as they are hatched, indeed in many amniotes before hatching an egg-tooth at the tip of the premaxilla is used to cut open the eggshell. Young mammals are fed on milk, and eruption of their first teeth is delayed. It is not known when the milk glands first evolved, but the youngest known specimens of cynodonts already have erupted teeth. Exceptional among mammals are the bats, which have hooked deciduous incisors used for clinging to the mother (Fig. 12.2), and the guinea-pig, which is born at a surprisingly advanced stage of development, with teeth already erupted.

The deciduous dentition has to perform the same functions as the permanent dentition, but in shorter jaws in which there is room for fewer teeth. The last deciduous tooth always functions as a molar and is molariform in pattern; the more mesial deciduous teeth are like premolars. Thus the human infant has one 'premolar' (D) and one 'molar' (E) in short jaws, which function like the two premolars and three molars of the permanent dentition in long jaws. In young carnivores the carnassials are $Dm^3$ and $Dm_4$, one place forward from the permanent carnassials, $P^4$ and $M_1$ (Fig. 10.20), but in relation to the length of the jaw the deciduous carnassials stand in the same position as the permanent carnassials: $Dm^4$, is molariform, biting against the talonid of $Dm_4$.

Sometimes the deciduous teeth fail to develop. Marsupial young remain for some time in the pouch, attached to a nipple, and nearly all their deciduous teeth are rudimentary; only the most posterior one, which (as always) is molariform, becomes functional. In seals the rudimentary deciduous teeth are shed before birth, and in shrews they do not develop beyond the epithelial bud stage. The rat and mouse have no premolars and so (by definition) no deciduous molars; the deciduous incisors are embryonic rudiments.

**The mixed dentition**

As the animal grows it needs more cheek teeth, and at the same time its jaws are getting longer; additional teeth develop distally to the deciduous dentition. These are the permanent molars, but they function for a time with the deciduous teeth, so they can be regarded as late-developing members of the deciduous dentition. Replacement of the deciduous molars by (permanent) premolars takes place after the eruption of the second molars (man is an exception) and sometimes of the third molars. In primitive insectivorous mammals the deciduous molars are replaced from behind forwards: Dm 4 – Dm 3 – Dm 2. Dm 1 is usually not replaced, but persists into the permanent dentition.

The first lower permanent molar begins by occluding with the last upper deciduous molar

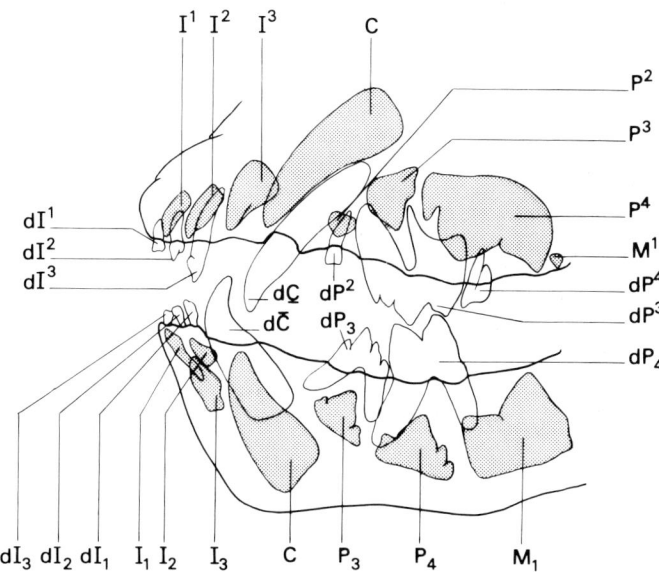

Fig. 10.20. Dentition of a lion cub, with deciduous teeth in place and permanent dentition ready to erupt. The deciduous carnassials ($dP^3$ and $dP_4$) are not the direct predecessors of the permanent carnassials ($P^4$ and $M_1$).

($Dm^4$), and when that is replaced it occludes with the last premolar ($P^4$). Hence the distal part of $P^4$ needs to resemble the distal part of $Dm^4$. However in carnivores $P^4$ is a carnassial but $Dm^4$ is a molariform tooth; the eruption of $M_1$ is therefore retarded till $Dm^4$ has been replaced, and $M_1$ can assume its carnassial function with $P^4$ (Fig. 10.20).

**Longevity**

Once the permanent dentition is in position it has to last for the rest of the animal's life. The length of life therefore depends upon the durability of the teeth. The smallest mammals live for only a year or two, but man and the elephant can survive for half a century or more.

The elephant has the largest molars of any mammal. They are so large that not more than two teeth can be in use in the jaw at any one time. Instead of the 'vertical' replacement seen in nearly every vertebrate, the teeth are replaced 'horizontally'. Each tooth, as it wears down, moves towards the mesial end of the jaw, the place it occupied being gradually taken over by the next more distal tooth (Fig. 10.21). The process goes on

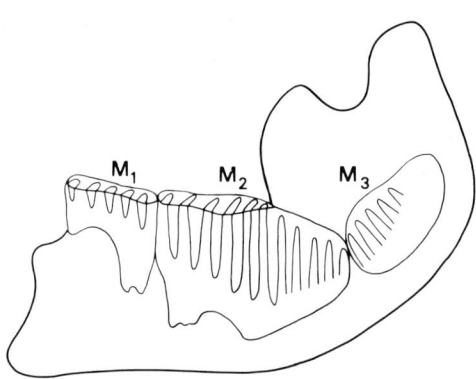

Fig. 10.21. Jaw of an elephant, with the fourth cheek tooth ($M_1$) mainly worn away, $M_2$ moving forward to take its place, and $M_3$ developing inside the ascending ramus. The teeth are represented as if sectioned mesiodistally. Note that $M_2$ while being worn at the front is still developing at the back. As well as moving mesially, the teeth are also erupting to keep the occlusal surface at a constant level.

continuously throughout life. Six teeth develop successively in each half-jaw, corresponding to the three deciduous molars and three permanent molars of other mammals. The continuous forward movement of the teeth seems to be an exaggeration of the process of mesial drift.

Horizontal replacement also occurs in the manatee, a marine animal (order Sirenia) distantly related to the elephant. Its molars are brachyodont, and an indefinite number of them develops, new ones being formed at the back throughout life while worn teeth fall out at the front.

Hypsodont cheek teeth, like those of the rabbit, that never develop roots, continue to grow as fast as they are worn, and so their wear does not limit the length of the animal's life; the life-span of rabbits must be controlled by other factors.

The long survival of man with his brachyodont teeth is less easy to understand. Human molars have low cusps, covered with very thick enamel which resists wear. After dentine is exposed, enamel ridges continue to function, even when only the marginal enamel wall remains. Though the cusps are low, the marginal ridges of human teeth are strongly developed. No doubt a major factor is that much of our food is softened by cooking.

## AGEING

In the previous section the evolution of mammalian molars has been described. The advantage of the mammalian dentition is that the teeth can slice and grind food into easily digested particles, a process which is not possible with the dentitions of most other vertebrates.

However, the action of grinding food leads to the loss of tooth substance. While this benefits the dentition by maintaining a good fit, and therefore free grinding movements, between opposing teeth it is possible for the wear to be so rapid and excessive that within a year no tooth substance is left (for example, in shrews) and the animal can no longer feed. Therefore, in describing age changes in the human dentition, we first consider attrition of the teeth and the response of the dentition to this attrition.

**Attrition**

The amount of attrition is related to the length of time a tooth has been functioning, the consistency of the food and the hardness of the teeth. For example, Aborigines and Eskimos put their teeth to such vigorous use that in some old individuals they may be worn down to the gum margin. But most European diets contain little roughage with the result that, even in the oldest members of the community, the majority of the tooth crown is still present although the cusps may have been worn flat. Because it has been longest in the mouth the first permanent molar is nearly always the most heavily worn of the permanent molars. It is possible to assess the coarseness of a diet by studying the difference in attrition between the first and third molars of a young adult. With a very coarse diet the occlusal surface of the first molar may have been completely flattened before the third molar has fully erupted. The coarser the diet the greater is the difference between the attrition of these teeth.

Obviously the cusps, the high points on an occlusal surface, are the first to wear. The cuspal dentine becomes exposed and is surrounded by a rim of enamel. The exposed (softer) dentine wears more than the (harder) enamel with the result that a worn cusp is surmounted by a shallow dentine crater rimmed by higher enamel. After considerably more wear the original pulp horn might be exposed were it not for the fact that secondary dentine is laid down (Fig. 6.10). This secondary dentine readily picks up stains and often appears as a dark brown core within the exposed primary dentine which is denser and less easily stained. Similar appearances can be seen on heavily worn incisors and canines.

With the loss of several millimetres of tooth substance the jaws can be brought closer together before the teeth come into contact. In some individuals this increased closure, together with wear of the biting edges of the incisors which eliminates the normal overbite, allows the mandible to slide forward so that during chewing upper and lower incisors may be edge to edge. In other individuals the loss of tooth substance is compensated by active eruption of the teeth so that the jaws are not 'overclosed'.

Because each tooth is 'independently suspended' in its socket, touching teeth rub against each other during chewing and the (mesiodistal) contact points of the young become worn into contact areas. The resultant potential separation between adjacent teeth is compensated by mesial drift (Fig. 9.24).

Due to their soft diets, the teeth of Europeans are often little worn with the result that the cusps and fissures of the upper and lower cheek teeth do not become ground down into accurately matching surfaces. The inaccuracies hinder free movement between cusps during chewing. A minority consider that this cuspal interference is an important cause of pathologies of the periodontal ligament and temporomandibular joint. In their view our 'civilized' diet is the ultimate cause of the diseases: a coarse diet would produce sufficient tooth wear to allow free grinding movements. However, this interpretation may not take sufficient account of the fact that each tooth is independently suspended in the jaws. Teeth which are under little or no strain erupt and twist into new positions whereas those which are most heavily loaded are pushed into positions where they take less strain. Within limits, it seems probable that the teeth are constantly undergoing minor movements which tend to spread out the masticatory load more evenly.

**Enamel**

The most important age change in enamel is its loss due to attrition: unlike other tissues which are damaged by wear, the dental tissues cannot be naturally replaced. Much of the work in dentistry involves procedures for replacing lost dental tissues by artificial tissues. Apart from the biting and interstitial surfaces, enamel is also worn away from the buccal and lingual surfaces of teeth so that the perikymata are lost.

It seems probable that, due to its very low content of organic material, and its near isolation from the blood vascular system, age changes within the enamel would be almost entirely physicochemical with little or no opportunity for biological repair or modification of the changes.

Treated as a purely physicochemical problem, alteration in the structure and properties of enamel would be brought about by the diffusion of reactive materials into its substance. Diffusion is measured by permeability studies. Dyes or radioactive isotopes (for example) can be sealed on to the enamel surface or inside the pulp cavity of extracted teeth and their rates and directions of movement studied in ground sections. These studies have shown that small molecules and ions can slowly diffuse inwards and outwards through young human enamel. Larger molecules can diffuse through the dentine and only into tufts and lamellae of the enamel. With age the enamel rapidly becomes increasingly less permeable indicating that there must have been changes in either its structure or composition.

Little is known of any structural changes in ageing enamel. It has been suggested that the surface enamel may be different from the remaining enamel because of an effect similar to work-hardening in which the repeated compressions caused by mastication alter its molecular structure.

Changes in enamel composition have been studied by microanalysis. Unfortunately the results are often conflicting. However, there is agreement that with age there is an increase in fluoride in the surface enamel.

Finally, the enamel in old people often seems discoloured and may contain fine hairline fractures. The change in colour may be due to (a) an undetected change in composition (b) a darkening of the underlying dentine which is seen through the enamel or (c) a thinning of the enamel which renders the yellower dentine more visible. Hairline fractures could develop in the following way. With age the dentine may lose enough of its water content to contract away from the enamel: the now unsupported enamel splits and organic debris from the saliva fills and then stains the crack.

**Dentine**

Although dentine and pulp constitute a single functional unit it is easier to describe their age changes separately.

Many of the age changes associated with dentine have been described in the section on dentine structure: physiological (regular) secondary dentine, pathological (irregular) secondary dentine, translucent dentine, dead tracts, and pulp stones are all found to increase with age but it is sometimes difficult to assess whether, at a given site, they are normal age changes or responses to abnormal stimuli.

Physiological secondary dentine which continues to be formed throughout life seems clearly to be related to normal ageing of the dentine. If attrition is normal then any response to attrition, be it the formation of secondary dentines, dead tracts or translucent dentine, must be considered a normal age change. But these reactions also develop in response to caries, for example. This suggests that the pulp (a truly vital tissue) has a selection of reactions which are seen as changes in the dentine but which may be activated either in response to the normal 'stimulus' of age or to abnormal stimuli. It should be noted that physiological secondary dentine is thickest on the floor and roof of the pulp chamber and that translucent dentine gradually spreads from the root apex towards the crown. It is not known whether the formation of translucent dentine is biologically controlled by the pulp or whether it is a physicochemical reaction of the dentine. The spread of translucent dentine may make the root more brittle and account for the clinical observation that it is sometimes very easy to fracture the teeth of the elderly during extraction. The narrowing of the periodontium also contributes to extraction difficulties.

**Pulp**

Because dentine continues to be formed throughout life it is clear that the size of the pulp decreases. It is sometimes necessary to remove the pulp of a tooth and fill it with an inert material, a process known as 'root filling'. This procedure can be very difficult in elderly patients who, due to age changes, have a tiny, constricted pulp chamber and a thread-like pulp canal, all that is left of the plump, richly vascular pulp cavity of the young tooth. The apical foramina also become constricted with age both by secondary dentine and by cement.

Histologically, the old pulp tissue looks very different from the delicate network of reticulin fibres interspersed with plump stellate fibroblasts seen in the young. The proportion of mature collagen increases with a reciprocal decrease in the number of fibroblasts and odontoblasts. The odontoblast layer often contains intra- and intercellular vacuoles ('wheatsheafing' of the odontoblasts) (Fig. 6.29d). With increasing age the whole pulp contains more and larger vacuoles separated by a reticular network of collagen fibres—the condition of reticular atrophy. The number of vessels and nerve fibres is reduced, the latter accounting for the observed decrease in tooth sensitivity.

For a few years after it has erupted, the pulp continues to possess a sub-odontoblast layer of cells which seem to be some form of satellite layer aiding the odontoblasts during dentinogenesis. Later, this cell layer is either lost or displaced, its position in the normal adult tooth being taken by the cell-free layer of Weil beneath which is the cell-rich layer (Fig. 6.29).

It seems reasonable to argue that many of the above changes in the ageing pulp are the result of changes in its blood supply. The apical foramen becomes constricted by the continued deposition of dentine and cement. This narrowing of the vascular lifeline may progressively restrict the blood supply to the pulp and could account for the marked reduction in pulpal vessels which takes place with age: this reduction can be demonstrated by injection techniques (Fig. 10.22).

Alternatively, the reduction in blood supply could be the result of arteriosclerosis, a condition whose onset is related to ageing and which has been demonstrated in pulpal vessels. As the next link in the chain of events, the reduced number of pulpal vessels can support fewer cells and less active metabolism of the remaining cells. The reduced metabolism leads to a slowing down in collagen turnover, particularly collagen degrada-

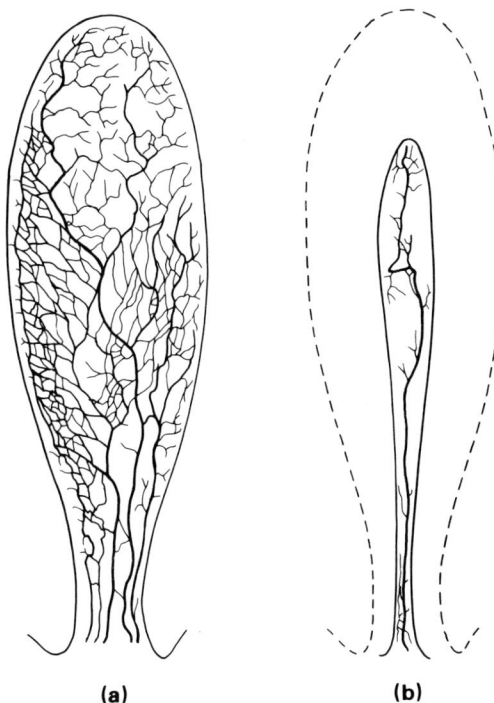

**Fig. 10.22.** Comparison between (a) young pulp and (b) old pulp.

tion, with the result that the pulp becomes increasingly fibrous. If the above explanation for pulpal changes is correct, we might expect a progressive decrease in the rate of secondary dentine formation and in the ability of the pulp to respond to external stimuli.

The wretched histological appearance of reticular atrophy seen in an elderly pulp can partly be produced in a young pulp by poor fixation. Because the apical foramen is small it may take so long for fixatives to penetrate into the pulp chamber that many cells die giving a false appearance of sparse cellularity and moribund cells.

Diffuse calcific changes and the number of pulp stones increase with age so that they may be considered as age changes although young pulps can be severely affected. Both have been described earlier (p. 173).

**Dental supporting tissues**

For developmental and functional reasons it is normal to consider the pulp and dentine as the two parts of a single unit. For the same reasons cement and the periodontal ligament (at least its inner layers) can also be considered to be two parts of a single unit; the dentally derived supporting tissues (as opposed to those derived from the jaws).

There seems to be an optimum width of the periodontal ligament (about 0.15–0.35 mm). Too wide a ligament allows the tooth too much movement during chewing with the result that the soft tissues are damaged and the hard tissues cannot be kept in good repair. However, in a very narrow ligament a slight movement of the tooth causes a much greater compression of tissues (with resultant damage) than would the same movement in a thicker periodontium. The optimum thickness may be a balance between the two extremes.

The width of the periodontal ligament is locally controlled by its cells, probably in response to masticatory forces. It can be narrowed by the deposition of either bone or cement but, generally speaking, it can only be widened by the resorption of bone. Cement seems to be protected from resorption.

Cement continues to be formed throughout life and therefore, because it is only infrequently resorbed, the root of a tooth becomes increasingly more stout. Although for large numbers of teeth it is possible to demonstrate a linear relationship between cement thickness and age, the thickness by itself is not a reliable guide to age because the deposition of cement is too much influenced by functional stresses applied to the tooth and by periodontal disease.

It seems probable that the intermittent but continued deposition of cement is necessary in order to maintain a sufficient number of viable Sharpey fibres for tooth attachment. Obviously, these can only be incorporated into newly formed cement layers where they become part of the cement matrix. However, most teeth show one or two isolated small patches of cement resorption and subsequent repair (equivalent to reversal lines in bone; Fig. 6.45). They are probably regions in which a previous injury has been healed.

Due to active eruption in response to occlusal attrition the tooth moves out of the alveolar bone. It is in those parts of a tooth which erupt directly away from the bone (as opposed to sliding past the bone), its root apex and interradicular dentine, that cement is normally thickest.

Permeability studies have shown that young cement is only barely permeable to dyes sealed in the pulp cavity: subsequently it becomes impermeable from this direction. However, young cement is readily permeated through its full thickness by dyes sealed on to the surface of the root but as the cement thickens so its deeper layers become increasingly impermeable. This suggests why the lacunae in old cement do not appear to contain viable cells: the deep cementocytes die because food and metabolites can no longer diffuse into and out of the deeper layers. Either the main diffusion channels, the canaliculi, become blocked, or it requires too long for materials to diffuse to and from the periodontal ligament through a thick layer of cement.

Continued and heavy stress on a tooth leads to a thickening of the periodontal ligament followed by loosening and ultimate loss of the tooth. However, within the limits which can be tolerated by the attachment tissues, the heavier the stresses the thicker is the ligament. In studies of large numbers it has been shown that the older an individual, the narrower is the ligament. It can therefore be argued that the narrower periodontal ligament usually seen in elderly people is related to a reduction in the forces which they apply during mastication. Perhaps the actual width is the result of a balance between, on the one hand, an inherent tendency to form bone and cement thereby narrowing the ligament and, on the other hand, biting forces which move the tooth in its socket thereby inhibiting the formation of mineralized tissues and sometimes promoting their resorption with a consequent widening of the ligament.

Throughout life the junctional epithelium continues to creep apically over the root surface. The movement is due to both active eruption which compensates for occlusal attrition and passive eruption which may be brought about in the following way.

Even in the apparently healthiest gingiva there are many inflammatory cells: they indicate a continuing reaction to oral bacteria and their toxins. Since these bacteria are normal the reactions which they evoke may be considered to be normal rather than pathological. The bacterial toxins. Since these bacteria are normal, the reformation of new collagen necessary to compensate for its normal turnover. The loss of the coronal periodontal fibres allows the downgrowth of junctional epithelium which is characteristic of passive eruption.

**Forensic**

Being the most durable of all biological tissues, teeth have proved to be exceptionally important in the recognition of decayed or mutilated bodies. The state of the dentition can be used to determine the approximate age of an individual.

Up to the age of about 20 years the state of the developing and erupting teeth gives a very good idea of an individual's age. In the young, radiographs are particularly valuable in making such estimates. After this time, when all the teeth have erupted and their apices have closed, a good estimate can be made of an individual's age by quantifying the extent to which the following five features differ from their appearance in a newly erupted tooth: (a) the amount of attrition, (b) the position of the epithelial attachment, (c) the thickness of secondary dentine, (d) the extent to which translucent dentine has spread coronally from the root apex, and (e) the thickness of cement. Of these, (c), (d) and (e) are best studied in longitudinal ground sections while (a) and (b) can be seen on any extracted tooth. Each feature is 'scored' from 0–3 where 0 is the score for a newly erupted tooth and 3 for a very aged tooth. Thus a single tooth might score 2 for attrition, 1 for epithelial attachment, 3 for secondary dentine, 1 for translucent dentine and 2 for cement, giving a total of 9. The age of a tooth with a score of 9 can be estimated from published tables. In practice, greater accuracy is achieved if a worker constructs personal tables from his own studies of a large number of teeth of a known age. The tables then take account of the particular bias he gives to measurements.

## FURTHER READING

MILES, A.E.W. (1976) Age changes in dental tissues. In *Scientific foundation of dentistry*, Eds. Cohen B. and Kramer I.R.H., London: Heinemann.

# CHAPTER 11

# Evolution of Man

## THE PRIMATES

The great Swedish naturalist, Linnaeus, knew nothing of evolutionary theory when he developed his hierarchical system for classifying animals and plants, published as *Systema Naturae* in 1758. Linnaeus had recognized that some animals resemble each other more than they resemble others and argued that the greater the resemblance, the closer the basic relationship. It was, therefore, no accident that he grouped the monkeys with man in a single order, Primates. Linnaeus' views on man's, and the monkeys', place in the scheme of things is reflected in his choice of ordinal name; 'primate' is derived from *primus* meaning first. This basic similarity between monkeys and men was not explained until a century later. Darwin published his treatise *The Origin of Species* in 1858. This not only propounded the fact of evolution but was the first scientific attempt to explain its mechanics. The inescapable inference that men and monkeys had a common ancestor caused a furore in Victorian society since the idea of 'special creation', at least for man, was then still widely accepted. The publication of the 'Origin' led to major changes in the philosophy of what were then new sciences, palaeontology and geology. In the last century the study of animals in their natural habitats was largely confined to the casual observations of explorers collecting specimens for the world's great museums. Today, two centuries after Linnaeus, we are beginning to understand the interrelationships between the structure of an animal, its behaviour and its environment. Even so, whilst the fossil evidence documenting the stages in the evolution of the primates and of man continues to accumulate, the nature of the selective pressures which produced the changes leading through each stage, remain almost entirely a matter for informed speculation.

### The order Primates

Living organisms have a distribution in both space and time. Primates are known to have evolved from a group of insectivorous early placental mammals between 70–80 million years ago (Fig. 11.1). Since then the distribution of the order has fluctuated widely with changes in equatorial and continental position.

Non-human primates are currently found in most vegetated equatorial and tropical regions of the world (Fig. 11.2). There is palaeoecological evidence which suggests that primates have always inhabited the warm forested and savanna areas of the earth's surface. It is recent man that has extended his range outside this basic primate habitat by his capacity to at least partially control his immediate environment.

When the earliest recognisable primates first evolved, or even shortly before, one group split away from the main stock and developed into the tree-shrews (Tupaiidae) (Fig. 11.1), which are now found only in South-east Asia. The exact status of these small insectivorous mammals is controversial. Some authorities consider they should be classified as Insectivora since their molars have the highly adapted dilambdadont pattern found in some members of that order (Fig. 10.14). Others consider the tree-shrews good 'living ancestors' for all other primates on the basis of their general anatomy. On the evidence of their blood proteins, the tree-shrews are no more closely related to the Insectivora than they are to the Primates. On balance, it seems more appropriate to consider them representative of the ancient primate stock and so to include them in the order.

There are two main divisions (suborders) of primates: the Prosimii and the Anthropoidea. In German the prosimians are called 'Halbaffen' which freely translates as 'half-monkeys', giving a clear idea of their status. The living members of the group (Fig. 11.1, Table 11.1) are the lemurs of Madagascar (Lemuriformes); the galagos and lorises of Africa and Asia (Lorisiformes); and the tarsier, a single genus *Tarsius*, found in the East Indies. Both lemurs and lorises are thought to have evolved from a group represented by *Adapis*, a well-known fossil lemuroid from Europe. The tarsier could well have evolved from another

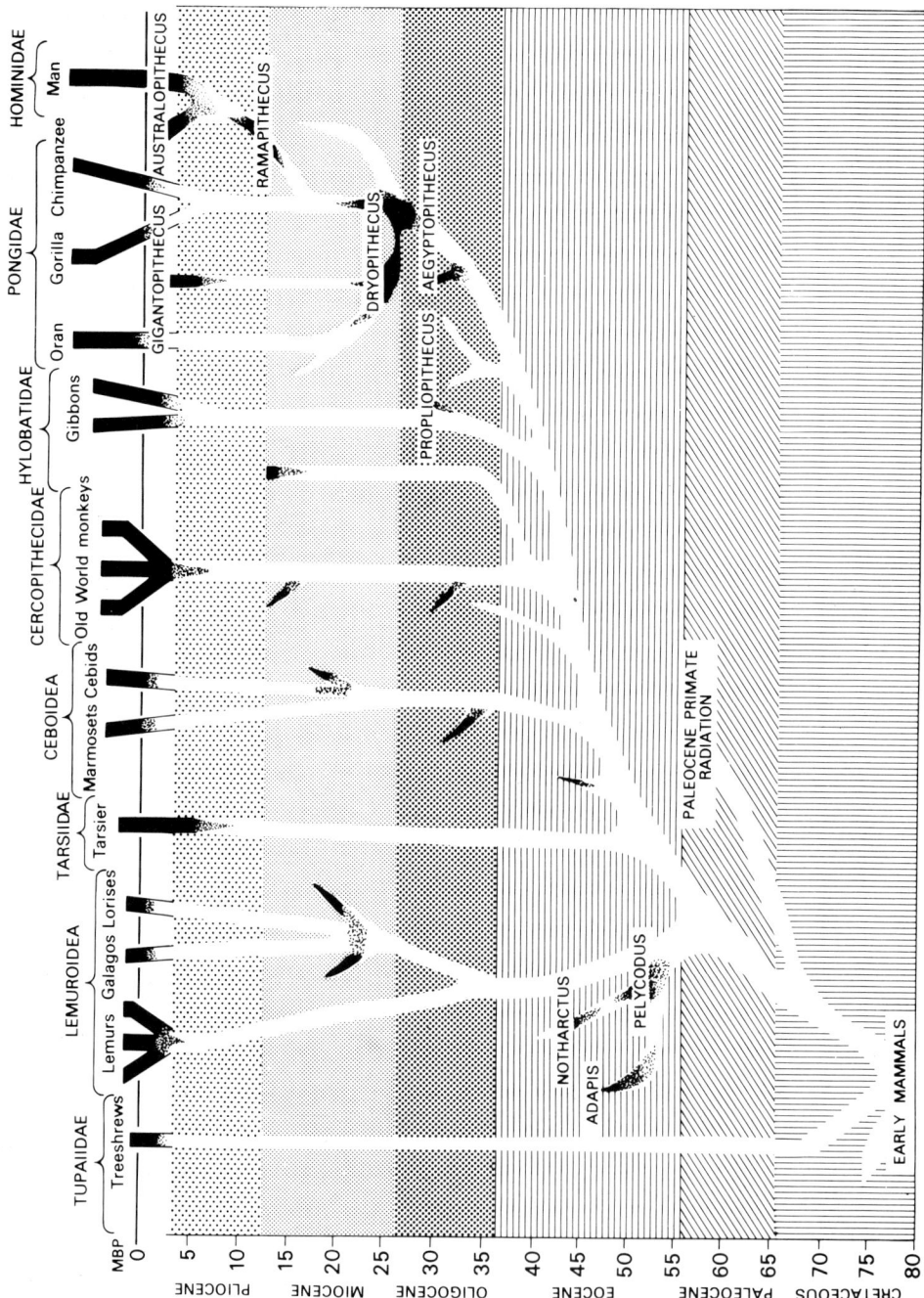

**Fig. 11.1.** The phylogeny of the primates. Living primates (top of figure) form a morphological sequence grading from the most primitive, the treeshrews, to the most advanced, man. (This is the so-called 'scala naturae'.) Each living group is however the product of its own evolutionary history (bottom part of figure) although all (save the treeshrews) have evolved from the same group of early Cretaceous mammals. Extant and major fossil forms are shown in black. Some possible alternative phylogenies are indicated: for example some authorities would regard the Eocene lemuroid forms (*Adapis*, *Pseudoloris*, *Notharctus* and *Pelycodus*) as a much more closely related group than shown here. (MBP, millions of years before present.)

# Evolution of Man

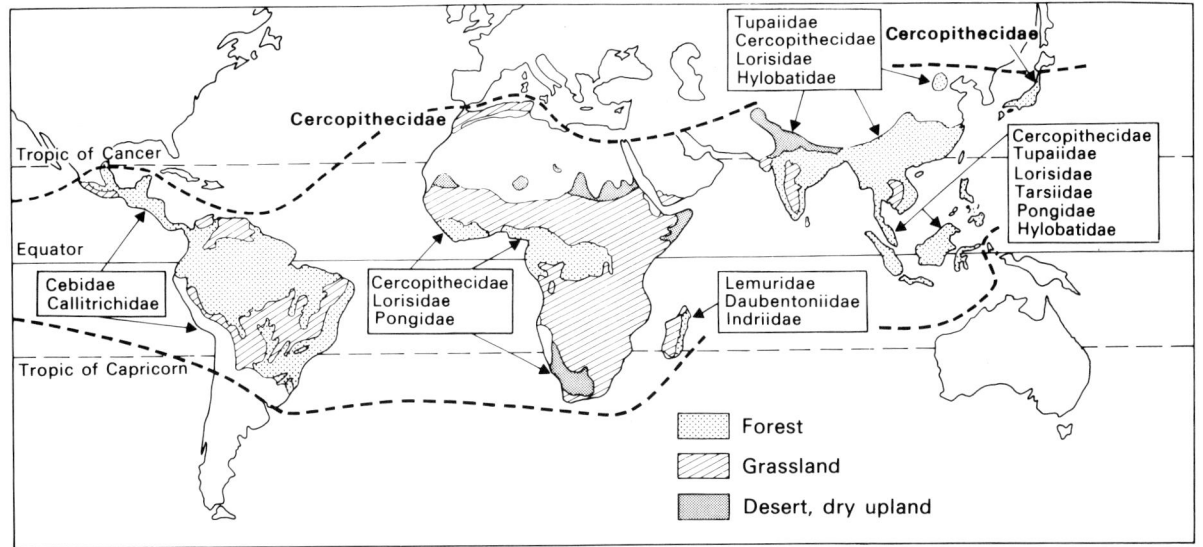

**Fig. 11.2.** The current distribution of non-human primates is restricted to areas within the equatorial, tropical and subtropical belts outlined by the heavy dotted lines, familial names (see Table 11.1) of the groups found in each major area are shown. Areas within the belts are desert, high mountains or otherwise uninhabitable by primates. *Forest* includes tropical rain forest, swamp forest, mangrove, secondary forest, deciduous forest (temperate and tropical), monsoon forest and montane forest. *Grassland* (Savanna and steppe) includes forest outliers, gallery forest, wooded steppe, thorn forest, Mediterranean scrub and montane meadow.

European form *Pseudoloris*. Little is known of the history of the lemurs until the Pleistocene. By this time the group were isolated on Madagascar where, free of competition from more advanced primates, three distinct groups evolved: the Lemuridae, including the small generalized quadrupedal lemurs which feed primarily on insects or fruit: the Indriidae, which are large long-legged and agile leaping forms feeding on leaves and, lastly, the single aberrant rodent-like aye-aye (*Daubentonia*) (see Table 11.1). There is evidence that there were also numerous large semi-terrestrial and arboreal forms which, like the dodo, became extinct in historical time as a result of human depredation.

The tarsier is considered the most 'monkey-like' of the prosimians since it closely resembles the anthropoids in a number of cranial and dental features: for example, the short snout, the front-facing orbits, the structure of the middle ear and in its brain/body size ratio. These resemblances could reflect a common ancestry for the tarsioids and anthropoids or, alternatively, result from convergent evolution, the two groups developing quite independently from lemuroid stocks. Which explanation is the correct one is not yet clear. However, several animals adapted for a nocturnal insectivorous habit like that of *Tarsius* are known from the Eocene of Europe.

There is little doubt about the independent origin of the New World (Ceboidea) and Old World (Cercopithecoidea) monkeys. The former, now found across Latin America from Panama south to Paraguay and Southern Brazil, almost certainly evolved from a North American lemuroid or tarsioid stock. In the Miocene the group split producing the two modern families; the Callithricidae and the more advanced Cebidae (see Table 11.1). Unlike their Old World counterparts, the cebids have never evolved a terrestrial form nor anything approaching the ape grade of primate organization (Fig. 11.1).

The history of the Old World monkeys is poorly understood. A few fossil cercopithecoids are known from the Oligocene and Miocene of Africa but not of Asia. On present evidence it appears that apes were very much commoner than monkeys in Africa between 20–30 million years ago (in a ratio of 20:1). This is the reverse of the present situation. It has been suggested that the cercopithecoids first evolved in Europe and then migrated into Africa and across southern Asia. A more likely explanation is that these monkeys evolved in Africa at about the same time as the first

**Table 11.1.** (continued)

| | Common name and typical genera | Present distribution | Habitat | Diet | Activity | Locomotion |
|---|---|---|---|---|---|---|
| CERCOPITHECOIDEA Colobinae | Colobines: *Colobus* | Africa | Tropical forest, upper and middle storey | Leaf-eaters | Diurnal | Arm swinging, leaping. Quadrupedal. |
| | Langurs: *Presbytis* | Asia | | | | |
| Hylobatidae (Lesser Apes) | Gibbon: *Hylobates* | S.E. Asia Philippines | Tropical rain forest | 80% fruit 20% leaves, buds, flowers. | Diurnal | Arboreal True brachiation. No leg movement, arm swinging. Bipedal on ground. |
| | Siamang *Symphalangus* | Malay Peninsula Sumatra | | Predominantly leaves | | |
| HOMINOIDEA Pongidae (Great Apes) | Orang: *Pongo pygmaeus* | Sumatra Borneo | Tropical rain forest | Fruit, some leaves, bark, birds, eggs | Diurnal | Modified braclination. Four-handed climbing. O much larger than O. |
| | Chimpanzee: *Pan paniscus Pan troglodytes* | Central Africa | Tropical forest | Fruit, leaves and wide range other items | Diurnal | 50–75% time in trees. Knuckle walk on ground. Modified brachiation in trees. |
| | Gorilla: *Gorilla gorilla* | Equatorial Africa (Highlands in East, Lowlands in West.) | Montane and Tropical rain forest | Wholly vegetation. (Leaves, bark, buds etc.) | Diurnal | 90% time on ground when knuckle walk. Young move in trees. |
| Hominidae (Man and his ancestors) | Man: *Homo Homo erectus Homo sapiens* | Now ubiquitous ? origin in East Africa. | Ubiquitous | Omnivorous | Diurnal | Terrestrial Bipedal |

apes but had a much later adaptive radiation, probably in the Pliocene. This resulted in the appearance of two main groups: the highly specialized colobines or 'leaf-eating' monkeys and the more diversified macaque group which includes many arboreal forms as well as the terrestrially adapted patas monkeys, baboons and geladas.

There are three extant 'great' apes (Pongidae): the chimpanzee and the gorilla, both found in equatorial Africa, and the orang utan, now restricted to Borneo and Sumatra. The gibbon and its close relative, the siamang, (Hylobatidae) are frequently referred to as 'lesser' apes. They have a wide distribution throughout South-east Asia. The earliest known unequivocal fossil 'apes' were found in the Fayum in Egypt and date from 25–30 MBP (millions of years before present). Of these some authorities consider *Propliopithecus*, on dental grounds, to be ancestral to the gibbons and *Aegyptopithecus* to the great apes and man. About 5 million years later the descendants of the '*Aegyptopithecus* stock' had developed into a group of apes of various sizes all classified in a single family, Dryopithecidae. Dryopithecines have been found in Miocene beds in Africa, Eurasia and in the Indian subcontinent. *Dryopithecus* had most of the dental characteristics associated with the great apes (Table 11.3). In contrast, *Ramapithecus*, a slightly more recent fossil (9–12 MBP), possibly descended from an as yet unknown member of the *Dryopithecus* group, had teeth sufficiently unlike those of the pongids and like those of man and his immediate ancestors (Hominidae) for it to be, arguably, the earliest known member of the human lineage (Fig. 11.1).

PRIMATE HABITATS

With few exceptions, primates are arboreal. Tropical forests contain a number of distinct primate habitats, each with its own food sources. This explains why different types of primates eating the same type of diet, as well as primates of the same group but with slightly different diets, can inhabit the same geographical area without direct competition (Table 11.1, Fig. 11.3). All forested areas have two main 'habitat strata': the forest floor

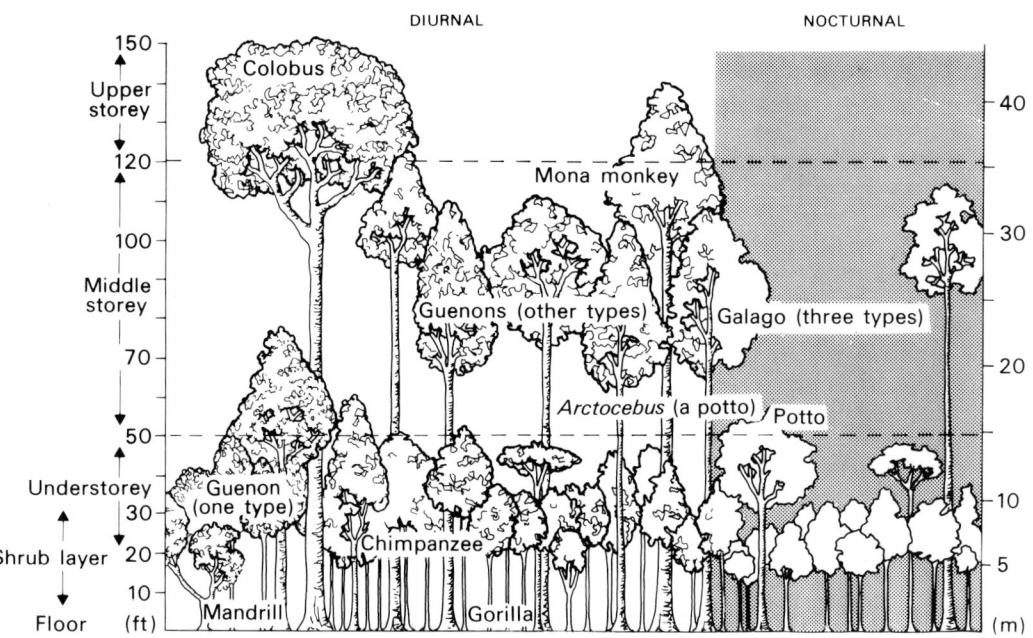

**Fig. 11.3.** To illustrate how the horizontal stratification of tropical rain forest creates sufficient different habitats or 'ecological niches' to support a number of primates each with slightly different diets and behaviour within the same area. The forest has four main levels: the floor, the shrub layer (up to 30 ft) overlaps the continuous layer of the understorey (25–50 ft); lateral contact occurs between trees in the middle storey (50–120 ft) but the upper storey (120–150 ft) contains only isolated trees. Colobus monkeys will move through the forest by coming down into the middle storey. The other primates will also move between storeys but spend most of their time in the one indicated. (Diagrammatic section of forest based on Richards (1957) *Tropical Rain Forest*. Cambridge University Press.)

with its covering shrub layer and the canopy formed by the crowns of the trees. The borderline between these two zones is at about 30 ft. In the true tropical forest of West Africa, the canopy itself contains three main zones each with its own population of both diurnal and nocturnal primates (Fig. 11.3). Arboreal primates are found in most types of forest, whether the secondary forest growing on abandoned but once cultivated land, gallery forest along the banks of rivers, or the mangrove swamps along sea coasts. The gorilla, chimpanzee and some cercopithecoids are found in the montane forest extending high up the slopes of East African mountains. Although the apes spend much of their time on the forest floor, only the macaques, patas monkeys and baboons (amongst non-human primates) have fully adapted to life on the ground. Their habitats range from the open forest on the edge of savanna through the grasslands and even into arid semi desert where there are no trees, only thorn bushes.

PRIMATE DIETS

Very small mammals eat insects. They were the diet of the earliest primates and are still a major food source for the smaller members of the order. The 'insectivorous' prosimians, some lemurs, lorises and the tarsier, supplement their diet with tree frogs, birds' eggs, small birds and fruit. Most primates rely on the fruits, shoots and leaves of the forest trees for their food. It has recently been shown that there is a fairly wide separation between the size range of predominantely insectivorous (small: about 115 g) and predominantly folivorous primates (larger: range 850 g to 200 kg and commonly weighing about 6300 g). Primates of all sizes eat fruit, the smaller group with a weight of 300 g also eat insects, the larger, weighing about 6300 g supplement their diet with leaves. Field studies in which groups of primates have been observed over a full year and, in some cases their stomach contents analysed, have shown that the balance of food items in the diet usually shifts with the seasons. Crops are a handy food source for ground-living monkeys but where the easy pickings of the farm cannot be had, then the terrestrial monkeys have to rely on insects, fruit, leaves and small vertebrates. In the drier savanna and steppes, this diet is supplemented by grubs, corms and rhizomes.

There is well-documented evidence that both baboons and chimpanzees are sometimes carnivorous but fresh meat is a very unusual element in the diet of these primates and most monkeys never eat mammalian flesh. Man is the only member of the order regularly feeding on animal protein, and then in large quantities only in developed countries (with newly recognized pathological consequences). Whatever their diet, all primates use their hands to collect their food and transfer it to the mouth.

PRIMATE CHARACTERISTICS

Most of the characters which distinguish primates from other mammals have developed in response to the demands of an arboreal life. Early mammals were small and quadrupedal, running up and down trunks and creepers and along branches. As primate body size increased so new locomotor patterns developed: better muscle coordination and improved vision were needed for safe movement through the trees and a new posture for safely resting in them. These changes are reflected in the skull and skeleton, making it easier to assess the status and habits of fossil primates by comparing them with appropriate living forms.

It has been suggested that the reproductive behaviour and social organization of primates are also an adaptation for arboreal life. All living primates, even the most primitive, have a longer gestation period than do other mammals of comparable size. They also produce fewer offspring. Young primates have a long infancy (from birth to the appearance of the first permanent molar) and a long 'juvenile' period (from the end of infancy to sexual maturity). This means that the young experience increased mother–child bonding and have a longer learning period than other mammals. Experiments in which baby monkeys were deprived of all 'maternal' contact, whether natural or from an artificial surrogate, produced emotionally deprived and developmentally retarded infants: a situation comparable to that found in similarly treated children. Inevitably the long infancy of primates affects the social organization of the primate 'group' or 'family'.

Primates have been and continue to be intensively studied. Living primates form a structural series from the most 'primitive' (tree-shrews) to the most 'advanced' (man) but it must be remembered that each member of the series is in fact the present product of its own evolutionary history (Fig. 11.1). The primates in the zoo are not living examples of the stages in the evolution of man! The behaviour of living primates is the only direct evidence for the evolution of primate behaviour. Nevertheless the development of, for example, the social behaviour and organization of primate groups seen in the living members of the order does

# Evolution of Man

not necessarily reflect the development of human behaviour and social structure.

## PRIMATE ADAPTATIONS

The main adaptations evolved in primates from the basic mammalian pattern are found in the limbs and axial skeleton (locomotor), in the special senses, and in the brain and the nervous system. All but the first are reflected in changes in the proportions of the skull. Primates have been dentally conservative by comparison with other animals, but they do show adaptations which can be correlated both with diet and social behaviour.

### Locomotor system

The manner in which animals move through trees depends on their size. All primates have retained the generalized pentadactyl limb and increased the mobility of the shoulder girdle and clavicle. In general the forelimb is adapted for grasping or swinging (*cf.* man) and the hindlimbs for support. The proportions of the fore and hindlimbs vary, the former reaching their greatest length in the brachiating (in which the arms are used to propel the animal through the trees, the legs are not used) and semibrachiating forms (in which the arms are used for swinging but also the legs in leaping through trees) (Table 11.1). The thumb (which is often very reduced in pongids) and big toe can be rotated or opposed towards the palmar surface of the hand or foot (but not in man), making it possible to grasp large objects (power grip) or small items (precision grip). The accuracy and control of the grip is increased by the great tactile sensitivity of the pulps of the fingers and toes. These are supported by nails (not the more primitive claws), another arboreal adaptation since claws impede rapid movement through trees. Primates use a wide range of locomotor patterns (Table 11.1) but spend a surprisingly large percentage of their time sitting (up to 75% in arboreal and 30% in terrestrial forms). During these periods they may be feeding, grooming themselves or each other or just 'socializing'—an important feature of primate as well as human life. The resting posture in almost all primates, including the lemurs, is normally vertical. The animal sits on its rump with its spine more or less erect. This habit, which can be considered preadaptive for a vertical posture in motion, is also reflected in a progressive shift of the foramen magnum from the back of the skull (Fig. 11.4) towards the base. As the cranium becomes positioned more vertically on the cervical vertebral column so the nuchal area tends to move

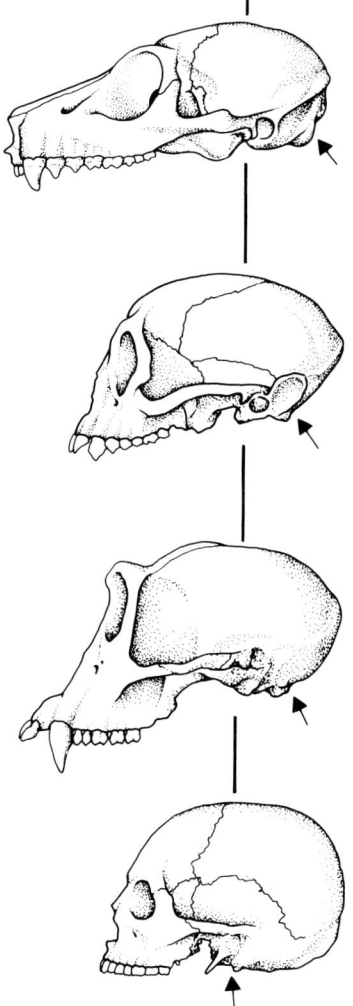

**Fig. 11.4.** The skulls of *Galago*, *Cebus*, *Pan* and modern man to illustrate the changing proportions of the face and cranium and the shift in the position and axis of the foramen magnum. The skulls are aligned on the glenoid fossa of the mandibular joint. The arrow indicates the axis of the foramen magnum. (Not to scale.)

onto the base of the skull. A later development, found in hominids, is the appearance of a true mastoid process projecting downwards behind the external auditory meatus.

The general trend towards increased verticality of the body culminated in the development of true bipedalism some 2.5–3.0 MBP. The swinging human stride depends not only on a specialized foot structure allowing the load to pass from heel to big toe through the lateral margin of the foot and then across its ball, but also on a rearrange-

Table 11.2. Some characteristics of primate skulls.

| | Lemurs and lorises | Tarsier | New World monkeys | Old World monkeys | Apes | Man |
|---|---|---|---|---|---|---|
| *The orbits* | | | | | | |
| Orbits face forward | No | Yes | Yes | Yes | Yes | Yes |
| Post-orbital closure | No. Postorbital bar | Partial. Postorbital bar expanded. | Fully closed posteriorly | | | → |
| *The middle and external ear* | | | | | | |
| 1 Tympanic bulla | Large, inflated in lemurs, small in lorises (Fig. 11.5) | Large inflated | Inflated | | | |
| 2 Tympanic ring | Within tympanic cavity in lemurs. Attached to outer wall in lorises | On outer wall of bulla (Fig. 11.5) | Outside but attached to bulla | Absent (Petrous temporal almost level skull base) Outside tympanum | | |
| 3 External auditory meatus | No | Short | No or short | Short in infants, long in adults | | |
| 4 Mastoid process | No | No | No | No | Irregularly, size variable | Yes |
| *The lower jaw* | | | | | | |
| 1 Symphysis menti | Yes, mobile | Yes, ? mobile | No, fused | Yes | Yes | No (chin) |
| 2 Simian shelf | No | No | Sometimes | Multiple, very close to lower border of mandible | Often multiple | Usually single |
| 3 Mental foramen | Usually multiple | | Usually single | | | ↑ |

ment of the pelvis and its associated muscles as well as the development of spinal curvatures to facilitate axial load distribution.

*The special senses*
Primates have few predators but a potentially hazardous habitat: healed fractures have been found in wild gibbons. Survival on the open plains depends on good hearing and an acute sense of smell but life in trees depends much more on superb vision and highly developed senses of touch and balance (Table 11.2).

*The ear—hearing.* Amongst mammals, only some carnivores have more acute hearing than primates. Rather than develop discrimination over a wide frequency range (e.g. the dog whistle), primates have evolved the capacity to detect patterns in sound, for example music. It has been suggested that this ability to discriminate between sound patterns played a large part in the evolution of speech.

The large mobile external ear of most mammals acts as a directional sound receiver and as a thermoregulator. The external ear of primates is generally small but the pinna of prosimians varies in size. Some nocturnal forms have larger ears to improve hearing and some diurnal types have larger pinnae to increase their capacity to lose heat. All anthropoids have small ears with limited mobility but the vestiges of the ear muscles can still be found in man.

Whilst the structure of the cochlea and spiral organ of Corti is much the same in all primates, there are taxonomically useful differences in the structure of the tympanic cavity (Fig. 11.5).

*The eye—vision.* Primitive, and many extant, mammals, have small eyes on the side of the face with little or no overlap of the visual fields. The orbits are open posteriorly and a fascial septum and lateral 'postorbital bar' formed by processes from the frontal and maxillary bones separate them from the temporal fossa (Fig. 11.4). Higher primates have evolved perfect colour and stereoscopic vision, their orbits face forwards to give the almost complete overlap of the visual fields necessary for full stereoscopic vision and are also completely walled-off posteriorly. *Tarsius* and the anthropoids, including the nocturnal cebid *Aotus*, have also lost the *tapetum lucidum* or reflecting layer of cells found in other nocturnal mammals, which is thought to maximize the utilization of all available light. During embryological development the eyes, first developed as optic placodes on the sides of the head, rotate bringing the optical axes into parallel (all anthropoids including man) or near parallel (New World monkeys).

*The nose—smell.* As the primate system grew in

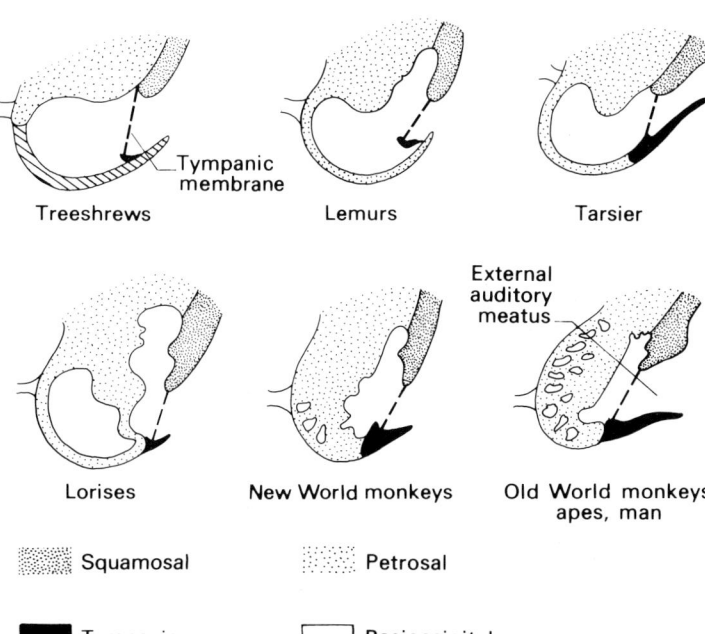

**Fig. 11.5.** Diagrammatic cross-section through the tympanic cavity of primates showing the position of the tympanic membrane and tympanic bone. In treeshrews the floor of the tympanic bulla is formed by the entotympanic (hatched), in all other primates it is formed by the petrosal bone (or petrous part of temporal). The tympanic membrane is supported by a ring formed from the tympanic bone and within the bulla in treeshrews and lemurs; the ring is attached to the edge of the bulla in lorises and New World monkeys and expanded to form a tube in the tarsier, Old World monkeys, apes and man.

importance, so that of the olfactory system diminished. Most mammals, including all prosimians except *Tarsius*, have their nostrils surrounded by moist glandular skin (the rhinarium) which extends into an almost fixed upper lip. The rhinarium is thought to act as an 'odour direction sensor'. Its loss in the tarsier and anthropoids not only reflects the diminishing importance of smell in that group but also permitted the development of a face and mobile upper lip. This in turn made possible a whole range of facial expressions so increasing patterns of communication and, later, the development of the labial sounds ('b', 'm' etc) which have become so important in speech. Primates also show a progressive reduction of the complex turbinate system of most mammals; represented in man by three barely curved conchae (p. 000) and at the same time have reduced the anteroposterior length of the nasal cavity. The latter trend may have little to do with the reduced importance of olfaction as such but could be associated with the general, and as yet inadequately explained, reduction in facial length found in the more advanced members of the order.

*The nervous system*
Safe arboreal locomotion depends on fine muscular coordination. Primate feeding patterns, as well as activities such as mutual grooming, depend on the precise use of fingers and thumbs. None of these are possible without the control effected by a well-developed motor cortex based on information supplied by a rich cutaneous and proprioceptive sensory system and sorted by an equivalently developed sensory cortex (Fig. 11.6).

Visual acuity depends not only on retinal structure and position but also on the correlated development of the visual components of the central nervous system. A flexible response to an environmental change in the widest sense depends on the coordination of the immediate visual image with the memory of comparable circumstances and the consequences of the action taken. All this requires enhanced capacity for 'memory' and 'association'.

The net effect of the expansion of these parts of the CNS is an enlargement of the brain as a whole: the brains of primates are relatively larger (as a proportion of body weight) than are those of other mammals. They also show a progressive tendency to folding of the cerebral cortex leading not only to complicated sulcular patterns but also to a greater volume of grey matter (neurons) per unit volume overall (Fig. 11.6). It is however important to appreciate that an increase in brain size as such does not necessarily mean an increase in 'intelligence' however that term may be defined. The two are to some extent independent although there is a fundamental relationship between brain size (or cranial capacity) and body weight. It is the absolute and the relative increase in size of the cerebral hemispheres in higher primates and particularly in man, which has led not only to the expansion of the cranium and the development of its 'egglike' shape but also to the appearance of a forehead. The combination of facial shortening, cranial expansion and increasing flexion of the cranial base has produced the skull profile characteristic of modern man (Fig. 11.12).

*The jaws and teeth*
What are possibly the earliest primates are known only from isolated teeth. It is however likely that the form of their jaw apparatus was very similar to that of other early mammals, particularly the insectivores. As primates evolved, increasing in body size and so shifting from a predominantly insectivorous to a frugivorous or herbivorous diet, so changes occurred in the shape of the jaw apparatus as well as in the form of individual teeth. The jaws and teeth of living primates are described in the Appendix (p. 399–439), the general trends in the evolution of the primate jaw apparatus and dentition are described here (Table 11.3).

Perhaps the first development was a reduction in the number of teeth from the primitive formula of $\frac{3143}{3143}$ to, first, $\frac{2133}{2133}$ in prosimians and New World Monkeys and then to $\frac{2123}{2123}$ in Old World monkeys, apes and man (Fig. 11.8, see Appendix). In some prosimians there is only a single lower incisor. It has always been assumed that the reduction in incisor number stemmed from the loss of the third tooth in the series ($I_3^3$) but that the first ($Pm_1^1$) and second ($Pm_2^2$) premolars were lost, leaving the third and fourth ($Pm_3^3$, $Pm_4^4$) as the 'first' and 'second' premolars in man.

*Incisors.* Primitive mammals use their incisors for collecting, grasping and holding material, not for biting. These teeth are small, subconical and may barely project above the oral mucosa. The upper incisors of prosimians are in most cases very small (missing in *Hapalemur*) but otherwise similar to those of animals such as the opossum (Fig. 12.17). Prosimians do, however, have a highly specialized lower anterior dentition: the lower incisors and the lower canine are elongated, narrowed mesiodistally and aligned across the front of the jaw to form a 'comb' (Figs. 11.7, 11.8). The teeth are also proclined, in some cases so sharply that the crowns are almost horizontal (e.g. *Lemur mongoz*, Fig. 11.7). The upper incisors, separated

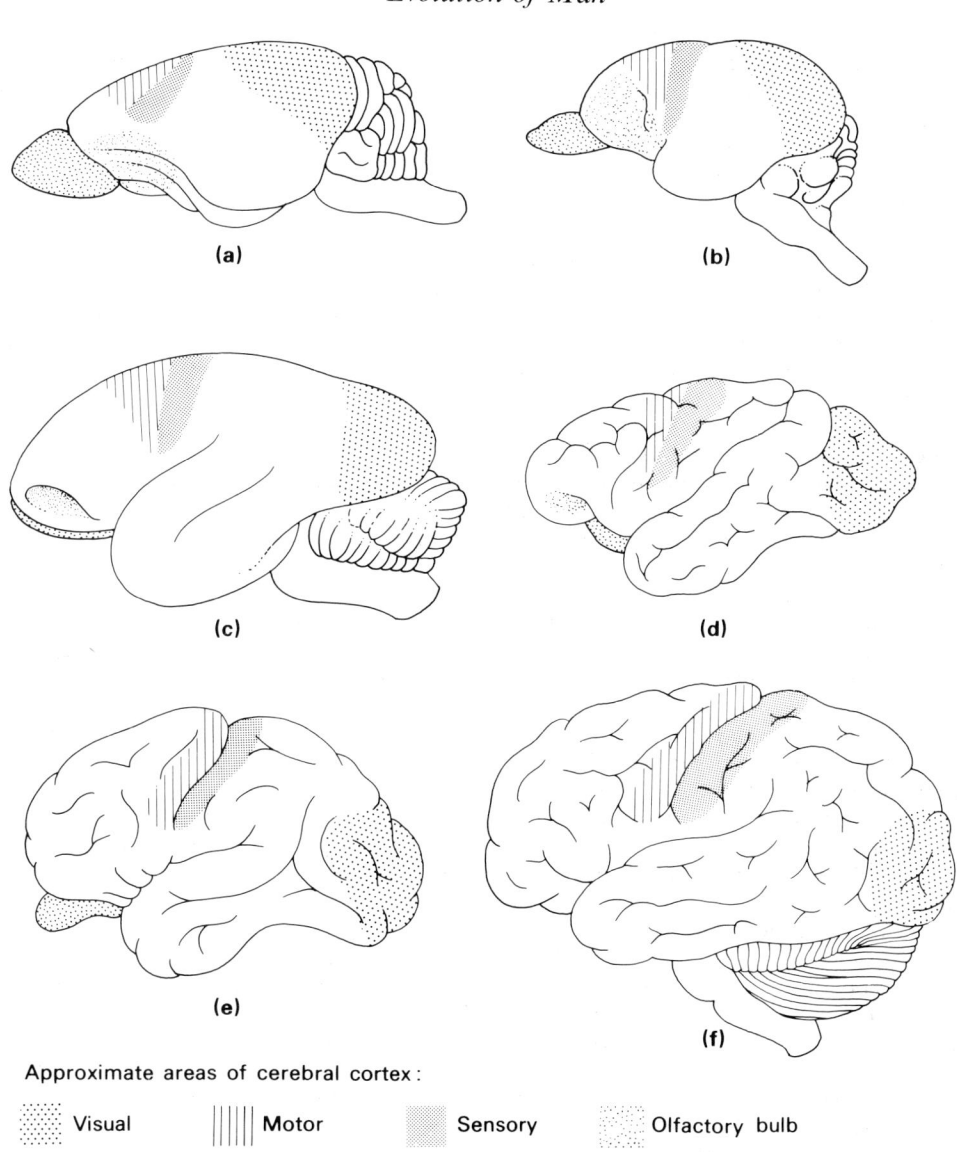

**Fig. 11.6.** The brains of some representative primates which show the progressive reduction in the size of the olfactory bulb (too small to be seen in lateral view in man); the increasing folding of the cerebral cortex and the development of sulcal patterns; the expansion (both absolutely and relatively, note the magnifications at which the brains are figured), of the motor, sensory and visual cortical areas. In contrast note the increasing area associated with other cerebral functions including 'general memory' or 'association'. (a) Tree-shrew, × 2.00; (b) tarsier, × 1.66; (c) marmoset, × 1.50; (d) macaque, × 0.66; (e) gorilla, × 0.33; (f) man, × 0.33.

by a wide median diastema, occlude with the distal edge of the comb. The comb is now known to be used in grooming the fur. (Grooming may have some physiological importance and not be a matter of simple cleanliness.) Some lemurs have also been observed using it as a 'resin scraper': they make a daily circuit of selected trees, scraping up the nutritious resin oozing from clefts in the bark.

*Propithecus* has been observed to use its lower incisors to gouge holes in succulent plants to obtain water.

Some early primates, like other Cretaceous and Paleocene mammals, developed a rodent-like specialization of the incisors. The aye-aye (*Daubentonia*) is the only living primate to have this adaptation; the deciduous incisors are shed

Table 11.3. Characteristics of primate dentitions.

| | Lemurs & Lorises | Tarsier | New World monkeys | Old World monkeys | Apes | Man |
|---|---|---|---|---|---|---|
| Dental formula | $\frac{2133}{2133}$ except (a) Indriidae $\frac{2123}{1123}$ (b) *Daubentonia* $\frac{1013}{1003}$ | $\frac{2133}{1133}$ | Cebidae $\frac{2133}{2133}$ Callithrichidae $\frac{2132}{2132}$ | $\frac{2123}{2123}$ →→→→ | | |
| Shape of arch | V-shaped | V-shaped | Variable: V-shaped parabolic rectangular | Variable, generally rectangular | Rectangular | Parabolic Continuous |
| | Median diastema between upper central incisors | | Diastema between I² and upper canine for occlusion lower canine →→→ | | | |
| Occlusal plane | Flat in both anteroposterior and transverse planes | | Generally flat both axes | Generally flat both axes | Generally flat both axes | Curved: Antero-posteriorly (Curve of Spee) Transverse (Curve of Monson) |
| Incisors | Uppers: small subconical Lowers: comb (with canines) | Subconical | Spatulate →→→→→→→→→→→→→→→→→→→→ | | | Incisiform |
| Canines | Uppers: large, project Lowers: incisiform (comb) | Pointed, caniniform | Large. Caniniform. Usually project. Some sexual dimorphism | Large, caniniform. Sexual dimorphism esp. baboons | Stout, large project. Sexual dimorphism | |
| Premolars | Lower first caniniform. Conical with lingual cingulum | Last molariform | Bicuspid. Lower first often sectorial | Upper first: canine fossa on mesial surface Lower first: sectorial | Bicuspid →→→ | |
| Molars | Uppers: tribosphenic incipient hypocone or four-cusped Lowers: tribosphenic with reduction/loss paraconid. | Tribosphenic | Four-cusped Uppers: oblique ridge Lowers: paraconid lost. | Bilophodont | 'Dryopithecus' pattern Uppers: Four cusps, oblique ridge Lowers: Four or five cusps. | |
| | | | | $M_{\overline{1}}^{\underline{1}} < M_{\overline{2}}^{\underline{2}} \gtrless M_{\overline{3}}^{\underline{(3)}}$ | $M_{\overline{1}}^{\underline{1}} < M_{\overline{2}}^{\underline{2}} > M_{\overline{3}}^{\underline{3}}$ | $M_{\overline{1}}^{\underline{1}} > M_{\overline{2}}^{\underline{2}} > M_{\overline{3}}^{\underline{3}}$ |

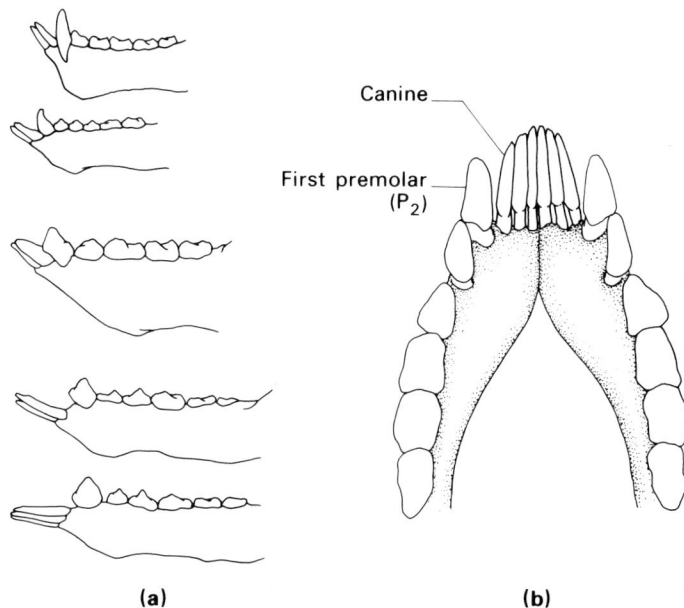

Fig. 11.7. The prosimian dental comb. (a) In lateral view; the angulation (or proclination) of the teeth varies from near vertical (*Galago*, top) to near horizontal (*Lemur mongoz*, bottom). (b) Viewed from above in *Galago* showing the incisiform canine and caniniform first premolar.

and replaced by large persistently growing incisors. The canines and all but one premolar are also lost.

The third major specialization in primate incisors occurred with the evolution of the anthropoids: spatulate incisors with a cutting edge are found in New World and Old World monkeys, apes and man. The mobile mandibular symphysis of prosimians which allows some independent movement of the two halves of the lower jaw, became fused (this takes place shortly after birth in Anthropoidea) at about the same time as the spatulate incisors evolved. Whether the development of incisors which are subjected to considerable masticatory force in biting necessitated the fusion of the symphysis to 'strengthen' the front of the jaw is not yet clear. The two developments are, however, likely to be connected.

The size of the incisors in Old World monkeys and apes is correlated with diet: they are relatively larger in the more frugivorous forms (e.g. in the chimpanzee as compared with the gorilla). Although in normal human occlusion, the upper incisors occlude with their edges in front of (overjet) and below (overbite) those of the lowers, this has not been thought the usual condition in anthropoids. Monkeys are described as having an 'edge-to-edge' bite. It is now known that some groups of 'leaf-eating' monkeys have a very high incidence (up to 95%) of an 'underbite' (Class III incisal occlusion in man, Fig. 9.7) so that the lower incisors bite in front of the uppers. This observation means that in some monkeys selection for a type of incisal occlusion regarded as abnormal in man has occurred. High incidences of 'underbite' are found in some South American as well as in African and Asian colobines and it is therefore likely that this type of incisal occlusion is an adaptation for the improved ingestion of leaves.

*Canines.* Man is unique among primates in having small 'incisiform' canines: they are strong, variably projecting, slashing and often markedly sexual dimorphic teeth in other members of the order.

The upper canines of prosimians are stout, conical teeth and in some (e.g. *Galago*) the first upper premolar is also caniniform. These teeth occlude with the caniniform lower first premolar (Fig. 11.8). There is no concrete evidence as to how most prosimians use their canines, however the 'functional replacement' of the incisiform lower canine by a modified lower first premolar indicates the importance of a stabbing or slashing element in the dentition. Whether this is used predominantly in feeding or as a potential or actual weapon in social behaviour is not yet clear in prosimians, although the latter is almost certainly the case in anthropoids. Although all monkeys have strong and projecting canines, these reach their greatest development in the terrestrial forms such as the baboons (Figs. 11.8, 11.9). All primates with lower

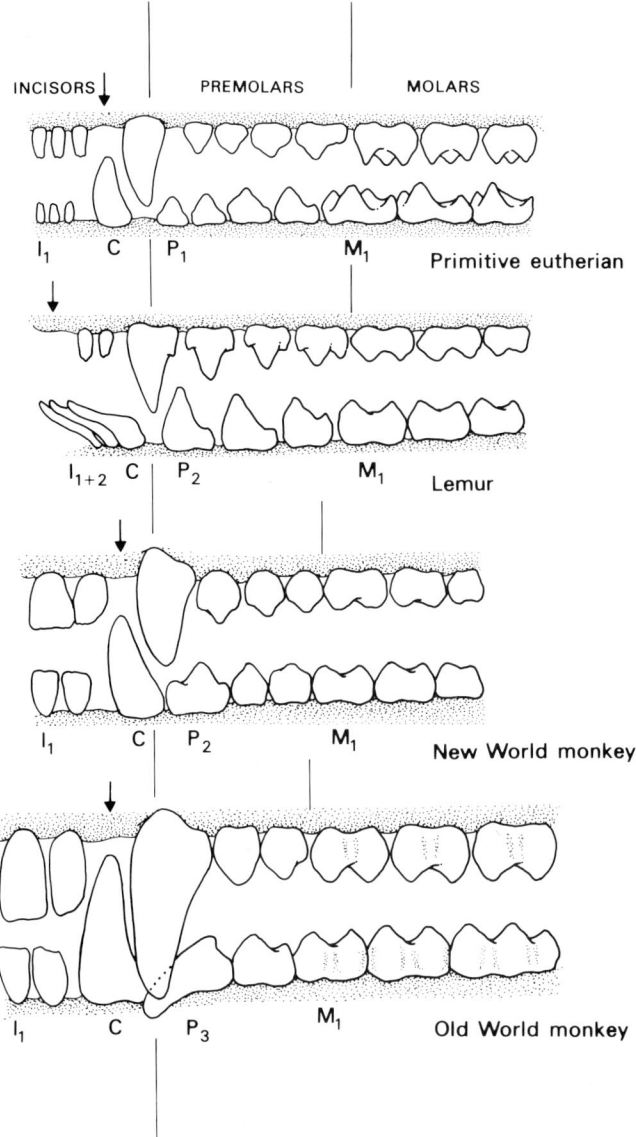

**Fig. 11.8.** The characteristics of the dentition in a primitive mammal and the main primate groups. There is a progressive reduction in the number of incisors and premolars but the occlusal relationships remain constant. The proportions of each part of the dentition differ (shown by the distance between the vertical lines through the centre of the upper canine and the contact point between the last upper premolar and the first upper molar). A diastema (arrowed) between the upper lateral incisor and the upper canine for the occlusion of the lower canine is present in all but the lemurs where the canine is incorporated into the comb. This group have a median diastema (arrowed). The molar series reduces in size from front to back in all the groups shown except Old World monkeys.

canines projecting above the occlusal plane have a diastema between the upper lateral incisor and upper canine into which the lower can occlude (Figs. 11.7, 11.8). The even larger upper canine flares slightly laterally and overlaps the mandibular bone when the jaws are closed. As upper and lower teeth converge on a 'bite', the lower canine cuts past the upper as does the lower first premolar. This produces two distinct wear facets on the upper tooth; one mesiolingually from the lower canine and one distolingually from the lower first premolar (Figs. 11.8, 11.9).

It is not surprising in view of these occlusal relationships, that the lower first premolar shows a characteristic modification in Old World monkeys and apes. The distal half of the tooth is similar in shape to the second premolar but the mesial part is extended into a long cutting blade (or sectorial tooth). In Old World monkeys this frequently overlaps the distolingual cingulum of the lower canine so that they combine to form a strong curved bar cutting against the upper canine (Fig. 11.9). Due to the mesial extension of the lower first premolar, the long axis of the crown of this tooth runs mesiodistally. This is quite different from the situation in man where its long axis runs buccolin-

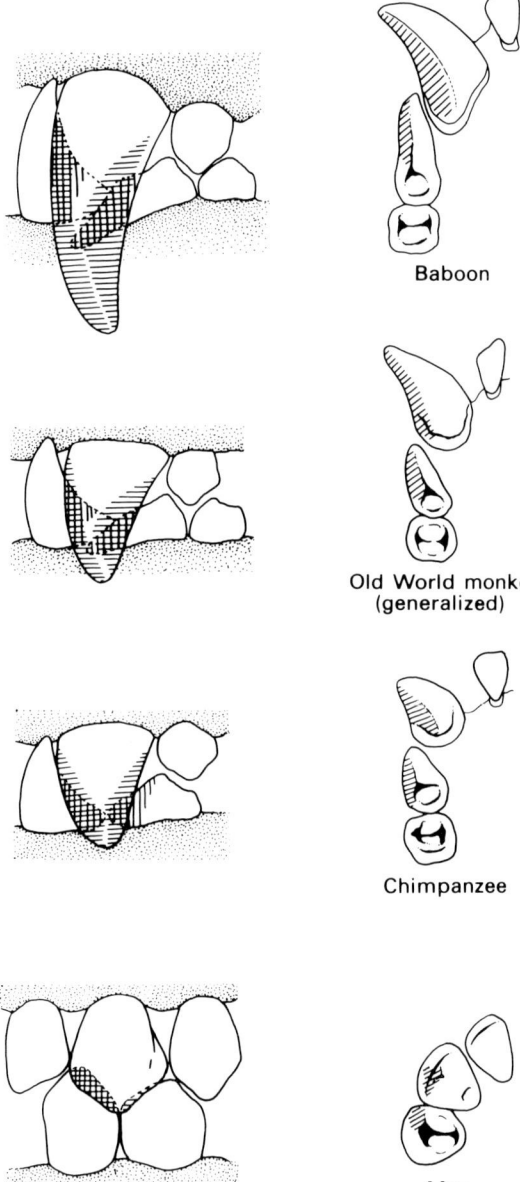

Fig. 11.9. The occlusal relations (left) and the occlusal view of the lower canine and first premolar (right) in Old World monkeys, an ape and man. The wear facets produced by the lower canine and lower first premolar cutting past the upper canine are hatched. In all but man, the lower first premolar is elongated anteriorly in front of its main (buccal) cusp to form a cutting edge.

gually. Further, the mesial extension is supported by a second root. It follows that, even in the absence of the canine, it is not only possible to recognize a fossil specimen as a pongid (or Old World monkey, see molars below) or as a hominid on the basis of the premolar shape but also, and this has proved important, on the position of its roots within the alveolus. It is also possible to gauge the size of the canine.

The fundamental difference in the proportions and shape of the canines (and lower first premolars) between pongids and hominids (Fig. 11.9) raised the question of whether the human line has shown a tendency to reduce the canine. (It has been suggested that the long stout root of the human canine is indicative of its having, at some time, been a much larger crowned and therefore projecting tooth.) It seems likely that the common ancestor of the extant great apes and of man had a slightly projecting canine. This became enlarged in the former, and somewhat reduced in the latter.

In both Old World monkeys and apes (as well as some cebids, see Appendix), the inner lower border of the mandible is strengthened in the symphyseal region by a bony buttress, the 'simian shelf'. This is best developed in the long-snouted, large-canined forms such as baboons amongst the cercopithecoids and gorillas amongst the apes. Like the fusion of the symphysis, the development of the shelf may be correlated with the development of large canines capable of withstanding large loads. It can, perhaps, be regarded as comparable to the human 'chin' which is an external buttress for the symphyseal region.

*Cheek teeth.* In primitive mammals, the main masticatory effort is concentrated in the post-canine teeth (particularly the molars). They act to crush, cut, grind and pulp the food ready for swallowing. The premolars, which increase in size from before backwards are simple teeth with, usually, a single pointed cusp elongated mesiodistally and a lingual cingulum. The last premolar may have subsidiary cusps. The insectivorous and frugivorous prosimians have retained this pattern. However primates with spatulate incisors tend to have molariform premolars: they are bicuspid (with the exception of the lower first) rather than sectorial. This change may be linked to the shift of the main cutting function of the dentition from premolars to incisors. Some prosimians have retained the simple tribosphenic molar but even the earliest known primates had already begun to convert this tooth into one with four cusps and at the same time to reduce the height of the cusps.

The early evolution of the primate upper molar involved the addition of a fourth cusp, the hypocone to the distolingual aspect of the trigon (Fig. 11.10). The ridge connecting the protocone and metacone persisted and in some cases became

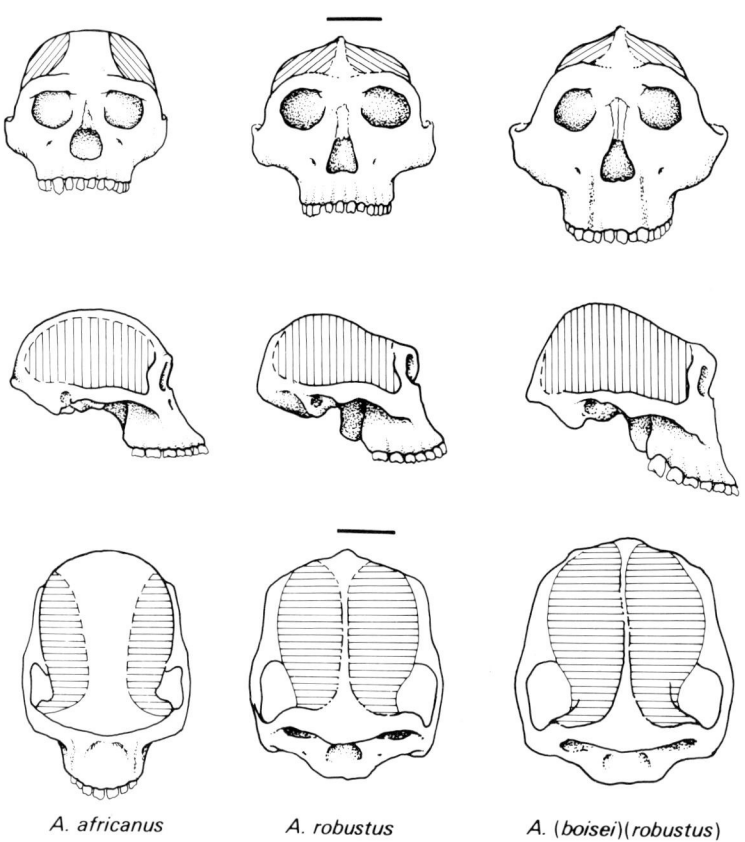

**Fig. 11.18.** Frontal, lateral and dorsal views of the skulls of the three species of *Australopithecus*. The cranial volume is much the same in all three groups; the difference in appearance can be attributed to a progressive expansion in the jaw apparatus. This is reflected by the relative expansion of the attachment area for temporalis (shaded) which extends to the development of sagittal crests in *A. robustus* and *A. boisei*. (The black bar corresponds to a 5 cm length.)

masseter and also the need to buttress the face against powerful masticatory forces.

AUSTRALOPITHECUS BOISEI

The original specimen was found at Olduvai in 1959 but since then more material has been recovered from Omo and Koobi Fora (Fig. 11.13). Mandibular fragments from the Far East, classified as *Meganthropus* indicate that a very large and deep-jawed hominid was also present in the Far East. *A. boisei* was large, weighing upwards of 150 lbs, but even so the skull is massive largely due to the expansion of the jaws (Fig. 11.18). The cranial capacity of the Olduvai specimen is estimated at between 500–550 cm$^3$. The face is very deep and heavily buttressed. A reconstructed jaw, based on an isolated mandible from Lake Natron, has a very high rectangular ramus (Fig. 11.19). The incisors and canines of *A. boisei* were the same size or smaller than those of other australopithecines and even of modern man but the premolars and molars are enormous (Fig. 11.19).

It has been suggested that the increasing disproportion between anterior and cheek teeth found in the australopithecines could be the result of progressive adaptation to a more 'herbivorous' diet (specifically foods which had to be thoroughly chewed, such as the graminivorous element of the diet of *Theropithecus*). Whatever the explanation 'Zinj' was not exclusively vegetarian, the remains of a selected variety of small mammals were found so close to the skull that it can only be reasonably concluded that they had recently been eaten.

'Homo'

In 1960 the Leakeys found an almost complete set of foot bones and a mandible at a site slightly lower (older) and about 300 yards away from the living

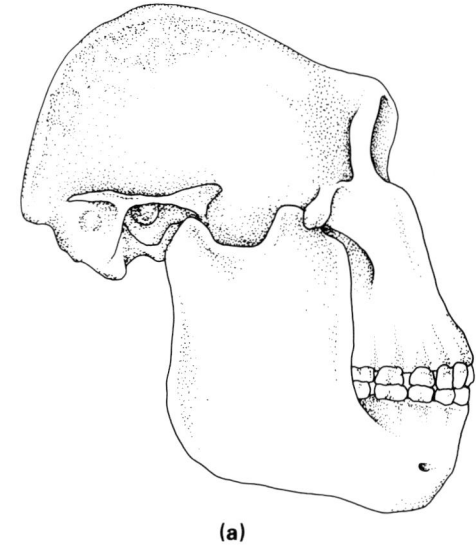

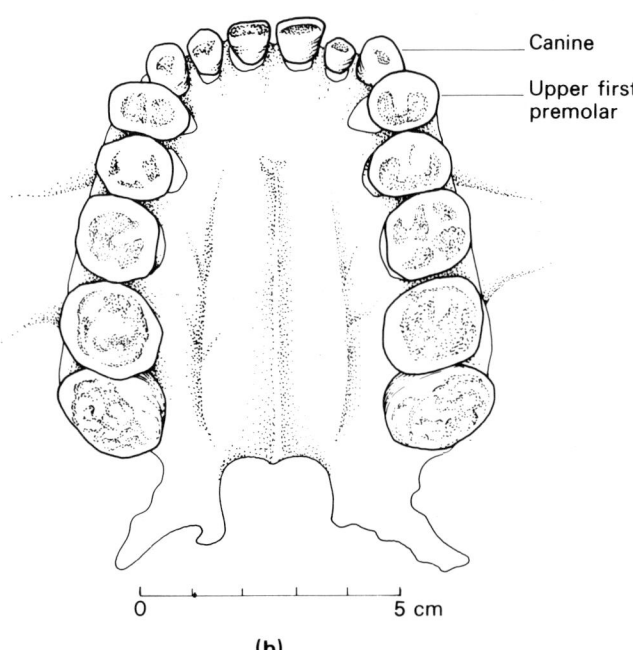

**Fig. 11.19.** (a) The skull of *Zinjanthropus (Australopithecus boisei)* based on the cranium found at Olduvai and the Peninj mandible. (b) Occlusal view of the upper dentition of the Olduvai specimen. The third molars have just erupted (giving the specimen a 'human equivalent age' of 18–21 years) and are covered with 'crinkled' enamel. Heavy wear has occurred on all the other teeth exposing dentine (shaded) and in some cases leaving an enamel ridge corresponding to the position of the original fissures between the cusps. The extreme disproportion between the anterior and posterior dentitions is shown by the relative size of the canine and upper first premolar.

floor where 'Zinj' had been discovered. Skull fragments including a lower jaw, most of two parietals and an occipital bone as well as parts of the skeleton of a hand were also recovered. These remains, from a juvenile and an adult have been described (not without some criticism) as the type specimens of *Homo habilis*.

The designation *Homo* was felt justified primarily by the structure of the foot which has both transverse and longitudinal arches, the cranial volume (estimates vary from 642–723 cm$^3$), the structure of the hand bones and the proportions and form of the dentition (which lacks the marked disproportion between anterior and posterior teeth found in australopithecines). Stone tools were found in association with the remains, but similar tools had also been found close to '*Zinjanthropus*'. Whether these remains belonged to

Homo or not, it was clear that an 'advanced' tool-making hominid had lived at Olduvai before or at the same time as *A. boisei*.

*Homo habilis* dates from about 1.75 MBP. The systematic exploration of the area to the east of Lake Turkana during the 1970s has yielded a large collection of hominid fossils and fossil fragments. Amongst these is a partial skull (KNM-ER 1470) with a long ovoid cranium, a broad face but no significant development of a supraorbital ridge and with little or no maxillary/premaxillary prognathism. This specimen has been dated at at least 1.60–1.82 MBP by one radiometric method and confirmed by stratigraphic evidence. It is therefore at least as old, if not older than the Olduvai specimen. Other fragments showing similar characteristics have also been found.

There is a growing consensus of opinion based on the remains found at Koobi Fora, Olduvai and in Ethiopia that a comparatively large-brained hominid with a relatively unspecialized (as compared with the australopithecines) dentition was living in the Rift Valley area between 2.5 and 1.75 MBP. The geographic range of this form may have extended into South Africa: an 'advanced' mandible, ascribed to '*Telanthropus*' and found at Swartkrans could belong to this general group or to *Homo erectus* (see below). It is possible that this form, currently designated *Homo sp.*, evolved from an early 'australopithecine' type. The two groups then diverged by adapting to slightly different diets but lived in the same general habitat: the australopithecines became progressively more heavily jawed or 'herbivorous', the hominines rapidly advancing into the next and generally recognized grade of *Homo erectus*.

**Pleistocene hominids**

The transition from the Ramapithecine grade of human evolution to that of *Homo habilis* or *Homo sp.* as known from East Africa involved the development of bipedalism, the reduction of the face, particularly the anterior dentition, and the development of a tool-making culture. At the same time there was a small but significant expansion in brain size and almost certainly some differential cerebral expansion and reorganization. The group of fossils collectively known as *Homo erectus* contains a range of forms from 'primitive' to more 'advanced', the oldest dating from 1.5 MBP and the youngest from about 0.4 MBP (400 000 years). The evolving human lineage reached an '*erectus*' stage in both Africa and Asia and was, obviously, widely distributed. As *Homo erectus* evolved, so *Homo sapiens* appeared, probably about 0.3 MBP although quite possibly earlier. There appears to have been a simple progression from an *erectus* to a *sapiens* grade of *Homo* rather than an abrupt transition since advanced forms of *H. erectus* had *sapiens* features. The transition may have happened more than once. It is likely that populations of advanced *H. erectus* became more or less isolated at a time when much of the northern hemisphere was intermittently covered by great sheets of ice. These 'localized' groups could well have continued their development into 'archaic man' (*Homo sapiens*). Indeed the distinction between advanced *H. erectus* and early *H. sapiens* is based largely on the single criterion of brain size (Table 11.4). Modern man (*H. sapiens sapiens*) is a recent development, the oldest known specimens date from about 40–50 000 years BP. During the 200 000 or so years between the first appearance of archaic man and that of modern man, a number of human 'types' appeared One, 'Neanderthal man', is well-known from Europe and has been considered a distinct subspecies (*Homo sapiens neanderthalensis*). Its 'primitive' cranial characters (heavy brow ridges, 'bunning' of the cranium) are reminiscent of *Homo erectus* but its cranial capacity was in the upper range for modern man (three classic Neanderthal specimens have a cranial volume in excess of 1600 $cm^3$, see Table 11.4). Other fossils differing in some craniofacial respects from modern man have been found in Africa (Broken Hill, Saldanha) and in Asia. It may be that *Homo sapiens* should be considered a single polytypic species rather than as a single modern subspecies (*Homo sapiens sapiens*) with at least one extinct subspecies.

**Homo erectus**

First discovered in Java by Dubois, specimens of early *H. erectus* are known from Europe, North and East Africa and mainland China (Fig. 11.13). As a group the *H. erectus* specimens are characterized by a rounded but anteroposteriorly flattened cranium which extends backwards to give an angulated profile in the occipital region (Fig. 11.20). *Homo erectus* had thick heavy supraorbital ridges projecting well forwards and a marked postorbital constriction. Unlike *Homo habilis* and the other Homo specimens from East Africa, *Homo erectus* had very thick cranial bones. Why this trait developed has not yet been explained. Cranial capacity in early *erectus* was little greater than that of *habilis* ranging from 750 to 800 + $cm^3$ in the younger Javanese specimens (Table 11.4).

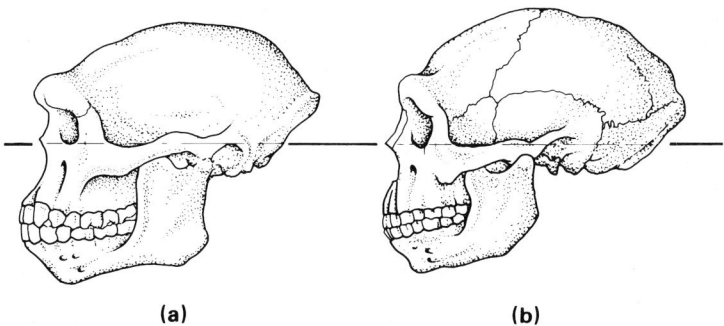

Fig. 11.20. The reconstructed skulls of *Homo erectus* from (a) Java (Trinil) and (b) China (Choukoutien). The reduction of the face and relative expansion of the cranium which occurred during the development of *H. erectus* are clearly shown when the skulls are aligned on the Frankfort plane.

Oddly the face (maxilla and associated bones) was not preserved in all but one of the earlier *erectus* specimens from Java, but a beautifully preserved specimen at Lake Turkana (Pith. VIII, 3733) has recently been found with the facial bones present. The lower jaw is well known, the teeth were smaller than those of the australopithecines and very similar to those of modern man. There was no chin.

*Homo erectus* was a fully adapted biped reaching an average height of 5 or more feet, i.e. within the range for modern man.

The best known group of *erectus* fossils were those from Choukoutien, although our present knowledge is based on the exquisite drawings and casts made from the originals rather than from the specimens themselves. Some fourteen crania and eleven mandibles were found at Choukoutien as were simple stone tools (Fig. 11.6) and unequivocal evidence of the use of fire. The faunal evidence suggests that these people had become efficient big game hunters. The general pattern of the skull is similar to that of the earlier Javanese specimens (Fig. 11.21) but the expansion of the brain from the 700–800 cm$^3$ level to an average of 1000 cm$^3$ had resulted in a more rounded cranial dome. The face was also less prognathic but still heavily buttressed. The teeth are robust when compared with those of modern man but arranged in a typically parabolic arch. The African examples of *H. erectus* (from Olduvai and North Africa, Fig. 11.13) differ only slightly from the Choukoutien specimens although fairly advanced stone tools were found near the Olduvan specimen. Remains of *H. erectus* have also been found in Europe (Mauer, Vértészöllös, Bilzingsleben in East Germany). The specimens from Vértészöllös and Swanscombe have been alleged, on the basis of occipital bone, to have sapient features.

The steady increase in brain size found in the succession of *erectus* specimens was probably associated with the development of increasingly complex social and cultural behaviour and a progressively (at least in East Africa) more sophisticated tool-making technology. It is likely that *H. erectus* was using language, it has been suggested that the use of fire at Choukoutien might have involved more than merely keeping warm and roasting meat, it could have had symbolic or ritual significance. Without a basis in language, symbolism and ritual are impossible.

### Homo sapiens

Advanced *Homo erectus* forms evolved into or were succeeded by early *H. sapiens* or 'archaic man'. The distinctions are blurred. Although in most respects similar to modern man, the archaic forms had generally longer, lower and broader skulls (although their cranial capacity reached contemporary levels) and heavy faces (Fig. 11.21). The teeth were slightly larger than those of modern man. Much has been made of subtle differences in occipital shape, supra-orbital ridge development and the degree of facial prognathism found in each specimen. What does seem clear is that over the period from about 0.25 MBP to about 50 000 years ago, groups of *Homo* in various parts of the world were undergoing local evolution (Fig. 11.21). There is evidence, for example, of two 'populations' with different cranial characteristics developing in, for example, Eurasia ('Neanderthal man' and modern man). Despite differences in facial form and cranial profile (long and low as opposed to short and high cranial vaults), the cultural attainment of at least the two European groups appears to have been comparable.

During this period the typical 'human' face finally developed. Brow ridges were reduced, the jaws became less prognathic and the definitive chin appeared. In pongids the symphyseal region is buttressed internally, in modern man externally by the mental protuberance (Fig. 11.22). The cross-sectional profile of the symphysis was, for a long time considered to be of major taxonomic

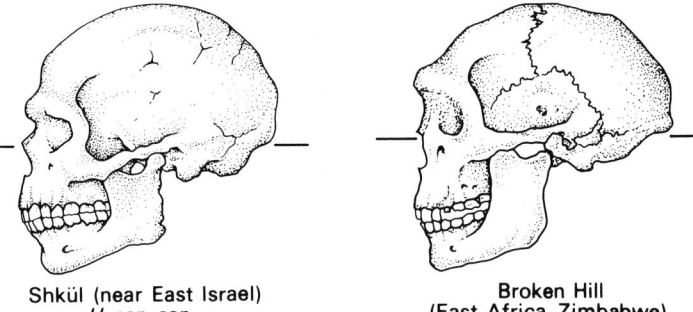
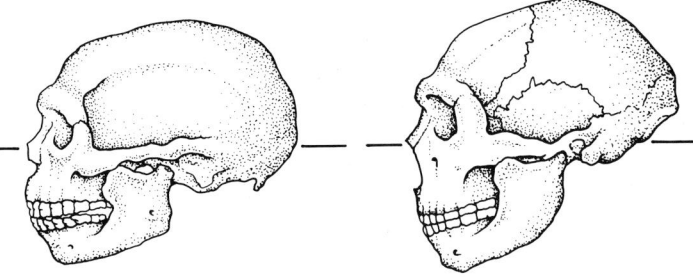
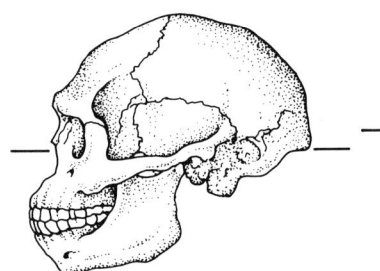

**Fig. 11.21.** *Homo erectus* from Choukoutien (bottom) and examples of crania from 'archaic man'. There are grounds for accepting that the differences between these types are the result of local evolution. The Monte Circeao specimen is regarded by some authorities as a 'classic' Neanderthal. The Solo specimen is thought to represent a local (Javanese) development from the Javanese form of *Homo erectus*. The variability in skull form in early *Homo sapiens* is best illustrated by the Shkül and Tabun specimens, these were found in two caves on Mount Carmel which, if not contemporaneous, are separated by no more than 10 000 years (Tabun being the older).

significance. However recent studies have shown that it is, in fact, highly variable even within pongid populations. Nevertheless the progressive shortening of the face and the concomitant conversion of the dental arcade from a 'V-shape' into a parabola has been associated with first the reduction and then the elimination of the internal buttresses, a more vertical orientation of the bone, and then the development of the chin as a new external buttress.

One feature observed in some populations of early man, particularly the 'Neanderthals' known from Krapina in Yygoslavia, is the presence of grossly enlarged pulp chambers in the teeth and an associated low level of root bifurcation in the postcanines. This condition has been alleged to be an adaptation for heavy tooth wear: the longer and larger the pulp chamber, the greater the opportunity for secondary dentine deposition and so the longer the life of the tooth.

## MODERN MAN

### Race

All human beings, at least over the past 10 000 years, have belonged to a single but polymorphic species, *Homo sapiens*. Yet men live in a wide range of habitats and are exposed to varied climates, diets and pathogenic factors.

Certain physical differences among groups of human beings are striking. A part of man's evolutionary success stems from this variability and its associated capacity to exist in a variety of climatic and environmental conditions (Fig.

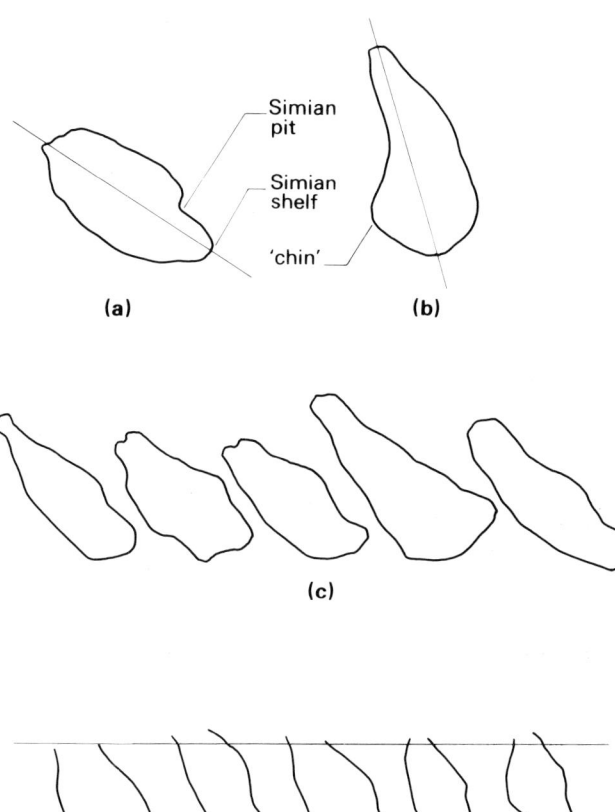

**Fig. 11.22.** Sagittal sections through the mandibular symphysis of (a) gorilla and (b) modern man (long axes shown as thin lines). (c) Sagittal sections through the symphyses of a number of gorillas showing the variation in its form and therefore the unreliability of the section as a taxonomic indicator. (d) Sections through the symphysis of some examples of fossil man: 1, Sangiran B; 2, Choukoutein G; 3, Maver; 4, Rabout; 5, Mountmaurien; 1–4, *H. erectus* and 5, *H. sapiens*.

11.23). Practically all human populations for which adequate records are available exhibit approximately the same degree of variability; it is high compared with that for a number of other animals.

The study of human variability is the study of human races. However, 'pure races' have never existed; population hybridization, race mixture and invasions have been going on during the whole of history. The notion of racial 'purity' depends more on emotionally conceived opinions than on the results of impartial scientific analysis.

To a biologist, a race is just a group of individuals or populations which form a recognizable subdivision of the species. A race is identified by the fact that the individuals within it share characteristics which distinguish them from other races of the species. A biological species itself is usually defined as that set of individuals which includes all those who could (and do) mate with each other and produce fertile offspring. This means that matings between members of different races within a species are just as fertile as matings within races. The members of a race (or subgroup) are, however, most likely to find their mates within their own race (or subgroup). This results in the races (or subgroups) becoming separated from one another so far as reproduction is concerned. Because such groups mate among themselves, rather than with other groups, they tend to become more and more distinct. The more distinct they become and the more they are separated from each other, the less likely it becomes that individuals marry outside their own group. This tends to make the groups become increasingly distinguishable from each other.

Four major poles of differences among peoples have been recognized:
1 Negroids, who possess genes for dark skin, kinked hair, broad noses and thick everted lips.

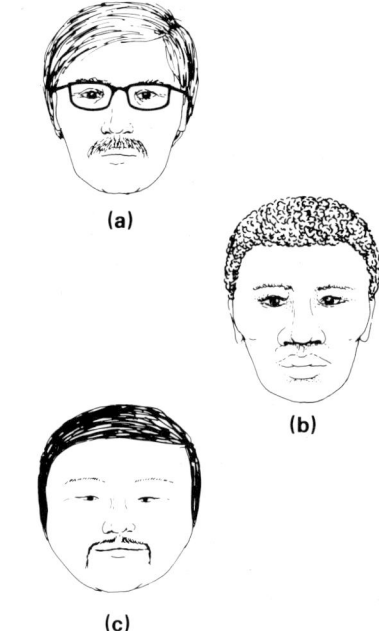

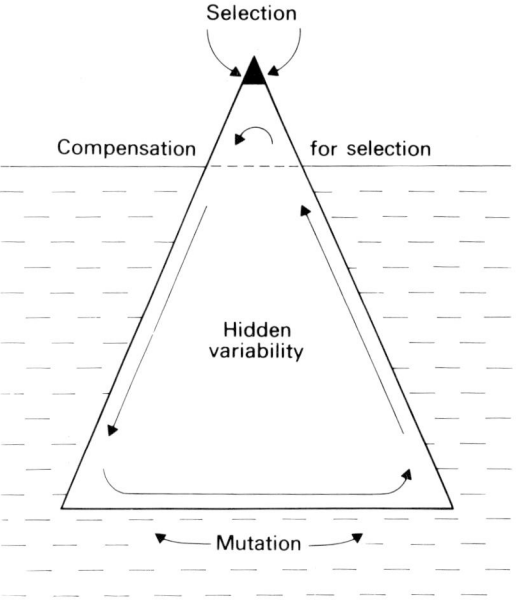

**Fig. 11.23** (a) Caucasoid, (b) negroid, and (c) mongoloid.

**Fig. 11.24.** Diagram to show the degree of variability in man.

2  Caucasoids, who possess genes for fair skin, long wavy hair, thin noses and thin lips.
3  Mongoloids, who possess genes for yellow-red skin, slanted eyelids, straight black hair and sparse body hair.
4  Australoids, who possess genes for dark skin, but otherwise the features characteristic of caucasoids.

These categories, however, represent only an approximate outline of genetic groupings that are presently regarded as 'races'. Nevertheless, they are not discrete entities, as there are fine gradations (clines) between extreme racial characteristics or even between one population sample and another from the same 'racial' group. Indeed there may be more variation within a 'racial' group than between different 'racial' groups, e.g. dental arch shape.

Although human diversity consists of morphological, physiological, biochemical and pathological variations subject mainly to genetic control, it is impossible to segregate the effects of genetic and external environmental factors, since they often interact one with another (Fig. 11.24). Moreover, when considering the craniofacial skeleton, some features, e.g. the cranial base, may be predominantly subject to genetic control whereas others, e.g. nasal form, may be mainly affected by environmental factors. Further the question as to whether the factors affecting different attributes vary between different population samples has yet to be resolved. Human genotypes (as in all sexually reproducing organisms) are also in a constant state of flux, raising the problem of the selective forces which coerce such a change. Selective forces operate in man to change his genotype even though such forces do not necessarily lead to uniformity. Some human communities remain distinct today because they contain individuals whose genes provide them with very different physical capabilities, e.g. Australian aborigines. Indeed human diversity within a community may well constitute a polymorphism maintained by selection.

The effect of environmental factors is also complex. For instance, climatic extremes stimulate the inhabitants to find ways of isolating themselves from heat or cold. Indeed it may be that the searching of ways to combat the rigours of a cold climate during the last Ice Age possibly provided the stimulus which elicited the development of the human brain that produced *Homo sapiens sapiens* (Cromagnon). Man's diversity may also be further complicated by the action of his cultural and social attributes, although it is difficult to subject these to critical scientific analysis.

BODY SIZE

Among the many 'racial' differences, variation in body size (e.g. body weight) is particularly conspicuous. In adults, the weight–climate relationship reflects differences in whole body morphology; the warmer the environment the greater the lengths of the arms and legs relative to the trunk, the lower the girths and transverse diameters of the body and hence the lower the weight per unit stature. Indeed, as the mean annual temperature rises, so the mean weight drops. Weight also increases with increasing altitude.

Adjustment to hot climates involves a small body mass, attenuated extremities, little fat and a great number of sweat glands per unit body surface. By contrast, adjustment to a cold environment involves a large body mass, short extremities and much fat. Although both tall and short people live in most of the major regions, investigation of the distribution of the cormic index (ratio of sitting height to stature, hence an indication of leg length) reveals that this index decreases from north to south, Chinese, Eskimo and American Indian values reaching from 54% while those of Africans lie nearer to 45%.

Despite variation in his proportions, man exhibits a similar size and shape (Fig. 11.25). Because it is related to volume, body weight is proportional to the cube of the linear dimensions; therefore, man could not be very much heavier and maintain the same proportions. For similar reasons, man could not be very much smaller than at present, i.e. very much smaller than pygmies. Height is in fact controlled by many genes and is influenced by many physiological processes.

Even with modern therapeutic measures, selection may eliminate any mutations which produce extremes, e.g. dwarfs and giants, and may also remove individuals who have a fortuitous combination of polygenes which produces extremes. Nevertheless, this still leaves an immense reservoir of the same genes in other individuals, where, unless complicated by dominance, they are balanced by genes working in the opposite direction. The actual variability conveyed by a polygenic system is vast.

*Growth*

The 'racial' differences seen in the adult build are produced by differences in the rates and patterns of growth. Some of these differences are genetically determined, others are nutritional in origin. Although climate has little direct effect on the growth rate, the growth period is prolonged and maturation somewhat delayed in warmer regions. The Africans are ahead of Europeans in skeletal maturity at birth and during the first 2 years; this most likely reflects genetic differences. Probably because of inadequate nutrition, this advance disappears by about the 3rd year. From the effects of famine resulting from war or natural calamities it is well known that malnutrition delays growth. Children have great recuperative powers, however, provided the adverse conditions are not carried too far or continued for too long. During the past century, there has been a worldwide trend towards greater size and earlier maturation. In Europe, stature is increasing by about 1 cm per decade whilst the menarche is getting earlier by approximately 4 months per decade. Such changes are also evident for the timing of tooth eruption, and tooth and dental arch size.

Examination of fetuses, neonates and infants of Asian, African and European populations, reveals obvious great similarities, whilst the adult representatives of these groups present certain characteristic differences. Somewhere between immaturity and maturity, therefore, the distinctive features become established. Up to the age of 5 years, there is an acceleration in skull growth which then tails off and proceeds more slowly. This change in the pattern of skull growth coincides with the end of the period of the deciduous dentition. It may be that direct genetic control of growth predominates up to about 5 years of age and thereafter the hormonal factors play an increasingly important role.

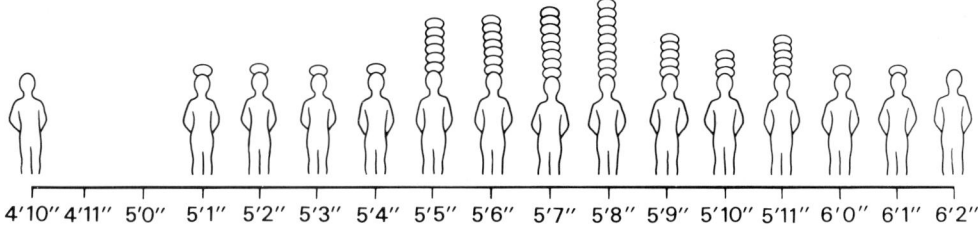

**Fig. 11.25.** Distribution of stature in a sample of 180 male dental students.

## Head size

There have been many investigations into the shape of the head (Fig. 11.26). This is assessed by measuring the breadth and length of the head and expressing it as a percentage ratio—the cephalic index. Head shape is classified into three types: dolichocephalic (long headed, <74.9), mesocephalic (intermediate, 75.0–79.9) and brachycephalic (broad headed, >80.0) (Fig. 11.27). At one time, it was considered that broad-headed people such as the Swiss and Austrians in Europe and certain Mongolians in Central Asia represented remnants of older populations that had been driven from the plains into the security of the mountains. Nevertheless, one must not neglect the fact that there have been the great Mongolian invasions into Europe and the Middle East, and these have undoubtedly contributed to an increase in brachycephaly in eastern and central Europe. Indeed, this phenomenon is on the increase all over the world. Archeological evidence shows that there is a tendency for modern populations to be more brachycephalic than their ancestors. This is termed brachycephalization. Today, the broadest heads are found among the Mongolians and the narrowest in parts of Africa. The underlying cause or mechanism for this change remains controversial, although it is known that brachycephaly is genetically dominant. Various factors have been considered to underly this increasing brachycephalization, such as domestication, cradling, endocrine and nutritional influences, but none of these have as yet clarified this phenomenon.

In modern man, variation in skull form is not reflected in the dimensions of the braincase or nose, but in more general differences in certain functional regions, e.g. facial height. This suggests that the analysis of cranial variation must depend upon a whole host of cranial dimensions, rather than single dimensions or simple indices that formed the bases of past analyses. Indeed, variation in cranial form is now regarded as so complex that sophisticated forms of statistical analysis are required in their investigation. Only in this way will it be possible to discriminate between the interaction of genetic and environmental factors.

## Face

Among caucasoids, vertically 'long' and vertically 'short' facial types exist (Fig. 11.28). The latter are characterized by a rounded head form and a more vertical cranial base. This contrasts with the longer skull form, which has a more angled cranial base. The latter are characterized by a more retrognathic facial profile due to a relative forward placement of the nasomaxillary complex by the more open cranial floor flexure and the downward and backward rotation of the mandibular ramus caused by the relatively long vertical midface and open cranial floor flexure.

The key feature among long-faced caucasoids that tends to offset the characteristic population tendency toward retrognathia is a horizontally wide ramus. This feature provides dimensional compensation that partially or entirely balances the effect produced by the more obtuse flexure of

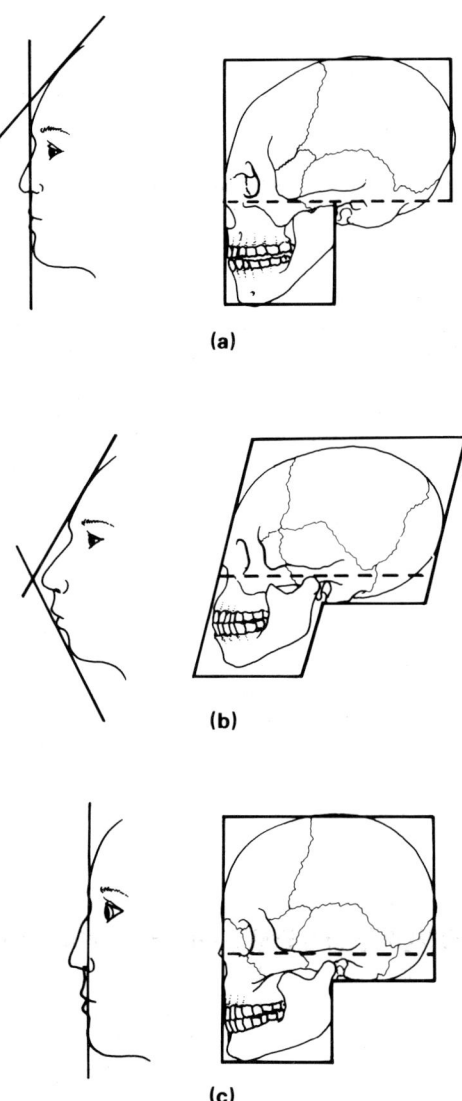

**Fig. 11.26.** (a) Dolicho-; (b) brachy-; (c) meso-cephalic heads.

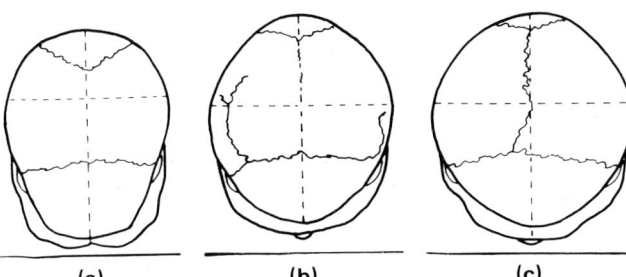

Fig. 11.27. (a) Dolicho-; (b) brachy-; (c) meso-cephalic skulls in norma horizontalis.

the cranial floor, the relatively long midface and the resultant backward and downward rotation of the whole mandible.

Negroids, like many caucasoids, have a dolichocephalic (long) head form, with consequent forward (and downward) placement of the maxilla. Also they have a wide horizontal ramus that serves to balance the forward position of the maxilla. The wide ramus exceeds the equivalent cranial floor (middle cranial fossa) dimension and produces a resultant protrusion of the mandibular body. This in turn produces a displacement (tipping) of the anterior maxillary region by the mandibular incisors and a consequent bimaxillary protrusion that is distinctive of this craniofacial combination. Thus, dolichocephaly is associated with (and may result from) a wide mandibular ramus.

While the headform and cranial base angle of negroids are similar to those of caucasoids, their upper ethmomaxillary pattern is more mongoloid. In negroids and mongoloids the dimensions of the upper face and anterior cranial floor produce a more vertical forehead, smaller frontal sinuses, low nasal bridge, short nasal protrusion and prominent cheekbones.

It has been suggested that the Mongolian face exhibits features specially adapted to a cold climate; reduction of the browridges and the concomitant decrease in the size of the frontal sinuses coupled with flattening and widening of the facial region. These features help to conserve heat. The epicanthic fold around the eye is also considered a protective adjustment to cold and arid environments that are subject to great temperature fluctuations and against glare.

Regarding the nose, generally, the further north one goes, the narrower the nasal aperture on the skull, and the further south toward the equator one goes, the broader is this aperture. The shape of the nose can be described by the nasal index (the ratio of breadth to height). The greater the index the wider the aperture. Most African populations, Melanesians and Australian aborigines have a high index while the Eskimos have low values and those of Mongolians and American Indians are intermediate. The nasal index rises markedly as temperature and humidity rise. The high nasal index of tropical populations appears to be related to the vascular condition of the mucous membrane of the nasal passages which facilitates the evaporation of water so that inhaled air is moistened. Functionally, the nasal shape is more related to moistening the inspired air than to heat exchange. This explains why narrower nasal apertures are found in regions of excessive dryness, such as hot and cold deserts. The Mongolian noses tend to look squat, due to a forward shift of the zygomatic bones which reduces the nasal projection. At the same time,

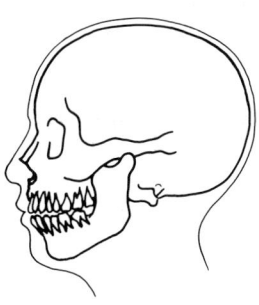

Figure 11.28. Skulls of (a) caucasoids and (b) negroids, illustrating constrasting proportions and relation between facial skeleton and braincase.

their orbits and eyeballs have also moved forward, and for extra protection, the cheek and eye regions are well padded with fat.

*Tooth size*

Tooth size also has an adaptive significance. In addition to mastication, the teeth are utilized for many manipulative functions including holding and grasping. Most of these functions involve the anterior rather than posterior teeth; the latter are primarily adapted to withstand occlusal wear; e.g. attrition and abrasion. Indeed, the major function of the premolars and molars is to masticate food and this requirement exerts the greatest selective influence on the size of these teeth.

Tooth size varies between different 'racial' groups and between different samples from the same 'racial' group. But the degree of discrimination between different samples depends upon the tooth dimensions actually included in the analysis. When comparing two population samples, different degrees of discrimination can be obtained depending upon whether the dimensions of the anterior rather than posterior teeth are compared, or whether cusp heights rather than cusp widths are compared. Thus the interpretation of variation in tooth size is far more complex that traditionally assumed.

During the evolution leading to modern man, a general reduction in tooth size is apparent. There is controversy, however, as to the causes of this dental reduction. Some contend that dental reduction occurred at the time of facial shortening concomitant with the evolution of a bipedal posture. Others contend that it occurred with a change from a predominantly vegetable to a mixed diet. The fundamental problem, however, is whether the predominant control over tooth morphology results from genetic or environmental factors. Various models have been proposed for the genetic control of tooth size, whereas family studies indicate that environmental factors also affect this biological structure. Furthermore, the effect of cultural changes on selection for tooth morphology are difficult to elucidate, although such factors possibly affected the anterior rather than posterior teeth.

Anatomical variations exist in different populations, and these vary in frequency or degree of manifestation. For example, congenital absence of the third permanent molar is not uncommon in Asian and European peoples (particularly Eskimos), but infrequent in others, although this trait may be interrelated with dental arch length and the size of the remaining teeth. Similarly, the Carabelli anomaly exhibits varying degrees of manifestation in different 'racial' groups, although recent research suggests that it may merely reflect variation in tooth size. Thus when considering a morphological trait, cognisance must be taken of the fact that rather than being a discrete entity, it may be associated with other poorly investigated or unrecognized traits.

Certain morphological features which at one time were considered to be important 'racial' variations have proved to be the results of malnutrition, e.g. the anteroposterior flattening of the upper part of the femoral shaft. Socioeconomic factors are also important. Disease and catastrophes, e.g. famine, floods and war, have all contributed to differential growth of populations. Apart from nutrition, population overcrowding also affects body growth, along with susceptibility to infection, although whether this affects craniofacial forms as well as general body form has yet to be elucidated.

Investigations during the last century have shown that in Europe, USA, Australia and Japan, there has been in general an increase in body weight, brachycephalization, an earlier eruption of both the deciduous and permanent dentitions as well as an earlier occurrence of the menarche and

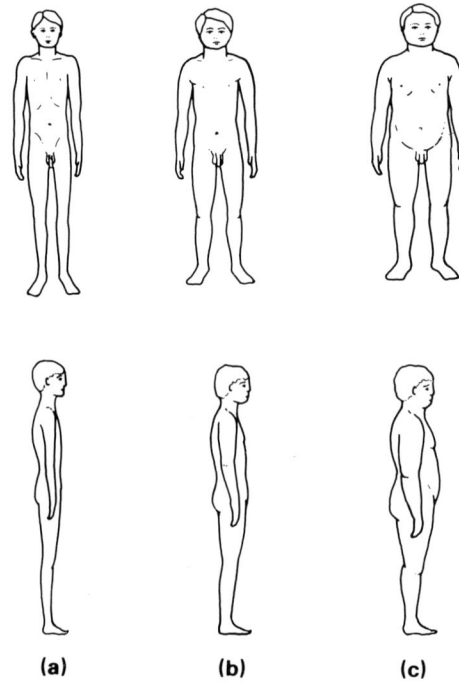

**Fig. 11.29.** (a) Ectomorph, (b) mesomorph and (c) endomorph men.

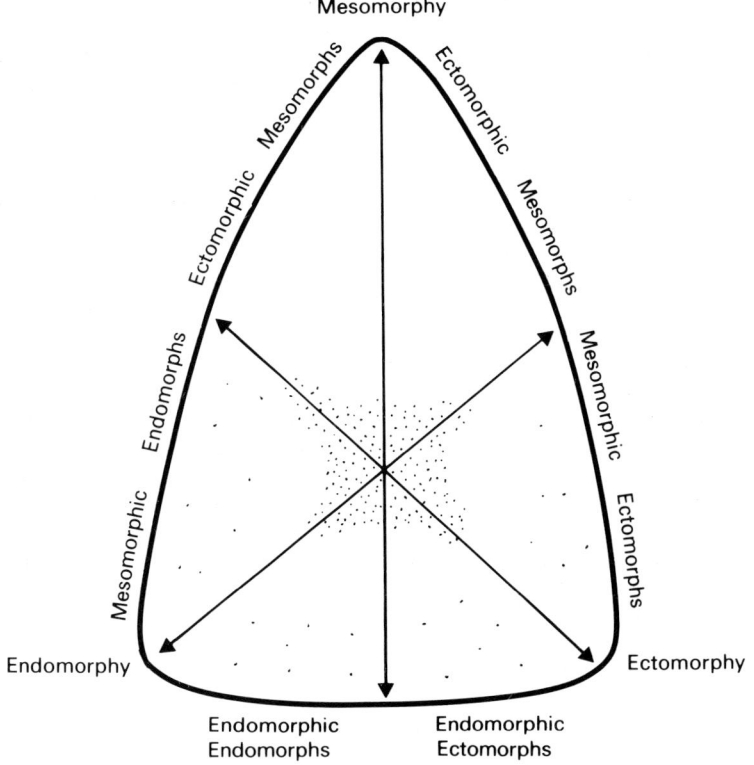

Fig. 11.30. Distribution of mesomorphy, endomorphy and ectomorphy in groups of 80 British male dental students.

later appearance of the menopause concomitant with an increase in stature. This is most likely due to the better living conditions, though contribution by hormonal and genetic influences cannot be excluded. Socioeconomic factors undoubtedly are going to be of increasing influence in the evolution of man.

BODY FORM

In order to facilitate the investigation of body form, three main categories have been defined: ectomorphy, mesomorphy and endomorphy, to which can also be assigned a variety of other attributes (Fig. 11.29).

1 An endomorph: characterized by a round, fat body associated with large livers, gut and lungs. These individuals tend to be relaxed, aimiable, sociable, but tend to suffer from diabetes and manic depression.

2 A mesomorph: defined as muscular bony bodies with a large heart. These individuals tend to be adventurous, aggressive, extrovert and dominating, but suffer from coronary thrombosis, hysteria and depression.

3 An ectomorph: defined as long thin individuals with large brains and narrow chests. These individuals tend to be secretive, inhibited, introvert and intelligent, but suffer from tuberculosis, schizophrenia, anxiety, hysteria and depression.

These categories represent only very broad generalizations, and obviously there are an infinite number of gradations between one category and another (Fig. 11.30). Nevertheless, such a classification has greatly helped in the elucidation of the factors influencing body form, although there is as yet little dental evidence in this respect.

**Conclusion**

Modern man has marked morphological, physiological, biochemical and cultural variability. The majority of these attributes are multifactorial, continuous and overlapping. In fact, the characteristics that 'races' share in common are much more significant than those which divide them.

## FURTHER READING

BAKER P.T. & WEINER J.S. Eds. (1966) *The Biology of Human Adaptability*. Oxford: Clarendon Press.

BISHOP W.W. & MILLER J.A. (1972) *Calibration of Hominoid Evolution*. Toronto: University of Toronto Press.

DARLINGTON C.D. (1969) *The Evolution of Man and Society*. London: Allen & Unwin.

DAY M. (1977) *A Guide to Fossil Man*, 3rd Edition. London: Cassell.

*DAY M.H. (1970) *Fossil Man*. London: Hamlyn.

HARRIS H. (1970) *The Principles of Human Biochemical Genetics*. Amsterdam: North-Holland Publishing Co.

HARRISON G.A., WEINER J.S., TANNER J.M. & BARNICOT N.A. (1964) *Human Biology: an introduction to human evolution, variation and growth*. Oxford: Clarendon Press.

PILBEAM D. (1972) *The Ascent of Man: an introduction to human evolution*. New York: Macmillan.

SIMONS E.L. (1972) *Primate Evolution: an introduction to man's place in nature*. New York: Macmillan.

*TATTERSALL I.A. (1970) *Man's Ancestors: an introduction to primate and human evolution*. London: John Murray.

There are many 'popular' texts on the general field of primatology and human evolution. The scale of recent new discoveries is such that any text cited at the present time will be out of date in at least some of the coverage. Those texts indicated by * can be read for pleasure. The remainder are more detailed and authorative.

# CHAPTER 12

# Comparative anatomy of dentition

## THE DENTITION OF MAMMALS

### THE ORDERS OF PLACENTAL MAMMALS

**Insectivora**

The order Insectivora contains the least modified descendants of the early Tertiary mammal radiation. They are all small animals and apart from spines (hedgehogs), stinkglands (shrews) and venom (some shrews and *Solenodon*), they are defenceless. Most are nocturnal, sheltering in nooks and crannies during the day; some are fossorial (moles), others are aquatic (otter shrews). Their diets usually include insects but the majority of species are by no means exclusively insectivorous and subsist on a variety of small animals, both invertebrate and vertebrate. Adaptively, the Insectivora are best described as 'small-time carnivores', as were the majority of the primitive Therian mammals of the Mesozoic era.

In number of teeth, most extant species are at or close to the primitive eutherian 'maximum' of 44. The most extensive adaptive modifications have been in the anterior teeth; the incisors are specialized as 'forceps' for picking up and immobilizing small prey, the lower incisors often being reduced in number and procumbent (leaning forward). The canines of some species are so reduced as to be indistinguishable from incisors or anterior premolars. The molars of the Insectivora are more like basic tribosphenic molars (Fig. 10.12) than are those of all other modern orders.

MOLES

$$I\frac{3}{3} C\frac{1}{1} P\frac{4}{4} M\frac{3}{3} = 44 \text{ (Fig. 12.1a)}$$

The lower canine is incisiform and joins the procumbent lower incisor group. The prominent upper canine therefore occludes in front of the apparent lower 'canine', which is a modified $P_1$.

The remaining dentition is basic eutherian. *Talpa europaea* prefers to eat earthworms, which are immobilized by biting and are stored alive in the burrow, but insect larvae and other soil invertebrates are also eaten.

HEDGEHOGS

$$I\frac{3}{2} C\frac{1}{1} P\frac{3}{2} M\frac{3}{3} = 36 \text{ (see Fig. 10.14)}$$

The first incisors are larger than the others: the procumbent lower pair occlude into a median diastema between the vertically implanted upper pair. The upper canine is small, the lower is procumbent and incisiform. $P^4$ has a very large mesiobuccal cusp supporting a crest which cuts against the mesial shearing edge of $M_1$. The molars are carapace-crushers; high-pointed cusps and opposing deep basins are exaggerated, shearing crests are reduced. Hedgehogs eat anything; most invertebrates, small invertebrates (grass-snakes, frogs, young birds, mice), vegetable matter, seeds and fruits. *Erinaceus europaeus* (the common hedgehog) prefers a diet of millipedes.

SHREWS

$$I\frac{3}{1} C\frac{1}{1} P\frac{3}{1} M\frac{3}{3} = 32$$

(Fig. 12.1b; see Fig. 10.1)
With over 200 species the shrews are the largest family of the Insectivora. *Sorex araneus*, the common shrew, has a very small and delicate skull which lacks a zygomatic arch. The single lower incisor is large and procumbent with a tricuspid distal edge which occludes with two large hooked cusps on the upper first incisor. The remaining upper incisors, both canines and anterior premolars are small and simple. $P^4$ is molariform. Upper molars are dilambdadont; having a W-shaped buccal cusp pattern (Fig. 10.14). The cusps of all teeth are coloured orange-red by an iron

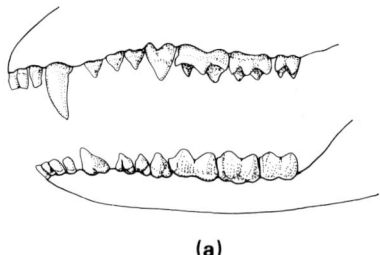

(a)

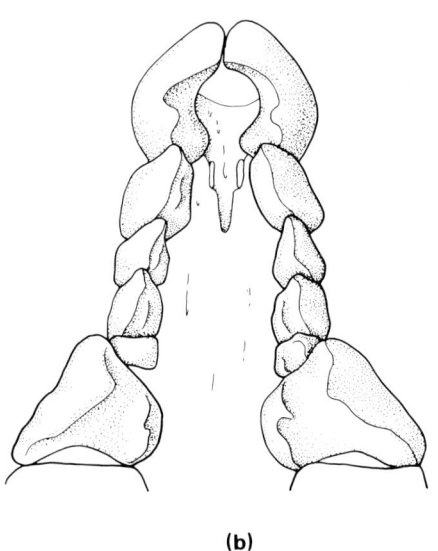

(b)

**Fig. 12.1.** (a) Dentition of the common mole. (b) Upper dentition of the white-toothed shrew, *Crocidura*.

pigment contained in the enamel (cf. rodents). Diet includes many small invertebrates, often woodlice, together with seeds and fruit. Since the small body can only store sufficient food reserves to keep it alive for about 1–2 hours, feeding is almost continual. The life span (about $1-1\frac{1}{2}$ years) appears to be limited by wear of the molar teeth, death being due to starvation. The deciduous dentition is formed and shed *in utero* (as in many Insectivora).

CAPE GOLDEN MOLES

$$I\frac{3}{3} C\frac{1}{1} P\frac{3}{3} M\frac{3}{3} = 40$$

In addition to the above dilambdadonts, the Insectivora contains a number of species (mostly confined to Madagascar and South Africa) which have zalambdadont molar teeth with a single V-shaped cusp pattern (Fig. 10.14) not unlike those of Jurassic pantotheres. The molars are very high, narrow and wedge-shaped. Upper molars have one lingual and one buccal cusp; the lowers lack a talonid. The first and second incisors are enlarged. Canines are no larger than the third incisors and anterior premolars. The posterior premolars are molariform. *Chrysochloris* is superficially very similar to the talpid moles, through convergent adaptation. Its diet also is similar to that of *Talpa*.

**Dermoptera**

This order contains only the two species of *Cynocephalus*, the so-called 'flying lemurs' of South-east Asia. Since they glide rather than fly and are now known to be but distantly related to the lemurs, their local familiar name 'Colugo' is now commonly used. The upper incisors are missing, the four specialized procumbent lower incisors and the lower canines are pectinated (Fig. 12.2a); each is elongated mesiodistally and flattened buccolingually with the crown being deeply divided, almost to its base, in to as many as twelve cusps arranged like the teeth of a comb. The diet is entirely vegetable; the specialized incisors are used for straining fruit and cropping leaves against a gum pad on the upper jaw (cf. cow). The front edge of the tongue is serrate and acts as a tooth-brush for the pectinate teeth. It is often assumed, but has never been observed, that these 'comb-teeth' are used for grooming as in lemurs. The molar teeth are dilambdadont.

**Chiroptera**

The bats are closely related to the ancestral insectivore stock. The Megachiroptera are large (up to 4 ft wing span) diurnal fruit-eaters of the tropics with well developed senses of sight and smell. The Microchiroptera, comprising the vast majority of species worldwide, are small (4–12 inch wing span) mostly nocturnal insect-eaters in which the sense of hearing is best developed. Nocturnal navigation and the ability to feed on the wing are facilitated by a phenomenon known as echolocation: as it flies the bat emits through its mouth or nose ultrasonic squeaks which are reflected back to the bat by obstacles or flying insects.

FRUIT BATS (FLYING FOXES)

$$I\frac{2}{2} C\frac{1}{1} Pm\frac{3}{3} M\frac{2}{3} = 34 \text{ (Fig. 12.2b)}$$

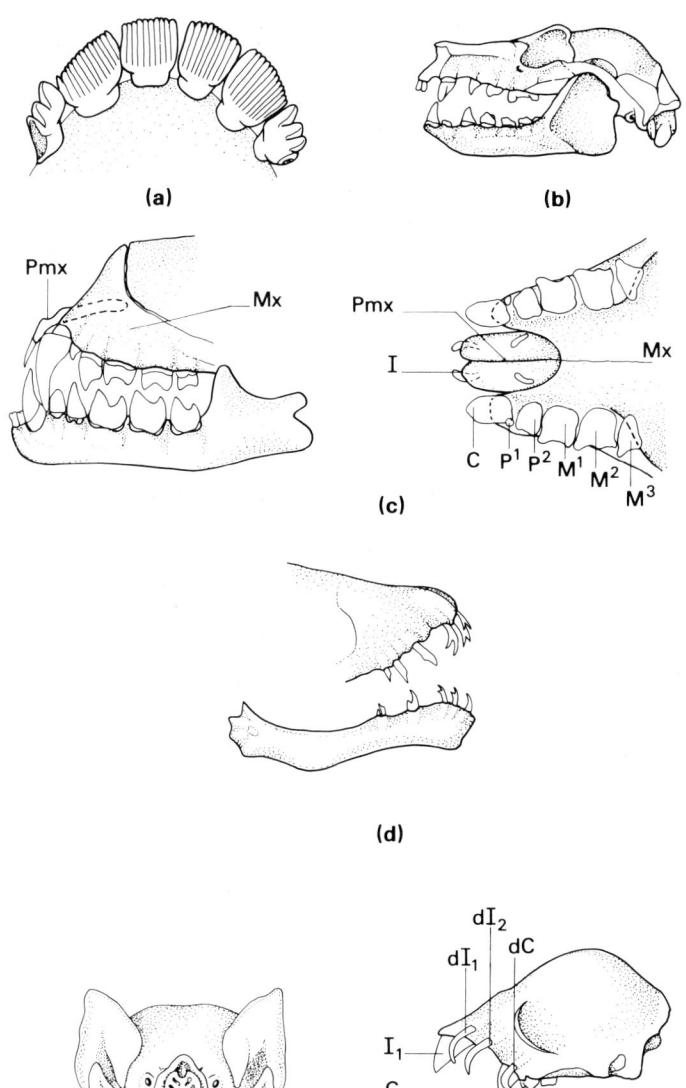

**Fig. 12.2.** (a) Lower anterior dentition of the colugo. (b) Skull of the fruit bat, *Pteropus*. (c) Dentition of an insectivorous bat: left, lateral view; right, palatal view. (d) Deciduous dentition of an insectivorous bat. (e) Face and dentition of the vampire bat, *Desmodus*. The deciduous anterior dentition is still in place.

Most species of Megachiroptera feed on fruit and flowers and are gregarious. Soft fruit is squashed by the tongue against pronounced palatal rugae and indigestible fibrous material spat out. Harder fruits are first chewed by the molar teeth which are spaced out and low crowned with few prominent cusps. Incisors are small (reduced to $I\frac{1}{0}$ in the tube-nosed species); the canines are large and in some species show sexual dimorphism of size.

INSECTIVOROUS BATS

$$I\frac{0-2}{2-3} C\frac{1}{1} P\frac{1-3}{2-3} M\frac{3}{3} = 26\text{--}38$$

In the Microchiroptera there are sixteen families of living species, some of which are extremely numerous. This suborder contains the smallest known mammal species. The extreme reduction, in some species, of the upper anterior dentition and premaxillae is related to the development of a specialized nose 'leaf' (Fig. 12.2c). The canines are large and prominent in both sexes of most species. The post-canine tooth row is shortened by the reduced number of premolars. The three dilambdadont molars are well developed. In some species of Phyllostomatidae (American leaf-nosed bats) the molars are shaped like those of the Megachiroptera. Although most species are insectivorous, some are carnivorous or even piscivorous and there are also nectar and pollen feeders. Young bats (there is usually only one offspring per year) hook on to their mother's fur when flying, by means of their specially adapted deciduous teeth (Fig. 12.2d).

VAMPIRE BATS

$$I\frac{1}{2} C\frac{1}{1} P\frac{2}{3} M\frac{0}{0} = 20 \text{ (Fig. 12.2e)}$$

The three species constituting the New World family Desmodontidae of the Microchiroptera are true vampires, feeding exclusively on fresh blood. *Desmodus* alights on or near an exposed area of the prey's skin and makes a shallow incision with its anterior teeth. The exuding blood is either lapped up or sucked from the wound by the tongue which can be rolled up into a tube. Their saliva contains an anticoagulant. A vampire will feed on any birds or mammals which are not alerted by the high frequency sounds emitted during echolocation. Although the canines are large the incision is made by the extremely specialized V-shaped and razor-edged upper incisors. The post-canine dentition is reduced and functionless.

## Edentata

These animals are the relics of a once numerous group which evolved in isolation in South America during the Tertiary (Fig. 4.17). Although Edentata means 'without teeth', only the anteaters are entirely toothless. Sloths and armadillos have cheek teeth but these lack enamel.

ANTEATERS

(Fig. 10.2)
Their skulls are extremely long and lack a zygomatic arch; their jaw muscles are very weak and they have no teeth. Giant anteaters tear open termite or ant colonies with the powerful recurved claws on their hands and then collect the insects with their long sticky tongues (the tongue of the giant anteater can be protruded up to 2 ft beyond the nose); the prey is swallowed whole. The Old World scaly anteater (*Manis*, order Pholidota) has convergently evolved similar masticatory structures and feeding behaviour. The adult pangolin is toothless but, unlike the New World anteaters, the embryo forms a few rudimentary teeth which can be regarded as evolutionary vestiges.

SLOTHS

Unlike the huge extinct ground sloths of the South American Pleistocene, living sloths are adapted for a life in the trees of rain forests and are quite helpless on the ground; some individuals have been observed to spend their entire lives hanging from the branches of a single tree. Tree sloths are obligate herbivores, often eating leaves exclusively. This is a diet for which they seem poorly equipped dentally. The skull is short and rounded; the teeth number $\frac{5}{4} = 18$ of which (in the two-toed sloth) the first are sharp-edged 'canines', triangular in section. The remaining cheek teeth are smaller and of uniform size and shape. Each tooth consists of a cement-covered cylinder of dentine, occlusally infilled by secondary dentine. Tooth wear is compensated by continuous formation of dentine and persistent eruption. The two-toed sloth (*Choloepus*) wears its teeth into a zig-zag occlusal plane. In the three-toed sloth (*Bradypus*) the occlusal surfaces are flat. Some masticatory benefit may be obtained from differential wear of the softer secondary dentine which is surrounded by a raised rim of primary dentine. Tree sloths have an extremely low metabolic rate (hence their laziness and their name) which accounts in part for their lack of elaborate masticatory equipment normally regarded as mandatory for herbivores.

ARMADILLOS

These are ground living or burrowing animals, rat to pig-sized, which feed on invertebrates, especially ants and other insects, small vertebrates and plants. The skull is flattened and the elongated jaws bear numerous peg-like, persistently growing, teeth along their margins. There is usually a total of 36 such teeth, but as many as 90 have been noted in one individual.

## Rodentia

Rodents are the most numerous (about 3000 species) and one of the most widespread and variably adapted mammalian orders, and yet they share a remarkable uniformity of structure, especially of the skull and dentition. In their adaptive radiation rodents have become fossorial (rodent moles; *Spalax*, bathyergids), arboreal (squirrel), aerial ('flying' squirrel), aquatic (beaver), armoured (porcupine), cursorial (agouti), saltatory (American 'kangaroo' rat) and 'elephantine' (capybara). Their adaptive radiation has been particularly extensive in South America, which was an isolated continent during most of the Tertiary, and rodents entered niches occupied by other mammalian groups in the rest of the world. Other mammalian orders have produced similar radiations but these have often involved quite extensive dental modifications to suit the peculiarities of the diet in each different niche and in some cases the modification is so great as to initiate a new order (e.g. Carnivora and Pinnepedia). Rodents have evolved a peculiar dentition which can do almost anything by only minor modifications between different adaptive types.

The key to the success of rodents is undoubtedly the continuously forming incisor (Fig. 12.31). These are used universally in attack and defence, for nibbling or gnawing food and for carrying the young and sometimes used as tools for digging (rodent moles) and gnawing. The absence of canines can be explained in two ways: (a) the canine region is occupied by the developing incisor; and (b) the functions of the canine have been usurped by the incisor (Fig. 12.3a). The diastema is extended by loss of the anterior premolars. The cheeks can be drawn medially through the diastema to isolate the incisors from the rest of the mouth cavity when the animal is using its incisors as a tool; that is, for gnawing through material which is not to be eaten. Rodents have from two to six cheek teeth (usually three or four) and depending upon crown height these may be brachydont through hypsodont to a complete absence of anatomical roots. Cusp patterns vary correspondingly from bunodont to lophodont. Most rodents can stand on their hind feet and use their hands in feeding. In many species, the surface of the incisor enamel is coloured yellow or orange by an iron pigment.

The four sub-orders (represented by the examples below) are distinguished by the form of the molar teeth and by the attachment position of the anterior deep masseter. This division of the masseter muscle is peculiar to rodents; it provides power for gnawing once the mandible has been protruded by the superficial masseter (Fig. 12.4a; see Fig. 10.18).

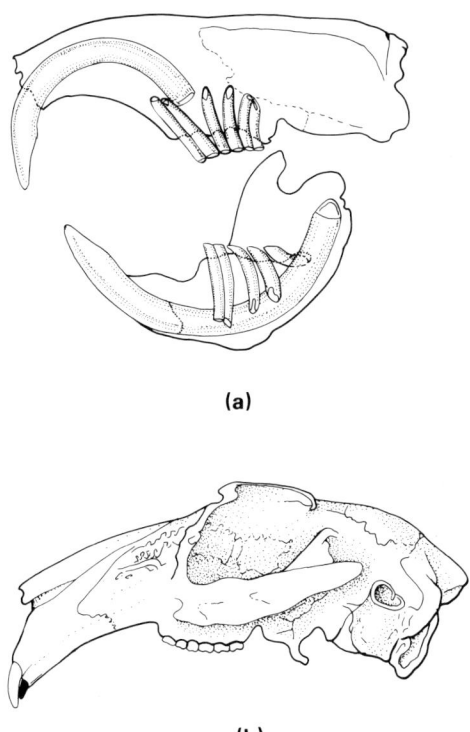

**Fig. 12.3.** (a) Skull outline and dentition of the pocket gopher, *Geomys*. (b) Skull of the hare, *Lepus*. The small second incisor is shown in black.

SQUIRRELS

$$I\frac{1}{1} \, C\frac{0}{0} \, P\frac{2}{1} \, M\frac{3}{3} = 22 \text{ (Fig. 12.4b)}$$

In sciuromorphs, the attachment of the anterior division of the deep masseter is extended forward on the face in front of the eye on to an expansion of the zygomatic process of the maxilla. The first premolar is frequently lost before maturity. Molar teeth are brachydont, the uppers with four transverse ridges, the lowers with basins ringed by cusps. Squirrels proverbially eat nuts, seeds and other plant material but they also devour insects and other small animals.

MICE AND RATS

$$I\frac{1}{1} \, C\frac{0}{0} \, P\frac{0}{0} \, M\frac{3}{3} = 16 \text{ (Fig. 12.4c)}$$

Mice and rats are monophyodont: they have no replacement teeth. The forward extension of the anterior division of deep masseter (as in the sciuromorphs) is retained but some of the deepest

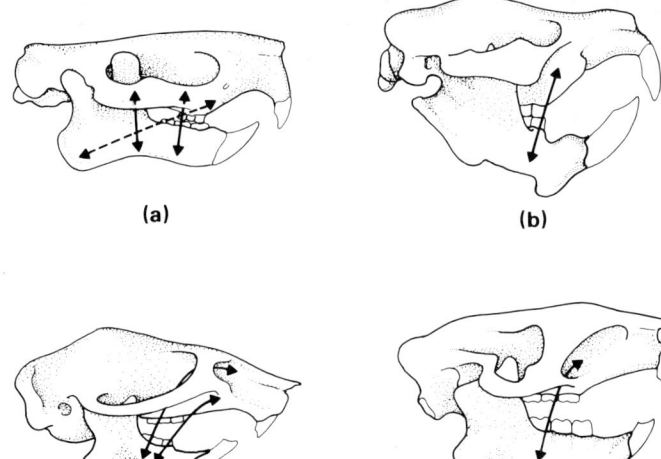

**Fig. 12.4.** The anterior deep masseter of rodents (for explanation see text). (a) Primitive condition, also showing orientation of superficial masseter (dotted line). (b) Advanced sciuromorphs. (c) Myomorphs. (d) Hystricomorphs and caviamorphs.

fibres pass through the infraorbital foramen and are attached to the lateral wall of the maxilla close to its suture with the nasal. Upper and lower molars are brachydont and (initially) bunodont. The failure to develop enamel on the tips of the molar cusps leads to the rapid formation of raised enamel ridges which are more effective in grinding. Some mice have lost their third molars. Most species feed on plant material and invertebrates.

PORCUPINES

$$I\frac{1}{1} C\frac{0}{0} P\frac{1}{1} M\frac{3}{3} = 20 \text{ (Fig. 12.4d)}$$

In the hystricomorph rodents, there is no expansion of the zygomatic process (*cf.* anteaters and sloths). Instead the anterior deep masseter muscle passes entirely through the expanded infraorbital foramen. The premolar is molariform. The four cheek teeth are hypsodont with late-developing roots. Deep infolding of the enamel produces multiple ridges on the occlusal surface through differential wear of the dental tissues. Cement covers the tooth including the infolded regions of the crown. Diet is usually vegetable (roots, bulbs and tree bark) but includes carrion (e.g. the marrow of long bones and even dental pulp of elephant tusks which is reached by gnawing through the dentine).

GUINEA PIGS

$$I\frac{1}{1} C\frac{0}{0} P\frac{1}{1} M\frac{3}{3} = 20$$

In most caviamorphs (New World rodents, regarded as the most advanced rodent forms) the cheek teeth permanently grow and erupt, and lack anatomical roots altogether. Each of the four cheek teeth usually has a VI-shaped pattern of enamel ridges with the vertically arranged component plates joined firmly together by cement. In some species (e.g. *Dinomys*, lit: 'terrible mouse') many of these plates are jointed together to form anteroposterior ranks in each tooth position. The enamel ridges on such teeth form extremely efficient grinding files. Masseter attachment is similar to that of hystricomorphs. Most caviamorphs eat plant material of various kinds.

## Lagomorpha

Once grouped with the Rodentia, the similarities between lagomorphs and rodents are now recognized to be the result of parallel evolution rather than of common ancestry.

RABBITS AND HARES

$$I\frac{2}{1} C\frac{0}{0} P\frac{3}{2} M\frac{3}{3} = 28 \text{ (Figs. 12.3b, 12.30)}$$

These are readily distinguished from rodents by dental characteristics. The incisors are persistently growing but, unlike the Rodentia, enamel is not confined to the labial surface. A small second upper incisor lies immediately behind the principal one and because it lacks a cutting edge may function as an occlusal stop for the single lower incisor. The cheek teeth, including molariform premolars, are lophodont and do not have anatomical roots: enamel is formed throughout life. Jaw mechanism is similar to rodents. The diet is strictly vegetarian; grasses and herbaceous plants being preferred. They re-ingest their nocturnal faeces (refection).

## Cetacea

There are two suborders; (a) Odontoceti: toothed whales, dolphins and porpoises and (b) Mysticeti: baleen or whalebone whales.

### SPERM WHALE (Fig. 12.5a)

Large odontocetes are adapted for low-speed surface travel and deep diving (up to 1 km). Aquatic adaptation has greatly influenced their head structure; e.g. the dorsal positioning of a single (fused) nostril and the telescoping of the skull by a backwards shift of maxillae so that the external nares, the blow hole, lies over the frontals and even the parietal. The dentition is homodont with the 30–60 functional teeth confined to the lower jaw and 'occluding' into keratin-lined sockets in the palate. They are large (1–6 inch diameter) and single rooted, often with a wide apical foramen, and erupt persistently. A small enamel cap is quickly worn off the crown. Rudimentary teeth are formed in the upper jaw but fail to erupt. These whales mainly eat pelagic (offshore) cephalopod molluscs (squid, cuttlefish) which live in the oceanic depths; their diet may be leavened by bony fish or sharks.

Most odontocetes locate their prey by sonar; ultrasonic squeaks are focussed and directed by an acoustic lens in the form of an oil-filled sac (the 'melon') above the upper jaw. Reflected sound is received by the lower jaw which functions as an ear trumpet.

Unfortunately, sperm whales have been slaughtered for a number of substances useful to man. Ambergris, a waxy material secreted to cover the indigestible beaks of squid to prevent irritation to the stomach lining, is prized as a perfume fixative. Spermaceti, once erroneously believed to be the sperm of the male whale, is a white wax used in ointments and sperm oil is an industrial machining lubricant with unique properties. Up to 1 ton of spermaceti and 30 barrels of sperm oil are found in the enormously developed melon of the sperm whale.

### DOLPHINS (Fig. 12.5b)

By contrast, small odontocetes are adapted for high speed surface travel (up to 25 knots) and do not dive deep. Their homodont dentition consists of up to 260 small sharp conical teeth, upper and lower rows interdigitating. There are no interdental septa and so the teeth occupy a continuous longitudinal groove in the jaw bone, being attached only loosely by periodontal connective tissue. Diet is principally bony fish. Killer whales are related to dolphins but have a different dentition, the teeth being much larger and only numbering ten to fourteen in each jaw quadrant.

The narwhal (*Monodon*) (Fig. 12.5c) is an unusual species of small odontocete which has only two teeth. One of these (the upper left 'incisor' of the male) forms a greatly elongated spirally twisted tusk, the horn of the mythical unicorn.

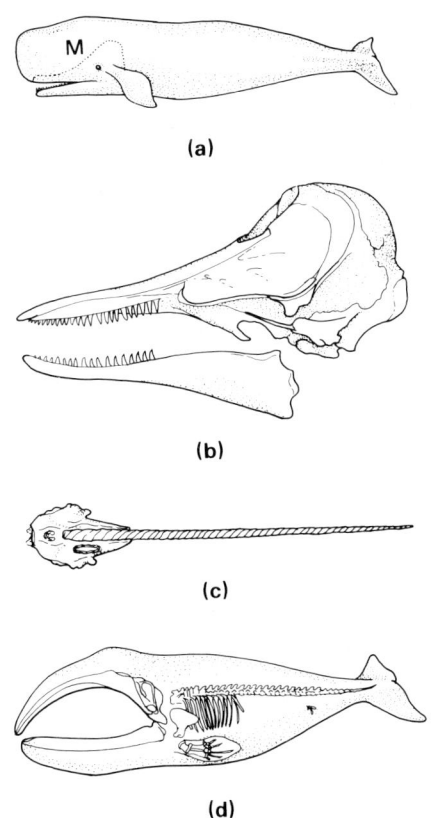

**Fig. 12.5.** (a) Sperm whale, *Physeter*, showing position of the melon (M) above the upper jaw (skull outline dotted). (b) Skull of a dolphin, *Delphinus*, showing the secondarily homodont dentition. (c) Dorsal view of the narwhal, *Monodon*, with superficial bone removed to show the root of the spiralling left incisor and the unerupted right incisor. The blowhole lies immediately behind the tusk. (d) Skeleton and body outline of the right whale, *Balaena*.

Usually the right tooth is small and remains unerupted. Neither tooth erupts in females. The narwhal eats cephalopods and fish. The function of the tusk is unknown but appears to represent an extreme expression of sexual ornamentation.

RIGHT WHALE (Fig. 12.5d; see Fig. 10.2)

Baleen whales are giant carnivores which can engulf entire populations of small invertebrates at a single gulp. The feeding apparatus occupies up to one-third of the body, the remainder of the skeleton being very reduced. There are no functional teeth (small teeth are formed and resorbed in the fetus); instead up to 350 plates of matted cemented hair (baleen or whalebone) derived from the palatal rugae hang from each highly arched upper jaw and function as a sieve-trap for planktonic animals (brit and krill). The whale swims slowly through the surface waters allowing the steady stream of water which enters the front of its mouth to pass between the fringed baleen plates and out at the sides. This traps the small crustaceans and molluscs on the inside of the plates. When a sufficient amount has accumulated, the mouth is closed and the plates are cleared by an enormous tongue whose keratinized papillae preen through the interstices of the baleen. The order Mysticeti includes the largest animal ever to have evolved on this planet, the blue whale, which can be over 100 ft in length and weigh as much as 130 tons.

## Carnivora

The order Carnivora is composed of two well-defined natural groups, the dog-like Canoidea (families Canidae, Ursidae, Procyonidae and Mustelidae) and the cat-like Feloidea (Viverridae, Hyaenidae and Felidae). Not all members of these families are carnivorous; e.g. otters are piscivorous, the aardwolf is insectivorous, bears and badgers are omnivorous, the giant panda is herbivorous. With the exception of the totally carnivorous cats and dogs the order contains so many animal species which have adapted to such a great diversity of diets that their collective name Carnivora can be quite misleading. However, they all share a relatively recent common ancestry from the Eocene miacids whose particular dental adaptations are still recognisable in even the most divergent of modern species. A full complement of simple or slightly trilobate incisors ($\frac{3}{3}$) and prominent canines have been inherited from Palaeocene insectivores with little modification other than an increase in size. The most obvious 'adaptive shift' has been the development in each jaw quadrant of a specialized shearing cheek tooth, the carnassial (see Fig. 10.13), which effectively slices flesh and bone. These teeth, $P^4$ and $M_1$ have greatly exaggerated the shearing planes of the tribosphenic molar and reoriented them parallel to rather than normal to the edge of the jaw while the crushing regions have in most cases been greatly reduced. Crushing and chewing functions are usually confined to molar teeth behind the carnassials.

DOGS, WOLVES AND FOXES (CANIDAE)

$$I\frac{3}{3} C\frac{1}{1} P\frac{4}{4} M\frac{2}{3} = 42$$

(Figs. 12.6a, 12.7a; see Figs. 10.13, 10.18)
The dog family is the most primitive group of the Carnivora and the genus *Canis* in particular, having changed little since Eocene times, can be taken as representative of the primitive type.

The incisors are used for seizing and tearing flesh and for carrying the young. Canines are for killing; they are very large, slightly recurved and deep rooted and are supported by an expansion of the maxilla. Occlusal space for the lower canine is provided by a diastema between the upper canine and $I^3$. Premolars are smaller at the front. P1 erupts with the deciduous dentition and is probably an unreplaced Dm1. With the exception of $P^4$ the upper and lower premolars do not meet when the mouth is closed. They fill in the space between the 'business ends' of the dentition and are used for holding or carrying objects. $M^1$ is a large crushing tooth which occludes with the talonid of $M_1$ and most of the smaller $M_2$. $M^2$ and $M^3$ are smaller crushing teeth which often fail to meet. The carnassials are used for shearing flesh, the molars for crushing bones and chewing. It should be noted that a primitive tribosphenic molar combines both these functions.

Canids are social creatures, often hunting in packs. Most species eat small animals; some (e.g. African hunting dogs) kill large prey; others (e.g. jackals) are carrion feeders, following lions, leopards or hyenas for remains of their kill.

BEARS AND GIANT PANDAS (URSIDAE)

$$I\frac{3}{3} C\frac{1}{1} P\frac{4}{4} M\frac{2}{3} = 42 \text{ (Fig. 12.7b, c)}$$

Bears have specialized the crushing elements of the dentition while the carnassials although still recognizable are greatly reduced in size and

# Comparative anatomy of dentition

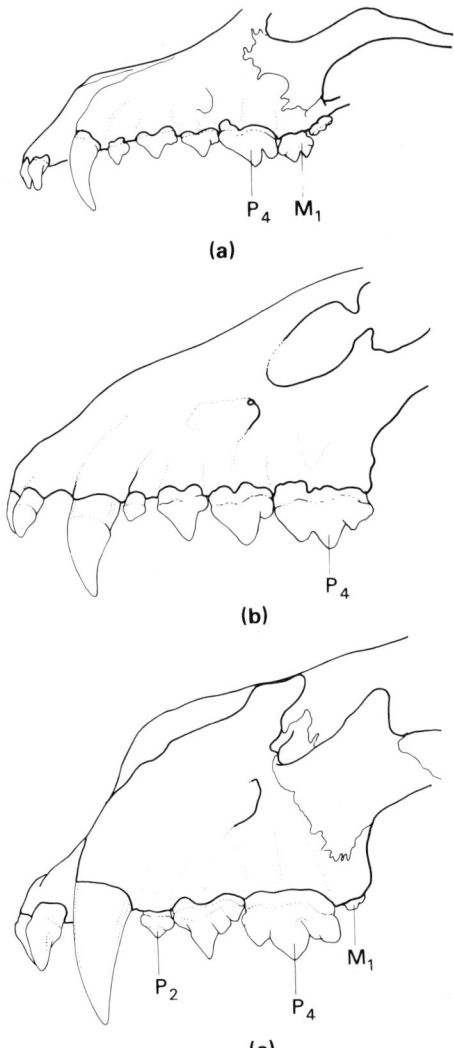

Fig. 12.6. Upper dentition of Carnivora: (a) dogs, *Canis*; (b) hyaena, *Crocuta*; (c) cat, *Panthera*.

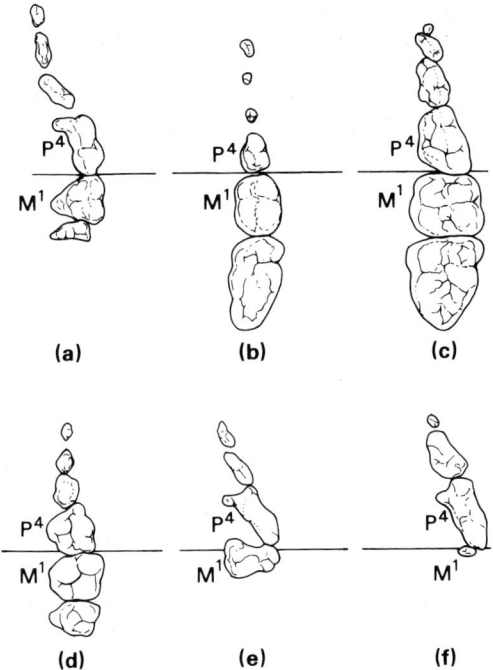

Fig. 12.7. Upper postcanine dentitions of Carnivora showing relative development of premolars and molars: (a) dog; (b) bear; (c) giant panda; (d) racoon; (e) weasel; (f) cat.

importance; $P^4$ has relatively rounder cusps and smaller crests than its counterpart in the dog. $M^1$ and $M^2$ are elaborately expanded bunodont crushing teeth. The first three upper premolars are reduced to the point of uselessness and are often lost early in life. Bears eat a great variety of food, both animal and vegetable. Only the polar bear is primarily carnivorous although other species have a preference for fish. The giant panda *Ailuropoda* (Fig. 12.7c) feeds almost exclusively on bamboo plants in its native territory, the mountains of western China. Unlike the other bears all the cheek teeth (except $P^1_1$) are expanded to form a crushing battery.

## RACOONS, COATIMUNDIS AND LESSER PANDAS (PROCYONIDAE)

$I\frac{3}{3} \ C\frac{1}{1} \ P\frac{4}{4} \ M\frac{2}{2} = 40$ (Fig. 12.7d)

The procyonids are primarily arboreal animals in many ways similar to diminutive bears. Their cheek teeth are similarly adapted for crushing and chewing, rather than shear. The cusps are more pointed than in bears. Racoons and coatimundis are omnivorous; the lesser panda, like his giant cousin, has a preference for bamboo shoots and leaves.

## WEASELS, BADGERS, SKUNKS, OTTERS, ETC. (MUSTELIDAE)

$I\frac{3}{3} \ C\frac{1}{1} \ P\frac{3}{3} \ M\frac{1}{2} = 34$ (Fig. 12.7e)

Most members of this family are small and feed on flesh or fish. Carnassials are prominent and the postcarnassial dentition always consists of a single pair of well-developed molars; the upper is a broad, transversely oriented tooth which crushes against a small $M_2$ together with the talonid region of $M_1$. $P^4$ is smaller and $M^1$ is considerably larger in badgers.

CIVET CATS AND
MONGOOSES (VIVERRIDAE)

$$I\frac{3}{3} C\frac{1}{1} P\frac{4}{4} M\frac{2}{2} = 40$$

This is the most primitive group of the cat-like Carnivora: their dentitions are similar to those of Oligocene miacids. They are small, short-limbed long-bodied carnivores which occupy an ecological position in the tropics equivalent to that taken by mustelids in northern temperate latitudes.

HYENAS AND
AARDWOLVES (HYAENIDAE)

$$I\frac{3}{3} C\frac{1}{1} P\frac{4}{3} M\frac{0-1}{1} = 32-34 \text{ (Fig. 12.6b)}$$

Adapted for crushing bones, the jaws of hyenas are probably the most powerful, relative to their size, of any living mammal. The dentition is dominated by the carnassials which are greatly enlarged and located at the back of the jaws where maximum bite force can be exerted. Their function is slicing flesh. A very small $M^1$ lies transversely at the back of the shortened palate and bites against the talonid of $M_1$. In *Crocuta* (the spotted hyena) $M^1$ is frequently absent. Unlike the majority of carnivores, who crush food with large molar teeth, the hyenas have developed the anterior premolars, especially $P^3$ and $P_4$, for this function; the more anterior location gives the advantages of wider gape and cheek clearance for dealing with the carcasses of large ungulates. In all carnivores, the third upper incisors are larger than the others; in hyenas the difference in size is more exaggerated with the $I^3$ becoming caniniform in shape.

Hyenas have been largely misrepresented; they do feed on carrion but it seems that this, their conventional role, is largely secondary. They are extremely effective primary predators.

Closely related to hyenas is the curiously adapted aardwolf (*Proteles*) of East and South Africa. Although similar in appearance to its ferocious cousins the aardwolf, like the aardvark, is a burrowing nocturnal animal which feeds on termites. The anterior dentition is quite normal with well-developed canines but the cheek teeth are small, spaced out rudimentary pegs (Fig. 12.8).

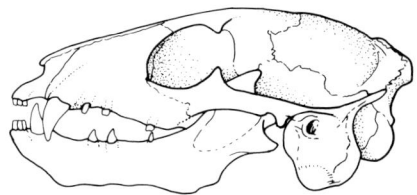

**Fig. 12.8.** Skull of the aardwolf, *Proteles*.

CATS (*Felis*) AND GREAT
CATS (*Panthera*) (FELIDAE)

$$I\frac{3}{3} C\frac{1}{1} P\frac{3}{2} M\frac{1}{1} = 30$$

(Figs. 12.6c, 12.7f; see Fig. 10.13)

Despite considerable differences in outward appearance, members of the cat family have remarkably similar dentitions. They are specialized for killing animals and slicing their flesh; they have no need for chewing equipment. The teeth are therefore even more reduced in number and are contained in such a short muzzle that the incisors make an approximately straight row across the front of the mouth. The canines form the anterior 'corners' of the jaws. Very much enlarged carnassial teeth are located at the back of the mouth. The lower which occludes with both $P^4$ and $M^1$ in hyenas has no talonid so that its crown consists only of a single V-shaped blade. $M^1$, lacking an opponent, is vestigial.

During the late Tertiary period some genera evolved greatly enlarged upper canines which were used like hatchets to penetrate the thick hides of contemporary herbivores (see Fig. 10.1). These sabre-toothed cats became extinct during the Pleistocene (with the demise of large pachyderms) leaving the modern smaller canined cats as their ecological replacement at the top of the food chain.

## Pinnepedia

Previously classified as a sub-order of the Carnivora, pinnepeds are now recognized to be sufficiently different through adaptation to an aquatic life to be regarded as a separate order: their dentitions differ radically from land (fissiped) Carnivora. As in most piscivores the jaws and dentitions of seals are adapted for grasping and tearing rather than for chewing; thus the cheek teeth tend to be homodont, without specialized carnassials.

# Comparative anatomy of dentition

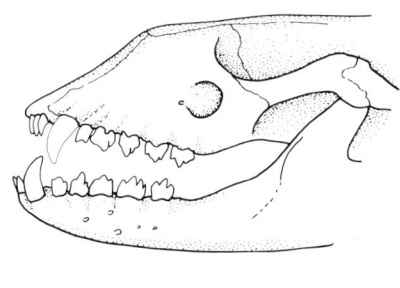

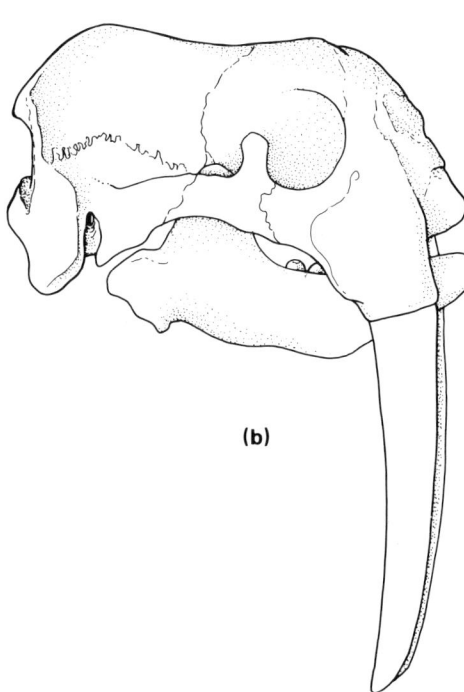

**Fig. 12.9.** (a) Dentition of the seal. (b) Skull of the walrus, *Odobenus*.

SEALS

$$I\frac{2-3}{1-2} C\frac{1}{1} PC\frac{4-6}{4-5} = 26\text{--}36 \text{ (Fig. 12.9a)}$$

Incisors have simple pointed crowns, the canines are larger and the postcanines are usually tricuspid. The 'crab-eater' seal (*Lobodon*) has more elaborate cheek teeth which are used as strainers of krill (small planktonic crustaceans).

WALRUSES

$$I\frac{1}{0} C\frac{1}{1} Pm\frac{3}{3} M\frac{0}{0} = 18 \text{ (Fig. 12.9b)}$$

The most prominent feature of the walrus is its enormous persistently growing upper canine tusks whose support considerably distorts the facial skull. They are present in both sexes (though not so large in females) and are used to dig in mud or gravel for bivalve molluscs and as picks for travelling over ice. The remainder of the dentition is very reduced. The lower canine is a small button-shaped tooth like the premolars. It is often supposed that these are used for crushing mollusc shells since they are exactly what one would expect in a molluscivorous animal; but the available evidence suggests that the walrus, like the carpenter, prefers to suck an oyster from its shell and discard the valves unbroken.

## Minor orders of the Ferungulata

AARDVARK (ORDER TUBULIDENTATA)

$$I\frac{0}{0} C\frac{0}{0} PC\frac{5-7}{4-5} = 18\text{--}24$$

This order contains the single species *Orycteropus afer*, the aardvark or 'earth pig' of southern Africa. The shape of the skull and position and extent of the dentition are similar to the armadillo, its New World analogue. Numerous deciduous teeth are formed but they are rudimentary and seldom erupt. There are no permanent anterior teeth. The cheek teeth vary in number between individuals and, like those of edentates, erupt continuously and lack enamel. Unlike edentates the cement-covered teeth consist of plicidentine (p. 160) which contains many vertical tubular pulp chambers (hence Tubulidentata) from each of which dentinal tubules radiate into polygonal columns of dentine. Occlusally the parallel pulp chambers are filled by secondary dentine. The aardvark is an extraordinarily powerful burrower: an ability used to advantage both in avoiding predators (cats, man) and obtaining food (mostly termites and ants).

HYRAXES (ORDER HYRACOIDEA)

$$I\frac{2}{2} C\frac{0}{0} P\frac{4}{4} M\frac{3}{3} = 38 \text{ (Fig. 12.10a)}$$

The incisors are enlarged gnawing teeth. The first upper incisor is persistently growing and triangular in section. Since enamel is restricted to the labial surface it becomes worn to a chisel shape by the lower incisors which are procumbent and initially pectinate. The second upper incisor and deciduous canines are lost early in life to leave a

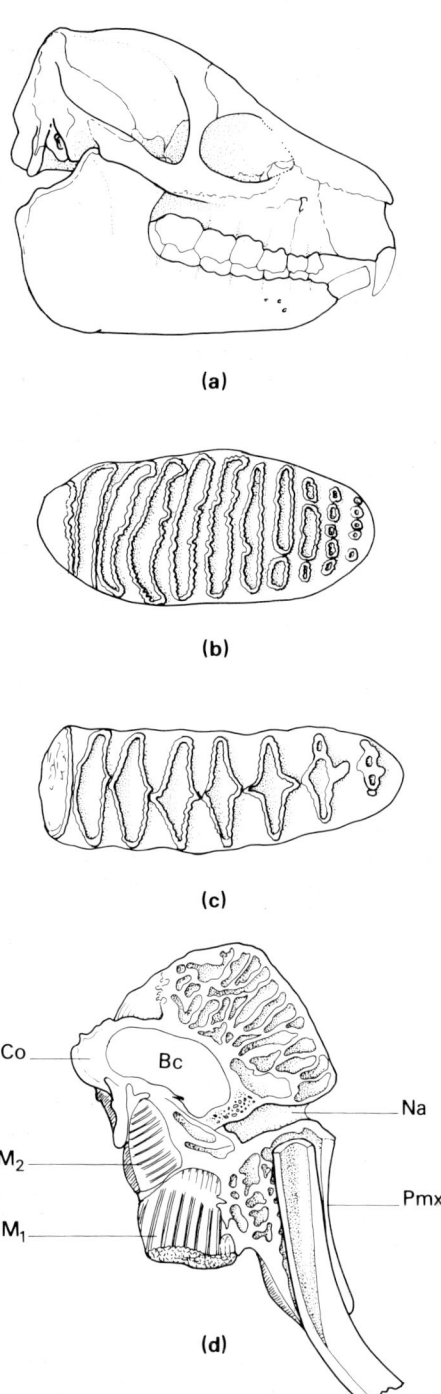

diastema between the incisors and the molariform premolars. The cheek teeth are brachydont and not unlike those of the primitive subungulates from which the hyracoids are thought to have evolved.

ELEPHANTS (ORDER PROBOSCIDEA)

$$I\frac{1}{0} \ C\frac{0}{0} \ Dm\frac{3}{3} \ M\frac{3}{3} = 24$$

The upper incisor is a persistently growing tusk which forms enamel only during its early development; the enamel cap is worn from the end of the tusk soon after eruption. The tusks (which are much larger in the African species—up to 10 ft) are thus composed of dentine (ivory) and an investing layer of cement. The cheek teeth are extremely hypsodont (see Fig. 10.21), the enamel organ being so deeply folded as initially to form separate transverse lamellae of enamel-covered dentine (Fig. 10.16). Later in development, with the spread of mineralization into the bottoms of the valleys, the lamellae become continuous one with another at the base of the tooth. The entire crown, including the spaces between lamellae is invested by cement which (a) rigidly connects the lamellae together and (b) provides attachment for periodontal ligament fibres. No premolars are formed. The molars erupt in horizontal succession moving into occlusion and then being lost over the front of the jaws. Since the jaws are short relative to the size of the teeth at most only two teeth at a time function in each quadrant. Each tooth erupts obliquely so that enamel ridges at its front edge are exposed by wear before the back lamellae, enclosed in a bony crypt, are even fused together by mineral. Mesio-occlusal eruption continues in pace with occlusal wear until the remaining lower posterior corner of crown and root is resorbed and the tooth is shed. The succeeding tooth is already in position with the erupted front of its occlusal edge biting against its opponent. Each successive tooth is of greater size than its predecessor. In *Elephas* (Indian elephant, Fig. 12.10b) the numbers of flattened lamellae per tooth (in sequence Dm2–M3) are 4, 8, 12, 13, 16, 24. In *Loxodonta* (African elephant, Fig. 12.10c) the broader, diamond-shaped lamellae are fewer in number; 3, 6, 7, 7, 8, 10. An elephant's skull is considerably larger than is needed to house the brain. This size is needed to provide adequate mechanical support for the tusks and cheek teeth, and sufficient surface area for the attachment of the trunk and neck muscles. Although the skull is large its mass remains relatively low due to the

**Fig. 12.10** (a) Skull of a hyrax, *Procaria*. (b) Upper molar of the Indian elephant, *Elephas maximus*. (c) Upper molar of the African elephant, *Loxodonta africana*. (d) Skull of *Elephas* cut parasagittally: Pmx, premaxilla; Na, nasal cavity; Co, occipital condyle; Bc, brain case.

development of air-filled cavities that occupy much of its volume (Fig. 12.10c). Elephants are exclusively vegetarian.

SEACOWS (ORDER SIRENIA)

The dugong (Indo-Pacific) and manatee (Atlantic) are the only herbivores among the fully aquatic mammals. They are related to the primitive ungulates with affinities to the Proboscidea. Sirenians are sluggish peaceful creatures living in rivers, estuaries and shallow coastal waters where they feed on water plants. They are extensively adapted for aquatic life; like cetaceans (to which they are completely unrelated) the hind limb is reduced and the tail is a horizontally flattened fluke; the nostrils are valvular. The dugong (Fig. 12.11a) has a densely-constructed skull which is characterized by large 'roman-nose' shaped premaxillae, bearing a pair of massively rooted incisor tusks in the male. Small unerupted tusks are found in the female. As in elephants, a dorsal shift of the external nostrils is as much related to the size of the tusk-bearing premaxillae as to any other factor. Behind the tusks there is a long diastema; the lingual surface of the premaxillae and anterior surface of the fused dentaries both support keratinized crushing pads. In the young, eight to ten small teeth are to be found beneath the crushing pad of the lower jaw but these are resorbed as the animal matures. It seems probable that horny plates developed because they proved more efficient in dealing with soft plant material than were the teeth in this position, but as yet the continued presence of functionless teeth has not been sufficiently disadvantageous for their complete repression. The cheek teeth number is $\frac{5}{5}$. Like those of edentates, they are persistently erupting, lack enamel, and are filled occlusally by secondary dentine as the cusps are worn. Their peculiarity is that the open roots have divergent sides, like a cone, so that as the teeth erupt in compensation for wear, the length of the tooth row is increased. This is a unique solution to the problem of growing jaws needing 'growing teeth' the occlusal surfaces of the teeth literally do grow! *Trichechus* (manatee, Fig. 12.11b) lacks tusks and its snout is only slightly depressed. Rudimentary incisors are formed but are buried under keratinized pads at the front of the mouth. Canines are absent. Unlike the dugong, the permanent cheek teeth are multicusped with a crown form similar to that of the tapir (q.v.), and multirooted. More than 20 such teeth are formed, in each quadrant, increasing in size from front to back. Only five or six of these are functional at one time, new teeth being added at the back and worn teeth being lost from the front. The components of the cheek tooth battery are constantly moving down the jaws (like the steps of an escalator) in a pattern of horizontal replacement similar to that already described in the elephant. The number of permanent teeth has increased from the eutherian 'maximum' of 44; this has also happened in toothed whales, *Otocyon* (the bat-eared fox) and some armadillos. The more elaborate dentition of the manatee (when compared with the dugong) can be related to its diet, which includes harder vegetable matter, seeds etc.

## Perissodactyla

The common term ungulate cannot be used to denote a natural taxon since ungulates (animals with hoofs rather than claws or nails) are of two evolutionarily distinct types: perissodactyls (odd-toed ungulates) and artiodactyls (even-toed or cloven-hoofed ungulates). It is because they share the adaptive role of 'large herbivore' that they have evolved similar structural characteristics in parallel. One of these is 'unguligrade' locomotion,

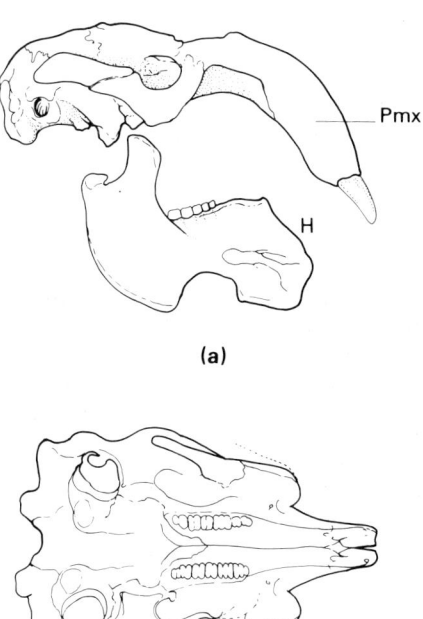

**Fig. 12.11.** (a) Skull of the dugong, *Halicore*: H, surface for the horny guiding plate. (b) Skull of manatee, *Trichechus*, in palatal view.

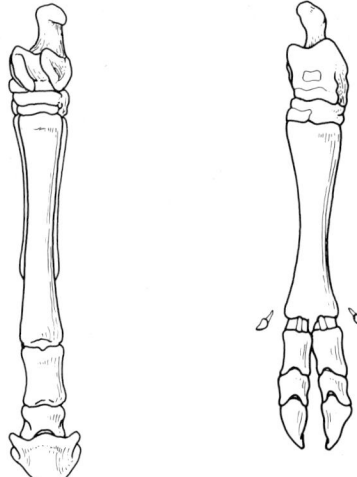

Fig. 12.12. Skeletons of hind feet of horse and cow.

an adaptation by which fast running has become a primary defence against predators. Advanced ungulates stand and run on the tips of their phalanges, the ankle joint being halfway up the leg. This change in limb proportions gives a longer stride for a given length of muscle contraction at the same time reducing the mass and inertia of the faster moving distal parts. Perissodactyls have enlarged the central digit of the pentadactyl limb and walk either on three digits (rhinoceros, tapir) or two (buffalo, cow) Fig. 12.12. Dental adaptations in both ungulate groups include lophodonty, hypsodonty and molarization of the premolars (p. 347).

HORSES AND ZEBRAS

$$I\frac{3}{3} C\frac{1}{1} P\frac{4}{4} M\frac{3}{3} = 44$$

(Figs. 10.16, 10.1)
The evolution of the above characteristics from the 'primitive insectivore condition' has been illustrated by a complete sequence of fossil horses through the Tertiary period.

The so-called $P_1^1$ are probably unreplaced $Dm_1^1$, as in all modern mammals. The canines are very small, uppers often being absent in females, and there is a diastema in front of the cheek teeth. Incisors meet in an edge-to-edge bite which leads to rapid attrition; they have invaginated crowns which wear to produce two concentric rings of enamel (see Fig. 10.1). Since the central pit (mark) tapers out towards the root, its size (or absence) on an incisor is used to tell an animal's age (the mark disappears from $I_1$ at 6 years, $I_2$ at 9 years, $I_3$ at 12 years). Although long-crowned, the incisors are not persistently growing. Molars are extremely hypsodont (see Fig. 10.16); the roots, when finally completed, are short and provide little attachment. The periodontal ligament is attached mainly to the crown which is correspondingly invested by cement. This also fills the deep valleys between lophs (crests) so as to support the high enamel crests. The unequal resistance to wear of the three component tissues leads to the maintenance of an efficient ridged grinding surface throughout the life of the tooth; the enamel edges being the operative element. Regions of the crown lophs can be homologized with the isolated cusps of the tribosphenic molar (see Fig. 10.16) which have, in the course of horse evolution, become 'fused' by the exaggeration of intervening crests. The premolars are molariform thereby increasing the effective grinding area of the dentition.

TAPIRS

$$I\frac{3}{3} C\frac{1}{1} P\frac{4}{3} M\frac{3}{3} = 42 \text{ (Fig. 12.13)}$$

The progressive development of both unguligrade locomotion and hypsodonty by horses of Miocene and later times can be related to the rapid and widespread advance of open grasslands during that epoch. For successful occupation of the new environments, enormous selective advantages would have been put on speed of running and on dental improvements; since grasses contain appreciable quantities of silica, grazing results in very high rates of abrasion of dental hard tissues. The tapir, however, staying within the retreating regions of forest has evolved little since Miocene times. Both the feet and the dentition are of similar grade to those of contemporary browsing horses (e.g. *Miohippus*, *Parahippus*). The cheek teeth

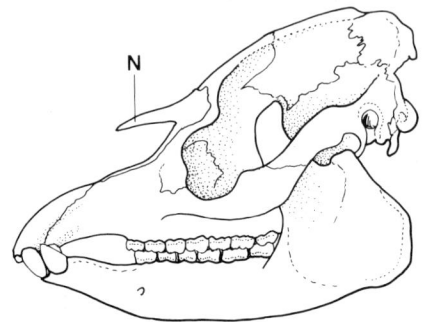

Fig. 12.13. Skull of the tapir, *Tapirus*: N, nasal bone.

(including molariform premolars) are brachydont and cement is not deposited on occlusal surfaces. The four principal cusps of the upper molar (protocone and paracone, hypocone and metacone) are joined by transverse ridges (paraloph and metaloph) forming a bilophodont tooth (see Fig. 10.17). There is a slight development of an ectoloph, connecting paracone and metacone; this is much larger in the otherwise similar teeth of *Rhinoceros*. Lower molars of *Tapirus* are also bilophodont.

## Artiodactyla

PIGS AND
HIPPOPOTAMI (BUNODONTS)

$I\dfrac{2-3}{2-3} C\dfrac{1}{1} P\dfrac{4}{4} M\dfrac{3}{3} = 40\text{--}44$ (see Fig. 10.1)

The omnivorous bunodonts are the least specialized group within the artiodactyls, both in limb structure (walking on four toes) and dentition. The premolar teeth are simple; the molars are brachydont and bunodont with no approach to the advanced adaptations seen in the horse (lophodonty) and ruminant artiodactyls (selenodonty).

The first two upper incisors are upright, their elongated incisive edges occluding against the lingual sides of their procumbent opponents. In both jaws the third incisors are small and variably positioned in relation to the canine. The canines of wild species are greatly enlarged tusks whose growth and eruption are continuous throughout life.

In both male and female the canines project outside the mouth cavity but they are considerably larger and more effective weapons in the male. Their size appears to be a secondary sex character since growth is slowed or arrested by castration. The upper canine is nearly horizontal and its growth describes a circle of tight radius—at first forwards and outwards, then, after clearing the upper lip, recurving upwards and inwards. The lower canine is a more slender tooth, triangular in section, and recurved upwards in front of the upper canine: the posterior surface, devoid of enamel, is worn away obliquely by the upper canine so as to produce a constantly sharpened point. The cheek teeth increase in size and complexity from front to back. P2 and P3 are simple cutting teeth, P4 is larger and M1 is a four-cusped tooth with slightly developed transverse ridges. M3 is as long as M1 and M2 put together, being lengthened by the distal addition of numerous small rounded cusps (hence bunodont).

*Babyrousa*, from the Indonesian islands of Buru and Celebes, is an unusual pig whose upper canines never enter the mouth cavity. They erupt upwards through the soft tissues of the snout and then curve back in front of the eyes, becoming coiled in old individuals (Fig. 12.14). According to

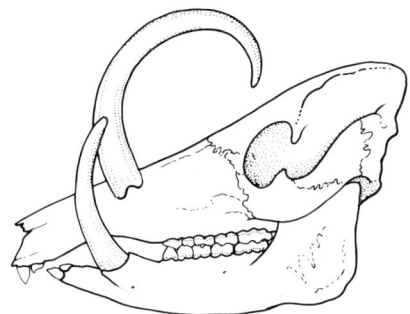

**Fig. 12.14.** Skull of *Babyrousa*.

folk legend, the tusks are used as hooks by which the *Babyrousa* hangs from tree branches. An alternative suggests that they protect the eyes from thorns when crashing through the undergrowth in search of food. Both these explanations are unsatisfactory because in the female, who must also rest and feed, neither pair of canines is prominent. For this reason these extraordinary tusks are usually consigned to the usefully vague categories of 'sexual ornamentation' or 'structures specialized beyond usefulness'.

In the African warthog it is the third molar that is peculiarly specialized (see Fig. 10.17). Its length is equal to the rest of the cheek teeth combined; these are quickly worn out and shed, leaving the hypsodont third molars to grind on alone. The occlusal surface of a newly erupted M3 is raised into about 25 prominent tubular cusps joined together occlusally by cement. When the tips of the cusps are worn away, the occlusal surface presents an 'organ pipe' appearance with the numerous separate rings of enamel cemented together. The canines of *Phacochoerus* are large in both sexes.

In the hippopotamus lower incisor implantation is similar to pigs but these teeth are large and of persistent growth. Together with the very large lower canines, the lower incisors are used to shovel plant material from the soil. The upper canines, though persistently growing, do not become excessively large. Their function seems to be restricted to keeping the lower ones sharp. Unlike the majority of pigs, there is little dimorphism in the sizes of the canines, a sexual equality which indicates either the importance of the canines in feeding, or more pronounced female aggression.

RUMINATING UNGULATES;
THE CAMELS AND
PECORA (SELENODONTS)

In the advanced artiodactyls, the tubercles of the bunodonts have become joined to form raised crescentic shearing edges—hence selenodont or 'moon-shaped' tooth (see Fig. 10.16). The curvatures of the half moons are opposed between upper and lower cheek teeth (in uppers, the concave side faces buccally: in lowers, lingually) so as effectively to shear fibrous plant material, mostly grasses, by medial jaw movements. In most modern selenodonts, the cheek teeth have become moderately hypsodont (see Fig. 10.16).

Camels and llamas ($I_3^1$ $C_1^1$ $P_2^3$ $M_3^3$ = 34) are the only selenodonts having teeth on the premaxilla. Initially there are three upper incisors on each side but the first two are lost early in adolescence and their place is taken by a fibrous pad against which bite the procumbent lower incisors. Canines are moderately well developed, the upper having a recurved hook shape.

In the lower jaw $P_1$ and $P_2$ are absent. In the upper jaw $P^2$ is absent but $P^1$ persists in the adult as a very small tooth behind the canine. In both jaws P3 is a small tooth which is frequently lost early in life. P4 is not molariform but forms a part of the cheek dentition, being separated from the anterior teeth by a long diastema. The molars are brachydont.

In all Pecora, upper incisors are absent. The lower incisors (together with an 'incisiform lower canine' (see Fig. 10.1); in all probability a fourth incisor) from an anterior procumbent group which crops against a thick keratinised gum pad on the premaxilla (Fig. 12.15a). This mechanism (used in conjunction with a large and mobile tongue) facilitates the rapid plucking of a huge quantity of vegetation which, in wild species, is chewed cursorily or not at all before being swallowed. It is stored in the rumen (a special anterior stomach chamber in which fermentation by ciliate protozoa takes place) and is regurgitated and thoroughly masticated when the animal reaches a resting place safe from predators. The premolars and molars form an uninterrupted battery of teeth. The premolars are molariform in shape (selenodont) but are only about half the size of the molars (cf. horse). Each genus of the Pecora is characterized by a distinctive variation in the selenodont pattern of the molar crowns.

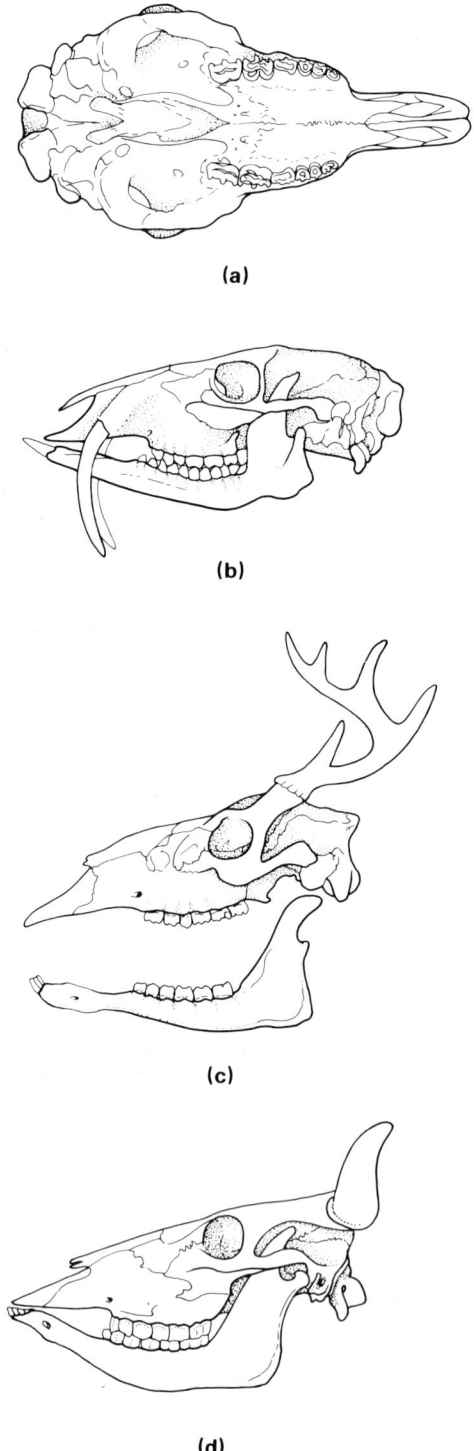

**Fig. 12.15.** (a) Skull of a sheep in palatal view. (b) Skull of the musk deer, *Moschus*. (c) Skull of a deer. (d) Skull of a cow.

In the Pecora (deer, giraffes, antelopes, sheep, cattle etc.) the dental formula $I^0_3 C^0_1 P^3_3 M^3_3 = 32$ is almost universal. Notable exceptions are the chevrotains, musk deer, and Chinese water deer; these species lack the horns or antlers of other pecorans and the males develop large persistently growing upper canine tusks (Fig. 12.15b). Lateral excursion of the mandible during chewing is unrestricted because the tusks are directed slightly outwards and are quite movable in their large sockets. The females of these species also develop canines but they are small and have closed roots. The antlers or enlarged canines of ruminants are weapons of defence (as are the large canines of pigs) but perhaps more important is their function in intraspecific selection as visual dominance–rank symbols. In the ritualized competition between males for dominance of the herd the largest antlers confer the highest status and the privilege of passing more genes into the next generation. Animals having horns or antlers rarely develop tusk-like canines and vice-versa, an example of the parsimony of nature known as concomitant variation. A solitary exception is the male of the muntjac deer (*Muntiacus*).

The Cervidae (deer) are characterized by the development of antlers (Fig. 12.15c). These are deciduous structures composed of a solid core of bone covered during the period of growth, spring and early summer, by fine-haired skin (velvet). Prior to the rutting season the blood supply is gradually cut down, the velvet dies and is rubbed off. During the winter and early spring a layer of bone between the antler and its permanent frontal pedicel is resorbed; the antler is pushed away from the skull by the growth of connective tissue beneath it and is shed. This process is extremely costly to the male animal; during a period of 4–5 months he has to consume sufficient quantities of vegetation to provide the several pounds of bone salt with which to build his antlers, only to throw them away and build a bigger set the next year. Red deer and caribou are known to chew shed antlers and the bones of dead animals; in incidence this behaviour is correlated with low-phosphorous soils and would appear to be a symptom of phosphate deficiency. The caribou is the only deer species in which the female also has antlers. In the Cervidae, the molar teeth are brachydont; the crowns are short and roots are formed soon after eruption. Small or rudimentary canines are often found in the upper jaw.

The Giraffidae (giraffes and okapis) have very short antlers which grow slowly throughout life in both sexes. Their molar teeth are brachydont with a characteristic rugosity of the enamel.

In the Bovidae (antelopes, sheep, cattle) permanent horns are formed by all species; in most by both sexes (Fig. 12.15e). Horns vary widely in size and shape between different genera but are basically of similar construction; they are composed of a frontally attached bony core covered by a thick sheath of hard keratinized material (horn). Upper canines are never formed. The molars of sheep and cattle are hypsodont; cement covers the sides of the crown for periodontal attachment. Molars of antelopes are moderately hypsodont being intermediate in height between those of deer and cattle.

## METATHERIAN MAMMALS

Marsupial mammals are geographically restricted to the Americas, Australia, Tasmania and the Malay Archipelago. This is a relic of a once wider distribution which was extensively reduced during late Mesozoic and early Caenozoic times presumably by unsuccessful competition with the reproductively superior placental mammals. Marsupials originated in North America during the Cretaceous period; by late Cretaceous or Palaeocene times they had spread to South America where they enjoyed an extensive adaptive radiation through the Tertiary period alongside various primitive placental types (e.g. edentates q.v.). Their success in South America is attributable to the fact that they were isolated from the majority of the contemporary placental orders by a water gap which separated the two American subcontinents from Palaeocene until Pliocene times. Rodents and primates managed to 'island-hop' or 'raft' their way to South America during the Oligocene epoch. Marsupials most probably colonized Australia in the Palaeocene when there were still land connections (or minimal water gaps) between Australia and South America. Antarctica, then apparently a warm vegetated continent, lay between the two and functioned as a 'stepping stone' (Fig. 12.16).

In late Pliocene times, the Panama land bridge emerged from the sea providing an entry for modern placental carnivores from the north who quickly upset the long established ecological balance of the South American fauna; with disastrous results for many forms of mammals, including the marsupials. Those marsupials that survived this massacre include a few mouse-like forms (the Caenolestidae) and the opossums (Didelphidae), which curiously not only survived but actually migrated across the land bridge back into North America. Fortunately the Australian

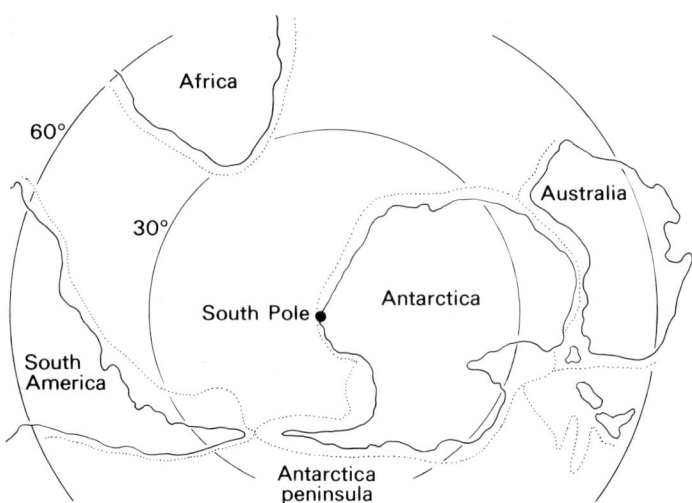

**Fig. 12.16.** Recent reconstruction of the relationships of South America and the Antarctic peninsula in the late Cretaceous and early Tertiary before their separation by continental drift. Dotted lines indicate the continental margins (1000 fathom contour). The existence of land connections or minimum water gaps between South America and Antarctica, and between Antarctica and Australia, in the late Cretaceous or early Tertiary could have permitted faunal interchange between these continents before the final breakup of Gondwanaland.

continental plate, long since separated from Antarctica and South America, had already drifted northwards with its cargo of variously adapted marsupials into its present position. It remains to be seen whether or not Australian marsupials, many of which are actively speciating, will eventually succumb in competition with placental mammals that have recently arrived, rabbit, dingo and most seriously, man.

In the discussion of marsupials, much is often made of their striking parallelism with the placentals—that is to say each marsupial species can be assigned a placental equivalent which, in becoming adapted to a similar niche elsewhere, has independently evolved similar features. This similarity ranges from superficial body form to the identity of single structures. Thus, there is a blind burrowing and marsupial mole, superficially very similar both to *Chrysochloris* and *Talpa*; there is a large wolf-like carnivore, the thylacine; the dentition of the wombat is remarkably like that of an advanced rodent; the Tasmanian Devil is both structurally and functionally a pouched hyena, and during the late Tertiary, both marsupials and placentals evolved sabre-toothed cats. In each case, the degree of parallelism depends both on the limits of genetic potential (i.e. what can be made) and the pressures of selection for the particular way of life (what needs to be made). But beyond these adaptive similarities there are characteristics unique to marsupials which unite them as a group and indicate their common ancestry from Cretaceous insectivorous stock. These conservative characteristics of a phyletic line are used to distinguish similarity due to true relatedness (where the characteristics have been retained from common ancestry) from that due to parallelism. The most obvious conservative feature of marsupials is their mode of reproduction, but more relevant to this account are the dental characteristics listed below:

**1** In all marsupials, apart from the wombat, the enamel contains a system of tubules.

**2** Only one tooth, a cheek tooth, is ever vertically replaced; clearly this tooth position alone possesses a deciduous tooth (Dm3) and a permanent replacement (P3). For the remaining teeth it is not always clear whether the deciduous teeth or their permanent replacements have been suppressed during evolution. Suppression is rarely complete; rudimentary teeth are often formed in several tooth positions and later resorbed. For the sake of simplicity, cheek teeth are numbered PC (postcanines) 1–7.

**3** Marsupials have different numbers of upper and lower incisors. The number of incisors is used in classification; polyprotodonts have $\frac{5}{4}$, $\frac{5}{3}$ or $\frac{4}{3}$; diprotodonts have $\frac{3}{1}$ or $\frac{1}{1}$ (very rarely $\frac{3}{3}$).

### Polyprotodontia

All have four or five equal sized peg-shaped upper incisors.

#### AMERICAN OPOSSUMS (DIDELPHIDAE)

$$I\frac{5}{4} C\frac{1}{1} PC\frac{7}{7} = 50 \text{ (Figs. 12.17a, b)}$$

*Didelphis* is a savage and wily little omnivore which has fitted well into man's world as a scavenger. The posterior upper cheek teeth look

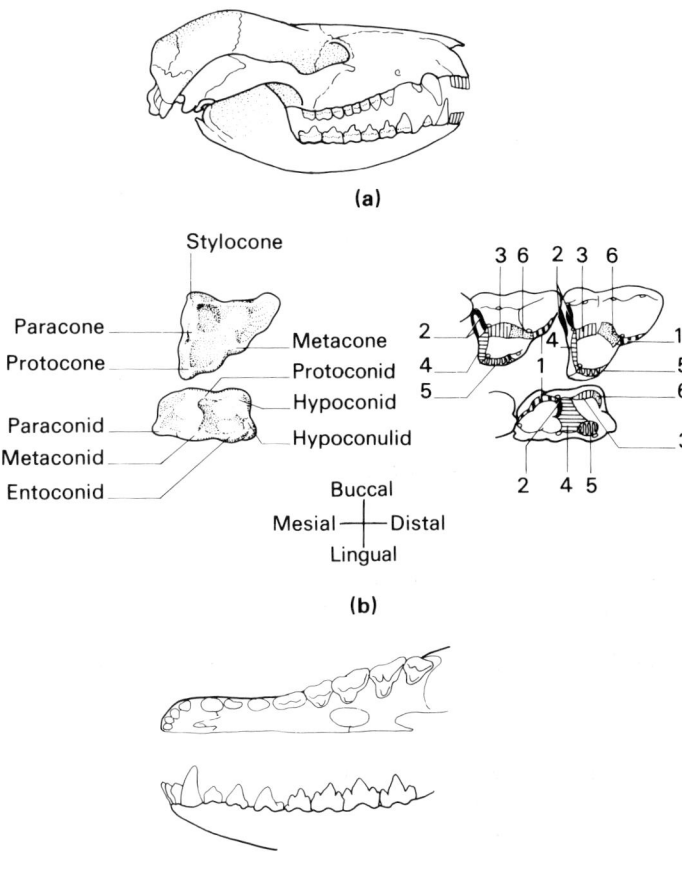

**Fig. 12.17** (a) Skull of the American opossum, *Didelphis*. (b) Tribosphenic molars of the American opossum. Upper figures: occlusal view of upper molars; lower figures: occlusal view of lower molars. Triangle of upper molar (paracone, protocone, metacone) termed trigon; triangle of lower molar (paraconid, protoconid, metaconid) the trigonid; posterior heel (bounded by entoconid, hypoconulid, hypoconid) the talonid. Right-hand diagram showing matching shearing facets on the occlusal surfaces. (c) Upper dentition (palatal view) and lower dentition (buccal view) of the Tasmanian 'wolf', *Thylacinus*.

like primitive tribosphenic molars and have extended metastylar shearing crests similar to that of the carnassial $P^4$ of eutherian carnivores.

DASYURIDAE

$I\frac{4}{3} C\frac{1}{1} PC\frac{7}{7} = 46$ (Fig. 12.17c; see Fig. 10.13)

*Dasyurus* (native 'cat'), *Sarcophilus* (Tasmanian devil) and *Thylacinus* (Tasmanian 'wolf') are Australian carnivores which have elaborated on the opossum dentition. The canines are large and intimidating; the first three cheek teeth are simple sectorial teeth similar in appearance to the premolars of a dog; the posterior four cheek teeth are sharply pointed and of the 'carnassial' type with elongated shearing crests. There are no exclusively crushing teeth

$$\left(\text{cf. } \frac{M^1}{M_1} \frac{M^2}{M_2} \text{ in the dog}\right),$$

this function being performed by cusp–basin apposition between all the posterior cheek teeth. Some of the smaller animals in this group are insectivorous; marsupial 'mice', pouched 'rats' (and the bandicoots, family Peramelidae) have long slender snouts with a similar dentition to the above although the cusps of the cheek teeth are more accentuated and the crests between them are lower.

*Myrmecobius* (the numbat or marsupial anteater) has increased the number of postcanines. Like the Old and New World eutherian anteaters, the numbat has a long tongue and feeds on termites; unlike most of them it has retained a full anterior dentition $I\frac{4}{3} C\frac{1}{1} PC\frac{8}{9} = 52$.

NOTORYCTIDAE

$I\frac{4}{3} C\frac{1}{1} PC\frac{6}{6} = 42$

In *Notoryctes*, the marsupial 'mole', the incisors,

canines and first two cheek teeth are simple blunt teeth; the posterior cheek teeth are multicusped. Implantation is feeble and teeth are frequently lost. Those that remain are quite rapidly abraded by the intake of sand with the food which is mostly soft-bodied insect larvae. Marsupial moles dig shallow furrows rather than deep burrows.

## Diprotodontia

The lower and first upper incisors are large and have cutting edges; the second and third upper incisors are variable in size, sometimes absent. Lower canines are absent; upper canines, when present, are small.

### PHALANGERIDAE

The members of this family are arboreal; most are nocturnal. They range through chipmunk-like, squirrel-like (also with gliding variants) and lemur-like possums of Australia and the Malay archipelago to the native 'bear' or koala. Many of the smaller species are insectivorous or omnivorous, the larger ones are herbivorous. The dentition of the koala is $I\frac{3}{1} C\frac{1}{0} PC\frac{5}{5} = 30$ (Fig. 12.18a). The procumbent lower incisors are persistently growing and superficially resemble those of rodents. However, enamel is initially present over the whole crown surface and is not made throughout life. The upper lateral incisors are reduced to pegs and there is a diastema both in front of and behind the small upper canine. Cheek teeth are quadritubercular and, by forming curved ridges, resemble a primitive selenodont pattern. The natural diet of the koala is almost completely restricted to the leaves and bark of eucalyptus trees.

### WOMBATS (PHASCOLOMIDAE)

$$I\frac{1}{1} C\frac{0}{0} PC\frac{5}{5} = 24 \text{ (Fig. 12.18b)}$$

Dental convergence with rodents is taken further by the wombats. The single pairs of upper and lower incisors are chisel-edged and persistently growing, resembling those of rodents in every way except that they are much shorter and do not grow back behind the cheek teeth. Cement invests both the enamel and the lingually exposed dentine. The cheek teeth also resemble those of advanced caviamorph rodents in being of persistent growth; but they are simply lobed and lack the complex enamel folding of the rodent type. Wombats are active burrowers and regularly construct quite complex underground homes. Diet is entirely vegetable.

### KANGAROOS, WALLABIES AND 'RAT' KANGAROOS (MACROPODIDAE)

$$I\frac{3}{1} C\frac{1}{0} PC\frac{5}{5} = 30$$

Kangaroos (e.g. *Macropus* Fig. 12.18c) are adapted for a grazing diet. The persistently growing

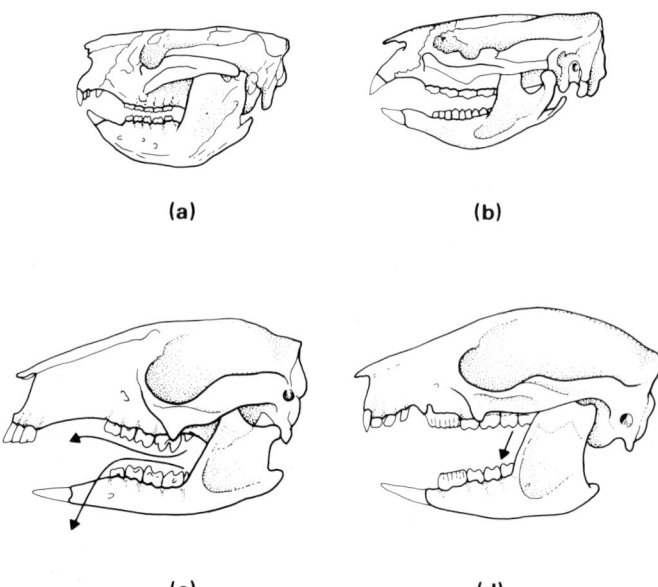

**Fig. 12.18.** Diprodont marsupials: (a) koala bear, *Phascolarctos*; (b) wombat, *Lasiorhinus*; (c) kangaroo, *Macropus*; (d) 'rat' kangaroo, *Bettongia*.

procumbent lower incisors have long sharp distal edges which occlude against the incisive edges of six vertically implanted upper incisors. The upper canine is small and often fails to erupt. The cheek teeth are bilophodont (cf. tapir); the first two are replaced together in young animals by PM 3. With increasing age teeth are lost from the front of the cheek series until it becomes reduced from $\frac{5}{5}$ to $\frac{2}{2}$ in old individuals. As each tooth is lost the remainder move along the jaw in manner similar to the manatee and elephant (q.v.). The 'rat' kangaroos differ from the other members of the kangaroo family in size (most are rabbit-sized) and nature of the dentition, e.g. *Bettongia* (Fig. 12.18d). Both the lower and first upper incisors grow persistently. The second and third upper incisors are small. The first lower cheek tooth ($P_3$) is a large serrate blade, replacing two teeth as in *Macropus*. These peculiarly specialized teeth are used for slicing up vegetable matter. The remaining cheek teeth are similar in form to those of *Macropus* but have a fixed position in the jaw.

## THE ORDER PRIMATES

The order Primates is divided into two suborders, Prosimii and Anthropoidea, each of which can be divided into six natural groups or 'families' (see Table 11.1a).

### Prosimii

TREESHREWS (TUPAIIDAE)

$$\frac{2133}{3133}$$ (Fig. 12.19)

These small squirrel-like animals are widely distributed throughout the Far East. They have an elongated skull, with a small braincase and long snout. The foramen magnum is well back on the skull base. There is almost no flexion of the basicranial axis. The large auditory bulla contains the tympanic ring (see Fig. 11.5). The orbits face laterally and are incomplete posteriorly: there is a post-orbital bar. A distinctive feature of the zygomatic arch is the oval fenestration of the zygoma. The mandible is slender and the ascending ramus short: the coronoid process is elongated and the angular process hooked.

The stout upper incisors are widely spaced along the premaxilla, the steeply proclined lower incisors form a comb. The small upper canine is well back but the lower is a stout projecting tooth and, unlike lemurs, does not form part of the comb. The premolars become progressively more molariform front to back. The molars are dilambdadont (see Fig. 10.14) and are much wider buccolingually in the upper jaw than in the lower.

MADAGASCAN LEMURS (LEMURIDAE)

$$\frac{2133}{2133}$$

This group of lemurs (there are two others) includes the more primitive survivors of the lemuriform radiation on Madagascar and some of the Comoro Islands (see Fig. 11.2). There are six genera (see Table 11.1), two are predominantly insectivorous, the rest eat flowers, fruit and leaves as well.

The proportions of the skull vary with snout length (normally long) but all have a rounded braincase, with the foramen magnum well back, and large auditory bullae. There is a post-orbital bar. The body of the mandible is long, the ramus generally appears somewhat triangular.

The most characteristic feature of the dentition is the dental comb incorporating both the lower incisors and the lower canine (Fig. 11.7). There is a wide median diastema between the small peglike upper incisors (the permanent upper incisors are lost in *Lepilemur*, the sportive lemur). The maxillary canines are large, stout and usually sexually dimorphic teeth occluding in to a diastema behind the incisiform lower canine. The enlarged and caniniform lower first premolar shears against the back of the upper canine. In some members of the family (e.g. *Phaner* 'forkmarked' dwarf lemurs) the upper first premolar is also caniniform. The upper molars are three-cusped or, if the hypocone has developed four-cusped. The lower molars have four cusps (the paracone has been lost) and are somewhat bilophodont.

LONG-LEGGED MADAGASCAN
LEMURS (INDRIIDAE)

$$\frac{2123}{1123} \text{ or } \frac{2123}{2023}$$

*Avahai*, *Indri* and *Propithecus* (the sifaka) are large herbivorous lemurs with large ovoid braincases, short muzzles and forward facing orbits. The foramen magnum faces as much downwards as backwards reflecting their upright posture both in locomotion and at rest (see Table 11.1). The stout lower jaw has a wide high ramus, well-developed coronoid process and expanded angle.

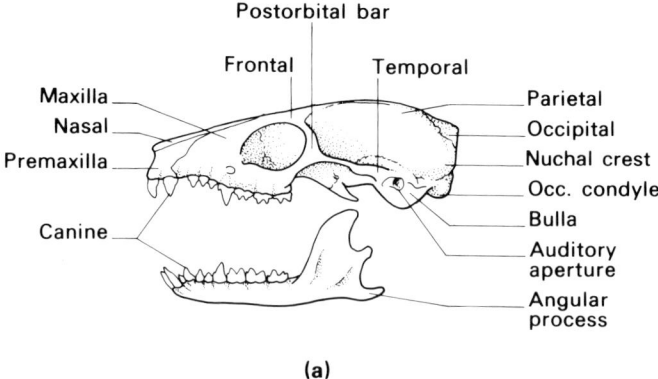

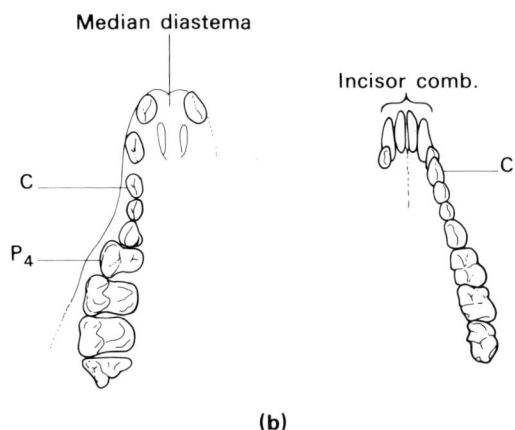

**Fig. 12.19.** (a) lateral view of the skull and lower jaw of the most primitive of the treeshrews *Ptilocercus* (left) and (b) occlusal views of upper and lower dentitions. The snout lies in front of rather than below, the cranium. The orbits face laterally and are ringed posterolaterally by a post-orbital bar. There is a median diastema between the caniniform upper incisors. The upper molars are simple teeth with a developing hypocone. The lowers have distinct trigonids and talonid basins. The zygomatic arch is not fenestrated in this representative.

The Indriids have a comb but there is controversy as to the teeth involved (see formula above). The comb occludes into a diastema between the small slightly spatulate upper incisors. The short, stout upper canines occlude with caniniform lower first premolars. The upper and the lower second premolars are mesiodistally elongated blade-like teeth markedly different from the somewhat 'bilophodont' four-cusped molars.

THE AYE-AYE (DAUBENTONIIDAE)

$$\frac{1013}{1003}\left(\frac{Di2}{2}, \frac{Dc1}{0}, \frac{Dm2}{2}\right)$$

The aye-aye is the only member of the group: the peculiarities of this animal, its rodent-like dentition, dramatically lengthened stick-like middle finger with a long pointed claw (as opposed to a nail), have been correlated with its habit of feeding on wood-boring insects. There are, in fact, distinct similarities between the mechanics of its skull and that of the woodpecker! Recent fieldwork on this exotic and almost extinct primate suggests that it is by no means exclusively insectivorous or 'grubivorous' but actually feeds quite extensively on fruit.

The skull is ovoid, with a postero-inferiorly directed foramen magnum (Fig. 12.20). The orbits face forward and are ringed laterally by a postorbital bar. The face is short and deep as is the mandible which has a mobile symphysis and is 'rodent-like' save that the coronoid and angular processes are short by comparison with true rodents (Fig. 12.4).

The huge, long anterior teeth, normally described as persistently growing incisors but thought by some authors to be canines, wear into the typical chisel shape associated with a gnawing habit and dominate the adult dentition. There are no canines (or incisors!) and only a single peglike upper premolar. The small rounded molars have a tribosphenic pattern on eruption but rapidly wear flat. In contrast the deciduous dentition consists of two upper and one lower incisor of 'conventional' shape, a deciduous canine in the upper jaw and

# Comparative anatomy of dentition

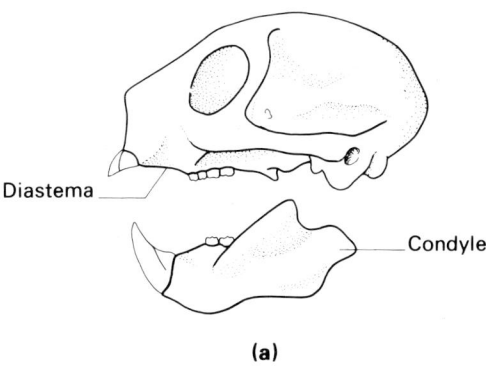

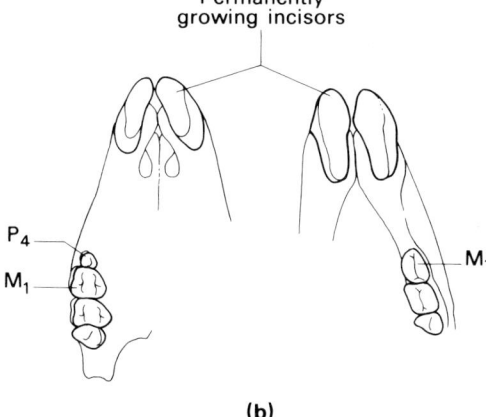

Fig. 12.20. *Daubentonia* (Daubentonidae). (a) Lateral view of the skull and (b) occlusal views of the upper and lower dentition. Note the rodent-like persistently growing incisors, the long diastema and short cheek tooth row, and the very simple form of the molars. (Compare with typical rodents, Fig. 12.4).

either a second incisor or canine in the lower jaw and two deciduous molars. Of these the incisors are replaced by the single permanent incisor, the canines are not replaced nor are all but one of the deciduous molars.

LORISES, POTTOS AND
GALAGOS (LORISIDAE)

$$\frac{2133}{2133}$$ (Fig. 12.21)

This family is distributed in both Africa (south of the Sahara) and in Asia (see Table 11.1). All the lorises have rounded crania, the foramen magnum faces both backwards and downwards, and lies between the large auditory bullae. The tympanic ring is attached to the bulla forming a very short auditory tube (see Fig. 11.5). Snout length varies but is longest in the galagos. In *Loris* and *Arctocebus* the premaxillae project beyond the incisors to form a keel-like support for the projecting nose. The mandible is short and strong in the lorises but slender in the longer-faced galagos.

All the lorises have a comb in the lower jaw but this is usually more vertically set than in lemurs: the teeth are shorter and less procumbent. The caniniform lower first premolar occludes between the stout projecting upper canine and caniniform upper first premolar. The remaining premolars increase in size from before backwards and have well-developed cingula. The four-cusped upper molars have an oblique ridge, except in the galagos where the large hypocone projects sharply backwards behind the trigon. The lower molars are also four-cusped although the third and smallest has a hypoconulid.

TARSIER (TARSIIDAE)

$$\frac{2133}{1133}$$

This nocturnal rat-sized primate, distributed throughout the Malay archipelago, has enormous eyes, dramatically elongated legs (its name is derived from the elongated tarsal bone of the foot) and long thin digits with expanded tips. The foramen magnum is well forward on the base of the rounded cranium. There is a short auditory tube leading to a prominent tympanic bulla. Although the snout is moderately prognathic, this is masked by the greatly expanded, front-facing orbits (Fig. 12.22) which are bordered posteriorly and laterally by a greatly expanded postorbital bar. The lower jaw is slender, with a mobile symphysis and short ramus.

The dentition is quite different from that of other prosimians. The large pointed upper incisors are in mesial contact and are flanked by the small lateral incisors. The single lower incisor is small and almost vertically implanted. The upper canine is smaller than the central incisor. The large lower canine occludes into the diastema. The premolars increase in size from before backwards in both jaws, the uppers having a well-developed palatal cingulum, the lowers a distolingual cingulum. The tribosphenic upper molars have a small hypocone and are much wider buccolingually than mesiodistally. The lower molars have four cusps except the third, the largest, which has a hypoconulid. All the lower cheek teeth have a buccal cingulum.

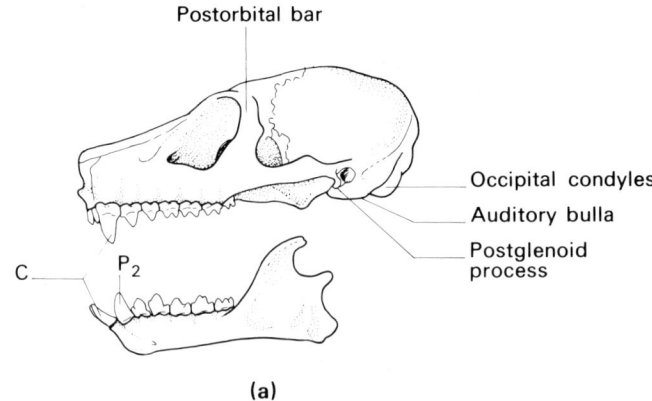

**Fig. 12.21.** *Galago* (Lorisidae). (a) Lateral view of the skull and (b) occlusal views of the upper and lower dentition. The lower comb occludes with the median diastema in the upper jaw. The upper molars have a well-developed hypocone (distolingual cusp). The lower molars have lost the paraconid. The appearance of the skull and dentition is very similar in lemurs.

## Anthropoidea

There are six families of Anthropoidea: two in the 'New World monkeys'; one large group of 'Old World monkeys'; and the three groups of Hominoidea, the lesser apes, great apes and man (see Table 11.1). 'Old' and 'New World' monkeys were originally classified by the shape of their nostrils: the former have forward facing external nares with a narrow median septum (the 'catarrhine' condition) whilst the South American monkeys have laterally facing nostrils with a wide central septum (the 'platyrrhine' condition). These terms are now rarely used by primatologists but do appear in the older zoological and in 'popular' primate literature.

### MARMOSETS AND TAMARINS (CALLITHRICIDAE)

$$\frac{3132}{3132}; \text{except } Callimico \frac{3133}{3133}$$

The marmosets are the most primitive of the Latin American monkeys and one genus, *Cebuella* (the pygmy marmoset), is also the smallest. Although small (overall length about 2 in) the skulls of this group are all long in relation to the body length (dolicephalic; see Fig. 11.27). The large ovoid braincase (marmosets have a high brain/body size ratio, even for primates) projects well back behind the foramen magnum producing a sharply angled nuchal area. The tympanic ring is attached to the outer margin of the auditory bulla as in all New World monkeys (see Fig. 11.5). The short face is dominated by the large forward facing orbits which have a complete posterior wall. The V-shaped mandible has a slender body and somewhat square ramus, and the coronoid process and angle vary in size but the latter is usually well developed. The marmosets can be distinguished from other New World monkeys by the shape of the skull and the number of molars.

All the group have two molars except *Callimico* (Goeldi's marmoset) which retains a very much

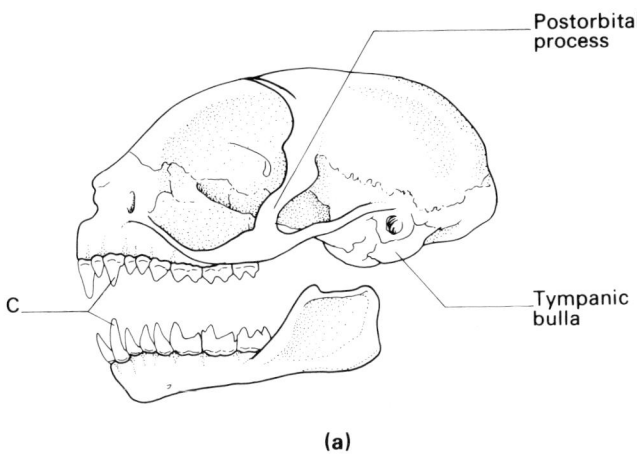

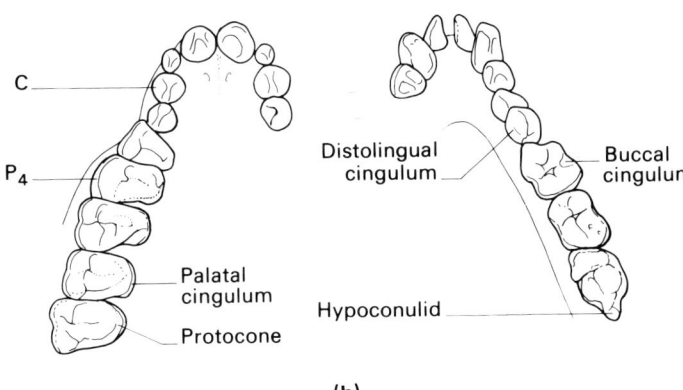

Fig. 12.22. *Tarsius spectrum*. The skull is dominated by the greatly enlarged orbits which make the tarsier appear short-faced. the dentition has no dental comb, the pointed upper incisors abut mesially and occlude with the single pointed lower. The upper molars are tricuspid with a well-developed lingual cingulum, the lowers have three cusps on the trigonid and a large talonid basin. There is a marked discrepancy in the buccolingual dimensions of upper and lower postcanines.

reduced third molar. Marmosets are described as 'short-tusked' (where the incisors are as large as the canines) or 'long-tusked' (the canines project above the occlusal plane). Both upper and lower incisors are narrow, slightly procumbent, spatulate teeth. The lower canine occludes into a diastema between the lateral incisor and the upper canine. The premolars are bicuspid. The upper molars have only the smallest suggestion of a hypocone, the lower molars are four-cusped. The last molar ($M^2_2$ or $M^3_3$) is always the smallest and the first is the largest of the series.

NEW WORLD MONKEYS (CEBIDAE)

$$\frac{2133}{2133}$$

All the cebids have forward facing orbits which are complete posteriorly, a tympanic bulla with an external tympanic ring fused to the bulla (see Fig. 11.5) and three premolars in each jaw quadrant. Some have a prehensile tail which serves as a fifth limb: *Ateles* (spider monkey), *Brachyteles* (woolly spider monkey), *Lagothrix* (woolly monkey) and *Alouatta* (howler monkey); others have evolved a method of vocalization which has resulted in a massive laryngeal expansion and modification of the shape of both the skull and lower jaw [*Callicebus* (titi) and *Alouatta*]. On the basis of their dentitions cebids can be divided into three broad groups but these do not necessarily have any taxonomic significance.

*Aotus* (night monkey), *Cebus* (capuchin), *Saimiri* (squirrel monkey), *Callicebus* and *Alouatta* (Fig. 12.23)

The first three are short-faced and have an anthropoid mandible; the lower dental arcade is U-shaped and the ramus rectangular with a moderately developed coronoid process and a slightly expanded angle. In contrast, the laryngeal enlargement found in *Callicebus* and *Alouatta* has led to the development of a mandible with a ramus very much like that of the horse: the coronoid

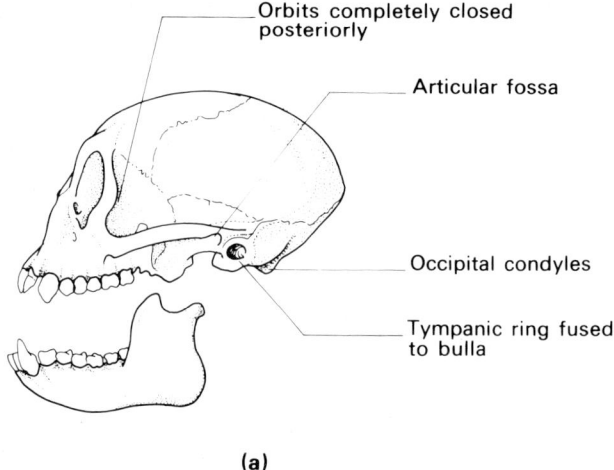

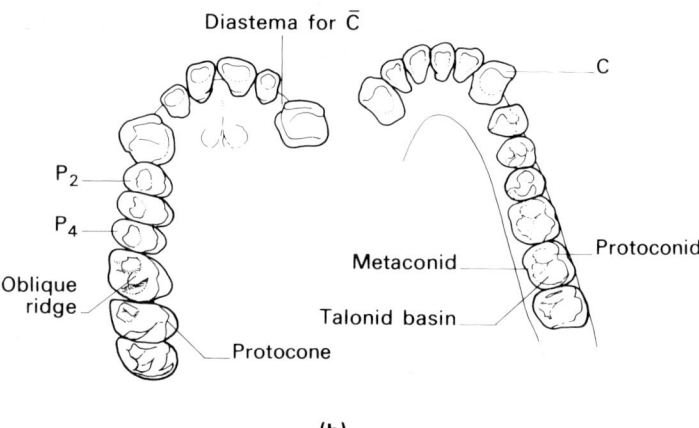

**Fig. 12.23.** (a) The skull of *Cebus*, a generalized New World monkey. Note the expansion of the neurocranium (compare with Figs 12.20, 12.22), the complete postorbital closure and the high mandibular ramus. (b) The dentition of *Ateles*, the spider monkey: the incisors are spatulate and there is a lateral diastema involving the premaxillary–maxillary suture for the lower canine. The upper molars have an oblique ridge, the lowers have lost the paraconid and have a wide deep talonid basin.

process is small, the condyle is high above the tooth row and the angle is greatly expanded.

The dentition is similar in all five monkeys. The upper incisors are spatulate and slightly procumbent, the laterals separated from the canine by a diastema. The lower incisors are fan-shaped and the laterals are larger. Both upper and lower canines are large and projecting (least in *Callicebus*) and show marked sexual dimorphism in *Cebus*. All the premolars are bicuspid but the lingual cusp of the lower first premolar is very small. The molars of both jaws have four cusps, the uppers have an oblique ridge, the first molar is the largest and the third may be so small as to be considered vestigial.

*Ateles, Brachyteles and Lagothrix*
The members of this group have fairly long faces with well-developed jaws. The mandible has a large angle (biggest in *Brachyteles*).

The dentition is similar to that of the first group save that a hypoconulid is often developed on $M_3$ and although $M^3$ is the smallest of the molars, all these teeth are of similar size.

*Cacajao (uakari), Pithecia (saki) and Chirpotes (bearded saki)*
These monkeys have a highly specialized anterior dentition whose selective advantage is poorly understood. The upper incisors are spatulate and project forwards so sharply as to be almost horizontal. They occlude with long, mesiodistally compressed lower incisors. Both upper and lower incisors are separated from the tusk-like laterally flaring canines by a large diastema. The postcanine teeth conform to the general cebid pattern of bicuspid premolars and four-cusped molars but appear small in comparison to the anterior dentition.

OLD WORLD MONKEYS (CERCOPITHECIDAE)

$$\frac{2123}{2123}$$

Like the Cebidae, this family can be divided into three main groups: 'generalized' Old World monkeys (macaques, mangabeys and guenons), 'terrestrial' monkeys (the baboon group and patas monkeys) and the 'leaf-eating monkeys' (colobines and langurs).

Although the neurocranium is large, in contrast to the situation in cebids and hominids it appears small by comparison with the often prognathic face. The foramen magnum is at the junction between the flattened basicranium and steeply raked nuchal area and faces downwards and backwards (cf. Fig. 11.4). The tympanic ring is extended into a tube, as in man. There is no mastoid process but rather a 'mastoid area' containing air cells. The orbits face forwards, are closed posteriorly, and have thickened lateral and superior margins. The latter often form a marked ridge or shelf, known as the 'supraorbital ridge' or 'supraorbital torus'. There is no forehead comparable to that found in man: the frontal bones curve gently backwards from the supraorbital ridge towards the coronal suture. The temporal fossa is widest anteriorly, immediately behind the orbits where the 'postorbital constriction' of the neurocranium is found (cf. Fig. 11.12). The face is prognathic in all cercopithecids, extremely so in baboons. There is no anterior nasal spine. A complete suture separates the maxilla and premaxilla (cf. man). The mandible has a long body and a somewhat squat but rectangular ramus. The coronoid and condylar processes are generally at the same level and are separated by a shallow sigmoid notch. The condylar process does not have a distinct neck and the condyle is flattened. The articular fossa is also flat and there is no articular eminence but there is a distinct post-glenoid process. The fused mandibular symphysis slopes sharply backwards and is buttressed internally by a shelf of bone formed by an expansion of the lower borders of both halves of the mandible. Similar buttresses are found in some cebids (e.g. *Pithecia*) and in the apes but the shelf (see Fig. 11.22) is best developed in the Old World monkeys, especially the baboons. The genial muscles (genioglossus and geniohyoid) are attached to the mandible on the inner surface of a simian pit above the shelf.

Cercopithecoid incisors are spatulate but longer crowned than those of cebids or hominoids. Even if they do not erupt into an edge-to-edge bite, wear rapidly produces this occlusion and with further wear the edges become flat ovoid surfaces (the original body of the crown). The canines are stout projecting teeth which show distinct sexual dimorphism, greatest in the terrestrial group. The lower canine occludes into a diastema between the upper canine and upper lateral incisor. The distal edge of the upper occludes with the blade-like anterior part of the lower first premolar (the canine–premolar complex; see Fig. 11.9). The remaining premolars are biscupid. The molars of cercopithecoids are frequently described as 'bilophodont' (see Fig. 11.10) as the four cusps are aligned to form mesial and distal transverse ridges. This appearance is enhanced by 'waisting' of the buccal and lingual surfaces between the two ridges. The lower third molar frequently has a large hypoconulid which forms a third 'ridge' on that tooth (there is no oblique ridge on the upper molars). In all Old World monkeys the upper and lower first molars are the smallest, the third molar is usually the largest.

*'Generalized Group': Macaca (macaques), Cercocebus (mangabeys), Cercopithecus (guenons), Cynopithecus (Celebes 'ape')*

This group is exemplified by the macaques. One species *Macaca fasciailaris* (the crab-eating macaque) is commonly used as a human analogue in dental research. All the members of the group have a skull and dentition conforming to the general description given above. There is marked canine sexual dimorphism: the canines barely project above the occlusal plane in the female but they are much longer, particularly the upper canine, in the male. Guenons can be distinguished from the other members of the group by the poor development of the talonid on the $M_3$ and the related 'reduction' in the size of $M^3$. The second molar is therefore the largest. Like the 'Barbary ape' of Gibraltar and Morocco which is a macaque, the Celebes black 'ape' (*Cynopithecus*) is misnamed. This fruit-eating monkey shows affinities with the macaques but has developed baboon-like features, notably a long snout and heavy facial bone structure.

*'Terrestrial group': Erythrocebus (patas monkeys); Mandrillus (mandrills), Papio (baboons), Theropithecus (gelada baboon)* (Fig. 12.24)

The ground-living monkeys all show marked sexual dimorphism of body size: the adult female weighs approximately half as much as the male. This difference extends to the skull and dentition.

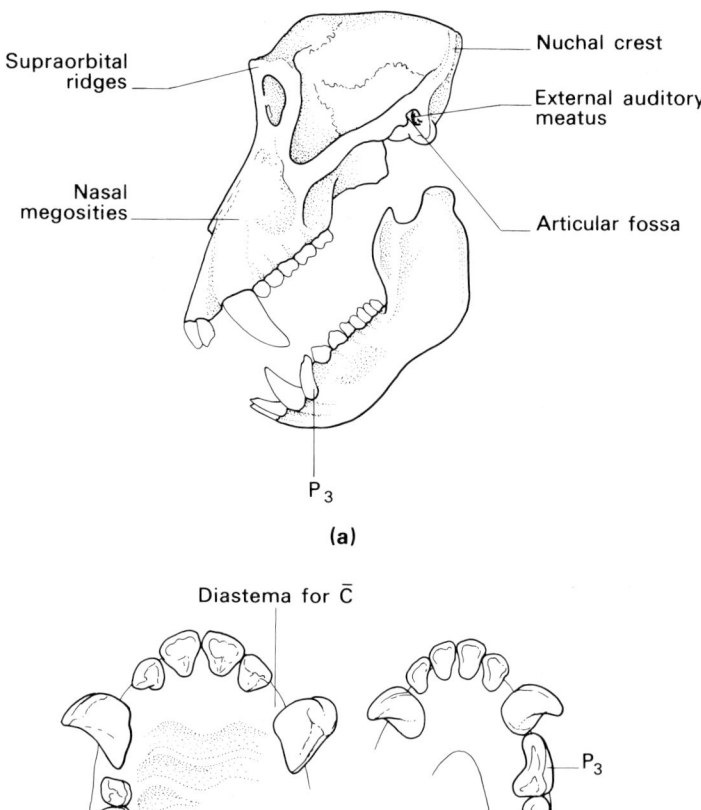

**Fig. 12.24.** the skull of a male baboon, *Papio*, orientated in the Frankfurt plane (see p. 81). Although these terrestrial Old World monkeys are long-snouted the face does not, in life, project in front of the orbits but rather below. The dentition ($\times 0.8$) shows the most extreme development of the canine-premolar complex seen in higher primates.

All the group are long-snouted; least in *Erythrocebus* and *Theropithecus* (although this is a secondary adaptation), most in *Papio*. The size, weight and bony development of the male skull is much greater than in the female, the males having large supraorbital ridges, nuchal, and often sagittal, crests. The canines, large in both sexes, become long and dagger-like in the males. The canine–premolar complex (see Fig. 11.9) is at its most exaggerated in this group and associated with it there is a marked depression in the lateral surface of the mandible below the lower premolars and first molar. The molars are bilophodont and increase in size from before backwards; the third molars are much the largest. The mandrills are perhaps best known for the brightly coloured skin covering the rugosities (bony expansions) on the outer surface of the maxilla which run parallel to the nose in the male. However, the anterior teeth are very large and the cheek teeth unusually small; the first molar is barely larger than the second premolar in the mandrills. The postcanine tooth rows converge sharply posteriorly (they are parallel in other members of the group) and the occluded plane is curved so that it appears concave on the maxillary teeth in lateral view. This is quite different from the flat occlusal plane of the baboons proper and the convex curve of man (curve of Spee, p. 305).

*'Leaf-eating monkeys'*: *Colobus* (*guerezas*), *Presbytis* (*langurs*), *Pygathrix* (*Douc langurs*), *Rhinopithecus* (*snub-nosed langurs*), *Simias* (*Mentawai Island langurs*) and *Nasalis* (*proboscis monkeys*) (Fig. 12.25)

The 'leaf-eating monkeys' are grouped together in

# Comparative anatomy of dentition

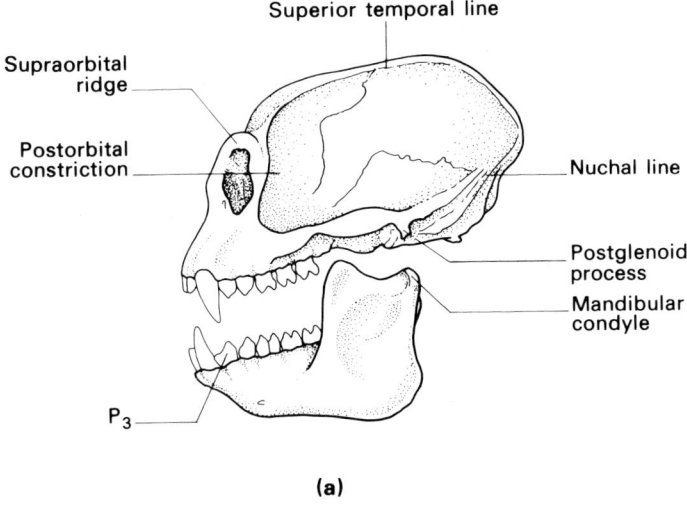

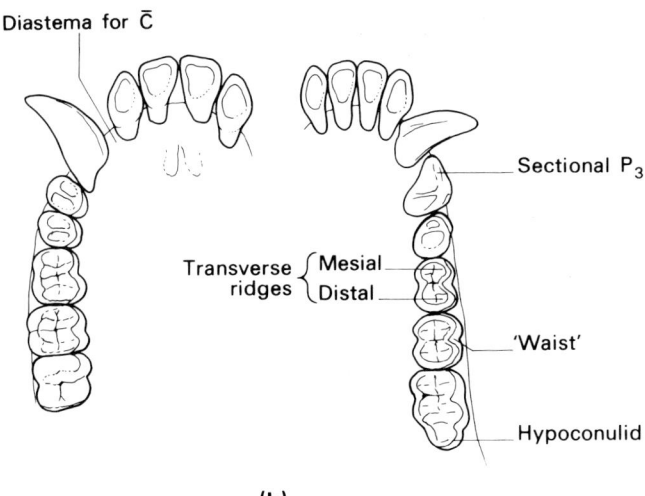

Fig. 12.25. The skull of *Presbytis* (Colobinae), a short faced Old World monkey. Compare with Fig. 12.23, noting the different appearance of the glenoid fossa, postglenoid process and external auditory meatus (see Fig. 11.5). The dentition includes large canines (this is a drawing of a male, in the female the canines would be smaller), a sectorial anteroposteriorly enlongated lower first premolar and bilophodont molars.

a single family, the Colobinae, one section found in Africa (the colobus monkeys), the other in Asia (the langurs). The distinctive features of these monkeys, including a sacculated stomach, have been associated with a herbivorous diet. For example, the mandibular ramus is high, with a corresponding distance between the level of the mandibular joint and that of the occlusal plane (see herbivores, Fig. 10.18). In some, but not all, members of the group the lower incisors occlude in front of the uppers. This condition is called 'underbite' and may be an adaptation for the more efficient ingestion of leaves. In other respects the dentition follows the cercopithecoid pattern save that the molars are particular lophodont.

## GIBBON AND SIAMANG
## HYLOBATIDAE (LESSER APES)

$$\frac{2123}{2123} \text{ (Fig. 12.26)}$$

The 'lesser apes' are found in the tropical rain and montane forest of S.E. Asia; *Hylobates* throughout mainland Indo-China, Malaya, Sumatra, Borneo and Java; *Symphalangus* only in the Malaya Peninsula and Sumatra. Of the two the siamang is the larger with a weight range of 9–12 kg compared with 4–8 kg for the gibbon (a healthy adult cat weighs about 3 kg). Both use an overarm swinging type of locomotion (brachiation) and

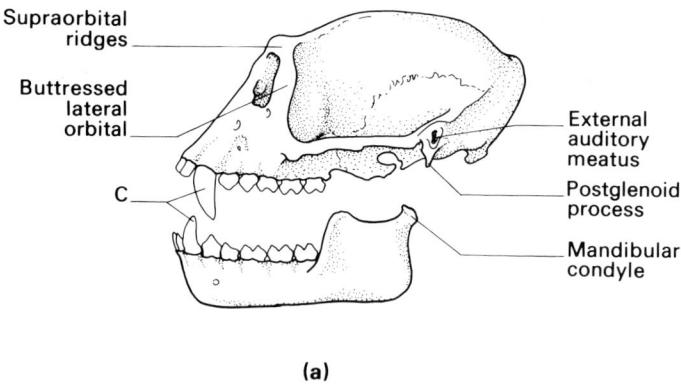

Fig. 12.26. The skull and dentition of the siamang *Symphalangus*, the larger of the two gibbon (hylobatid) genera. Although both sexes have large canines, the lower first premolar is only moderately sectorial (cf. Figs. 12.24, 12.25, 12.27). The upper molars have an oblique ridge and the lowers the 'Dryopithecus' pattern.

move rapidly through the trees with their legs folded against the abdomen; gibbons can however run bipedally for short distances. The group show negligible sexual dimorphism either in the skull or the dentition: both sexes have large projecting canines (not the case in other anthropoids).

The lightly built skull has an ovoid neurocranium with a cranial capacity ranging from 82–115 cm³ for *Hylobates*. There is a well-defined nuchal area but no nuchal crest, the occipital condyles are placed well behind the external auditory meatus in the adult. There are mastoid air cells but no mastoid process. A sagittal crest may develop in adult male siamangs but rarely in male gibbons. The large orbits face forwards and have a buttressed lateral margin and well-developed supraorbital ridges but these do not meet in the midline. There is a well-marked postorbital constriction. The palate in gibbons is exceptionally long (reaching 50–54% of total skull length) and broad. The lightly built mandible has a near vertical symphysis, a long slender body and a short square ramus. There is no distinct condylar neck, the posterior border of the mandibular notch merges into the condyle proper. The fossa has no distinct articular eminence although there is a post-glenoid process.

The incisors are heteromorphic: the upper centrals are weak and spatulate, the lateral small and often pointed. The lower incisors are fan-shaped. Both male and female gibbons have long narrow sabre-like canines projecting (especially the uppers) well beyond the occlusal plane and terminating in sharp points. The lower first premolar is sectorial, the remainder are bicuspid although the lower second is expanded distally. The upper molars are simple four-cusped teeth with an oblique ridge, the lowers have the 'Dryopithecus' pattern (see Fig. 11.11) also associated with the Pongidae. A Y-5 pattern is commonly found on $M_1$. The second molar is the largest cheek tooth in both jaws, the third is often very reduced. *Symphalangus* shows a tendency to develop supernumerary molars (13% of skulls in one sample), extra cusps or cusplets being common on all hylobatid molars.

GREAT APES (PONGIDAE)

$$\frac{2123}{2123}$$

There are three 'great apes', the chimpanzee (*Pan*), the orang-utan (*Pongo*) and the gorilla (*Gorilla*). They have different distributions, habits, locomotor patterns and skulls but very similar dentitions.

The general form of the dentition is the same in all three great apes. The incisors are spatulate, especially the upper centrals. The lower incisors are also large but fan-shaped. The canine is a stout almost conical tooth projecting well beyond the occlusal plane in both jaws. The lower occludes into the diastema between the upper lateral incisor and the canine, the upper canine with the lower and the slightly sectorial lower first premolar. There is a marked canine sexual dimorphism in the permanent dentition although, surprisingly, no equivalent dimorphism in the length of the blade on $P_3$. Although this tooth does have an elongated anterior ridge extending forwards from the buccal cusp, it is not as exaggerated as in either the terrestrial cercopithecoids or the hylobatids. The lower second premolar is expanded distally. Both upper premolars are bicuspid and have three roots. Like man, the upper molars have four cusps and an oblique ridge. The upper third molar is the smallest, the first and second may be of equal size or the latter slightly larger. The lower molars have the '*Dryopithecus*' pattern with a hypoconulid (see Fig. 11.11). In all the pongids the molar cusps are placed more peripherally on the crowns of the teeth than are those of man so the teeth appear less bulbous and have vertical rather than rounded buccal and lingual surfaces. The pattern of cusps and fissures may be obscured in *Pan*, and frequently in *Pongo*, by crinkled enamel. This trait is by no means confined to the great apes but is commonest in that group.

*The juvenile skull and deciduous dentition*
The juvenile pongid skull is much more 'human' in appearance than that of the adult and resembles that of *Australopithecus africanus* (see Fig. 11.19). This is due to the early development of the brain and neurocranium and the much later growth of the face. The heavy crests found especially in male *Pongo* and *Gorilla* develop with the eruption of the permanent dentition.

The deciduous dentition ($Di\frac{2}{2}$, $Dc\frac{1}{1}$ $Dm\frac{2}{2}$) is the same in all cercopithecoids and pongids. In the apes, the first molar is the first tooth in the permanent dentition to erupt followed by the incisors, second molars, premolars and then the canine. As in man the shape of the second deciduous molar closely resembles that of the first permanent molar.

*Chimpanzee (Pan)* (Fig. 12.27)
There are two species of chimpanzee, *Pan troglodytes* which is widely distributed across equatorial Africa and *Pan paniscus*, the pygmy chimpanzee, which is restricted to the area between the Congo and Lualaba Rivers of central West Africa. Both live in rain forest but *Pan troglodytes* is also found in montane rain forest to heights of 10 000 ft and in areas where forest and savanna mingle (forest–savanna mosaic). Chimpanzees have been much studied in the field. They spend 50–75% of daylight hours on the ground but sleep in tree nests normally at least 15 ft above ground which are freshly built each night. Although chimpanzees can 'run' across ground with a bipedal 'lope', they normally 'knuckle-walk' using the soles of the feet and the knuckles of the hands. This is a reflection of the much greater length of the arms than of the legs, also seen in the gorilla, and thought to have resulted from adaptation to a brachiating or semibrachiating habit (see p. 365 and Hylobatidae). Chimpanzees are primarily vegetarian with a diet of fruits, leaves, palm nuts, bark-seeds and stems but also galls, termites, cultivated fruit crops and fish. The observation that these animals used straws to catch termites first confirmed the deliberate use of tools by animals other than man. Unlike other great apes, chimpanzees do not show any marked sexual dimorphism in body weight. There are cranial differences in that a small sagittal crest is occasionally found in large males (but it can, rarely, be found in large old females!).

The rounded neurocranium (cranial capacity 290–500 $cm^3$ in a sample of 74 adults) has the foramen magnum well back on the base so that the occipital condyles are behind the external auditory meatus. If present, the mastoid process is very small. The orbits face forwards with their longest dimension in the transverse axis (cf. *Pongo*) and are surmounted by a continuous and prominent supraorbital crest. There is a postorbital constriction. The face is prognathic with a long premaxilla (the premaxillary–maxillary suture persists). The mandibular body although but-

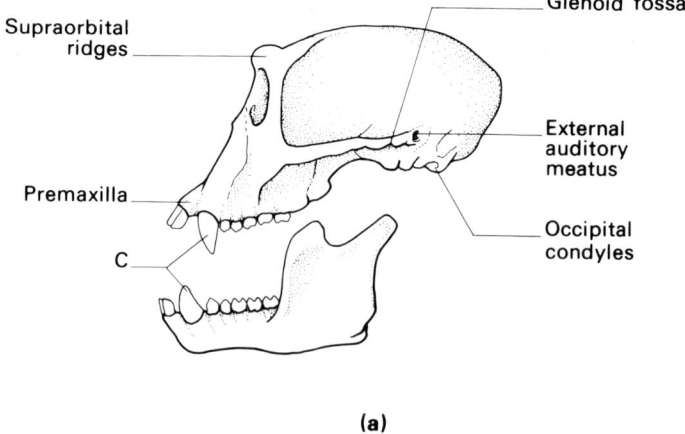

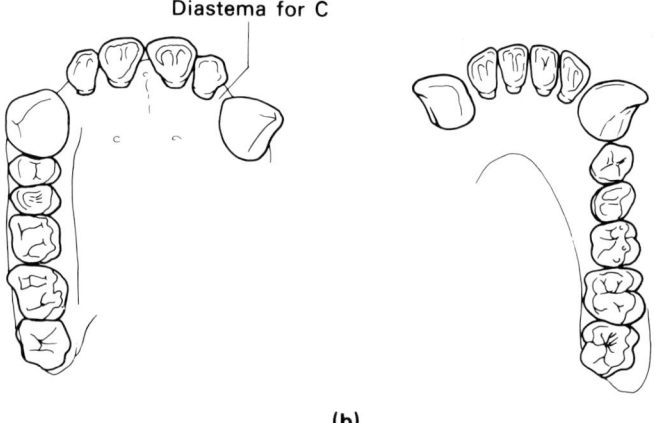

**Fig. 12.27.** The skull of a male chimpanzee (*Pan*). Note the pronounced supraorbital ridges and the protrusion of the premaxilla and upper incisors. The dentition is also that of a male. In the female the canines are smaller.

tressed by a narrow simian shelf in the symphyseal region, is deepest near the canine where there are often multiple mental foramina. The ramus is rectangular, with large areas for the attachment of masseter and temporalis, although the coronoid process is short and the mandibular notch shallow. The gently rounded condyle articulates with an almost flat glenoid fossa.

The dentition conforms to the description given above.

*Orang-utan (Pongo)* (Fig. 12.28)
There is a single species, *Pongo pygmaeus*, but there are slight differences between the form found in Borneo and the even rarer Sumatran type. The orang is completely arboreal, living at all forest levels from the canopy down (see Fig. 11.3) and feeding mainly on the fruit found on the smaller branches although it does eat leaves, bark and birds' eggs. The orang sleeps in a nest at heights anywhere from 6–24 m above ground.

The orang shows marked sexual dimorphism in body weight, the female attains only about half the male body size. Some old males develop enormous fatty and pendulous cheek flanges which almost completely obscure the face. The sexual dimorphism extends to the skull: male cranial capacity ranges from 405–540 cm$^3$ (sample size of eleven) and female from 320–400 cm$^3$ (sample of nine). Adults of both sexes have nuchal crests, seven out of ten males develop a sagittal crest which can reach a height of 12 mm. The foramen magnum is well back and the nuchal area steeply raked. The mastoid process is not, usually, well developed. In a prepared skull the close-set orbits have their long axis vertical (cf. *Pan*) and look rather like spectacles. The supraorbital ridges may be very large in old males, but do not normally extend evenly across the midline. The face is moderately prognathic and set both in front of and below the cranium. The large heavy mandible has a broad ascending ramus, a shallow mandibular

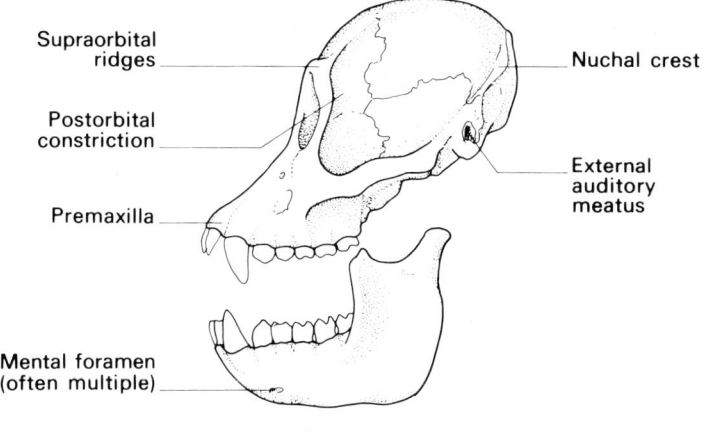

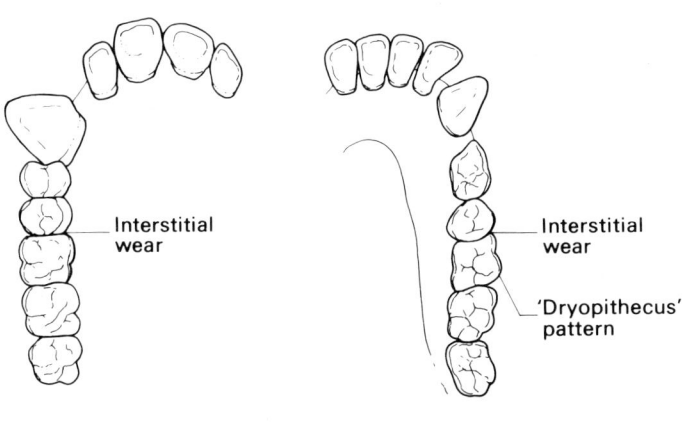

Fig. 12.28. The skull and dentition of a female orang-utang (*Pongo*). The cranium of the orang is comparatively short and domed (there is the suggestion of a forehead, compare Figs. 12.27 and 12.29). The dentition does not, in this case, show the heavy wrinkling of the enamel often found in this genus, but does show heavy interstitial wear (e.g. between the upper premolars and first molar, and the lower second premolar and first molar).

notch and a shallowly curved condyle. There is a simian shelf.

The dentition has the same general form as in the chimpanzee. The upper canine is much larger in the male although prominent in the female. Oddly there is no parallel sexual dimorphism in the size of the lower first premolar. In both jaws the second molar is normally the largest and the third the smallest. Supernumerary molars are common. The roots of the teeth are long, which partly accounts for the depth of the mandibular body.

### *Gorilla (Gorilla)* (Fig. 12.29)

The gorilla is the largest of the pongids: a mature male can stand 2 m high, weighs 300–400 lbs and has an arm span of at least $2\frac{1}{2}$ m. Females are about half as heavy as males. Gorillas are found in western (lowland gorilla) and eastern equatorial Africa (highland gorilla). The two ranges do not overlap. They spend 90% of their day on the ground although females and especially juveniles make brief forays up the trees. Gorillas are reported to be wholly vegetarian.

Both the neurocranium and facial skeleton are large. Cranial capacity ranges from 340–685 $cm^3$ in adult males. The largest ever recorded, 752 $cm^3$, is only slightly below the minimum figure for man. A nuchal crest is always present. A sagittal crest is found in males and about 30% of females. The mastoid process may be absent or can grow throughout life to become very large. The rectangular orbits are surmounted by a continuous heavy supraorbital ridge which is deeply excavated by the frontal air sinus. The very prognathic face has a rectangular hard palate extending backwards behind the third molars. The long lower jaw is strong and heavy with a sloping symphysis braced by a simian shelf. The rectan-

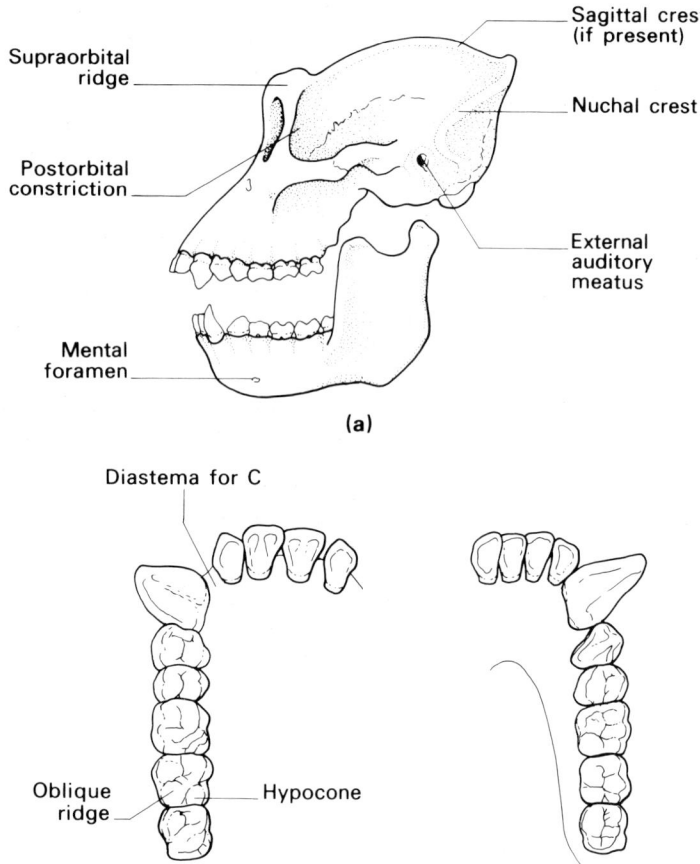

**Fig. 12.29.** The skull of a female *Gorilla* and the dentition of the male. Although large, with a robust and prognathic face, the female does not usually develop the heavy cresting of the skull (sagittal and nuchal crests) found in the male. Similarly the canines are smaller. The lower molars of this specimen show a typical '*Dryopithecus*' pattern.

gular ramus often shows strong muscle markings. The mandibular notch is shallow.

The dentition conforms to the general pattern although the teeth are large. Both canines show marked sexual dimorphism: in the female the lower barely projects above the occlusal plane. The lower first premolar is sectorial, the others bicuspid although the lower second has a distal cingulum. The upper molars have an oblique ridge and the lowers have the '*Dryopithecus*' pattern but both have very sharply pointed cusps when newly erupted. Lingual cingula are common in upper molars and buccal cingula in the lowers: they are most frequently developed on first molars and are rarest on the last which is also the smallest.

HOMINIDAE

The best known member of this group is modern man, *Homo sapiens sapiens*, the other members are his immediate ancestors (see Chapter 11).

## THE DENTITION OF LABORATORY RODENTS AND LAGOMORPHS

In most mammals, as in man, the teeth are of limited growth; that is, each tooth reaches its full size shortly after eruption. During life, enamel and dentine are worn from the occlusal surface. In compensation for this, the tooth slowly erupts from its socket thereby maintaining contact with the opposing tooth during mastication. This process, active eruption during tooth function, is more marked in the hypsodont teeth of ungulates, where tooth wear is extensive, than in modern man where tooth wear is relatively slight. In a number of mammals, however, some or all of the teeth retain the capacity to grow throughout life; the root apices remain open and new enamel, dentine and cement are laid down continuously. The teeth involved may be incisors (the narwhal, hippopotamus, elephants, all rodents and lagomorphs), canines (walruses, some pigs) or cheek teeth (edentates, the aardvark, all lagomorphs and some rodents, e.g. the guinea pig). The continuous growth of these teeth is coupled with continuous eruption. This sometimes results in a progressive lengthening of the tooth, as in walrus and elephant tusks, but when the teeth come into functional occlusion, more often results in the maintenance of tooth size. In the latter instance, at least in the adult animal, the attrition rate and eruption rate balance each other. Continuously growing teeth are put to a variety of uses, being used by different animals for gnawing, grinding, as weapons or as tools.

The teeth of rodents and lagomorphs are of immense importance in dental research. The animals are not difficult to maintain and breed in the laboratory, and are small enough for convenience in handling. In the teeth of continuous growth, each stage of hard tissue formation can be studied in a single specimen. Moreover, in these teeth, the eruption process, being continuous and relatively rapid, is accessible to a wider range of experimentation. The molars of rats, although of limited growth, are nevertheless also of great value in research.

The dental formulae of common laboratory rodents are shown below:

Rat and mouse: $I\frac{1^*}{1^*}$ $C\frac{0}{0}$ $P\frac{0}{0}$ $M\frac{3}{3}$

No replacement teeth

Guinea pig: $I\frac{1^*}{1^*}$ $C\frac{0}{0}$ $P\frac{1^*}{1^*}$ $M\frac{3^*}{3^*}$

Premolars are the only replacement teeth.

Rabbit: $I\frac{2^*}{1^*}$ $C\frac{0}{0}$ $P\frac{3^*}{2^*}$ $M\frac{3^*}{3^*}$

The incisors and premolars have deciduous predecessors.

Teeth of continuous growth are marked by an asterisk.

## Continuously growing incisors

The description given here concentrates on the incisors of the rat, but the remarks apply to a large extent to the incisors of the other species.

### ONTOGENY

The rat incisor first appears at about the 14th day *in utero* and begins to mineralize at or just before birth, on the 21st day after fertilization. The incisor erupts into the mouth at about 10 days after birth, coming into function about 6 days later. At first, the tooth is white but the enamel acquires pigment (see below) when the rat is about 25 days old.

### ANATOMY

Rodents have a single incisor at the front of each jaw quadrant, the upper pair working against the lower. Rabbits have an additional pair of small incisors lying directly behind the first pair in the upper jaw. The form of the incisors and their relation to the cheek teeth in the rat and rabbit are shown in Figs. 12.30a,b and 12.31.

Each incisor in the rat is curved, the shape being

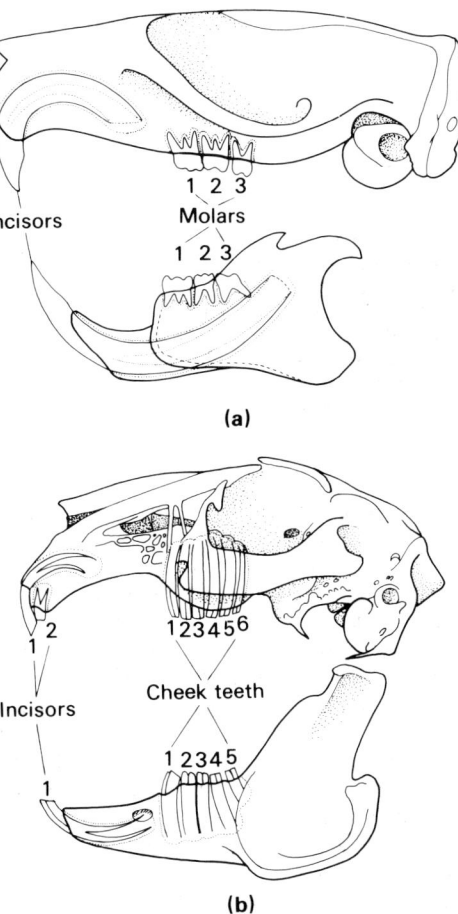

Fig. 12.30. Skulls of the rat (a) and the rabbit (b) to show the form of the incisors and molars and their relationships. Note the differences in dental formula and in the position of the incisors. The open roots of the continuously growing rabbit molars contrast with the closed apices of the rat molars.

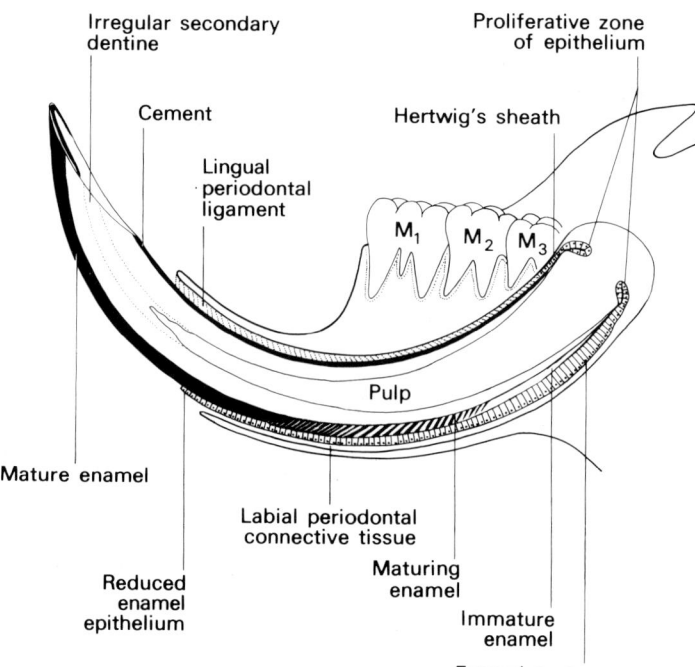

**Fig. 12.31.** Diagrammatic longitudinal section through the mandibular incisor of the rat, to show the arrangement of the soft tissues associated with the tooth, and the pattern of hard tissue formation.

that of a logarithmic spiral. This spiral shape, which is more pronounced in the lower incisors, means that although the bases of the teeth diverge the functional tips lie together. It also complicates life for the dental researcher, for it is not possible to cut a section through the incisor which is in a truly parasagittal plane, so that a series of sections needs to be examined to gain a picture of the structures along the length of the tooth. The curvature of the upper incisors of the rat is greater than that of the lower, so that the bases of the incisors lie in front of the cheek teeth in the upper jaw and behind them in the mandible. The lower incisors in the rabbit, however, have their bases further forward.

Each incisor has a core of dentine. Enamel covers only the labial (convex) surface, the rest of the tooth surface being covered by cement. (Figs. 12.31 and 12.32). All three hard tissues are exposed at the incisal edge and the more rapid

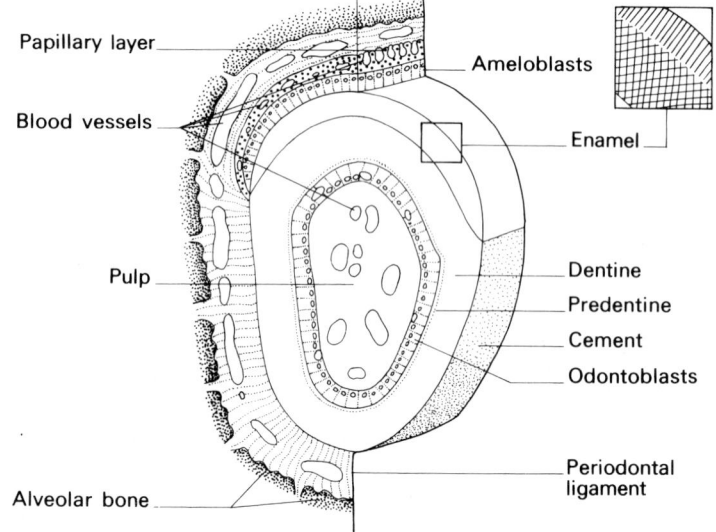

**Fig. 12.32.** A slice cut transversely through a rat incisor *in situ*, at the level of the maturing enamel. The structure of the enamel organ, including the papillary layer, is shown, as is the disposition of the hard tissues and the general arrangement of the fibres of the periodontium.

wear of the relatively soft dentine and cement behind the hard enamel leads to the production and maintenance of a sharp chisel edge used for gnawing. Exposure of the pulp by attrition is prevented by deposition of secondary dentine towards the incisal end (Fig. 12.31).

In conformity with the distribution of the cement, the tooth is attached to bone by a true periodontal ligament only on its lingual and lateral surfaces; between the enamel-covered labial surface and the neighbouring bone, there is a space filled with fibrous connective tissue of a different structure (Figs. 12.31, 12.32).

Growth of the tooth takes place at the basal end, which is encircled by epithelium. On the labial aspect, the epithelium differentiates into an 'enamel organ' and on the remaining surfaces into Hertwig's sheath, which breaks down after the initial formation of dentine (Fig. 12.31). Cell proliferation occurs in both the epithelium and mesenchyme at the basal end and the daughter cells are recruited into the epithelium and pulp or periodontal region respectively.

The great demand for nutrients by the growing tissues of the rat incisor is met by a rich vascular supply. In the mandible, the incisor region is supplied by the mental and mandibular arteries and by smaller arteries from the labial surface (Fig. 12.33). The incisal two-thirds of the cement-covered surfaces of the tooth are supplied by the mental artery. This artery may also run posteriorly and curve round the base, giving off branches to the pulp and basal third of the whole outer surface of the tooth. Alternatively, the basal region of the incisor may be supplied by branches of the mandibular artery, as in Fig. 12.33, this artery also being the source of the molar blood supply. The incisal two-thirds of the enamel-covered labial surface of the tooth is supplied by small arteries entering the periodontium by way of separate foramina in the bone. Efferent blood is drained from the incisor region by venous networks on the cemental and enamel aspects, which in turn connect with large venous trunks running longitudinally, level with the enamel–cement junction. The arteries and veins are concentrated on the bone side of the periodontium. From here, vessels cross over to the tooth side and form a capillary bed. This is particularly extensive in the papillary region of the enamel organ (see below), where the capillaries form a ladder-like network embedded in the outer layers of the enamel organ.

Innervation of the rat incisor has not been investigated fully. In the mandible, the inferior dental nerve enters the jaw near the base of the incisor and then runs beneath the molars, giving off branches of these teeth. The periodontal ligament of the incisors contains numerous myelinated and unmyelinated nerves. Mitochondria-rich bodies, perhaps representing sensory nerve endings, have been described. The incisor pulp contains only non-myelinated nerve fibres.

HISTOLOGY

The enamel of the incisors of rodents and lagomorphs is characterized by elaborate patterns of prism decussation. In the rat, the pattern is very regular, but is not completely elucidated. The enamel may be divided into two zones. In the inner two-thirds, the enamel is made up of single decussating rows of prisms running transverse to the tooth axis, the prisms sloping alternately left and right in successive rows. In the outer enamel the prisms are parallel to each other and run out straight to the surface. The appearance of the enamel in transverse section is indicated in the inset of Fig. 12.32. The total thickness of the enamel is about 150 $\mu$m. A widespread feature among rodents is a brown pigmentation of the incisor enamel. Lagomorph incisors are not pigmented and neither are those of some rodents, notably the guinea pig. The pigmentation is due to

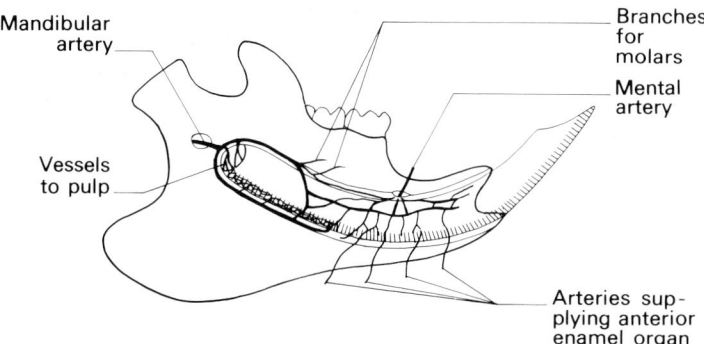

Fig. 12.33. Rat mandible to show the principal arterial vessels supplying the lower incisor. In this figure, the mandibular artery supplies the basal portion of the tooth but in many specimens, this function is performed by a posterior extension of the mental artery. In either pattern, there is anastomosis between branches of the two arteries (after Kindlová & Matena).

the presence of iron in the superficial layers of the enamel. The concentration in the outer enamel of the rat incisor is on average 10% by weight, although it reaches 30% in places. The iron is present in the ferric-state, probably as ferric hydroxide, but neither the true chemical form of the iron nor its structural relationship to the apatite lattice have so far been elucidated.

The primary dentine, which makes up the bulk of the tooth, has a very regular structure which differs only in detail from human dentine. Peritubular dentine is lacking, possibly as a result of the very rapid rate of formation. There are mantle and hyaline layers, as in man, but no granular layer. Towards the incisal end, the pulp is obliterated by a plug of secondary dentine. In the prefunctional incisor, the tip is made up of a spongy mineralized tissue which is anomalous in its trabecular structure, its mode of formation and in the pattern of mineralization. Because of its spongy structure it has been called osteodentine but its resemblance to other osteodentines (Fig. 6.5) may be only superficial.

The cement covering the rat incisor is uniformly about 4 $\mu$m thick and is acellular. The associated periodontal ligament (Fig. 12.52) is organized into collagen sheets running from cement to bone. It has been suggested that the middle region of the periodontium has a special structure, known as the 'intermediate plexus', concerned with tooth movement, but this is probably an artifact resulting from the appearance of the ligament in oblique sections. On the labial side, where the tooth is not attached, the periodontal space is filled with connective tissue fibres, running mainly parallel with the tooth surface, numerous blood vessels and abundant ground substance.

GROWTH AND DEVELOPMENT

Throughout life, the incisors of a grown rat erupt at a constant rate of about 400 $\mu$m/day (slightly less in the upper incisors) and the same amount of hard tissue is worn away at the functional tip. The teeth erupt even if they are not subjected to attrition; thus, if a tooth becomes misaligned or lost, the opponent of that tooth continues to spiral out into the mouth and, if not prevented, ultimately leads to the death of the animal by bracing the mouth open and interfering with feeding. Sometimes, the tooth grows so far as to pierce the soft tissues and bone of the oral cavity.

The rapid growth rate obviously necessitates intense cellular activity in forming hard tissues. The demand is highlighted by the following calculation: in a rat weighing 250 g, the lower incisor is about 25 mm long. At an eruption rate of 400 $\mu$m/day, hard tissue formed at the base takes about 62 days to reach the incisal edge, so that this tooth is replaced completely about six times per year. The base of the incisor is enclosed by a sheath of epithelium (Fig. 12.31) and for descriptive purposes the part of the sheath on the labial surface can be called the enamel organ and that covering the remaining surfaces Hertwig's sheath. However, these terms do not have quite the same meaning as in human tooth development because the rat incisor is not polarized into root and crown in the same way as in most teeth.

At the base of the incisor, the cells of the epithelial sheath and the enclosed mesenchyme form a stem-cell population (Fig. 12.31); there is a high frequency of mitosis and the daughter cells migrate anteriorly and differentiate into ameloblasts, odontoblasts, pulp cells, cementoblasts and fibroblasts.

*Amelogenesis*

The basal region of the enamel organ consists of inner and outer enamel epithelia (Fig. 12.31) enclosing a stratum intermedium and stellate reticulum. With the differentiation of the inner enamel epithelial cells into ameloblasts, the stellate reticulum is lost and the ameloblast layer becomes covered by a layer of closely packed cells. In the first stage of their differentiation, the ameloblasts are elongated cells engaged in secreting enamel precursors. When the immature enamel reaches its full thickness, the ameloblasts shorten and begin to absorb protein and water from the matrix, simultaneously secreting additional mineral. As the enamel nears its mature state, the ameloblasts accumulate considerable quantities of the iron-bearing proteins ferritin and haemosiderin and secrete iron into the superficial 5–10 $\mu$m of the enamel. The state in which the iron leaves the ameloblasts is unknown. Finally, the ameloblasts shorten further and the incisal portion of the enamel organ consists of a reduced enamel epithelium which merges with the attachment epithelium.

Blood vessels are in close contact with the enamel organ during the matrix secretion phase of amelogenesis and the contact becomes more intimate during the absorption (or maturation) phase; capillaries become embedded in transverse indentations in the outer epithelial layers and are separated from the ameloblasts only by two or three cell widths. This vascularized layer of the postsecretory enamel organ is known as the papillary layer (Fig. 12.32). The cytology of the epithelial cells around the vessels suggests that the papillary layer is adapted to facilitate the transport of ions, and possibly water as well, between the capillaries and the ameloblasts.

*Dentinogenesis*
This process is little different from that described in Chapter 8. The stem cells differentiate into pre-odontoblasts and then into fully active odontoblasts. After the completion of the primary dentine, the plug of secondary dentine is laid down.

*Cement and periodontal ligament*
The epithelial sheath away from the enamel covered surface has the typical two-layered structure of Hertwig's sheath which, after the deposition on its inner surface of a small amount of dentine, breaks up and allows access of cells which form the cement and periodontal ligament fibres (Fig. 12.31). Cement formation is soon complete but the fibroblasts of the ligament are active throughout the length of the tooth. At first, these cells are concerned with building up the system of principal fibres but even in regions where the ligament is fully formed the rate of protein turnover is extremely high, turnover time being only a few days. This rapid turnover is presumably related largely to remodelling of the attachment fibres in response to changing functional demands and/or with the continuous eruption of the tooth, so that proper support is maintained; it has been speculated that it may be part of the mechanism providing the eruptive force (p. 317). The rate of turnover is not raised over the middle region of the ligament; an important piece of evidence that an intermediate plexus does not exist.

**Experimental applications of the rat incisor**

HARD TISSUE FORMATION

Because the hard tissues of the incisor are being continuously generated, all stages of hard tissue formation are represented in a single specimen. This feature has proved to be of great value for histological, histochemical and ultrastructural studies of amelogenesis and dentinogenesis. Experiments in which the pattern of cell division has been studied, using tritiated thymidine or mitosis-arresting drugs such as colchicine, have provided much information about the way in which ameloblasts and odontoblasts are recruited from the stem cell population at the base.

A different approach to the problems of amelogenesis has used the techniques of chemical analysis on a microscale. The incisors are removed from a freshly killed rat, the enamel organ is stripped away and the enamel dissected from the dentine in pieces 1 mm long. Each fragment is then analysed chemically. This ingenious technique has provided detailed information about the levels of important constituents such as calcium, magnesium, phosphate and protein in enamel at different stages of development. Recent work has even succeeded in plotting the changes in amino acid composition of the matrix protein during enamel mineralization. The rat incisor is thus providing valuable insights into the molecular basis of amelogenesis.

EFFECTS OF DRUGS AND
OTHER AGENTS

Because the rat incisor contains a varied population of cells in all stages of differentiation, it provides a useful model for studying the effects of various agents. Sometimes the studies are concerned with specific dental effects but often the results are more widely applicable. Among the agents studied have been actinomycin D, cyclophosphamide and ionising radiations. In conformity with their effects on other tissues, these agents interfere with tooth formation indirectly, by damaging the proliferative stem cells, but some results have been unexpected; the cytotoxic drug cyclophosphamide, for instance, appears to affect the odontogenic mesenchyme more than the epithelium.

STUDIES OF ERUPTION

The great majority of studies on tooth eruption have used the rat incisor because of the constancy and rapidity of eruption rate; changes induced in the rate by experimental treatments are easily detected. Daily eruption rates can be measured simply by making a mark in the enamel and plotting the movement of this mark over a period of days or weeks with reference to some relatively fixed point such as the gingival margin or the alveolar crest. An alternative approach often used is to cut one lower incisor back to the gingiva and use a mark on the adjacent uncut incisor as the reference point. Cutting an incisor out of occlusion results in an approximately doubled eruption rate; the tooth moves out of the socket at about 1 mm/day. The increased distances moved by the tooth improves the accuracy of daily measurements. Moreover, the measurements are an indication of the rate of eruption in the absence of occlusal forces which tend to intrude the tooth. This is useful in circumstances where a treatment affects the quality of tooth support without altering eruption rate; such a treatment would appear spuriously to slow down eruption if studied with the incisor in occlusion.

Cutting an incisor out of occlusion has a number of other effects, which are due to the eruption rate increasing without a corresponding increase in other processes. Although the rate of cell division at the basal end increases, the rates of differentiation and hard tissue formation by ameloblasts and odontoblasts appear to be more or less fixed. This results in incomplete amelogenesis and dentinogenesis. Thus, the enamel, while reaching the normal level of mineralization, does not become pigmented because of insufficient time for the final stages of amelogenesis. Similarly, the pulp frequently becomes exposed because the plug of secondary dentine does not form.

It is possible to prevent eruption by wiring the incisor to the bone. The cellular changes resulting from this block, and by later releasing the tooth, provide additional information about the eruptive force.

The methods mentioned above, used in conjunction with techniques such as administration of drugs or surgical manipulation, have yielded large amounts of data. However, theories of eruption still abound (chapter 9) and the mechanism is far from solution. The methods so far considered are essentially long term because accurate measurements can be made only over days or weeks. Currently there is interest in the development of methods for recording tooth movement over minutes or hours, to enable study of the immediate effects of treatments, such as alteration of blood flow, which cannot be maintained over long periods. At present, these methods use either photographic or electronic devices. The latter approach involves cementing the two halves of a capacitor to the tooth and the bone and recording the change of capacitance caused by separation of the plates as the tooth erupts. This device records continuously and is extremely sensitive, detecting movements in the order of micrometres. However, because of technical considerations, it has so far been applied only to the larger incisors of the rabbit.

**Molar teeth of the rat**

Many of the experimental studies mentioned in connection with the incisor have been duplicated on the molars of the rat, although, in the case of amelogenesis, for instance, not all stages may be present in a single specimen. The value of work on the molars lies in the fact that the teeth are of limited growth and can thus be considered more directly comparable to human teeth than the incisors. One of the most important applications of the molars, for which the incisors are unsuitable, is in the field of dental caries since, using special diets rich in refined carbohydrates, caries-like lesions can be produced. Much useful information concerning, for example, the role of specific bacteria in the caries process has been obtained using gnotobiotic techniques. The effect of agents such as trace metals and fluorine which influence caries incidence have also been profitably studied in rats. The use of rats in caries research is subject to certain difficulties, however. First, the susceptibility of the molars to caries is to some extent dependent on the strain of rat employed. Second, the pattern of carious attack is not strictly comparable to that seen in man; most of the lesions produced affect the deep fissures on the crowns, while smooth surface caries in the interproximal regions is much less common.

**Table 12.1.** Chronology of development of the mandibular molars of the rat: the maxillary molars pass through the various stages approximately 1 day afterwards.

| Developmental stage | First molar | Second molar | Third molar |
| --- | --- | --- | --- |
| Initial appearance of tooth germ | 13 | 14–15 | 20 |
| Onset of mineralization | 20–21 | 1–2 | 13–14 |
| Completion of crown | 11 | 13 | 21 |
| Emergence into oral cavity | 19 | 22 | 35 |
| Functional occlusion | 25 | 28 | 40 |

(Figures above the dotted line are days *in utero*; those below days *post partum*)

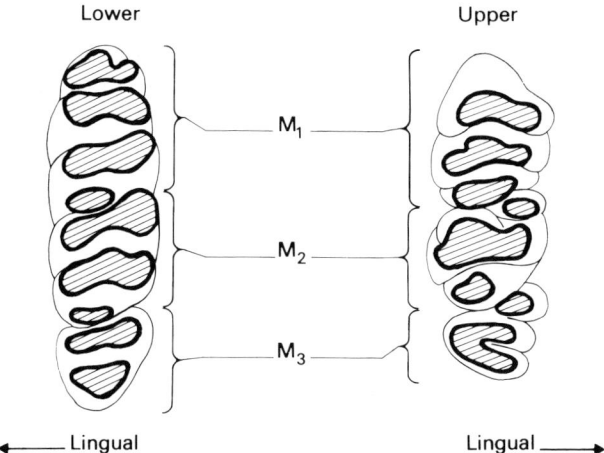

**Fig. 12.34.** Occlusal view of the molars of a rat, to show the pattern of attrition facets, indicated by hatching (exposed dentine) encircled by thick lines (enamel). In this specimen, attrition is moderate; the facets enlarge and partly coalesce with more prolonged use.

The chronology of development of the molars of the rat is shown in Table 12.1. The crowns of the upper first molars have five cusps, those of the lower first molars four; the second and third molars have four and three cusps respectively. At the tips of the cusps, enamel does not form. Pairs of cusps are joined by transverse ridges and attrition leads to the appearance on the occlusal surface of elongated islands of dentine each surrounded by a rim of enamel (Fig. 12.34). In each tooth, there are as many roots as cusps, except in the second lower molar, where there are only three roots. The roots are all covered with a thick layer of cement, which contains cells, unlike that on the incisors.

In the rabbit and the guinea pig, the crowns of the continuously growing molars possess a covering of cement. In the rabbit this forms a continuous layer, but in the guinea pig it is distributed as numerous small islands. The molars of the rabbit are deeply folded longitudinally and the groove is filled with a variety of cement commonly called 'cartilage-cement'.

## FURTHER READING

ADDISON W.H.F. & APPLETON J.L. (1915) The structure and growth of the incisor teeth of the albino rat. *Journal of Morphology* **26**, 43.

BERKOVITZ B.K.B. (1975) Mechanism of tooth eruption. In *Applied Oral Physiology*, p. 99, ed. Lavelle C.L.B. Bristol: Wrights.

GARANT P.R. (1968) The fine structure of the papillary region of the mouse enamel organ. *Archives of Oral Biology* **13**, 1167.

HALSE A. & SELVIG K.A. (1974) Incorporation of iron in rat incisor enamel. *Scandinavian Journal of Dental Research* **82**, 47.

KINDLOVA M. & MATENA V. (1959) Blood circulation in the rodent teeth of the rat. *Acta Anatomica* **37**, 163.

MATENA V. (1972) The periodontium of the enamel aspect of the rat incisor. *Journal of Periodontology* **43**, 311.

NESS A.R. (1964) Movement and forces in tooth eruption. In *Advances in Oral Biology*, Vol. 1, ed. Staple P.H. London: Academic Press.

NESS A.R. & SMALE D.E. (1959) The distribution of mitoses and cells in the tissues bounded by the socket wall of the rabbit mandibular incisor. *Proceedings of the Royal Society, London Series B.* **151**, 106.

REITH E.J. (1959) The enamel organ of the rat's incisor, its histology and pigment. *Anatomical Record* **133**, 75.

ROBINS M.W. (1967) The proliferation of pulp cells in rat incisors. *Archives of Oral Biology* **12**, 487.

SCHOUR I. & MASSLER M. (1949) The teeth. In *The Rat in Laboratory Investigations*, 2nd Edition, p. 104, ed. Farris E.J. & Griffiths J.Q. Philadelphia: Lippincott.

SUGA S. & GUSTAFSON G. (1963) Studies on the development of rat enamel by means of histochemistry, microradiography and polarized light microscopy. *Archives of Oral Biology* **8** (suppl.), 223.

TAKUMA S. & NAGAI N. (1971) Ultrastructure of rat odontoblasts in various stages of their development and maturation. *Archives of Oral Biology* **16**, 993.

# Index

Aardvark, dentition, 409
Aardwolves, dentition, 408
Abrasion of teeth, 305, 326, 335, 375
Abscesses, dental, 216, 217, 244
Actinopterygii, evolution and adaptation, 98, 99–100
Age
  dental, 66
  effects on teeth, 149, 172–3, 356
  estimation of, from human teeth, 149, 172–3, 356
  gestational, and crown-rump measurements, 17–18
  morphological, 66–7
  skeletal, 65–6
  see also Ageing; Longevity
Ageing, 81–2, 352–6
  causes, theories on, 85–6
  changes associated with, 82–5 172–3, 188
  factors affecting, 82
  see also Longevity
Agnathans
  dental tissue, 160
  evolution and adaptation, 88–91
Alimentary tract, development of, 15–16, 21–4
Allantois, 10, 16
Alleles, 47, 48, 49–52
  frequency, 59–61
  mutation, 49–50
  and patterns of inheritance, 52–6
Alveolar bone, 119–20, 215
  development, 215
  and eruption of teeth, 74, 312
  histology, 218
  lamina dura, 215, 218
  mechanics, 218
  resorption, 293
  structure, 215–17
Alveoli, 119, 120, 215
Ameloblasts, 155, 165, 184, 260, 269–77, 279–80
Amelodentinal junction, 118, 184–5, 260
Amelogenesis, see Enamel, development
Amelogenesis imperfecta, 295

Amelogenin, 207–8, 271, 272, 273, 274
Amnion, 9, 10, 16
Amniotic cavity, 9, 16
Amniotic fluid, 16
Amphibians
  dental tissues, 156, 159, 164
  evolution and adaptation, 102–6
  sense organs, 103–5
  tooth support, 213
Anaesthetization of teeth and associated structures, 243
Angle's classification of malocclusion, 308, 318, 371
Angulation of teeth, 305–7
Ankylosis in tooth support, 210, 211, 212, 213, 233
Anodontia, 215, 254, 295, 297
Anomalies
  in tooth development, 294–7
  in tooth morphology, 149
Anteaters, anatomy and feeding, 402
Anthropoidea, 357, 367, 368
  dentition, 371, 422–32
Antrum
  maxillary, 216–17
  nasal, 80
Anura, dentition, 105–6
Aorta, development of, 18, 19, 20–1
Apatite, 164, 166, 168, 173, 264
Apes
  great, 363, 365
    dentition, 371–3, 375, 381–4, 429–32
  lesser, 363
    dentition, 427–9
Arch, dental, adaptation in mammals, 375–7
Archosaurs, 109–10
Armadillos, dentition, 402
Arteries, development of, 18–21
Artiodactyla, dentition, 411, 413–15
Atherosclerosis, and ageing, 82–3
Atrophy of organs with advancing age, 82
Attrition of teeth, 149, 173, 305, 326, 333–6, 352–3, 375

*Australopithecus*, 384–6, 388
  *afarensis*, 384
  *africanus*, 378, 379, 384–5
  *boisei*, 384, 386, 388
  *robustus*, 379, 384, 385–6
Autoimmunity, and ageing, 86
Aye-aye, 359
  dentition, 160, 369–71, 420–1

*Babyrousa*, dentition, 413
Baleen whales, 406
Bats, dentition of, 400
  fruit, 400–1
  insectivorous, 401–2
  vampire, 402
Bears, dentition, 406–7
Bennett movement, 303
'Bilophodont' molar, 375
Birds, evolution and adaptation, 112–13
Blastocyst, 9–10
Blastomeres, 8–9
Blood supply to teeth and periodontium, 189–90, 226–8, 243–5
Bone
  formation, mechanisms of, 35–7
  growth, 65–6, 71–2
Bone of attachment, 212
Bovidae (antelopes, cattle, sheep), dentition of, 415
Brachycephaly, 394, 396
Brachyodont teeth, 347, 348, 352, 403
Branchial arch arteries, fate of, 20, 35
Branchial arches, development of, 23, 26–7
  and face and nasal cavities, 27–31
  and mesodermal derivatives, 35 (Table 1.2)
  and mouth and tongue, 31–2
Branchial clefts, derivatives of, 34–6
Branchial pouches, derivatives of, 34
Buccopharyngeal membrane, 12, 14, 15, 22, 27
Bulbus cordis, 18, 19
Bundle bone, 218

# Index

Bunodont teeth, 403, 404, 407, 413, 414

Calcospherites in dentine, 168, 264–5
Calculus (tartar), 205, 282
Calvaria, 37–9
Camels, dentition, 414
Canine rise, 305
Canines
  adaptation in primates, 371–3
  morphology, human, 128–32, 147
Cape golden moles, dentition, 400
Carabelli, tubercle of, 138, 139, 148, 153, 396
Cardiovascular system, embryology of, 17, 18–21
Caries, 149, 173, 187, 208
Carnassials in carnivores, 341–2, 349
Carnivora, dentition, 341–2, 406–8
Cartilage
  of mandible, 45, 76–8
  Meckel's, 39, 43, 44, 45, 94, 117
  primary, 35, 71
  quadrate, 39
  secondary, 37, 71
  of skull, 71
Cats (*Felis*), dentition, 408
Cats, great (*Panthera*), dentition, 408
Cells
  and ageing, 83, 86
  differentiation, 1–3, 62–3
  and embryogenesis, 5–11
  germ, 5–7
  growth of, 62–3
  and morphogenesis, 3–5
  somatic, 47, 48
Cement, 118, 119
  and age, changes due to, 149, 355–6
  coronal, 281, 282, 283
  development, 286–8, 437
    afribrillar, 288
    extrinsic fibre, 288–9
    intrinsic fibre, 292
    mixed fibre, 289–92
  in human teeth, 193–5
    afibrillar, 198
    biochemistry of, 205–9
    chemical characteristics, 197–8
    distribution, 195–7
    exposed, 204–5
    fibres in, 198–204
    incremental lines, 198–9, 201
    intermediate, 202
    physical characteristics, 195–7, 198
    structure, 198–204
  repair, 294
  resorption, 292–4
Cement–dentine junction, 118, 196, 287–8

Cement–epithelial junction, 204–5
Cementoblasts, 198–203, 224, 283, 287, 288–9
Cementoclasts, 224
Cementocytes, 118, 202–3
Cementogenesis, 286–92
Central nervous system, changes due to ageing, 85
Cervidae (deer), dentition, 415
Cetacea, dentition, 405–6
Chalones, 82
Chemotaxis in morphogenesis, 4, 5
Chewing, 116, 300, 302–5, 319–20, 331–6, 344–5
Chimpanzee, 363, 364
  dentition, 429–30
Chiroptera, dentition, 400–2
Chondrichthyes, evolution and adaptation, 92–8
  head, segmentation, 92–6
  jaw attachment to cranium, 96
  neurocranium, 93–4
  teeth of, 96–8
  viscerocranium, 94–6
Chorion, 9, 10, 16
Chondrocranium, 37, 92
Chromatids, 6
Chromosomes, 5–7
  abnormalities, 6, 49
  autosomal, 47, 48
  diploid number, 5, 6, 7, 8, 47–8
  and genes, 47–8
  haplid number, 6, 7, 47
  independent assortment, 48–9, 50
  loci on, 47, 48
  non-dysjunction, 49
  recombination of segments, 48–9, 50
  sex, 7, 47, 48, 53–4
  translocation, 49
Cingulum, 123
  canine, 129, 130, 147
  incisor, 125, 126, 145
  molar, 148, 338
Civet cats, dentition, 408
Cleavage of cells in embryogenesis, 8–10
Cloaca, 24
Cloacal membrane, 12, 15, 22, 24
Clone unit in dentition, 255, 257
  and tooth shapes, 257–60
Coatimundis, dentition, 407
Coelacanths, 98, 101, 164
Coelom, 14, 24
Collagen, 254
  in cement, 197–8, 288, 289
  contraction theory of eruption, 317
  in dentine, 155, 167, 170, 262–3, 264
  in enameloid, 155
  in gingiva, 235
  in periodontal ligament,

Collagen (*continued*)
  219–22, 224–5, 229–30, 232
  in pulp, 266
  and tooth attachment, 210, 211
Comb, prosiminian dental, 368–9, 420, 421
Concrescence of teeth, 255
Congenital abnormalities, 19–20, 31, 254–5
  *see also* Anomalies
Connecting stalk of embryo, 9, 11
Corona radiata, 6, 8
Coronal cement, 281, 282, 283
Craniofacial development, 35–7
  cranial base, 37
  cranial vault, 37–9
  face, 39–46
  mandible, 27, 39, 43, 44–6
  maxilla, 39, 40, 42, 43–4, 45
  origin of the bones, 37
Crocodiles, 107, 109–10, 156, 213, 214
Crossopterygii, evolution and adaptation, 98, 99, 101–2
Crown–rump measurement, and gestational age, 17–18
Cusps, 123
  entoconid, 340, 341, 344, 375
  hypocone, 344, 373, 375
  hypoconid, 339, 340, 341, 344, 375
  hypoconulid, 340, 344, 347, 375
  metacone, 340, 341, 344, 373, 375
  metaconid, 340, 341, 375
  metaconule, 341
  metastyle, 341
  paracone, 340, 341, 342, 375
  paraconid, 340, 344, 375
  paraconule, 341
  parastyle, 340, 341
  protocone, 339–41, 344, 373, 375
  protoconid, 340, 341, 375
Cuticles, 280–3
  dental, 281–2, 283
  primary, 281, 283, 321
Cyclostomes, evolution and adaptation, 88–90
Cynodontia, 299, 331, 333, 350, 351
Cysts, dental, 255, 261

Dasyuridae, dentition, 417
*Daubentonia* (aye-aye), 359
  dentition, 160, 369–71, 420–1
Decidua of uterus, 9
Dental tissues, separation of, for analysis, 206
Dentary bone, 113, 117, 333
Denteons, 160
Denticles, 173
Dentine, 90
  circumpulpal, 166, 263–4, 266

Dentine (*continued*)
  development, comparative, 155-6
  formation, 260-6
  histology, comparative, 158-61
  in human teeth, 118, 166
    ageing, 172, 354
    biochemistry of, 205-6, 208
    composition, 166-7
    dead tract in, 173
    denticles, 173
    opalescent, hereditary, 295-6
    primary, 166, 173, 262
    properties of, related to function, 173-4
    and pulp stones, 173
    sclerosis, 173
    secondary, 166, 171-3, 262
    sensory mechanisms, 190-3
    structure, 167-73
  line markings in, 171, 265
  mantle, 166, 168, 262-3
  mineralization, 264-6
  peritubular, 170-1, 265
  and roots, 266
  tubules in, 158, 166, 168-71, 172, 264, 265
Dentine-cement junction, 118, 196, 287-8
Dentinogenesis imperfecta, 295-6
Dentition
  development of, 246
    anomalies, 294-7
    bell stage, 247-53, 260
    bud stage, 246
    cap stage, 246-7
    cement, 286-94
    clinical considerations, 254-5
    congenital abnormalities, 254-5
    controls, 255-60
    cuticles, 280-3
    dentine, 260-6
    enamel, 267-80
    epithelial/mesenchymal interactions, 253-4
    functional aspects, 349-52
    periodontium, 283-6
    pulp, 260-7
    tooth shapes, 249, 257-60
    tooth succession, 255-7
  human, 120-1, 318-28
  *see also* Teeth, human, form of
Dentogingival junction, 237-8
Deoxyribonucleic acid (DNA), 1, 5, 6, 62, 230
  and ageing, 85, 86
Dermoptera, dentition, 400
Developmental defects in tooth morphology, 149
Diastema, 347-8
Diet and ageing, 82
Dilambdadont teeth in insectivores, 342-4, 399
Dinosaurs, 107, 109, 110-2

Diphyodonty, 120, 299, 318, 350
Dipnoi, evolution and adaptation, 98, 99, 100-1
Dogs, dentition, 406
Dolichocephaly, 394, 395
Dolphins, dentition, 405-6
Down's syndrome, 49
Drift of teeth, 309-10
  approximal, 326
  mesial, 309, 310, 326-7, 328, 376
  and periodontal ligament, 230-2
'*Dryopithecus*' pattern molar, 375, 381-3, 428, 429, 432
Ductus arteriosus, 21
Ductus venosus, 21
Durodentine, 156

Ear
  in amphibians, 104
  in mammals, 113-16
  in reptiles, 109, 115
Ectoderm, 9, 11, 12
  structures developing from, 17 (Table 1.1)
Ectopic pregnancy, 10
Edentata, dentition, 402
Elasmobranchs, 98, 103
  dental tissues, 156, 159, 160
  tooth support, 210, 211, 212
Elastin fibres, 263
  in periodontal ligament, 224
Elephants, dentition, 410-1
Enamel
  and cuticles, 280-3
  development, 246-52, 267-80, 436-7
    comparative, 155-6
  epithelium of
    external, 247-8, 269, 270
    internal, 247, 249-50, 254, 260, 269, 270-1
  glycoproteins, 175, 272, 273
  histology, comparative, 164-5
  in human teeth, 118
    ageing, 353-4
    biochemistry of, 205-9
    clinical considerations, 187
    and enamel-dentine junction, 184-5
    fissures in, 184
    hypoplasia; acquired, 295; hereditary, 295
    increment lines, 181-3
    lamellae in, 183
    living or dead tissue?, 185-7
    pearls, 196
    physical properties, 173, 174 (Table 6.2), 174-5
    pits in, 184, 185
    prisms *see under* Prisms in enamel
    spindles in, 184
    surface of, 185
    tufts in, 183, 184

Enamel (*continued*)
    interprismatic region, 275-6
    maturation of, 273-4
    prisms, *see* Prisms in enamel
    proteins, 206-8, 273-4
    ridges (lophs), 345, 403
    tubules, 165
Enamel-cement junction, 196
Enamel cord, 250-1
Enamel-dentine junction, 118, 184-5, 260
Enamel knot, 250
Enamel niche, 251
Enamel organ, 246-54, 260, 262, 281
  functions, 267-8
  prisms of, 269, 270-5
  structure of, 269-70
Enameloid
  development, comparative, 155-6
  histology, comparative, 161-3
Endocrine system, changes due to ageing, 84
Endoderm, 9, 11, 12
  structures developing from, 17 (Table 1.1)
Enteron, 15-16, 21-4
*Eozostrodon*, and occlusion, 299, 333, 338
Epithelial cells of periodontal ligament, 225-6
Epithelial cuff, *see* Epithelium, gingival, junctional
Epithelium, gingival, 233, 235, 238
  junctional, 120, 186, 204-5, 233, 236-7, 320-1, 356
  oral, 233, 235-6, 238
  oral sulcular, 233, 235, 236
Eruption of teeth, 66, 309-10
  clinical features, 318
  dentition, establishment of, 318-19
    deciduous, 319-22
    permanent, 322-5
  mechanism, theories of, 310-12
    alveolar bone deposition, 312
    periodontal ligament, tensions within, 316-17
    pulp cell proliferation, 312-14
    root growth, 312-14
    tissue fluid pressure, 314-16

Face
  development, 27-31, 39-46
  evolution
    in modern man, 394-6
    in primates, 376-7
Feeding, and functions of teeth, 329-36
Fertilization of ovum, 6, 7-8, 47-8
Ferungulata, dentition, 409-11
Fetal circulation, 21

Fibroblasts
  contraction/motility theory of eruption, 317
  in periodontal ligament, 224–5, 230, 288, 289
  in pulp, 188, 266
Fillings, dental, 187, 354
Fishes
  dental tissues, 155, 159, 160, 161–3, 211–12
  evolution and adaptation
    Agnatha, 88–91
    Chondrichthyes, 92–8
    Osteichthyes, 98–102
    Placodermi, 91–2
Fluoride, 185, 186
  in enamel, 208
  and mottling, 209
Fluorosis, dental, 209
Flying foxes, dentition, 400–1
Follicle
  dental, 247, 248, 250, 260, 283–4, 285
  ovarian, 5, 6
Foramen
  apical, 119, 187–8, 189
  cacumen, 125, 126
  caecum, 32, 33
  mental, 79, 240
  ovale, 18, 20, 21
Forebrain, embryonic, 15
Foxes, dentition, 406
Functional matrices in skull growth, 72
Functions of teeth, 329–31
  chewing, 116, 300, 302–5, 319–20, 331–6, 344–5
  and dental development, 349–52
  and jaw joints, 348–9
  and jaw muscles, 348
  and mammalian evolution, 336–48
Fused teeth, 255

Gametes (germ cells), 5–7, 47, 48
Geminated teeth, 255
Genes, 47–8
  and characters, 50–1, 56
  frequency, 59–61
  interaction, 52
  mutation in, 49–50
  penetrance, incomplete, 51
  pleiotropic, 51
  in populations, 56, 58–61
  X-linked, 48, 54
Genital system, development of, 25–6
Genotype, 50–9
Germ cells (gametes), 5–7, 47, 48
Gibbon, 363
  dentition, 427–9
Gingiva, 31, 32, 119–20, 233
  effects of age on, 149
  attached, 234–5

Gingiva (continued)
  biochemistry, 238
  blood supply, 243–5
  clinical features, normal, 234–5
  dentogingival junction, 237–8
  epithelium, see Epithelium, gingival
  free, 234
  lymphatics, 245
  nerve supply, 241
  physiology, 238
  protection of, by dental features, 149–50
  structural features, 235–7
Giraffidae (giraffes and okapis), dentition, 415
Glycosaminoglycans
  in dental papilla, 250, 252
  in dentine, 263, 264
  and enamel, 175, 247, 249, 252, 270, 274
  in pulp, 188, 189, 266
Gomphosis, 110, 213, 233, 299
Gorilla, 363, 364
  dentition, 429, 431–2
Grinding in herbivores, 344–5
Growth, human, 62
  adolescent spurt, 65, 67
  allometric, 69
  assessment, 63–7
  body proportions, changes 66–7
  of bone, 65–6, 71–2
  curves, 63–4
  dental, 66
  factors affecting, 67–8
    climate, 68
    genetic, 68–9
    hormones, 68
    illness, 69
    malnutrition, 69
    race, 68
    seasons, 68
    socioeconomic class, 65, 69
  gnomonic, 69
  in height, 64–5
  of jaws, 74–9
  phases of, 63
  and prediction of adult size, 67
  processes, 62–3
  secondary sex characters, 67, 68
  of skull, see Skull, human, growth of
  in weight, 65
Gubernacular cord, 312
Guinea pigs, dentition, 404
Gut, 15–16, 21–4

Haplodont teeth, 101
Hardy-Weinberg law, 59–61
Hares, dentition, 404–5
Hassall's corpuscles, 34
Healing, retardation of, in ageing, 83

Heart
  congenital abnormalities, 19–20
  embryology, 17, 18–19
Hedgehogs, dentition, 399
Hemizygous males, 48, 52, 54
Herbivores, dentition of, 344–8
Heredity, and ageing, 82
Hertwig's root sheath, 211, 225, 260–2, 268, 283, 287
Heterodonty, 107, 108
Heterozygote, 48, 52
Hinged teeth, 212–13
Hippopotami, dentition, 413–14
Hominids, 363, 365, 373, 377–9, 432
  *Australopithecus*, 378, 379, 384–6, 388
  dating techniques with fossils, 379–81
  *Homo*, see *Homo*
  'man' defining of, 381
  of Pleistocene period, 388
  of Plio-Pleistocene periods, 384
  and pongids, 381–4
  *Homo*, 381, 386–8
    *erectus*, 379, 388–9
    *habilis*, 379, 387, 388
    *sapiens*, 388, 389–90
    *sapiens neanderthalensis*, 379, 388
    *sapiens sapiens*, 379, 381, 388, 392
Homodonty, 108
Homozygote, 48, 52
Hopewell-Smith, hyaline layer of, 166, 168, 266
Horses, dentition, 412
Hunter-Schreger bands in enamel, 180–1, 187
Hyaline layer (of Hopewell-Smith) in dentine, 166, 168, 266
Hydroxyapatite in dental tissues, 118, 205, 208
  in cement, 197
  in dentine, 167
  in enamel, 174–6, 273
Hyenas, dentition, 408
Hypercementosis, 197
Hypodontia, 254
Hypophysis cerebri, development of, 33–4
Hypsodont teeth, 214, 347, 352, 403
Hyraxes, dentition, 409–10

Immunity system, changes in, in ageing, 84–5
Incisive nerve, 240
Incisors
  adaptation in primates, 368–9, 371
  morphology, human, 123–8, 145–7
  in rodents, 187, 345, 347, 433–8

Indriids, 359
  dentition, 375, 419–20
Inheritance
  patterns of, 52–6
  quantitative, 56–8
Innervation of teeth and periodontium, 217, 228, 239–43
Insectivora, dentition, 342–4, 399–400
Ionizing radiation, and ageing, 82

Jaws
  and chewing, 331–3
  and evolution
    amphibians, 105–6
    birds, 112
    fishes, 92, 94–101
    mammals, 113–17
    primates, 368–77
    reptiles, 107, 109, 113–16
  human, growth of, 74–9
  in mammals, 113–17, 348–9
Joints, human, changes due to ageing, 84

Kangaroos, dentition, 418–19
Kuehneotherium, and functions of teeth, 333, 338

Labyrinthodonts, 101, 102, 105, 160
Lagomorphs, dentition, 404–5
  and laboratory research, 432–9
Lamina, dental, 246, 253
Lamina dura of alveolar bone, 215, 218
Lamina propria of gingiva, 235
Lemurs, 357, 359, 364
  dentition, 419–20
Lepidosaurs, 107–9
Ligament, periodontal, 119, 193–4, 215, 218, 219, 285
  and ageing, 355–6
  cells of, 224–6, 230
  clinical features, 232–3
  connective tissue, turnover of components, 228–32
  development, 284–6
  fibres of, 219–24
  functions, 232
  gel in, 224
  nerves of, 228
  tissue fluid in, 228
  vascular supply, 226–8
Lip, cleft, 31, 58
Lipofuscin, accumulation of in ageing, 83, 85, 86
Liquor amnii, 16
Lissamphibia, 102
Llamas, dentition, 414
Locus, chromosomal, 47, 48
Longevity, relationship to teeth, 352
Lophodont teeth, 345, 403
Lorisidae, dentition, 357, 364, 421

Lung fish, 98, 99, 100–1
Lymphatic drainage of dental tissues, 245

Macrodontism, 255
Malassez, rests of, 225–6, 261, 283, 287
Malocclusion, 300, 308–9, 318
Mammals
  dental tissues, 156, 160, 164–5
  evolution, 113–17, 336–48
  functions of teeth, 329–36, 349–52
  molar evolution, 336–48
  tooth support, 213–15
  see also named mammals and orders
Mammelons, 124, 125, 127, 129
Mandible, 215, 217
  development, 27, 31, 39, 43, 44–6
  growth, 74, 76–9
Markers, metal, in skull radiography, 70, 77
Marmosets, dentition, 422–3
Marsupials, dentition, 415–19
  diprotodontia, 418–19
  polyprotodontia, 416–18
Mast cells
  in gingiva, 235
  in periodontal ligament, 226
Maturity, assessment of, 63–7
Maxillae, 216–17
  development of, 39, 40, 42, 43–4, 45
  growth of, 73–6
Maxillary process, 27–9, 31, 43–4
Meckel's cartilage, 39, 43, 44, 45, 94, 117
Meiosis, 6–7, 48, 49
Mental nerve, 79, 217, 240–1
Mesocephaly, 394
Mesoderm, 9–10, 11, 12
  intermediate, 12, 14, 25
  lateral, 12–13, 14
  paraxial, 12–13
  structures developing from, 17 (Table 1.1)
Metatherian mammals, dentition, 415–19
  diprotodontia, 418–19
  polyprotodontia, 416–18
Mice, dentition, 403–4
Microdontism, 255
Misplaced teeth, 296
Missing teeth, 297
Mitosis, 48
Modern man, and evolution
  body form, classification, 397
  body size, 393–7
  face, 394–6
  growth, 393
  head shape, 394
  race, 390–8
  tooth size, 396–7

Molarization of premolars in herbivores, 347
Molars
  adaptation in primates, 373–5
  creation of space for lower third, 79
  mammalian, evolution of, 336–48
  morphology, human, 137–43, 147–8
Moles, dentition, 399, 400
Mongolism, 49
Mongoose, dentition, 408
Monson, curve of, 305–7, 326, 376
Morganucodonts, and molar function, 333, 338
Morphogenic field model and tooth shapes, 257–60
Morula, 8–9
Mosaicism, 48
Mottling of teeth, and fluoride, 209
Mouth, human, development of, 29–32
Movement of teeth, 212, 316
  and periodontal ligament, 230–2
  see also Eruption of teeth
Mustelids, dentition, 407–8

Narwhal, dentition, 405–6
Nasal capsule, 39, 40–2
Nasal cavities, development of, 27–31, 44
Nasmyth's membrane, 280–1
Nasolacrimal duct, formation of, 29
Neonatal line in enamel, 183
Nerve supply of teeth and periodontium, 190–3, 217, 228, 239–43
Neural crest, 17, 253, 260
Neural tube, 12, 17
Neurocranium, 37, 39, 73–4
New World monkeys, 359, 367, 422
  dentition, 368, 371, 375, 423–4
Nose, growth of, 79–80
Notochord, 12
Notoryctidae, dentition, 417–18

Occlusion, 299–300, 309, 310, 322–5
  and attrition, 305, 326
  axial deviation of teeth, 305–7
  balanced, 304–5
  in deciduous dentition, 307–8
  dynamic, 302–5
  and evolution, 299
  ideal, 300–2, 305
  intercuspal position, 300–2
  protrusive, 305
  see also Malocclusion
Odontoblasts
  and cement, 287

Odontoblasts (*continued*)
  and dead tracts, 173
  and dentine, 118, 155–6, 158, 160–1, 166, 170, 260–6
  and dentine sclerosis, 173
  and enamel, 165, 250, 267–71
  and enameloid, 156
  and pulp, 188, 190
  'wheatsheafing' of, in ageing, 354
Odontostichos unit in dentition, 255–6
Old World monkeys, 359–63, 364, 422
  dentition, 368, 371–3, 375, 425–7
Olfactory pit, 27, 29
Oocytes, 5, 6, 7
Oogonia, 5
Opossums, American, dentition, 416–17
Orang-utan, 363
  dentition, 429, 430–1
Orthodentine, 158–60, 166, 212
Osteichthyes, 98–102, 103, 162
Osteoblasts, 71, 72, 78, 224
Osteoclasts, 72, 186, 224, 293
Osteodentine, 97, 158, 160, 212
Osteoporosis, and ageing, 83–4
Ostracoderms, evolution and adaptation, 90–1
Overbite, 300, 305, 307, 308, 322, 371
  and ageing, 328
Overjet, 300, 307, 322, 328, 371
Ovulation, 5, 6
Ovum, 5–8
Owen, lines of, 171, 265
Oxytalan fibres in periodontium, 223–4, 235, 285

Pain, and human teeth, 190–3
Palate
  cleft, 31, 58
  development, 29–31, 39, 42, 44
  growth, 74
Pandas, dentition
  giant, 406–7
  lesser, 407
Pantotheres, and molar function, 338–9
Papilla, dental, 155, 247, 249, 250, 253–4, 260
Parathyroid glands, development of, 34
Pecora, dentition, 414–15
Pedicel, in tooth attachment, 210, 211–2, 213
Pellicle, acquired, 282, 283
Perikymata in enamel, 182–3, 185
Periodontium, 119, 193–5, 219
  development of, 283–6
Perissodactyla, dentition, 411–13
Phalangeridae, dentition, 418
Pharyngeal arches, see Branchial arches

Phenotype, 50–9
Pigments, accumulation of, in ageing, 83, 85
Pigs, dentition, 413–14
Pinnepedia, dentition, 408–9
Placenta, 10–11, 16
Placodermi, evolution and adaptation, 91–2
Plaque, 205, 282, 283
Plicidentine, 101, 158, 160
Polar bodies, 6–7
Polyphyodonty, 108, 213–14, 255, 350
Pongidae, 363, 365, 375, 381–4
  dentition, 371–3, 429–32
Porcupines, dentition, 404
Precement, 289, 292, 293
Prechordal plate of embryo, 11, 12
Premaxillae, 39, 40, 42–3
Premolars
  adaptation in primates, 373–5
  molarization of, in herbivores, 347
  morphology, human, 132–7
Primates, 357–63
  adaptations, 364, 365
  face, 376–7
  hearing, 367
  jaws, 368, 371–3, 375–6
  locomotor system, 365, 367
  nervous system, 368
  smell, sense of, 367–8
  special senses, 367–8
  teeth, 368–77
  vision, 367
  characteristics, 364–5
  classification, 360–2 (Table 11.1)
  dentition
    anthropoidea, 422–32
    prosimii, 419–22
  diets, 364
  habitat, 363–4
  see also Hominids, *Homo*, Modern man and evolution, *and named primates and groups*
Primitive knot of embryo, 12
Primitive streak of embryo, 12
Prisms in enamel, 118, 164–5, 175–83, 185, 280
  development, 269, 270–7
  in human teeth, 175–81, 185
    arrangement of, 178–81
    cross striations, 178, 181–2
    crystal orientation, 176
    decussation, 181
    incremental lines, 178, 181–3
    shapes, 176
    sheaths, 176
    size, 176
    terminology, 175–6
Prosimii, 357, 364, 367
  dentition, 368, 371, 373, 419–21
Proteoglycans
  and dentine, 173, 264

Proteoglycans (*continued*)
  and enamel, 252, 270, 272, 273
  and pulp, 188–9, 266
Pulp
  cell proliferation, and eruption of teeth, 312–14
  development, 266–7
  in human teeth, 118–19, 187–8
    ageing, 354–5
    blood supply, 189–90
    in canines: deciduous, 147; permanent, 129, 131
    in incisors: deciduous, 145; permanent, 125, 128
    lymphatics, 190
    mineralization, 173
    in molars: deciduous, 148; permanent, 139, 141, 143, 144
    nerve supply, 190–3
    in premolars, 133, 135, 137
    sensory mechanics, 190–3
    structure, 188–90
Pulp stones, 173, 355

Rabbits, dentition, 404–5
  and laboratory research, 432–9
Race
  and differences in human teeth, 149, 151–4, 396–7
  and evolution in man, 390–8
Racoons, dentition, 407
Radiography in skull growth measurement, 70
*Ramapithecus*, 363, 383–4
Raschkow, plexus of, 190, 192, 267
'Rat' kangaroos, dentition, 419
Rathke's pouch, 33
Rats, dentition, 403–4
  and laboratory research, 432–9
Rays, teeth of, 98, 160, 161, 212
Reptiles
  dental tissues, 156, 160, 164, 165
  evolution and adaptation, 106–16
    anapsid, 106–7
    diapsid, 107
    marine, 112
    synapsid, 113–16
  tooth support, 213
Respiratory passages, development of, 21, 24
Reticulin fibres, 263
  in periodontium, 219, 224, 235
Retzius lines in enamel, 182, 183, 269
Rhipidistia, evolution and adaptation, 101–2, 103, 104
Ribonucleic acid (RNA), 188, 247, 249, 250, 252, 254
  and ageing, 85, 86
Right whale, dentition, 406
Rodents, dentition, 402–4
  and laboratory research, 432–9

Roots, 118, 119
  development, 260-2, 266, 283-5, 286-7
  and eruption of teeth, 312-14
  short, 150-1

Salivary glands, development of, 32-33
Seacows, dentition, 411
Seals, dentition, 409
Secondary sex characters, 67, 68
Selenodont teeth, 345, 414-15
Septum
  nasal, 30, 40, 42
  primum, 18-19, 21
  secundum, 18, 21
  transversum, 12, 15, 23, 24
Serres' glands, 253
Sharks, teeth of, 98, 160, 161-2, 212
Sharpey's fibres, 198, 218, 221, 231, 356
Shearing function of teeth in early mammals, 336-8
Shrews, dentition, 399-400
Siamang, 363
  dentition, 427-9
'Simian shelf' on mandible, 373
Sinus venosus, 18, 21
Skates, evolution and adaptation, 98
Skeletal age, 65-6
Skeleton, changes due to ageing, 83-4
Skin, changes due to ageing, 84
Skull, human
  development, 35-9
    face, 39-43
    mandible, 27, 31, 39, 43, 44-6
    maxilla, 39, 40, 42, 43-4, 45
  growth of, 69-70
    antrum, nasal, 80
    and brain growth, 73-6
    and the eye, 74, 76
    mandible, 74, 76-9
    maxilla, 73-6
    measurement of, 70-1
    methods of, 71-2
    neurocranium, 73-4
    nose, 79-80
    palate, 74
    reference planes, 80-1
    reference points, 80-1
    zygomatic arch, 80
Skull of primates, adaptations, 365, 366 (Table 11.2)
Sloths, dentition, 402
Somites, 12-14
Spee, curve of, 305-7, 323, 376
Sperm whale, dentition, 405
Spermatids, 7
Spermatocytes, 7
Spermatozoa, 7-8
Squirrels, dentition, 403

Stellate reticulum of enamel organ, 247, 249, 254, 269, 270
Stomatodeum, 15, 22-3
Stratum intermedium of enamel organ, 247, 249, 269, 270
Submerged teeth, 296-7
Subodontoblasts, 188
Supernumerary teeth, 254-5, 297, 318
Sutures, and skull growth, 71-2
Synapsida, 331, 340

Talonid on mammalian molars, 336, 338-9, 340, 341, 344, 375
Tamarins, dentition, 422-3
Tapirs, dentition, 348, 412-13
Tarsier, 357-9, 364, 367, 368
  dentition, 421
Taurodontium, 295
Teeth, human, form of, 118-23
  contrasts between deciduous and permanent, 144-5, 324-5
  deciduous
    canine, lower, 147
    canine, upper, 147
    incisor, lower first (central), 145
    incisor, lower second (lateral), 147
    incisor, upper first (central), 145
    incisor, upper second (lateral), 145
    molar, lower first, 148
    molar, lower second, 148
    molar, upper first, 147-8
    molar, upper second, 148
  permanent
    canine, lower, 129-32
    canine, upper, 128-9
    incisor, lower first (central), 126-8
    incisor, lower second (lateral), 128
    incisor, upper first (central), 123-5
    incisor, upper second (lateral), 125-6
    molar, lower first, 140-1
    molar, lower second, 142-3
    molar, lower third, 143-4
    molar, upper first, 137-9
    molar, upper second, 139-40
    molar, upper third, 140
    premolar, lower first, 134-6
    premolar, lower second, 136-7
    premolar, upper first, 132-3
    premolar, upper second, 133
  racial differences in, 151-4
  ridges of, 123
  surfaces of, 121-3

Teeth, human, identification shorthand systems, 121
Teleosts, 98, 99
  teeth of, 99-100, 156, 160, 163
  tooth support, 212-13
Temporomandibular joint, 45-6, 113, 333, 348-9
Tetracycline lines, 70, 71, 171
Thegosis, 335-6
Thymus, development of, 34
Thyroid gland, development of, 33, 34
Tomes, layer of, 166, 266
Tomes' process of ameloblasts, 165, 271-7, 279-80
Tongue, development of, 31-2
Tooth germ, 155, 156, 246-53, 260
  biochemical studies, 251-2
Tooth support
  alveolar bone, 215-18
  attachment tissues, formation of, 211-2
  blood supply of dental structures, 243-5
  evolution, 210
  gingiva, 233-8
  innervation of dental structures, 239-43
  lymphatics of dental structures, 245
  periodontal ligament see Ligament, periodontal
  structures, adaptive radiation of, 212-15
  types of, 210
Toothless animals, 331
Treeshrews, 357
  dentition, 419
Tribosphenic mammalian molars, 339-41
  developments from, 341-8, 373
Trigeminal nerve, 239
Trigon on mammalian molars, 341, 373, 375
Trigonid on mammalian molars, 336, 338-9, 341, 344, 375
Trophoblast, 9, 10
Truncus arteriosus, 18, 20
Tubal pregnancy, 10
Tumours, dental, congenital, 255

Umbilical cord, 10, 16, 21
Umbilical hernia, fetal, 23-4
Underbite, 371, 427
Ungulates, ruminating, dentition, 414-15
Urinary organs, development of, 24, 25-6
Urodeles, teeth of, 106, 163

Vascular changes in ageing, 82-3
Vasodentine, 158-9, 160-1
Veins, development of, 18, 19, 21
Vertebrates, classification of 88, 89 (Table 4.2)

Vestibule of the mouth, 246, 252–3
Villi, in embryo development, 9–10
Viscerocranium, 37, 39
Vitrodentine, 156
von Ebner lines, 168, 171, 265
von Korff fibres, 189, 263, 264

Wallabies, dentition, 418–19
Walruses, dentition, 409
Warthog, dentition, 347, 413

Wave replacement of alternate teeth, 255–7
Wear of teeth, 333–6
  occlusal, 326, 327–8, 376
  in primates, 375–6
  proximal, 326, 336
  *see also* Abrasion; Attrition
Weil, cell-free zone of, 188, 192, 266, 354
Whales, dentition, 405–6
Wolves, dentition, 406
Wombats, dentition, 418

X chromosomes, 7, 48, 53–4
Y chromosomes, 7, 48, 53
Yolk sac, 9, 10, 15, 22

Zahnreihe unit in dentition, 256–7
Zalambdadonts, 344
Zebras, dentition, 412
*Zinjanthropus boisei*, 379, 386, 387
Zona pellucida, 6, 7, 8, 9
Zygomatic arch, growth of, 80
Zygotes, 8, 48